Register Now for Online Access to Your Book!

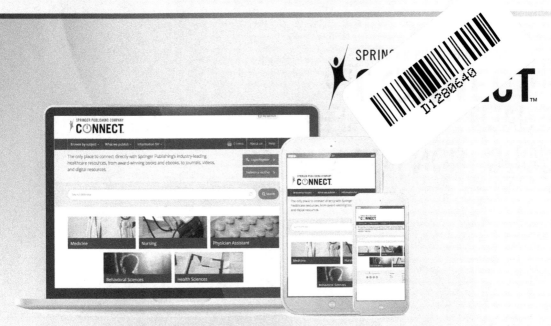

Your print purchase of *Introduction to Quality and Safety Education for Nurses, Second Edition,* **includes online access to the contents of your book**—increasing accessibility, portability, and searchability!

Access today at:

http://connect.springerpub
or scan the QR code at the r
and enter the access code b

TK417H7G

Scan here for quick access.

LS

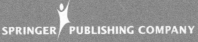

SPRINGER PUBLISHING COMPANY

View all our products at springerpub.com

INTRODUCTION TO QUALITY AND SAFETY EDUCATION FOR NURSES

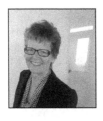

Patricia Kelly, MSN, RN, earned her diploma in nursing from St. Margaret Hospital School of Nursing, Hammond, Indiana; baccalaureate in nursing from DePaul University in Chicago, Illinois; and master's degree in nursing from Loyola University in Chicago, Illinois. She is Professor Emeritus, Purdue University Northwest, Hammond, Indiana. She has worked as a staff nurse, travel nurse, school nurse, and nurse educator. Patricia has traveled extensively in the United States, Canada, and Puerto Rico, teaching at conferences for the Joint Commission, Resource Applications, Pediatric Concepts, and Kaplan, Inc. She currently teaches nationwide National Council Licensure Examination for Registered Nurses® (NCLEX-RN®) review courses for Evolve Testing & Remediation/ Health Education Systems, Inc. (HESI), Houston, Texas. She also currently volunteers in a level one trauma center, emergency room, Advocate Christ Medical Center, Oak Lawn, Illinois and has been a nursing volunteer at the Old Irving Park Community Clinic in Chicago, a free clinic for patients without healthcare insurance.

Patricia was director of quality improvement at the University of Chicago Hospitals and Clinics. She has taught at Wesley-Passavant School of Nursing and Chicago State University. Patricia was program director of the Associate Degree Nursing Program and is Professor Emeritus, Purdue University Northwest, College of Nursing, Hammond, Indiana. Patricia has taught Fundamentals of Nursing, Adult Nursing, Nursing Leadership and Management, Nursing Issues, Nursing Trends, Quality Improvement, and Legal Aspects of Nursing. She has been a member of Sigma Theta Tau, the American Nurses Association, and the Emergency Nurses Association. She is listed in Who's Who in American Nursing, Notable American Women, and the International Who's Who of Professional and Business Women.

Patricia has served on the board of directors of Tri-City Mental Health Center, St. Anthony's Home, and the Mosby Quality Connection. She is a coeditor/author of *Introduction to Quality and Safety Education for Nurses, Core Competencies*, first edition, with coeditors/authors Beth A. Vottero and Carolyn Christie-McAuliffe. Patricia is also an editor/author of *Nursing Leadership and Management*, now in its third edition in the United States and Canada; *Essentials of Nursing Leadership and Management* (with Janice Tazbir, coeditor/author), now in its third edition; and *Nursing Delegation, Setting Priorities, and Making Patient Care Assignments* (with Maureen Marthaler, coeditor/author), second edition. She contributed a chapter, "Preparing the Undergraduate Student and Faculty to Use Quality Improvement in Practice," in *Improving Quality*, second edition, by Claire Gavin Meisenheimer. Patricia also contributed a chapter on Obstructive Lung Disease: Nursing Management in *Contemporary Medical-Surgical Nursing by Rick Daniels*. She has served as a national disaster volunteer for the American Red Cross and has also been a team member on healthcare relief trips to Nicaragua. Patricia has been a nurse for 50 years and currently lives in Chicago, Illinois, and in Fort Myers, Florida. She can be reached at patkelly777@aol.com.

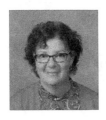

Beth A. Vottero, PhD, RN, CNE, earned a baccalaureate degree in liberal studies with a focus in business management from the University of Maine at Presque Isle; a baccalaureate degree in nursing from Valparaiso University; a master's degree in nursing from University of Phoenix; and a PhD in nursing education from Capella University. Previously, Beth taught in the undergraduate nursing at Purdue University North Central and the graduate nursing program at Bethel College. Beth currently is an associate professor of nursing at Purdue University Northwest, teaching courses including Evidence-Based Practice and Knowledge Translation at the doctoral level and Informatics and courses in the

Nurse Educator program at the graduate level. At the undergraduate level, she teaches Quality and Safety for Professional Nursing Practice, Informatics, and Evidence-Based Quality Improvement projects in the Capstone course.

Beth's background includes over 18 years as a staff and charge nurse. After completing her doctorate, Beth coordinated and led a successful Magnet redesignation for Indiana University Health La Porte Hospital in La Porte, Indiana. She brought a desire to instill quality concepts to academia where she created an undergraduate quality course at Purdue Northwest focused on quality and safety in healthcare. Beth is a research associate with the Indiana Center for Evidence-Based Practice in Hammond, Indiana, a Joanna Briggs Institute (JBI) Collaborating Center. Through this association, she has completed systematic reviews on various topics. In collaboration with Dr. Lisa Hopp, she assisted in developing an Evidence Implementation Workshop to train nurses in translation science using an evidence-based quality improvement focus. Beth is a certified Comprehensive Systematic Review Program Trainer with JBI and conducts weeklong training for healthcare providers nationally.

Beth has published chapters in Hopp and Rittenmeyer's *Introduction to Evidence-Based Practice: A Practical Guide for Nurses*; Bristol and Zerwekh's *Essentials of E-Learning for Nurse Educators*; and has developed case studies for Zerwekh and Zerwekh's *Nursing Today: Transitions and Trends*. She has published several articles on "Teaching Informatics" (*Nurse Educator QSEN Supplement*), "Conducting a Root Cause Analysis" (*Nursing Education Perspectives)*, and "3D Simulation of Complex Health Care Environments" (*Clinical Simulation in Nursing*). Beth is an active member of the QSEN Academic Task Force with multisite studies on quality and safety education for nurses (QSEN) teaching strategies. As a funded researcher through Purdue University, Beth has studied factors affecting medication errors in the clinical setting. Beth can be reached at bstarnes@pnw.edu.

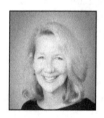 **Carolyn A. Christie-McAuliffe, PhD, FNP,** obtained her diploma in nursing from Crouse-Irving Memorial Hospital School of Nursing, Syracuse, New York; a baccalaureate and master's degree in nursing from the State University of New York, Health Science Center at Syracuse, Syracuse, New York; and a PhD in nursing from Binghamton University, Binghamton, New York. Her clinical experience has included staff nursing, home healthcare, oncology care, and private practice. She has functioned as an administrator primarily in clinical research and taught at the undergraduate and graduate nursing levels at Crouse-Irving Memorial Hospital School of Nursing, Syracuse, New York; the College of Notre Dame of Maryland, Baltimore, Maryland; State University of New York (SUNY) Institute of Technology, Utica, New York; and Keuka College, Keuka Park, New York. She has implemented multiple evidence-based practice and quality assurance programs and served as a compliance officer and Institutional Review Board chair at SUNY Institute of Technology. Carolyn's research interest and efforts have focused on primary prevention. The majority of her publications and speaking engagements have centered on topics of research, evidence-based practice, and leadership.

Currently Carolyn provides Integrative Medicine in her private practice in Syracuse, NY. In addition, she runs a clinic at the Syracuse Rescue Mission where she serves as a preceptor for undergraduate and graduate nursing students. Carolyn can be reached at cmcqsentext@gmail.com.

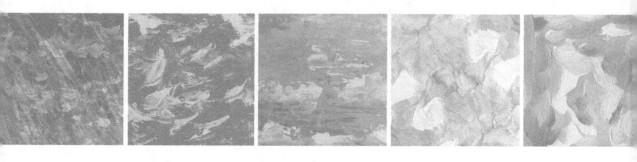

INTRODUCTION TO QUALITY AND SAFETY EDUCATION FOR NURSES

CORE COMPETENCIES FOR NURSING LEADERSHIP AND MANAGEMENT

Second Edition

Patricia Kelly, MSN, RN

Beth A. Vottero, PhD, RN, CNE

Carolyn A. Christie-McAuliffe, PhD, FNP

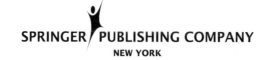

SPRINGER PUBLISHING COMPANY

NEW YORK

Springer Publishing Company, LLC
11 West 42nd Street
New York, NY 10036
www.springerpub.com

Acquisitions Editor: Joseph Morita
Managing Editor: Cindy Yoo
Compositor: diacriTech, Chennai

ISBN: 978-0-8261-2341-1
ebook ISBN: 978-0-8261-2385-5
Instructor's Manual: 978-0-8261-2565-1
Instructor's PowerPoints: 978-0-8261-2574-3

Instructor's Materials: Qualified instructors may request supplements by emailing textbook@springerpub.com.

18 19 20 21 22 / 5 4 3 2 1

The author and the publisher of this Work have made every effort to use sources believed to be reliable to provide information that is accurate and compatible with the standards generally accepted at the time of publication. Because medical science is continually advancing, our knowledge base continues to expand. Therefore, as new information becomes available, changes in procedures become necessary. We recommend that the reader always consult current research and specific institutional policies before performing any clinical procedure. The author and publisher shall not be liable for any special, consequential, or exemplary damages resulting, in whole or in part, from the readers' use of, or reliance on, the information contained in this book. The publisher has no responsibility for the persistence or accuracy of URLs for external or third-party Internet websites referred to in this publication and does not guarantee that any content on such websites is, or will remain, accurate or appropriate.

Library of Congress Cataloging-in-Publication Data

Names: Kelly, Patricia, 1941–editor. | Vottero, Beth A., editor. |
    Christie-McAuliffe, Carolyn A., editor.
Title: Introduction to quality and safety education for nurses : core
    competencies for nursing leadership and management / [edited by] Patricia
    Kelly, Beth A. Vottero, Carolyn A. Christie-McAuliffe.
Description: Second edition. | New York, NY : Springer Publishing Company,
    LLC, [2018] | Includes bibliographical references and index.
Identifiers: LCCN 2018012105| ISBN 9780826123411 | ISBN 9780826123855 (e-book)
Subjects: | MESH: Nursing—standards | Quality of Health Care | Patient
    Safety | Safety Management | United States
Classification: LCC RT73 | NLM WY 16 AA1 | DDC 610.73071/1—dc23 LC record available at
    https://lccn.loc.gov/2018012105

Contact us to receive discount rates on bulk purchases.
We can also customize our books to meet your needs.
For more information please contact: sales@springerpub.com

This book is dedicated by Patricia Kelly to her loving Dad and Mom, Ed and Jean Kelly (Dad was a Safety Engineer at Inland Steel Company); to her charming, wonderful fiancé, Ron Vana; to her super sisters, Tessie Kelly Dybel and Kathy Kelly Milch; to her dear aunts and uncles, Aunt Pat and Uncle Bill Kelly and Aunt Verna and Uncle Archie Payne; her nephew, John Milch; her nieces, Natalie Dybel Bevil, Melissa Milch Arredondo, and Stacey Milch Monks; her nephews-in-law, Tracy Bevil, Peter Arredondo, and Derek Monks; her grandnephew, Brock Bevil, and her grandniece, Reese Bevil. I love you all!

Beth Vottero would like to thank her support, her rock, and her hero . . . her ever-patient husband Dino. Thanks also go to her children Tom (Army Strong), Mitchell (ump extraordinaire), Micah (King of Games), Michelle (ever-patient educator), and Trisha (the beautiful mother); to her amazing parents Tom and Judy, Ray and Dolly; and to her dog Ben, who sat on a chair and stared at her for hours while she worked. To her super-human coworkers—you know who you are and how much you motivate me.

Carolyn A. Christie-McAuliffe would like to acknowledge all the patients she has been graced to know and work with. Her efforts on this book are dedicated to them: for the trust and honor they place in her; for the honesty and courage they exhibit; but most of all, for the privilege to hear, and see, and witness healing of mind, body, and spirit. For that privilege, she will always feel a sense of responsibility to do what she can to facilitate higher levels of safety and quality in healthcare.

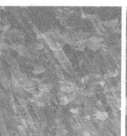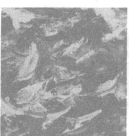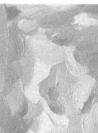

CONTENTS

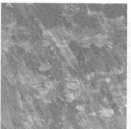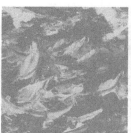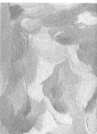

CONTRIBUTORS

 Catherine C. Alexander, DNP, RN   VA Quality Scholar, White River Junction, Vermont, Adjunct Faculty, MGH Institute of Health Professions, Boston, Massachusetts

 Gerry Altmiller, EdD, APRN, ACNS-BC   Associate Professor, Director, QSEN Institute Regional Center at The College of New Jersey, School of Nursing, Health, and Exercise Sciences, Ewing, New Jersey

 Gail Armstrong, PhD, DNP, ACNS-BC, CNE   Associate Professor, University of Colorado College of Nursing, Aurora, Colorado

 Amy J. Barton, PhD, RN, FAAN, ANEF   Associate Dean for Clinical and Community Affairs Professor, Daniel and Janet Mordecai Endowed Chair in Rural Health Nursing, University of Colorado College of Nursing, Aurora, Colorado

 Jodi L. Boling, MSN, RN, CNS   Core Faculty, American College of Education, Indianapolis, Indiana

 Kay Burke, MBA, BSN, RN, NE-BC   Chief Nursing Information Officer University of California, San Francisco Health, San Francisco, California

Carolyn A. Christie-McAuliffe, PhD, FNP Integrative Practitioners, Syracuse, New York

Melinda Davis, RN, MSN, CCRN, CNL Clinical Improvement Consultant, VHA QMS Consultative Division (10E2C3), Office of Quality, Safety and Value, Antioch, Tennessee

Anthony L. D'Eramo, MSN, RN, CPHQ ISO Consultant, Region 1, VHA ISO Consultation Division, Office of Quality, Safety, and Value, Coventry, Rhode Island, Providence VA Medical Center, Providence, Rhode Island

Ronda G. Hughes, PhD, MHS, RN, CLNC, FAAN Director, Center for Nursing Leadership, Director, Executive Doctorate of Nursing Practice, Associate Professor, University of South Carolina, School of Nursing, Columbia, South Carolina

Patricia Kelly, RN, MSN Professor Emerita, Purdue University Northwest, College of Nursing, Hammond, Indiana, Faculty, Health Education Systems, Inc. (HESI), Houston, Texas

Patti Ludwig-Beymer, PhD, RN, CTN-A, NEA-BC, CPPS, FAAN Associate Professor, Purdue University Northwest, College of Nursing, Hammond, Indiana

Jerry A. Mansfield, PhD, RN, NEA-BC Executive Chief Nursing Officer and Chief Patient Experience Officer, Medical University of South Carolina, Charleston, South Carolina

Maureen T. Marthaler, RN, MS Professor Emerita, College of Nursing, Purdue University Northwest, Hammond, Indiana

Theodore M. McGinn, JD, BBA, CPA   Managing Partner Lavelle Law, Ltd., Adjunct Professor, The John Marshall Law School, Chicago, Illinois

Peter D. Mills, PhD, MS   Director, VA National Center for Patient Safety Field Office, Veterans Affairs Medical Center, White River Junction, Vermont and
Adjunct Associate Professor of Psychiatry, The Geisel School of Medicine at Dartmouth College, Hanover, New Hampshire

Joanne Belviso Puckett, EdM, RN   Director, Quality and Risk Management, USAF 48th Medical Group, Royal Air Force, Lakenheath, United Kingdom

Christine Rovinski-Wagner, MSN, ARNP   National Transformational Coach Captain, VHA Office of Veterans Access to Care, Faculty Scholar, VA Quality Scholars Fellowship Program, White River Junction, Vermont and
Clinical Instructor in Community and Family Medicine, The Geisel School of Medicine at Dartmouth College, Hanover, New Hampshire

Danielle Scheurer, MD, MSCR, SFHM   Hospitalist and Chief Quality Officer, Associate Professor of Medicine, Medical University of South Carolina, Charleston, South Carolina

Jamie L. Vargo-Warran, DM/IST, MSN, BSN, LSSGB   Dean, Academic Affairs, Chamberlain University College of Nursing, Rancho Cordova, California

Beth A. Vottero, PhD, RN, CNE   Associate Professor of Nursing, Purdue University Northwest, College of Nursing, Research Associate, Indiana Center for Evidence-Based Nursing Practice, Joanna Briggs Collaborating Center, Hammond, Indiana

Kimberly J. Whalen, MLIS   Associate Professor of Library Services, Health Sciences Librarian, Valparaiso University, Valparaiso, Indiana

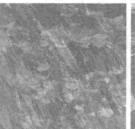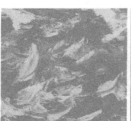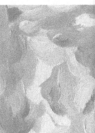

FOREWORD

Nurses are at the core of healthcare delivery and their role requires both competence and leadership to ensure that high quality and safe care is provided. It is exciting to see the publication of the second edition of *Quality and Safety Education for Nurses: Core Competencies for Nursing Leadership and Management*. Based on the Quality and Safety Education for Nurses (QSEN) competencies (Cronenwett et al., 2007) and emphasizing leadership and management principles, this book is a valuable educational resource that facilitates teaching contemporary nursing practice. Nursing students and faculty across the nation will benefit from the content of the book. It includes personal interviews, essential content, and study questions that promote reflection and critical thinking. The book is an essential resource to learning and applying the QSEN competencies.

Now is the time for nurses to have the knowledge, skills, attitudes, and leadership to provide consistent high quality and safe care. Although there is evidence that we have made some progress in the delivery of care (National Patient Safety Foundation, 2015) since the Institute of Medicine (IOM) report over 17 years ago (IOM, 2000, 2003), medical error remains the third leading cause of death (Makary & Daniels, 2016). This is due in part to the increasing complexity and dynamic nature of healthcare, the delivery of care by interprofessional teams that demands new types of communication strategies, and the challenge of integrating informatics and the electronic health record. The delivery of healthcare is not what it used to be and new educational strategies are needed to address these changes.

The QSEN competencies were developed over 12 years ago and schools of nursing continue to report that the QSEN competencies are not integrated into their curriculum (Altmiller & Armstrong, 2017). This is concerning as 24% of NCLEX® questions are directly related to quality and safety content. Since 2012, the QSEN Institute at the Case Western Reserve University Frances Payne Bolton School of Nursing has continued the QSEN movement by continuing to provide resources to integrate the QSEN competencies into the curriculum in the classroom, simulation lab, and clinical experiences. The qsen.org website provides ready-to-use teaching strategies, resources, and connections to QSEN experts. A monthly newsletter and annual conference connect nurse educators and nurse practice leaders to ensure that nursing students are quality and safety practice ready and that nurse preceptors and practicing nurses are ready to role-model quality and safety standards.

The QSEN movement includes a fundamental paradigm shift: a shift from nurses not just doing their work but improving their work. This requires nurses and other healthcare professionals to "systems think" and garner the power to change the systems in which they work (Dolansky & Moore, 2013). Systems thinking moves nurses to not just have the knowledge and skill to deliver care to their patients (e.g., use the five steps to safe medication administration) but to understand and value the connections of their actions to the systems of care around them (e.g., ask how many medication errors are occurring on my unit and what actions are being taken to reduce these errors). This paradigm shift to systems thinking requires nurses to embrace a philosophy of continuous improvement that facilitates learning from errors and designing new ways of providing care that ensure high quality and safe care.

Professor Emerita Patricia Kelly, Dr. Beth Vottero, and Dr. Carolyn Christie-McAuliffe bring the QSEN core competencies alive in this introductory book to improve student preparation. The addition of leadership and management to this second edition of the book is important as they are important at both the front line and the management level of patient care. Leadership and management are essential to move from traditional nursing care to nursing care that includes systems change to improve patient care. Leadership is the necessary ingredient to empower nurses to stand-up and speak out and say, "I am not going to do this workaround any longer as it violates my core value of delivering high quality and safe care." As Eleanor Roosevelt said, "With the new day comes new strength and new thoughts." Let us embrace these words and move quality and safety to new heights.

Mary A. Dolansky, PhD, RN, FAAN
Associate Professor and Director of the QSEN Institute
Frances Payne Bolton School of Nursing
Case Western Reserve University
Director of Interprofessional Integration and Education
Center of Excellence in Primary Care
VA Quality Scholars Program (VAQS) Senior Nurse Fellow
Louis Stokes Cleveland VA Medical Center

REFERENCES

Altmiller, G., & Armstrong, G. (2017). National QSEN faculty survey results. *Nurse Educator*, 42(5S), 1–6.

Cronenwett, L., Sherwood, G., Barnsteiner, J., Disch, J., Johnson, J., Mitchell, P., . . . Warren, J. (2007). Quality and safety education for nurses. *Nursing Outlook*, 55(3), 122–131.

Dolansky, M. A., & Moore, S. M. (2013). Quality and safety education in nursing: The key is systems thinking. *Online Journal of Issues in Nursing*, 18(3), 1.

Institute of Medicine. (2000). *To err is human: Building a safer health system*. Washington, DC: National Academies Press.

Institute of Medicine. (2003). *Health professions education: A bridge to quality*. Washington, DC: National Academies Press.

Makary, M. A., & Daniels, M. (2016). Medical error—The third leading cause of death in the US. *BMJ*, 353, i2139.

National Patient Safety Foundation. (2015). Free from harm: Accelerating patient safety improvement fifteen years after to Err is Human. A report from an expert panel. Retrieved from http://www.npsf.org/?page=freefromharm#form

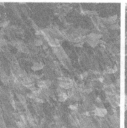
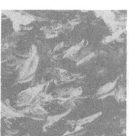

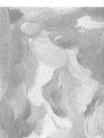

FOREWORD

Healthcare providers and consumers of care demand excellence. When that is not achieved, and less than optimal outcomes are realized, the competence of individual providers pushes to the forefront of discussions, complaints, and root cause investigations. Assuming or judging individual competence is complicated, particularly when other causes, such as organizational factors, are disregarded or not appreciated. In too many instances, particularly when care does not meet our expectations or an adverse event occurs, the key factors indicate troubles with the competency of not just one but many.

With the increasing complexity of healthcare and patient needs, there is a demand for qualified and competent healthcare providers for high-quality, safe patient care. The attainment of nursing quality and safety competencies begins during coursework and clinical preparation, is developed in practice, and is refined with experience. While we may agree that all healthcare providers need to demonstrate specific competencies in practice, we struggle with the definition, context, attainment, importance, and demonstration of competencies within various healthcare environments. A common understanding of the definitions, standards, and domains of competencies is essential and antecedent to potential associations with understanding and improving organizational, professional, and patient outcomes.

Each day, nurses fulfill many different expectations in different contexts with changing demands and multiple challenges. To do so, nurses apply and adapt their competencies as part of their professional practice performance. The application and adaptation of one's competencies are influenced by many factors, including attitudes, motives, and perceptions. Notwithstanding, perceptions of functioning competencies or levels of competencies may be intertwined with the performance of other nurses and healthcare providers. As such, there are challenges in measuring competencies and understanding the confluence of competencies across healthcare teams. It may be that differences in scope of practice among the professions do not necessarily indicate discipline-specific competencies. Instead, competencies are interdependent and practice specific.

Core competencies for quality and patient safety have been defined by the Quality and Safety Education for Nurses (QSEN) initiative, funded by the Robert Wood Johnson Foundation, to prepare the future nursing workforce with necessary knowledge, skills, and attitudes to be actively engaged in improving the quality and safety of healthcare. The approach in this book is based on QSEN and is structured to ensure that students will obtain the recommended competencies and knowledge necessary to provide care that is both high quality and safe in practice. Patricia Kelly, Beth A. Vottero, and Carolyn A. Christie-McAuliffe bring the QSEN core competencies together with leadership and management in an introductory book to improve student preparation. It is a book that will be an essential tool on our journey to realize the quality and safety of care we all demand.

Ronda G. Hughes, PhD, MHS, RN, CLNC, FAAN
Associate Professor/Director, Center for Nursing Leadership
College of Nursing, University of South Carolina
Member, Institute of Medicine Committee on Credentialing Research in Nursing
Editor, *Patient Safety and Quality: An Evidence-Based Handbook for Nurses*
Agency for Healthcare Research and Quality

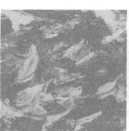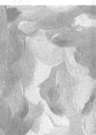

PREFACE

The 1994 Institute of Medicine (IOM) report, *America's Health in Transition: Protecting and Improving Quality*, highlighted the seriousness and pervasiveness of healthcare error rates and their effect on patient outcomes and morbidity and mortality rates. Then, in 2000, the IOM released the report, *To Err Is Human: Building a Safer Health System*. This IOM report instantly received national attention from policymakers, healthcare providers, and consumers. The IOM report stated, "At least 44,000 people, and perhaps as many as 98,000 people, die in hospitals each year as a result of medical errors that could have been prevented." This IOM report caused major ripples throughout the healthcare system and highlighted the need to change how healthcare is delivered. Shockingly, recent research by Makary and Daniel (2016) has found that more than 250,000 deaths each year are the result of errors within healthcare. That means that after heart disease and cancer, patient safety errors are the third leading cause of death in the United States (Makary & Daniel, 2016).

America has some of the best hospitals in the world but it is also the only large, rich country without Universal Healthcare coverage. About half of Americans have their health insurance provided by their employers. Healthcare costs can be financially ruinous for others. In 2016, America spent $10,348 per person on healthcare, roughly twice as much as the average for comparably rich countries. On average, both hospital cost and drug prices can be 60% higher than in Europe. The American Affordable Care Act expanded the health insurance system and cut the number of uninsured people from 44 million to 28 million but still left a gap among people not poor enough to qualify for Medicaid, but not rich enough to buy private insurance.

In the U.S., prices for the same service can vary enormously. Having your appendix removed, for example, can cost anywhere from $1,500 to $183,000 depending on the insurer. Add to this the fact that 9 of the 10 best-paid occupations in the U.S. involve medicine, and we see that doctors and other healthcare providers have little incentive to change the system.

The 2001 release of the IOM report, *Crossing the Quality Chasm: A New Health System* for the 21st century, spotlighted general problems in healthcare in an attempt to close the gap between what is known to provide quality healthcare and what is actually occurring in practice. This IOM report defined six principles for healthcare: Healthcare should be Safe, Timely, Effective, Efficient, Equitable, and Patient-Centered (STEEEP Principles). This IOM report also identified 10 rules for care delivery redesign (available at www.nap. edu/catalog/10027/crossing-the-quality-chasm-a-new-health-system-for-the). This IOM report spawned a series of other IOM reports on priority healthcare areas, for example, public health; biomedical and health research; diseases; quality and patient safety; health services, coverage, and access; select populations and health disparities; food and nutrition; veterans' health; healthcare workforce; environmental health; global health; substance abuse and mental health; women's health; aging; and education.

The IOM report, *The Future of Nursing: Leading Change, Advancing Health* (2011), recommended that nurses practice to the full extent of their education, improve nursing education, provide nursing leadership positions in healthcare redesign, and improve data collection for workplace planning and policy making. This IOM report further states that strong leadership is critical if the vision of a transformed healthcare system is to be realized. The nursing profession must produce leaders throughout the healthcare system. Everyone from the bedside to the boardroom must engage colleagues, subordinates, and executives so that together they can identify and achieve common goals (Bradford & Cohen, 1998). Nurses must understand that their leadership is as important to providing quality care as is their technical ability to deliver care at the bedside in a safe and effective manner.

Care has been provided to patients from early history, often by religious orders. More recently, Florence Nightingale led 38 women into Scutari Barrack Hospital in Turkey in 1854 to manage care for British casualties of the Crimean War. She went on to establish Saint Thomas Hospital and the Nightingale Training School for Nurses in 1860. Many other nurses have also led and managed patient care; some of them honored in the American Nurses Association Hall of Fame (see www.nursingworld.org/ Hall-of-Fame for a listing of ANA Hall of Fame inductees).

Every nurse is a nursing leader and manager, from the beginning frontline nurse who works directly with patients and takes action to ensure their safety and care quality to the advanced practice nurse clinician to the top federal nurse administrator in health services, scientific and academic organizations, and public health and community-based organizations. All of these nurses continuously demonstrate leadership and management and work with the interprofessional team to ensure patient-centered, high quality, safe, evidence-based care, utilizing informatics as appropriate.

The IOM reports also called for changes in how healthcare organizations provide safe, high-quality patient care services. Currently, the IOM and many others, including clinicians, healthcare organizations, employers, consumers, foundations, research agencies, government agencies, and quality organizations are working to create a more patient-centered, 21st-century healthcare system.

A primary movement for change in nursing academia toward the inclusion of more educational information on STEEEP Principles has been the Quality and Safety Education for Nurses (QSEN) initiative. QSEN followed the IOM lead and stated that changes in healthcare needed to focus on the development of nursing competencies in patient-centered care, teamwork and collaboration, quality improvement, evidence-based practice, and informatics. Because of nurses' unique position at the sharp end, front line of care in direct contact with patients, safety was added as a sixth QSEN competency. The QSEN initiative convened a national panel of experts to identify the core knowledge, skills, and attitudes (KSAs) required for each of the six competencies. Information about the KSAs is available at qsen.org. QSEN also sponsors nursing conferences including:

- An annual QSEN Forum to attract nursing leaders in academia and practice to share innovations and research in patient quality and safety.
- An annual Summit on Leadership and Quality Improvement to explore interprofessional and frontline leadership strategies that will help to accelerate organizational and systems cost, safety, and quality improvement performance in organizations (qsen.org/conferences/1st-annual-summit-on-leadership-and-quality-improvement-accelerating-change-through-positive-forms-of-leadership/).

Another significant movement for healthcare change comes from the Agency for Healthcare Research and Quality (AHRQ). This agency, with funding from the Robert Wood Johnson Foundation, published *Patient Safety and Quality: An Evidence-Based Handbook for Nurses* (2008), edited by Ronda G. Hughes, to provide all nurses with evidence-based techniques and interventions to improve patient outcomes. AHRQ also provides many other resources for Quality and Patient Safety at their website.

WHY THIS BOOK, QUALITY AND SAFETY EDUCATION FOR NURSES: CORE COMPETENCIES FOR NURSING LEADERSHIP AND MANAGEMENT, SECOND EDITION?

The idea for this book was born when two of the editors, Patricia Kelly and Dr. Beth A. Vottero attended the 2011 QSEN conference in Milwaukee, Wisconsin. Patricia and Beth, both from the Chicago area, invited Dr. Carolyn A. Christie-McAuliffe, from New York, to join them as the third editor to facilitate the development of a broad look at quality and safety. The three coeditors experienced the rapid evolution of quality and safety information in their clinical and academic practices and they identified the need for nursing students to receive an understanding of quality and safety in their basic nursing preparation. The three editors believed in the need to organize existing information about quality and safety into one basic, easily understood textbook. This need was recently emphasized with the publication of the Makary and Daniel report (2016), mentioned earlier. This report is *shocking* to us as nurses who have been delivering what we believe is safe high-quality nursing care for a combined total from the three editors of approximately 112 years! The purpose of this book is to provide a comprehensive overview of the essential QSEN KSAs about the six quality and safety competencies in nursing practice to beginning frontline leaders and managers of interprofessional patient care. These frontline nursing leaders and managers use informatics and work with interprofessional teams to deliver patient-centered, evidence-based, safe, high-quality patient care.

Many practical examples from real-life experiences are discussed in this text for students. The contributors to this text include nurse educators, nurse faculty, nurse researchers, library scientists, nurse administrators, nurse case managers, physicians, lawyers, nurse quality improvement practitioners, nurse practitioners, nurse entrepreneurs, psychologists, and others. The contributors are from all over the United States, emphasizing a broad view of quality and safety. There are U.S. contributors from Colorado, Florida, Illinois, Indiana, New Hampshire, New Jersey, Massachusetts, New York, Ohio, Pennsylvania, Rhode Island, South Carolina, Vermont, and Washington, DC, as well as an international contributor.

Each chapter includes interviews with experts in their respective healthcare field to provide an interprofessional team perspective. Interviewees include pharmacists, nurses, lawyers, physicians, library scientists, quality improvement nurses, radiology technologists, nurse practitioners, hospital board members, members from the Committee of Directors for Joanna Briggs Institute, patients, and others.

An important feature of this book is the listing of QSEN competencies and the associated KSAs found in Appendix B. Appendix B also identifies the chapter in which the QSEN competency's KSA information can be found in the text. This will help both students and faculty plan for the development of KSA competency in students.

ORGANIZATION

Quality and Safety Education for Nurses: Core Competencies for Nursing Leadership and Management, Second Edition, consists of 17 chapters. Each chapter provides nursing students and beginning nurses with a background and foundational knowledge of quality and safety to assist them in their role as sharp end, frontline leaders in today's healthcare environment.

- Unit I, "Introduction to Quality and Safety Education for Nurses: Core Competencies for Nursing Leadership and Management," includes eight chapters. They are "Overview of Patient Safety and Quality of Care," "Quality and Safety Education for Nurses," "Nurses as Leaders and Managers for Safe, High-Quality Patient Care," "Quality and Safety in High-Reliability Organizations," "Legal and Ethical Aspects of Quality and Safety," "Delegation and Setting Priorities for Safe, High-Quality Nursing Care," "Patient-Centered Care," and "Interprofessional Teamwork and Collaboration."
- Unit II, "The Use of Quality and Safety Education Concepts by Nursing Leaders and Managers" includes four chapters. They are "Informatics," "Basic Literature Search Strategies," "Evidence-Based Nursing Practice," and "Patient Safety."
- Unit III, "Nurse Leadership and Management for Quality Improvement," includes five chapters. They are "Essentials of Quality Improvement," "Tools of Quality Improvement," "Quality Improvement and Project Management," "The Future Role of the Registered Nurse in Patient Safety and Quality," and "Transition from Student Nurse to Leadership and Management of Your Future as a Registered Nurse."

CHAPTER FEATURES

Several chapter features are used throughout the text to provide the reader with a consistent format for learning. Chapter features include the following:

- Photos, tables, and figures to enhance student understanding
- Healthcare or nursing quotes and interviews to illustrate the chapter content
- Objectives that state the chapter's learning goals
- Opening Scenario, a mini entry-level clinical situation that relates to the chapter, with two or three critical thinking questions
- Key Concepts, a listing of the primary understandings the reader is to take from the chapter
- Key Terms, a listing of important new terms defined in the chapter and identified within the chapter by bold type
- Clinical Discussion Points for nurses, several questions to engage students in dialogue (guidelines for discussion are available online)
- Review Questions, several multiple-choice and alternate-style National Council Licensure Examination for Registered Nurses (NCLEX-RN) questions (answers to Review Questions available online)
- Review Activities, to help students apply chapter content to patient care situations (answers to Review Activities available online)
- Exploring Websites
- References
- Suggested Readings
- QSEN Activities

Special elements are sprinkled throughout several chapters to enhance student learning and encourage critical thinking and application of the knowledge presented. These include the following:

- Highlights of historical nursing leaders and managers, many of them in the American Nurses Association Hall of Fame
- Evidence From the Literature with a synopsis of key findings from nursing and healthcare literature

- Real-World Interviews with healthcare leaders and managers, including nursing staff, clinicians, administrators, risk managers, faculty, nurses, physicians, patients, nursing assistive personnel, lawyers, pharmacists, hospital administrators, and others
- Critical Thinking Exercises regarding a safety- or quality-related issue (answers to Critical Thinking exercises available to faculty online)
- Case Studies to provide the nursing student with a patient care situation calling for critical thinking to solve an open-ended problem (answers to Case Study questions available to faculty online)
- Answers to all questions, opening scenarios, and QSEN activities are available to faculty online

HIGHLIGHTS OF THE TEXT

New to the Second Edition is a robust online evolving clinical case study as an instructional supplement for faculty to guide teaching the content, with options for how to use the case study for student learning. The content includes discussion questions for each section of the case study or guidance for a written paper assignment. The evolving case study pulls content from the text into how to address an evidence-based quality improvement project as a new nurse.

- A strong foundation for evidence-based healthcare with attention to high quality, safe care is emphasized throughout the text.
- Chapters include new information from national, federal, and state healthcare and nursing organizations.
- Leadership and management for frontline nurses are highlighted throughout the text and within each topic.
- Teamwork and interprofessional collaboration is stressed throughout the text.
- The six QSEN competencies with their KSAs are highlighted in the chapters.
- There are many critical thinking activities, case studies, and clinical discussion points for nurses throughout the chapters.
- There is an additional set of critical thinking exercise in Appendix C (answers are available to faculty online).

INSTRUCTOR RESOURCES

1. PowerPoint lecture slides for each chapter serve as guides for faculty presentations in the classroom. These can be obtained for qualified instructors by emailing Springer Publishing Company.

Patricia Kelly
Beth A. Vottero
Carolyn A. Christie-McAuliffe

REFERENCES

Agency for Healthcare Research and Quality (AHRQ). (2008). *Patient safety and quality: An evidence-based handbook for nurses.* AHRQ Publication No. 08–0043. Rockville, MD: Author. Retrieved from http://www.ahrq.gov/professionals/clinicians-providers/resources/nursing/resources/nurseshdbk/index.html

Bradford, D. L., & Cohen, A. R. (1998). *Power up: Transforming organizations through shared leadership.* Hoboken, NJ: John Wiley & Sons.

Institute of Medicine (IOM). (1994). *America's health in transition: Protecting and improving quality*. Washington, DC: National Academy of Sciences. Retrieved from http://www.nap.edu/openbook.php?record_id=9147&page=R1

Institute of Medicine (IOM). (2000). *To err is human: Building a safer health system*. Washington, DC: National Academy of Sciences. Retrieved from http://www.nap.edu/openbook.php?record_id=9728&page=R1

Institute of Medicine (IOM). (2001). *Crossing the quality chasm: A new health system for the 21st century*. Washington, DC: National Academy of Sciences. Retrieved from https://www.nap.edu/catalog/10027/crossing-the-quality-chasm-a-new-health-system-for-the

Makary, M., & Daniel, M. (2016). Medical error—The third leading cause of death in the U.S. *British Medical Journal, 353*, i2139. doi:10.1136/bmj.i2139

Land of the free-for-all: America is a health-care outlier in the developed world. Economist. April 26th 2018, available at, https://www.economist.com/news/special-report/21740871-only-large-rich-country-without-universal-health-care-america-health-care-outlier.

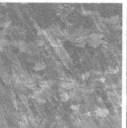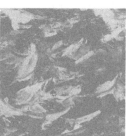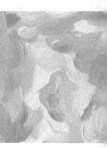

ACKNOWLEDGMENTS

A book such as this requires much effort and the coordination of many persons. Pat, Beth, and Carolyn would like to thank all of the contributing authors for their time and effort in sharing their knowledge gained through years of experience in both clinical and academic settings. All of the contributing authors on both editions within tight time frames to share their expertise. Thanks also to Jane Woodruff for her computer support and Jane A. Walker, PhD, RN, for her networking support.

We would like to acknowledge and sincerely thank the Springer Publishing Company team who worked to make this book a reality. Joseph Morita, senior acquisitions editor, and Chris Teja, assistant editor, are great people who worked hard to bring the first edition of this book to publication. We would also like to acknowledge and thank Cindy Yoo, Managing Editor, Nursing, Springer Publishing Company; Nandhakumar Krishnan, Key Accounts Manager, DiacriTech Technologies; and Kumeraysen Vaidhyanadhasamy, Project Manager, DiacriTech Technologies, for their hard work on the second edition.

The three co-editors would like to thank the following nursing, medical, and librarian authors for their contributions to the First Edition of this book:

Anne Anderson, DNP, MHSA, RN, CPHQ, NEA-BC (Winfield, Illinois)

Pauline Arnold, MSN, MSA, RN, HACP (LaPorte, Indiana)

Esther Bankert, PhD, RN

Lindsay Bonaventura, MS, RN, FNP, BC (Chesterton, Indiana)

Ashley Currier, MSN, RN, NE-BC (Chicago, Illinois)

Mary A. Dolansky, PhD, RN, FAAN (Cleveland, Ohio)

Mary Gillaspy, MLS, MS (Woodland Park, Colorado)

Corinne Haviley, RN, MS, PhD (Winfield, Illinois)

Joanne M. Joseph, PhD

Andrea Lazarek-LaQuay, MS, RN

Karen L. McCrea, DNP, FNP-C (Washington, DC)

Francia I. Reed, MS, RN, FNP-C (Utica, New York)

Kathleen Fischer Sellers, PhD, RN (Alfred, New York)

Donna L. Silsbee, PhD, RHIA, CTR, CCS (Utica, New York)

J. Scott Thomson, MLIS, AHIP (North Chicago, Illinois)

Cibele C. Webb, MSN Ed., RN (Mishawaka, Indiana)

Patrick M. Webb, MD (LaPorte, Indiana)

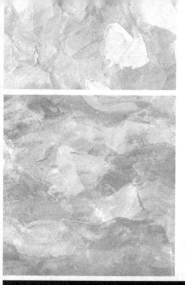

UNIT I.

INTRODUCTION TO QUALITY AND SAFETY EDUCATION FOR NURSES: CORE COMPETENCIES FOR NURSING LEADERSHIP AND MANAGEMENT

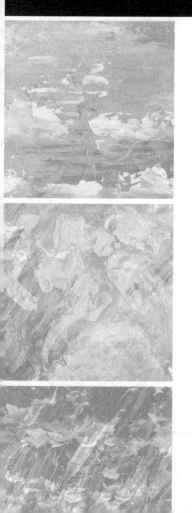

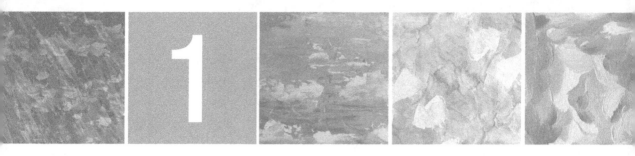

OVERVIEW OF PATIENT SAFETY AND QUALITY OF CARE

Ronda G. Hughes

It is, I guess, politically correct, widely believed, that to say that American health care is the best in the world. It's not. (Berwick, 2009)

Upon completion of this chapter, the reader should be able to

1. Define quality of care and patient safety.
2. Discuss key terms used to define quality of care and patient safety.
3. Identify national healthcare organizations influencing quality and safety.
4. Discuss measuring quality and safety.
5. Discuss core measures, sentinel events, and never events.
6. Discuss healthcare quality and safety in industrialized countries.
7. Describe the costs of achieving patient safety and quality of care.
8. Describe key programs that recognize hospital excellence.
9. Discuss the influence of the Institute of Medicine's (IOM) Quality Chasm series of reports.
10. Discuss the role of nurses at the "sharp" end of healthcare.
11. Discuss efforts to increase healthcare transparency, improve public reporting of healthcare, and reduce unwarranted variation in healthcare safety and quality.

A patient, Mr. R., was admitted to the hospital with uncontrollable pain from a kidney stone. He also had a history of sleep apnea. The nursing unit was short staffed that night and each nurse was busy, taking care of more patients than normal. Mr. R., who was a tall, overweight, 46-year-old man, kept asking for additional intravenous pain medication as he walked around the unit to try to ease the pain. The nurse called the physician to increase the dose of the pain medication. The physician ordered the increase and the nurse on the next shift proceeded to administer the higher dose without looking at how much pain medication Mr. R. had already received in the past 12 hours, nor did the nurse look at his health history. An hour later, Mr. R. told his nurse that he finally had some pain relief and he was going to his room to see if he could sleep for a few hours. His nurse, busy with other patients, went to check on Mr. R. 3 hours later. She found Mr. R. in his bed, cold to the touch with no respirations. He had been dead for 2 hours by the time the nurse went to check on him. With the combination of what ended up being too high of a dose of the pain medication (a medication known to be associated with life-threatening respiratory depression), the patient's history of sleep apnea, and the fact that the nurse did not assess her patient during a 3-hour period, the nurse, the physician, and the hospital were sued for malpractice by the family.

1. *What should the nurse have done prior to administering the last dose of the pain medication?*
2. *What should the nurse have done after administering the last dose of the pain medication?*
3. *What should the nurse, physician, and hospital have done to assist the nurse in avoiding the medication error?*

During the past 20 years, our nation has been focused on improving healthcare outcomes for patients and their families through improving the quality and safety of care. Concerns about rising healthcare costs, difficulty in accessing care, and healthcare research have highlighted the need for improving healthcare, and national initiatives have been implemented to accelerate change. However, improvements in quality and safety have been slow. These improvements can be slowed by the complexity of healthcare and the everyday challenges and opportunities of ensuring that the care available to and accessed by patients and their families reflects high quality and is safe. This slow improvement in quality and safety could be considered outrageous, especially considering how much is spent on healthcare in the United States, more than any other country in the world.

Frontline bedside nurses, as well as all nurses, have a significant leadership role to play in patient care. They have a significant influence on the incidence of patient falls, pressure ulcers, nosocomial infections, pain management, quality improvement (QI), and safety. Nurses influence patient satisfaction, mortality and morbidity rates, lengths of stay, complications, and so on. When a patient is at risk for a problem, it is often the bedside nurse who alerts the interprofessional team and begins the problem-solving process on behalf of patients.

This chapter provides an overview of the key concepts, drivers, and strategies for improving the quality of care and patient safety. Specifically, it begins with an overview of key terms used to define quality of care and patient safety, followed by key factors that influence healthcare safety and quality including the role of national healthcare accreditation organizations. The chapter then provides an overview of core measures, sentinel events, and never events. Since healthcare and patient safety issues are occurring worldwide, the chapter also includes an overview of quality and safety in industrialized countries. The chapter then provides a discussion of the costs of achieving patient safety and quality of care, and the key programs that recognize hospital excellence. This is followed by an overview of the influence of the Institute of Medicine's (IOM) Quality Chasm series of reports and how the role of nurses puts them at the "sharp end" of healthcare in direct contact with patients. The chapter concludes with an overview of efforts to increase healthcare transparency, improve public reporting of healthcare, and reduce unwarranted variation in healthcare safety and quality.

QUALITY OF CARE AND PATIENT SAFETY

The IOM considers patient safety both "indistinguishable from the delivery of quality health care" (Aspden, Corrigan, Wolcott, & Erickson, 2004), and the foundation of healthcare quality (Committee on the Quality of Health Care in America, 2001). Leaders in the United States have emphasized the need to redesign systems of care to better serve patients in the complex environment of our healthcare system. This has included efforts to inform policy through national policy reports, such as the IOM Quality Chasm series of reports (IOM, 1999, 2001), healthcare research and evaluation, and both federal and state policy changes to accelerate safety and QIs. Federal and state regulatory agencies have implemented new quality and safety requirements and financial penalties for poor quality care and care that has harmed patients. There have also been several national initiatives to improve quality and safety, such as the Institute for Healthcare Improvement's (IHI) *Transforming Care at the Bedside* (IHI, 2017a), *5 Million Lives Campaign* (IHI, 2017b), and the *Triple Aim* (IHI, 2017c). The Centers for Medicare and Medicaid Services (CMS) have also stopped reimbursement for extra healthcare costs associated with events that harm patients that are considered preventable. Yet, despite these many efforts, both government agencies, such as the Agency for Healthcare Research and Quality (AHRQ), and national healthcare quality organizations, such as the Leapfrog Group, report that there have been some improvements in quality and safety, but disparities and problems with quality and safety persist (AHRQ, 2011; The Leapfrog Group, 2017).

KEY TERMS USED WITH QUALITY AND SAFETY

Healthcare quality is defined as "the degree to which healthcare services for individuals and populations increase the likelihood of desired health outcomes and are consistent with current professional knowledge" (IOM, 2001). **High-quality care** is defined as care that is safe, timely, effective, efficient, equitable, and patient centered (also referred to as STEEEP) with no disparities between racial or ethnic groups (IOM, 2001). AHRQ expanded the definition of quality to include, "doing the right thing, at the right time, in the right way, to achieve the best possible results" (AHRQ, 2011). The IOM has recommended that quality can be improved on four levels:

- The patient level
- The health-delivery "microsystems" level, such as a surgical team or acute-care unit
- The organizational level, such as hospitals and healthcare systems
- The regulatory and financial environment level in which those organizations operate (IOM, 2001)

Errors are defined as "an act of commission (doing something wrong) or omission (failing to do the right thing) leading to an undesirable outcome or significant potential for such an outcome" (Wilson, Harrison, Gibberd, & Hamilton, 1999). Unfortunately, most errors in healthcare are viewed as a reflection of an individual's lack of knowledge or skill. Thus, when an error occurs, you will see efforts to blame or punish an individual. Yet, when considering the context in which healthcare errors occur, errors are usually a reflection of human failings within poorly designed systems. From this systems perspective, after an error occurs, we must try to identify factors that most likely led to the error and find solutions and changes to current healthcare processes so that we can reduce the possibility of a recurrence of the error or reduce the impact of the error on patients.

An **adverse event**, which may be considered either preventable or not, is defined as any undesirable experience in which harm resulted to a person receiving healthcare that "requires additional monitoring, treatment, or hospitalization, or that results in death" (IOM, 1999). Preventable adverse events are considered to reflect care that falls below the standard of care. Serious preventable adverse events are generally defined as an adverse event that is preventable and results in a patient death, loss of a body part, disability, or loss of bodily function lasting for more than 7 days or still present at the time of discharge. The U.S. Food and Drug Administration (FDA), expands this definition to focus on any undesirable experience associated with a medical product, such as a medication or medical device. In such instances, the undesirable experience is considered an adverse event and should be reported to the FDA when, for example, the patient:

- Dies
- Experiences a life-threatening reaction
- Has an initial or prolonged hospitalization resulting from the adverse event
- Experiences "significant, persistent or permanent change, impairment, damage or disruption" of normal function
- Needs a "medical or surgical intervention" because of an adverse event (FDA, 2016)

When there are problems or an adverse event occurs with any medication or medical device, health professionals and consumers/patients can report the event online via the FDA Adverse Event Reporting System (FAERS) (www.fda.gov/Drugs/GuidanceComplianceRegulatoryInformation/Surveillance/AdverseDrugEffects/default.htm) or MedWatch (www.fda.gov/Safety/MedWatch/default.htm). Adverse events can also be reported to the organization where the event took place through incident reporting systems, if appropriate, and/or to a state adverse event reporting system or health department, depending on the state.

Sentinel events (sometimes referred to "never events" or "serious reportable events") are defined as any unanticipated event in a healthcare setting that reaches a patient and results in any of the following:

- Death
- Permanent harm
- Severe temporary harm and intervention required to sustain life (The Joint Commission [TJC], 2017a)

When a sentinel event occurs that results in death or serious physical or psychological injury to a patient that is not related to the natural course of the patient's illness, it should be (but is not required to be) reported first within the organization according to policy because these types of events, which are rare occurrences, should never

TABLE 1.1 SENTINEL EVENT DATA, 2014 TO SECOND QUARTER, 2017

Retention of foreign body	400 sentinel events
Wrong-site surgery	325 sentinel events
Fall	300 sentinel events
Suicide	300 sentinel events
Delay in treatment	250 sentinel events
Operative/postoperative complication	150 sentinel events
Criminal event	100 sentinel events
Medication error	100 sentinel events
Perinatal death/injury	100 sentinel events

Numbers are approximate. The reporting of most sentinel events to TJC is voluntary.
Source: The Joint Commission. (2017). *Sentinel event data general information 2Q 2017 Update.* Retrieved from www.jointcommission.org/assets/1/18/General_Information_2Q_2017.pdf

happen. There are 29 types of sentinel events/serious reportable events (the full list is available at http://www.qualityforum.org/Topics/SREs/List_of_SREs.aspx), including:

- Surgery on the wrong patient, at the wrong site, or a wrong procedure surgery
- Suicide in a hospital or within 72 hours of discharge
- Falls
- Delay in treatment
- Medication errors
- Surgical instrument or object left in a patient after a surgery or other procedure (National Quality Forum [NQF], 2017)

When a sentinel event occurs, the healthcare organization is "strongly encouraged," but not required, to report the sentinel event to The Joint Commission (TJC) and is "expected to conduct thorough and credible comprehensive systematic analyses (e.g., root cause analyses), make improvements to reduce risk, and monitor the effectiveness of those improvements" (TJC, 2017b). Patients, family members, staff, and the media can also report patient safety events to TJC. Note that the reporting of most sentinel events to TJC is voluntary and represents only a small proportion of actual events (Table 1.1).

CAUSES OF ERRORS

Everyone can make mistakes. Errors in providing healthcare to patients and their families are caused by a variety of factors, such as incompetency, lack of education or experience, inaccurate documentation, language barriers, fatigue, and inadequate communication among clinicians (Weingart, Wilson, Gibberd, & Harrison, 2000). Errors are also associated with extremes of age, new procedures, urgent conditions, and the severity of the medical condition being treated (Palmieri, DeLucia, Ott, Peterson, & Green, 2008).

NATIONAL HEALTHCARE ORGANIZATIONS INFLUENCING QUALITY AND SAFETY

While the initial estimates in the IOM's *To Err Is Human* report proclaimed that each year there were about 98,000 preventable deaths, recent research by Makary and Daniel (2016) has found that more than 250,000 deaths each year are the result of errors within healthcare. That means that after heart disease and cancer, patient safety errors are the third leading cause of death in the United States (Makary & Daniel, 2016). Recognizing these and other challenges within healthcare, national healthcare organizations provide resources and incentives to improve quality of care and patient safety.

There are three key agencies within the U.S. Department of Health and Human Services that are influential in encouraging improvements in healthcare quality and patient safety. These agencies include AHRQ, CMS, and FDA. The AHRQ (www. ahrq.gov) is focused on producing evidence to make healthcare safer, higher quality, more accessible, and equitable, and working to make sure that evidence is understood and used. The CMS (www.cms.gov) has multiple roles in influencing the quality of care and patient safety. The CMS works with both public and private organizations to ensure quality care, promote efficient health outcomes, and make sure that CMS policies are used by healthcare organizations and clinicians to receive reimbursement payments for their services to improve patient outcomes. The FDA (www.fda.gov) is responsible for protecting the public health by ensuring the safety, efficacy, and security of human and veterinary drugs, biological products, and medical devices; and by ensuring the safety of our nation's food supply, cosmetics, and products that emit radiation (FDA, 2017).

Several organizations, particularly the organizations listed in the following section, have significant roles in influencing the quality of care and patient safety. These organizations influence healthcare safety and quality by working with government organizations, healthcare organizations, and healthcare clinicians, as well as accreditation organizations:

- The Institute for Safe Medication Practices (ISMP) is a private nonprofit organization that leads efforts to improve how medications are used by preventing medication errors and promoting safe medication use, through its national Medication Errors Reporting Program, which collects medication error reports from healthcare professionals, and the Medical Error Recognition and Revision Strategies program, where ISMP works directly and confidentially with pharmaceutical companies to prevent errors associated with confusing or misleading medication naming, labeling, packaging, and device design (www.ISMP.org).

- The National Academy of Medicine (NAM), formerly the IOM, provides peer-reviewed evidence-based information and advice concerning health and health policy issues. The NAM released a series of 11 reports on quality and patient safety, starting with its seminal report, *To Err is Human: Building a Safer Health System* (IOM, 1999), followed by *Crossing the Quality Chasm* (IOM, 2001). The IOM also released the report, *The Future of Nursing: Leading Change, Advancing Health*, which sets forth a series of recommendations for nursing to have a greater role in the complex U.S. healthcare system (IOM, 2013).

- The National Quality Forum (NQF) is a private nonprofit organization that conducts review processes and works with stakeholders to standardize healthcare performance measures. NQF has certified 34 separate healthcare practices and procedures to be effective in reducing the occurrence of adverse events. A National Priorities Partnership, convened by the NQF, has issued sets of specific actions to reduce healthcare costs in three important areas, i.e., avoiding hospital readmissions, reducing emergency department overuse, and preventing medication errors (www.qualityforum.org).

- IHI is a private nonprofit organization that motivates and builds the will for change, partnering with patients and healthcare professionals to test new models of care and ensuring the broadest adoption of best practices and effective innovations (www.ihi.org).
- TJC, formerly named the Joint Commission on Accreditation of Healthcare Organizations, is a private nonprofit organization that operates accreditation programs for a fee to subscriber hospitals and other healthcare organizations. Generally, TJC ensures that quality compliance requirements are met, including core measures, safe practice measures, and process improvement efforts to accredit a hospital. It is also known for its standards and tools aimed at ensuring quality of care and patient safety, such as the Sentinel Event Policy, Improving the Root Cause Analyses and Actions (RCA2) methodologies and techniques, and the National Patient Safety Goals (www.JointCommission.org).
- The Leapfrog Group is a private nonprofit organization that collects and reports its Leapfrog Hospital Survey on hospital performance to improve the value of care and, through its Leapfrog Hospital Safety Grade, assigns letter grades to hospitals based on how they perform on patient safety measures (www.leapfroggroup.org).
- Healthcare Financial Management Association (HFMA) represents leaders in healthcare finance with broad-based stakeholders in healthcare to provide education and coalition building to improve healthcare through best practices and standards. Through its Value Project, HFMA identified patient quality concerns including "access, make my care available and affordable; safety, don't hurt me; outcomes, make me better; and respect, respect me as person, not a case" (HFMA, 2015; Table 1.2)

There are also some efforts to collect and provide information on performance measurement data to consumers, physicians, and others. Data from CMS Hospital Compare provides information on the quality of care provided to patients at hospitals. The information that enables consumers to compare hospitals, which can be accessed at, www.medicare.gov/hospitalcompare, is organized into several categories, including

- Survey of patients' experiences (Hospital Consumer Assessment of Healthcare Providers and Systems [HCAHPS])
- Timely and effective care
- Complications
- Readmissions and deaths
- Use of medical imaging
- Payment and value of care (CMS, 2017a)

TABLE 1.2 PATIENT QUALITY CONCERNS

ACCESS	MAKE MY CARE AVAILABLE AND AFFORDABLE
Safety	Do not hurt me
Outcomes	Make me better
Respect	Respect me as person, not a case

Source: Healthcare Financial Management Association (HFMA). (2015). *Value in health care: Current state and future directions.* Westchester, IL: Healthcare Financial Management Association. Retrieved from http://www.hfma.org/valueproject/valuesourcebook/

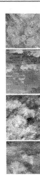

CASE STUDY 1.1

The case manager at a community hospital was reviewing occurrence report data trends over the last quarter. There appeared to be an increasing trend of patients who are not appropriate candidates for an MRI due to the patients having implanted metal devices. The lead MRI technologist is very concerned that these patients are not being correctly screened by the nurses on the unit.

The risk manager put together an interprofessional team from the nursing, medical, and MRI departments. After reviewing the MRI screening process, it was discovered that a new scheduling system that had been put in place in the radiology department was so efficient at getting patients an MRI appointment, the unit nurses did not have time to complete an MRI patient screening after the doctor had ordered it. A new MRI screening process was immediately implemented. The MRI order would now not be placed by the unit secretary until the RN communicated that the MRI patient screening was completed. Note that the problem reported by MRI staff led to the work process change. This protected patients from a potential injury.

1. *Why is it important that patients with implants be identified on the unit by the nurse rather than later by the MRI technologist?*
2. *How did the Risk Management process of reviewing the MRI screening process help with this patient safety issue?*

MEASURING QUALITY AND SAFETY

Work by the AHRQ, CMS, and NQF has led the development of measures for improving the quality of care and patient safety. Many of these measures depend on the occurrence of adverse patient outcomes or injury (measures of patient safety) while others raise the standard of care by ensuring that recommended care is available and used by all patients at the right time (measures of quality of care). When considered together, these measures can help healthcare organizations improve the value of care they provide to all patients.

There are several examples of quality care and patient safety measures that are used primarily in healthcare organizations, such as hospitals, nursing homes, and outpatient clinics. The major sets of measures include the CMS Core Measures, AHRQ Quality Indicators, AHRQ Patient Safety Indicators, NQF and American Nurses Association (ANA) Nurse Sensitive Indicators, and the National Committee for Quality Assurance (NCQA) Healthcare Effectiveness Data and Information Set (HEDIS) Measures (Table 1.3). Many professional organizations and other healthcare organizations also have quality of care and patient safety measures that can be found through websites of professional organizations and in peer-reviewed journal publications.

TABLE 1.3 EXAMPLES OF MEASURES OF PATIENT SAFETY AND MEASURES OF QUALITY OF CARE

MEASURE SET	A FEW EXAMPLES OF THE MEASURES	WHERE USED
Core Measures (CMS, 2017b) • Used to improve quality of care for common conditions • www.cms.gov/Medicare/Quality-Initiatives-Patient-Assessment-Instruments/QualityMeasures/Core-Measures.html • www.cms.gov/Medicare/Quality-Initiatives-Patient-Assessment-Instruments/QualityMeasures/Core-Measures.html	• Stroke: Received medication to prevent blood clots • Immunization: Assessed for flu vaccine • Heart failure: Received beta blocker therapy for left ventricular systolic dysfunction • Age appropriate screening colonoscopy • Readmission: All-cause readmission rate following elective total hip or total knee replacement	• Hospitals • Health plan/integrated delivery systems • Individual clinician level
Patient Safety Indicators (AHRQ, 2017a) • Used to improve the safety of inpatient care • www.qualityindicators.ahrq.gov/modules/psi_overview.aspx	• Rate of pressure ulcers • Retained surgical item or unretrieved device fragment count • Rate of central venous catheter-related blood stream infections • Rate of postoperative sepsis • Transfusion reaction count • Rate of accidental punctures or lacerations • Rate of birth trauma—injury to neonate	Hospitals
Quality Indicators (AHRQ, 2017b) • Used to improve quality of care • qualityindicators.ahrq.gov	**Prevention Quality Indicators** • Perforated appendix admission rate • Hypertension admission rate • Urinary tract infection admission rate • Uncontrolled diabetes admission rate • Bacterial pneumonia admission rate	Hospitals
	Inpatient Quality Indicators • Hip replacement mortality rate • Heart failure mortality rate • Acute stroke mortality rate • Laparoscopic cholecystectomy rate • Hysterectomy rate	Hospitals

(continued)

TABLE 1.3 EXAMPLES OF MEASURES OF PATIENT SAFETY AND MEASURES OF QUALITY OF CARE (*continued*)

MEASURE SET	A FEW EXAMPLES OF THE MEASURES	WHERE USED
	Pediatric Quality Indicators • Neonatal mortality • Pressure ulcers • Transfusion reactions • Postoperative hemorrhage or hematoma • Postoperative respiratory failure	Hospitals
Nurse Sensitive Indicators (ANA, 2010; NQF, 2004) • Used to improve the quality of nursing care • www.qualityforum.org/improving_care_through_nursing.aspx	• Falls with injury • Nursing care hours per patient day • Pressure ulcers • Rate of nosocomial infections • Staffing mix (ratios of RNs, LPNs, and unlicensed staff)	Hospitals
HEDIS (NCQA, 2017) • Used to measure performance in care and services • www.ncqa.org/hedis-quality-measurement/hedis-measures	• Childhood immunizations status • Colorectal cancer screening • Medication management for people with asthma • Controlling high blood pressure • Annual dental visit	• Outpatient clinics and offices • Other organizations (e.g., health insurance company)
URAC • Used to assess QI with organizations • www.urac.org/standards-and-measures-glance	• Patient and family member engagement • Effectiveness of communications and service coordination between providers and across providers and their patients • Errors and infections associated with harm and death	• Variety of healthcare programs (e.g., healthcare management programs, provider integration and coordination programs)

HEDIS, Healthcare Effectiveness Data and Information Set; LPN, licensed practical nurse; URAC, Utilization Review Accreditation Commission.

CRITICAL THINKING 1.1

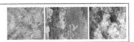

Each year, hospitals, healthcare systems, and healthcare providers report quality measures to national organizations. They also use these measures to assess their overall performance and they generally group these quality measures into several key strategic areas:

- Quality and safety of care
- Patient satisfaction/experience
- Workforce issues

(*continued*)

CRITICAL THINKING 1.1 (*continued*)

- Financial performance
- Strategic sustainability and growth)

Explore one of the websites in Table 1.3 for one of the measures described there. Think about how nurses can use these measures to improve nursing care and patient outcomes in these five key strategic areas.

1. How can nursing care and patient outcomes be improved by reviewing patient satisfaction measures?
2. How can nursing care and patient outcomes be improved by reviewing quality and safety of care?

UNWANTED VARIATION IN HEALTHCARE QUALITY AND SAFETY

Unwanted variation is variation in the use of medical care that cannot be explained on the basis of illness, medical evidence, or patient preferences, Wennberg, as reported by McCue (2003) has categorized four types of variation:

- Variations from the underuse of effective treatments or intervention that has been shown in clinical studies to improve health status or quality of life, for example, the use of beta blockers postmyocardial infarction
- Variations in outcomes attributable to the quality of care, for example, increased mortality following surgery
- Variations from the misuse of preference-sensitive services, for example, hysterectomy versus hormone treatment
- Variations from the overuse of supply-sensitive services, for example supplies that are overused because they are easily available to patients and healthcare practitioners, for example, medications and various technologies

There is variation in healthcare in various areas of the United States, variation provided by different healthcare providers and agencies, and variation in services available to different socioeconomic groups. There is also significant variation in what healthcare providers charge for different services. Nurses and the interprofessional team must work to reduce variation and improve healthcare service delivery to all patients.

TRANSPARENCY AND REPORTING PERFORMANCE

Healthcare clinicians, insurance companies, state and federal governments, patients and their families, and many others have the opportunity to improve patient safety and the quality of healthcare. National and state efforts to motivate improvements in healthcare have included financial incentives, regulation, accreditation, and public reporting. Of these, public reporting of performance is thought to be the best motivator for improving patient safety and quality of care. When organizations and clinicians are transparent in reporting their performance against quality measures, it is believed that they are being accountable, that they ethically respond to failures (Leape, 2010), and that they are informing consumer choice (Berwick, James, & Coye, 2003). In most instances, **transparency** is considered to include reporting not only the real cost of care, but also clearly reporting information about performance failures as well as successes (Pronovost et al., 2016). Major domains of healthcare transparency include the following:

- Clinical quality
- Resource use
- Efficiency
- Patient experience of care
- Professionalism
- Healthcare system/facility recognition and accreditations for meeting national standards
- Financial relationship of physicians and other healthcare professionals
- Financial relationship between physicians and other healthcare professionals, and industry
- Health insurance company processes (American College of Physicians [ACP], 2010)

Improvement of how care is delivered and improvement in patient outcomes from care received is a labor-intensive process that uses many staff and financial resources. Improvement processes include accurately looking at errors that occur from providing care; looking at areas where the quality of care can be improved through the early detection, prevention, and reporting of errors; and looking at improving performance on measures of quality care. Yet reporting errors or problems in quality of care is not straightforward. Federal and state governments, as well as private organizations have used mandatory reporting systems for errors and instances of poor quality of care, yet they are often not effective because of the fear that clinicians have of being punished, for example, with financial fines or punitive actions. As a result, errors continue to be underreported.

In many states, when a serious preventable adverse event occurs in a healthcare facility, for example, a hospital, nursing home, and so on, that is licensed by a state government, the facility is required by state law to report the event to their state government. However, it is important to note that while the majority of states have this requirement, not all states require this. TJC also has a voluntary reporting system.

Relatedly, it is also important to report successes and achievements in patient safety and quality of care within an organization. For example, reports of positive nursing sensitive indicators of high-quality care include achievement of appropriate self-care, demonstration of health-promoting behaviors, achievement of positive health-related quality of life, perception of being well cared for, and good symptom management. Mortality (i.e., death), morbidity (i.e., disease), and adverse events are considered negative outcomes by both clinicians and external organizations. Reporting successes can be helpful in understanding if an organization or clinicians are able to sustain and attain goals in safety and quality.

Patient safety and quality of care can improve in organizations committed to safety and quality throughout the organization. Unfortunately, not all organizations are committed to improving patient safety and quality. Nurses report that there is a lack of a blame-free environment and problems with leadership support to establish and maintaining a culture of safety (Wolf & Hughes, 2008). The barriers for attaining a culture of safety include lack of leadership, a culture where low expectations prevail, poor teamwork, and poor communication. Optimally, everyone, at all levels within an organization, would work in a culture of safety where there is

- Acknowledgment of the high-risk nature of an organization's activities and the determination to achieve consistently safe operations

- A preoccupation with safety
- An emphasis on systems improvement to support performance
- Organizational commitment of resources and encouragement of collaboration across ranks and disciplines to seek solutions to patient safety concerns
- Encouragement of collaboration to find solutions for patient safety problems
- Proactive reporting of unsafe conditions
- A just culture (or culture of justice) response to error, which includes frequent debriefing and sharing of "lessons learned," and which has an atmosphere of teamwork within a blame-free environment with mutual respect, which enables candid discussion among employees, where patient safety concerns are dealt with quickly (AHRQ, 2017c)

Safety culture is generally measured by surveys of providers at all levels. Available validated surveys include AHRQ's Patient Safety Culture Surveys (available at psnet. ahrq.gov/resources/resource/5333) and the Safety Attitudes Questionnaire (available at psnet.ahrq.gov/resources/resource/3601).

THE CONSEQUENCES OF WHEN THINGS GO WRONG

Errors in healthcare that harm patients cost approximately $17.1 billion each year (Van Den Bos et al., 2011). It has been estimated that, while hospitalized, about one in four patients experience one or more adverse events that result in a longer hospital stay, permanent harm, the need for a life-sustaining intervention, or death. Of these adverse events that resulted in injury, almost half were preventable (Office of the Inspector General [OIG], 2010).

Errors happen because of a multitude of factors, such as lack of education or experience, misdiagnosis, under-and over-treatment, urgency, and fatigue (IOM, 1999). Patient harm during a hospitalization is also impacted by nurses. The more times a hospitalized patient is exposed to below targeted nurse staffing levels, the greater the risk for patient mortality (Needleman et al., 2011). While nurses are capable of preventing the majority of errors from harming a patient, all errors need to be reported (Wolf & Hughes, 2008) by the members of the healthcare team, not just nurses. The team needs to work together to mitigate (or minimize the amount of) the effects of an error for the patient.

As part of national efforts to reform Medicare, and in an effort to encourage hospitals to improve the quality and safety of care, CMS and many private insurance companies require hospitals to report the occurrence of sentinel events and will apply a financial penalty to the hospital if and when sentinel events do occur. Sentinel events (e.g., mortality, readmissions within 30-days of discharge, and wrong-site surgery) are considered to be preventable and should not happen. When they do happen, the hospital will not be reimbursed for the cost of care associated with the cost of care for the aftermath of the sentinel event (e.g., longer hospital stays, a corrective surgical procedure) from CMS. CMS (and now many private insurance companies) will also not pay for conditions related to Never Events, including:

- Certain serious pressure ulcers
- Acquired urinary tract infections from catheter use
- Acquired blood stream infections from catheters
- Air embolism
- Giving the wrong blood type
- Foreign objects left in surgical patients (CMS, 2008)

In some instances, errors that cause patient harm result in a medical malpractice law-suit. Approximately $55.6 billion in 2008 or 2.4% of total U.S. healthcare spending is estimated to be spent on medical liability. Medical liability includes items such as malpractice payments to patients, attorneys' fees and other legal expenses for both sides, and defensive medicine costs, which are the costs of medical services ordered primarily for the purpose of minimizing the physician's liability risk (Mello, Chandra, Gawande, & Studdert, 2010).

PROFESSIONAL RESPONSIBILITIES FOR NURSES

Nurses are key to ensuring and improving quality of care and patient safety for patients and families, as well as for the organizations in which they work. Quality and Safety Competencies, developed as part of the Quality and Safety Education for Nurses (QSEN) initiative, that identify knowledge, skills, and attitudes that nursing students should achieve as part of their prelicensure programs and be able to exemplify in practice. They include the following:

- Patient-centered care
- Teamwork and collaboration
- Evidence-based practice (EBP)
- QI
- Safety
- Informatics (QSEN, 2014)

It is important to understand that the best way to exemplify these six competencies in practice is to apply each competency within the wider context of complex healthcare systems, which has not been the traditional approach for healthcare clinicians that have been educated to focus at the individual point of care (Dolansky & Moore, 2013). In other words, clinicians tend to focus on the individual patient and their family, not necessarily how that patient and their family affect and are affected by the larger population and system of care. As such, to effectively apply each of the six competencies within the wider context of complex healthcare systems, nurses need to think about how performance can be measured, how the strengths of each team member can be maximized to improve care delivery to patients and improve their outcomes, and what can be done in the healthcare system to assure quality and safety and prevent harm from unintended consequences from errors. To take this one step further, in some circumstances, it is important to think about how nurses can accomplish QI and patient safety within organizations that may not truly have a culture of safety. It can be very difficult to improve quality and patient safety within an organization that does not have a culture of safety.

CRITICAL THINKING 1.2

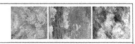

In thinking about what you are learning in nursing school about patient safety and quality of care, go to http://qsen.org/competencies/pre-licensure-ksas/ and explore the specifics of each of the six QSEN competencies.

(continued)

CRITICAL THINKING 1.2 (*continued*)

---

1. What specific ways do you see the QSEN competencies being used in your nursing courses?
2. What specific ways do you see quality and safety being practiced in your clinical experiences?

PREVENTING AND RESPONDING EFFECTIVELY TO ADVERSE EVENTS

Strategies to reduce unwarranted variation and ensure predictable and favorable patient-care outcomes have proven successful in improving healthcare quality and patient safety. These strategies include developing checklists and other standardized tools, using best practices, and working in an organization with a culture of safety and communication when an error does occur. Checklists have been proven successful particularly in operating rooms and other areas where multiple tasks need to be accomplished consistently to ensure quality and safety. Checklists have demonstrated that they protect against failure, they establish a higher standard of baseline performance, and they are only an aid if they are done right to begin with (Gawande, 2011).

Standardized communication tools such as the SBAR (Situation, Background, Assessment, Recommendation) technique (www.ihi.org/resources/Pages/Tools/SBARTechniqueforCommunicationASituationalBriefingModel.aspx), and using standardized order sets, protocols, and other best practices can be used by nurses and other members of the healthcare team to prevent errors, ensure quality care, and reduce variability in patient care and the potential for error.

It is important for nurses to work in organizations dedicated to a culture of safety and communication when an error does occur. Organizations that have a culture of safety are nonjudgmental, acknowledge the risk and error-prone nature associated with healthcare, and focus on improving healthcare systems and processes. In that quality and patient safety errors are often systems related and are not always attributable to individual negligence or misconduct, organizations that foster a culture of safety continuously strive to intercept errors before they happen, measure the quality of care processes and outcomes, and mitigate (or take action to minimize) harm involving patients. Organizations with a true culture of safety maintain an environment where nurses are not afraid to speak up and report errors or potential errors.

When something goes wrong and patients are harmed, it is difficult for clinicians, leadership, and patients. The first thing to remember is that when an adverse event occurs, it is important to respond in a timely manner, and as the Leapfrog Group recommends, do the following:

1. "Apologize to the patient and family
2. Waive all costs related to the event and follow-up care
3. Report the event to an external agency
4. Conduct a root-cause analysis of how and why the event occurred
5. Interview patients and families, who are willing and able, to gather evidence for the root cause analysis

6. Inform the patient and family of the action(s) that the hospital will take to prevent future recurrences of similar events based on the findings from the root cause
analysis
7. Have a protocol in place to provide support for caregivers involved in Never
Events, and make that protocol known to all caregivers and affiliated clinicians
8. Perform an annual review to ensure compliance with each element of Leapfrog's
Never Events Policy for each never event that occurred
9. Make a copy of this policy available to patients upon request" (Leapfrog Group,
2017)

One tool that health care organizations and providers can consider using to learn
more about being successful after an adverse event occurs is the Communication and
Optimal Resolution (CANDOR) kit. CANDOR is a communication and resolution process designed to open lines of communication between clinicians, patients, and their
families after patient harm occurs. The free program (available at www.ahrq.gov/
professionals/quality-patient-safety/patient-safety-resources/resources/candor/
introduction.html), includes eight training modules and also encourages clinicians to
report near misses and errors to better inform patients (AHRQ, 2016).

CRITICAL THINKING 1.3

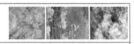

*During your shift, you discover that the wrong medication was given to the wrong
patient. Hospitals have policies and procedures that should be followed when a patient
is given the wrong medication.*

1. What are the policies and procedures at your clinical agency?
2. What do those policies state?

WHY IS IT WRONG TO BLAME AND POINT FINGERS?

When errors occur, we seem to traditionally blame the nurse as causing the error since
many of the roles of nurses in patient care often put the nurse in direct contact with
patients. In the past, we have even gone so far as to blame nursing leadership for
"allowing" nurses to cause errors. By being in direct contact with patients, nurses are
in a unique position to most likely be the only person in the room with the patient or
the last person able to stop a chain of events that may result in an error. If a nurse is
unable to stop an error from happening, the nurse is seen as literally at the sharp end
of the arrow of blame. The term **"sharp end"** has been used to identify the important
and significant direct contact role that nurses at the bedside, closest to clinical activities, play in recognizing the need for and potential impact of practice changes. Nurses
may see the sharp end effects on patients and others first when the right care is not
provided. Front line clinical nurses (as well as nurses in formal leadership positions)
often assume leadership at the "sharp end" of care in direct contact with patients to
assure safety and quality.

Nurses are qualified to offer invaluable insights and perspectives about what is
preventing effective and efficient care as well as how the quality and safety of care can
be improved based on their skills and experience. Other contributing factors, whether
individual or health system related (e.g., such as the physician who may have ordered

the wrong medication, or the design flaw in the infusion pump that malfunctioned), while maybe not in direct contact with the patient when the error occurred, also contribute to errors.

CAN HEALTHCARE BE PERFECT?

The quality and safety of care does not just spontaneously improve, and in many respects, it may not be possible to have error-free care that is of the highest quality at all times and in all places. Generally speaking, something needs to be done or someone needs to take action to either make improvements or ensure that a quality standard is maintained. A key goal of healthcare is to reduce unwarranted variation in healthcare safety and quality to ensure optimal patient outcomes. Yet even with the understanding that the quality of healthcare in the United States and throughout the world needs to improve, there is no consensus on how to best achieve consistent, high-quality care.

One of the challenges we have in improving healthcare is that nurses tend to be resilient—meaning that if something does not work well while they are providing care to a patient, they work around the "normal" way of doing things. These workarounds increase the opportunities for inconsistent care and inconsistent outcomes. Related to this, patients can also at times be resilient. For example, some patients can take the wrong medication at the wrong time and have no effects. Unfortunately, the resiliency of nurses coupled with the resiliency of patients does not guarantee the best possible outcomes nor does it ensure safe quality care.

Over the years, healthcare has become very complex. It involves multiple healthcare professionals and information from many sources. This complexity is closed linked with increased opportunities or increased risk for something going wrong and patients being harmed or the quality of care being compromised. Patients in hospitals and those that receive care from multiple healthcare providers at multiple sites of care are particularly vulnerable to safety and quality errors.

In an effort to ensure that safety is fundamental for every healthcare system, the IOM asserted that "Patients should not be harmed by the care that is intended to help them, nor should harm come to those who work in health care" (IOM, 1999).

IOM stated in its *Crossing the Quality Chasm: A New Health System for the 21st Century* (IOM, 2001) report that the healthcare system should focus on six aims (Table 1.4).

TABLE 1.4 SIX "STEEEP" AIMS OF THE HEALTHCARE SYSTEM

Safe	No one should ever be harmed by or as a consequence of receiving healthcare services.
Timely	Care should be obtained when needed with minimal delays.
Effective	The best available evidence should guide how healthcare is delivered to achieve the best possible outcomes.
Efficient	The quality of care should be maximized at the lowest, possible cost.
Equitable	Everyone should have equal quality of care even if patients may differ in personal characteristics other than their clinical condition or preferences for care.
Patient centered	A patient's culture, social context, and specific needs deserve respect, and each patient should have an active role in making decisions about their own care.

Source: Institute of Medicine (IOM). (2001). *Crossing the Quality Chasm: A New Health System for the 21st Century.* Retrieved from https://www.nap.edu/catalog/10027/crossing-the-quality-chasm-a-new-health-system-for-the

REAL-WORLD INTERVIEW

I live in the state of Georgia and up to this year, I have purchased individual coverage through Blue Cross and Blue Shield (BCBS) of Georgia. The cost has increased substantially in the last few years, but at least I was able to sign up for a preferred provider organization (PPO) plan. BCBS has notified me that they pulled out of the individual market for 2018. Thus, today I spent several hours looking for health insurance. None of the large companies (BCBS, United Healthcare, AETNA, Humana, etc.) offer individual health insurance coverage in Georgia. It looks like the best I can do is to sign up for a Health Maintenance Organization (HMO) with Kaiser Permanente HMO, which costs just under $900 per month. They do not offer PPOs for individuals in Georgia and only their Signature HMOs are available to me at all three **HMO levels (bronze, silver, and gold).** This offers a very limited number of doctors and hospitals near me. It is crazy, but it is the best I can do. The Kaiser Signature HMOs require me to find a general practitioner within their network of doctors that accept my plan. If I need a specialist, they will refer me to one in their network. However, for each HMO level, there are only a few doctors within 10 miles of my home and only one major hospital that accepts my HMO. This will be the first time in my life that I have an HMO. It is also the most I have ever paid for health insurance. The plan I am signing up for now will only cover 70% of expenses. I will have to pay 30% of expenses out of pocket. Going to an HMO means that I will not be able to go outside a prescribed network of HMO doctors in Georgia.

At present, the healthcare situation in the United States for middle class individuals like me that have to pay for our own health insurance is suboptimal. I have lived in several countries in Europe and Latin America and never found myself in this predicament. Usually, the healthcare is covered by some sort of national **insurance.** If you are middle class, you can afford to either purchase a private health insurance plan or simply pay out of pocket, since the cost of medical procedures and prescriptions is a lot more reasonable. In the United States, the costs of medical treatment and prescriptions are prohibitive without medical insurance. For example, if I were to get seriously sick and need treatment in a place like Spain or Panama, I could make an appointment with any specialist in a private clinic or hospital and pay out of pocket a lesser amount than the cost of my 30% insurance charges in the United States For instance, a doctor's visit in Spain or Panama costs less than $100. A specialist costs slightly more. You can get a full checkup including full blood and urine tests, Pap test, mammogram, and dermatologist check up from $500 to $700. Most common surgeries cost a few thousand dollars, not tens of thousands of dollars like in the United States. If you are a middle-class person there, you may not even need to have insurance. Medical tourism to other countries is growing fast in the United States, as you can obtain treatment in a foreign country, pay out of pocket, and it will cost you less than the out of pocket healthcare expenses in the United States, even with the travel expenses involved.

O. H.
Atlanta, GA

The 2001 IOM report further noted that by focusing on these six aims, a transformation will begin to occur in the healthcare system. In another report, the IOM stated that healthcare systems needed to be redesigned to improve quality of care and patient safety, but to do so, organizations needed to meet these six challenges:

1. Redesign care processes
2. Make effective use of information technologies
3. Manage clinical knowledge and skills
4. Develop effective teams
5. Coordinate care across patient conditions, services, and settings over time
6. Incorporate performance and outcome measurements for improvement and accountability (IOM, 2001)

INTERNATIONAL ADVANCES IN QUALITY AND SAFETY

Researchers and healthcare providers throughout the world have been actively involved in improving patient safety and quality of care. Significant research and practice innovations have been developed primarily in the United Kingdom, Canada, Australia, and the United States. Research across the world on strategies to understand and improve healthcare quality and patient safety can be found throughout peer-reviewed healthcare journals.

Even though some may consider the United States as the leader in healthcare or in efforts to improve healthcare quality and patient safety, comparative studies by the Organization for Economic Cooperation and Development (OECD), the United Kingdom, and The Commonwealth Fund, among others, have consistently found that the United States does not have better healthcare outcomes than other industrialized nations, including countries in Europe, Australia, Canada, and New Zealand (The Commonwealth Fund, 2014; The Commonwealth Fund, 2015; The Health Foundation, 2015; OECD, 2017). Poor U.S. healthcare outcomes do not make sense when you consider the fact that year after year, the United States continues to spend more on healthcare (per capita), than any other country in the world (OECD, 2017). Higher spending appears to be largely driven by greater use and cost of medical technology (Table 1.5) and higher drug and healthcare prices, rather than by more frequent doctor visits or hospital admissions (Table 1.6). Despite spending more on healthcare, Americans have poor health outcomes, including shorter life expectancy, greater prevalence of chronic conditions, and higher infant mortality rates (The Commonwealth Fund, 2017; Table 1.7).

TABLE 1.5 SELECTED COSTS OF MEDICAL TECHNOLOGY

MRI machine	$1,541,788
OR table	$65,263
Electric bed	$15,981
Stretchers	$7,618
Implantable pacemaker	$3,820
Knee implant—femoral	$1,970
Drug-eluting stent	$1,189
Hip implant—acetabular shell	$1,073

Source: Modern Healthcare. *Technology price index.* Retrieved from http://www.modernhealthcare.com/section/technology-price-index

TABLE 1.6 MEDICATION COSTS

	UNITED STATES	CANADA
100 mg of sitagliptin (Januvia)	$382	$105.03
1 inhaler of Advair Diskus 250 mcg/50 mcg	$386.97	$131.87
dimethyl fumarate (Tecfidera)	60-capsule package of 120 mg costs $6,805.76 or $113 per capsule	42 capsule supply of 120 mg costs $1,177.80, or $28.04 per capsule

Source: The Motley Fool. (2017). *5 drugs that are way cheaper in Canada*. Retrieved from https://www.fool.com/investing/2017/01/21/5-drugs-that-are-way-cheaper-in-canada.aspx

While organizations focused on improving the quality and safety of care have been previously mentioned in this chapter, there are similar organization outside the United States and even organizations within the United States that are focusing on either country-specific goals or global initiatives. For example, the European Medicines Agency and Health Canada have similar functions as the FDA in the United States The U.S.-based Joint Commission, has an international component that has established the International Patient Safety Goals that are used worldwide, including:

1. "Identify patients correctly
2. Improve effective communication
3. Improve the safety of high-alert medications
4. Ensure safe surgery
5. Reduce the risk of healthcare-associated infections
6. Reduce the risk of patient harm resulting from falls" (Joint Commission International [JCI], 2017)

Each of these international goals can be related to the U.S.-based Joint Commissions patient safety goals. The World Health Organization (WHO) also continues to lead worldwide efforts to improve patient safety (see www.who.int/patientsafety/en as an example). And since 1998, the Australian Patient Safety Foundation has also led key initiatives to improve patient safety (see apsf.net.au).

As these and other countries became involved in focusing on improving quality and safety of healthcare, inconsistency continued in how patient safety terms were used across nations, which hampered global advances to improve patient safety. The World Alliance for Patient Safety, a part of the WHO, developed the International Patient Safety Classification framework to facilitate a common understanding and use of definitions and preferred terms for patient safety (WHO, 2009; see www.who.int/patientsafety/taxonomy/icps_statement_of_purpose.pdf). Also, there has been inconsistency in how quality and safety of care is measured. The OECD developed a set of indicators for comparing the quality of health across OECD member countries through its Health Care Quality Indicator Project (see www.oecd.org/els/health-systems/health-care-quality-indicators.htm).

TABLE 1.7 U.S. HEALTHCARE FROM A GLOBAL PERSPECTIVE

	Total Healthcare Spending per Capita[a]	Infant Mortality per 1000 Live Births, 2013	CT Scanners per 1 Million Population	Price Comparisons for In-patient Pharmaceuticals, 2010 United States set to 100[b]	Life Expectancy at Birth	Percent of Population With Two or More Chronic Diseases, 2014
United Kingdom	$3,364	3.8	7.9	46	81.1	33
New Zealand	$3,855	5.2[c]	16.6		81.4	37
Australia	$4,115[a]	3.6	53.7	49	82.2[c]	54
France	$4,361	3.6	14.5	61	82.3	43
Canada	$4,569	4.8[c]	14.7	50	81.5[c]	56
Germany	$4,920	3.3	-	95	80.9	49
Netherlands	$5,131[d]	3.8	11.5	-	81.4	46
United States	$9,086[e]	6.1[c]	43.5	100	78.8	68

a   2012.
b   Price for basket of in-patient pharmaceuticals; lower number is lower price.
c   *Source, OECD Data, 2015.*
d   Current spending only; excludes spending on capital formation of healthcare providers.
e   Adjusted for differences in cost of living.

Source: The Commonwealth Fund. (2017). *U.S. health care from a global perspective.* Retrieved from http://www.commonwealthfund.org/publications/issue-briefs/2015/oct/us-health-care-from-a-global-perspective

EVIDENCE FROM THE LITERATURE

Citation

Marsa, L. (2017, September). *Take charge of your health care: Surgeries and side effects.* (p. 20).

Discussion

These are among the most common surgeries for Americans over 50 and the most common complications. In 2% to 4% of all cases, complications happen, and the patient needs to be readmitted to the hospital within 30 days.

SURGERY	COMPLICATION	OCCURRENCE
Cataract removal	Posterior capsule opacity	20%
Pacemaker implant	Hematoma	2.2% in patients over 70
Colectomy	Infection	12.4%
Coronary artery bypass	Atrial Fibrillation	24%
Hip replacement	Dislocation	2%
Knee replacement	Blood Clot	1%
Prostate removal	Bleeding	5.3%
Inguinal Hernia	Infection	0.3% Open surgery 0.2% Laparoscopic surgery
Cholecystectomy	Infection	7.6% Open surgery 1% Laparoscopic surgery
Appendectomy	Infection	4.3% Open surgery 1.9% Laparoscopic surgery

Implications for Nursing: Nurses must be aware of the higher incidence of complications in patients over 50 and, when possible, implement nursing care strategies to prevent complications.

WHAT IS THE COST OF ACHIEVING QUALITY AND SAFETY

From a systems perspective, the cost of providing safety and quality care comes at a cost (Table 1.8). Across types of healthcare organizations, there are many categories of costs, primarily including the costs of healthcare salaries (Table 1.9), costs associated with the technology used to provide healthcare services, and the cost of the physical space where healthcare is delivered. Hospitals also have significant costs when it comes to ensuring quality of care and patient safety. While some of these costs can be seen as high, the cost of poor quality of care far exceeds these amounts. The majority of hospitals in the United States (American Hospital Association [AHA], 2017) are required by the CMS to meet TJC accreditation requirements to be reimbursed for care received by Medicare and Medicaid beneficiaries, who represent the majority of hospitalized patients. There are over 4,000 hospitals and approximately 77% of them are currently accredited by TJC (2017). The accreditation process, which includes an expensive onsite survey, recurs every 3 years (JCI, 2017).

TABLE 1.8 SELECTED COSTS OF ACHIEVING QUALITY OF CARE AND PATIENT SAFETY

ORGANIZATION	REQUIREMENT	WHAT IS INVOLVED	AVERAGE ANNUAL COST
Hospital	Joint Commission Accreditation	• Meeting each of the standards • Planning for the survey • Staff time in record keeping and treatment planning • Conducting a mock survey • Actual survey	Approximately 0.03% to 1% of a hospital's operating budget. Annual fees are based on type of hospital, volume, and types of services provided (TJC, 2017c)
Home care agency	Joint Commission Accreditation	• Meeting each of the standards • Planning for the survey • Staff time in record keeping and treatment planning • Conducting a mock survey • Actual survey	Average of $1,500 for single-service home care providers, and onsite survey fee of $3,240 (TJC, 2015)
Healthcare organization	Director of QI	• Lead and direct process improvement activities to provide efficient and effective care	Average salary = $109,293 (range $95,713-$127,272) (Salary.com)
Healthcare organization	Nursing informatics specialist	• Manage information and communications (including documentation) for nursing	Average salary = over $100,000 (HIMSS, 2017)
Hospital	Magnet® Accreditation	• Performing a gap analysis to identify problems • Meeting each of the Magnet® requirements • Preparing and submitting an application and required documentation • Actual site visit survey	Average annual cost of $500,000 (total average investment of $2,125,000 over several years) (Robert Wood Johnson Foundation [RWJF], 2014)
Healthcare organization	Baldrige Award	• Meeting each of the criteria • Preparing and submitting an application and required documentation	Eligibility certification = $400 (initial cost) then the application fee = $10,560 to $19,800, supplemental section = $1,100 to $2,200, and site visit = $33,000 to $66,000 (National Institute of Standards and Technology [NIST], 2016)

Source: Glassdoor. (2017). Salary.com Salaries. Retrieved from https://www.glassdoor.com/Salary/Salary-com-Salaries-E35301.htm

TABLE 1.9 SELECTED HEALTHCARE SALARIES

ROLE	SALARY	SOURCE
CEO, Merck Pharmaceuticals	$24.2 million	www.usatoday.com/story/money/markets/2016/08/26/drug-money-pharma-ceos-paid-71-more/89369152/, Retrieved September 10, 2017
Anesthesiologist	Mean annual wage $269,600	www.bls.gov/oes/current/oes291061.htm, Retrieved September 10, 2017
General practitioner	Mean annual wage $200,810	www.bls.gov/oes/current/oes291062.htm, Retrieved September 10, 2017
Nurse practitioner	Mean annual wage $104,610	www.bls.gov/oes/current/oes291171.htm, Retrieved September 10, 2017
Pharmacist	Median annual wage $122,230	www.bls.gov/ooh/healthcare/pharmacists.htm, Retrieved September 10, 2017.
Dietitian	Median annual wage $58,920	www.bls.gov/ooh/healthcare/dietitians-and-nutritionists.htm, Retrieved September 10, 2017.
Registered nurse	Median annual wage, $68,450	www.bls.gov/ooh/healthcare/registered-nurses.htm, Retrieved September 10, 2017
Licensed practical nurse	Median annual wage$44,090	www.bls.gov/ooh/healthcare/licensed-practical-and-licensed-vocational-nurses.htm, Retrieved September 10, 2017.
Nursing assistant	Median annual wage $26,590	www.bls.gov/ooh/healthcare/nursing-assistants.htm, Retrieved September 10, 2017.

There are also costs and savings for outpatient organizations when it comes to improving quality of care. For example, improving a patient's glucose management would increase the average cost per individual with diabetes by $327 per year, but would save between $555 to $1,021 annually (Nuckols et al., 2011).

Preventing hospital-acquired conditions (HACs), such as adverse drug events, falls, pressure ulcers and healthcare associated infections, can avert death. For example, about 44% of HACs are considered preventable. Recent decreases in the number of HACs has resulted in billions of dollars of savings for national healthcare expenses (AHRQ, 2015).

RECOGNIZING HOSPITAL EXCELLENCE

The most recognized award for excellence within a hospital is the Baldrige Award. The Baldrige Health Care Criteria for Performance Excellence have been used by many healthcare organizations to improve quality. Recipients of the Baldrige Award are selected based on the following Criteria for Performance Excellence:

1. Leadership: How upper management leads the organization and how the organization leads within the community.
2. Strategy: How the organization establishes and plans to implement strategic directions.

3. Customers: How the organization builds and maintains strong, lasting relationships with customers.
4. Measurement, analysis, and knowledge management: How the organization uses data to support key processes and manage performance.
5. Workforce: How the organization empowers and involves its workforce.
6. Operations: How the organization designs, manages, and improves key processes.
7. Results: How the organization performs in terms of customer satisfaction, finances, human resources, supplier and partner performance, operations, governance and social responsibility, and how the organization compares to its competitors" (ASQ, 2017).

The Criteria for Performance Excellence is based on a set of core values. Award recipient organizations are considered to have a role-model organizational management system that continuously makes improvements in delivering products and/or services, demonstrates efficient and effective operations, and provides a way of engaging and responding to customers and other stakeholders.

RECOGNIZING NURSING EXCELLENCE

The American Nurses Credentialing Center's (ANCC, 2017) Magnet Recognition Program awards healthcare organizations that have achieved superior performance and is often referred to as the ultimate credential for high-quality nursing. The Magnet Recognition Program evaluates sources of evidence that create the foundational infrastructure for excellence, while its focus on results fosters a culture of quality and innovation. To achieve Magnet Recognition, organizations participate in a rigorous review process where organizations must demonstrate support of professional clinical practice, promote excellence in the delivery of nursing services to patients, and have processes to promote best nursing practices (ANCC, 2017).

Similar to the Magnet Recognition Program, but not as expensive and not requiring as extensive a process, is the Pathway to Excellence Program. To be nationally recognized and designated for the Pathway to Excellence Program, a healthcare organization must meet specific practice standards, including:

1. Shared decision making
2. Leadership
3. Safety
4. Quality
5. Well-being
6. Professional development (ANCC, 2017).

Organizations earn the award by demonstrating that their practices and policies help create a safe, positive work environment for nurses and high-quality, safe care for patients.

There are also numerous opportunities for individual credentialing, where licensed nurses complete a specific number of education hours and/or hours of experience and take a test to demonstrate mastery of a body of knowledge and acquired skills in a particular specialty (McHugh et al., 2014). The ANCC, among many other organizations, offers numerous certification for the various types of nursing care (see http://www.nursecredentialing.org/Certification).

NURSE LEADER AND MANAGER

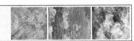

RADM Jessie M. Scott, DSc, RN, FAAN, was Assistant Surgeon General in the U.S. Public Health Service and led the Division of Nursing for 15 years. She was instrumental in the passage and implementation of the Nurse Training Act. Her career led her to address nursing shortages from Arkansas to Connecticut and later to work with nursing education programs in India, Egypt, Liberia, and Kenya. Read more about her at www.nursingworld.org/halloffame

ROLE OF NURSE LEADERS IN ENSURING QUALITY AND SAFETY

In 2010, the IOM released the report, *The Future of Nursing: Leading Change, Advancing Health* (IOM, 2010). The key message of the report was for nurses to take a greater leadership role across care settings in the increasingly complex U.S. healthcare system. As the population ages and becomes increasingly diverse and to effectively respond to the changes and complexity of healthcare, the report examines how the roles, responsibilities and education

TABLE 1.10 IOM RECOMMENDATIONS FOR THE FUTURE OF NURSING, 2010, AND 2015

IOM RECOMMENDATIONS—2010

- Remove scope of practice barriers
- Implement nurse residency programs
- Expand opportunities for nurses to lead and diffuse collaborative improvement efforts
- Double the number of nurse with a doctorate by 2020
- Build an infrastructure for collection and analysis of interprofessional healthcare workforce data
- Increase the proportion of nurses with a baccalaureate degree to 80% by 2010
- Ensure that nurses engage in lifelong learning
- Prepare and enable nurses to lead change to advance health

IOM RECOMMENDATIONS—2015

- Build common ground with other health professions groups around scope of practice and other issues in policy and practice
- Create and fund transition-to-practice residency programs
- Expand efforts and opportunities for interprofessional collaboration and leadership development for nurses
- Make diversity in the nursing workforce a priority.
- Promote nurses' pursuit of doctoral degrees
- Continue pathways toward increasing the percentage of nurses with a baccalaureate degree
- Promote nurses' interprofessional and lifelong learning
- Promote the involvement of nurses in the redesign of care delivery and payment systems
- Improve workforce data collection
- Communicate with a wider and more diverse audience to gain broad support for campaign objectives

Source: Institute of Medicine (IOM). (2010). *The future of nursing: Leading, changing, advancing health*. Retrieved from http://nationalacademies.org/HMD/Reports/2010/The-Future-of-Nursing-Leading-Change-Advancing-Health.aspx

of nursing should change to improve healthcare for everyone. In that nurses represent the largest segment of the healthcare workforce, the IOM recommended that nursing:

1. Be able to practice "to the full extent of their education and training
2. Improve nursing education
3. Assume leadership positions and serve as full partners in healthcare redesign and improvement efforts
4. Improve data collection for workforce planning and policy making" (IOM, 2010)

A few years later, the IOM released a report on the progress achieved on the IOM 2010 report recommendations (see Table 1.10), focusing on the areas of removing barriers to practice and care; transforming education; collaborating and leading; promoting diversity; and improving data. In this report, the IOM committee concluded that "no single profession, working alone, can meet the complex needs of patients and communities. Nurses should continue to develop skills and competencies in leadership and innovation and collaborate with other professionals in healthcare delivery and health system redesign. To continue progress on the implementation of The Future of Nursing recommendations and to effect change in an evolving healthcare landscape, the nursing community must build and strengthen coalitions with stakeholders both within and outside of nursing" (IOM, 2015).

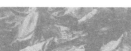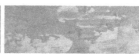

KEY CONCEPTS

1. **Healthcare quality** is defined as "the degree to which healthcare services for individuals and populations increase the likelihood of desired health outcomes and are consistent with current professional knowledge" (IOM, 2001).
2. Several organizations have significant roles in influencing the quality of care and patient safety;, for example, The ISMP, The NAM, The NQF, IHI, TJC, The Leapfrog Group, HFMA.
3. Data from CMS Hospital Compare provide information on the quality of care provided to patients in hospitals and includes information about patients' experiences (HCAHPS), timely & effective care, complications, readmissions and deaths, use of medical imaging, payment and value of care.
4. There are several examples of quality care and patient safety measures that are used primarily in healthcare organizations, such as hospitals, nursing homes, and outpatient clinics; for example, the CMS Core Measures, AHRQ Quality Indicators, AHRQ Patient Safety Indicators, NQF and ANA Nurse Sensitive Indicators, and the NCQA HEDIS Measures.
5. **Unwanted variation** is variation in the use of medical care that cannot be explained on the basis of illness, medical evidence, or patient preferences.
6. **Transparency** is considered to include reporting not only the real cost of care, but also clearly reporting information about performance failures as well as successes (Austin et al., 2016).
7. It has been estimated that, while hospitalized, about one in four patients experience one or more adverse events that result in a longer hospital stay, permanent harm, the need for a life-sustaining intervention, or death. Of these adverse events that resulted in injury, almost half were preventable (OIG, 2010).

8. Nurses are key to ensuring and improving quality of care and safety for patients and families, as well as for the organizations in which they work.
9. Strategies to reduce unwarranted variation and ensure predictable and favorable patient-care outcomes have proven successful in improving healthcare quality and patient safety; for example, developing checklists and other standardized tools, using best practices, working in an organization with a culture of safety, and communication when an error does occur.
10. Standardized communication tools such as the SBAR technique and using standardized order sets, protocols, and other best practices can be used by nurses and other members of the healthcare team to prevent errors, ensure quality care, and reduce variability in patient care and the potential for error.
11. The term **"sharp end"** has been used to identify the important and significant direct contact role that nurses at the bedside, closest to clinical activities, play in recognizing the need for and potential impact of practice changes. Nurses may see the sharp end effects on patients and others first when the right care is not provided. Front line clinical nurses (as well as nurses in formal leadership positions) often assume leadership at the "sharp end" of care in direct contact with patients to ensure safety and quality.
12. Workarounds may occur when something doesn't work well while nurses are providing care to a patient and they work around the "normal" way of doing things. These workarounds increase the opportunities for inconsistent care and inconsistent outcomes.
13. Even though some may consider the United States as the leader in healthcare or in efforts to improve healthcare quality and patient safety, comparative studies by the OECD, the United Kingdom, and The Commonwealth Fund, among others, have consistently found that the United States does not have better healthcare outcomes than other industrialized nations, including countries in Europe, Australia, Canada, and New Zealand (The Commonwealth Fund, 2014; The Health Foundation, 2015; OECD, 2017).
14. Poor U.S. healthcare outcomes do not make sense when you consider the fact that year after year, the United States continues to spend more on healthcare (per capita), than any other country in the world (OECD, 2017).
15. Higher U.S. spending appears to be largely driven by greater use and cost of medical technology and higher drug and healthcare prices, rather than by more frequent doctor visits or hospital admissions.
16. Despite spending more on healthcare, Americans have poor health outcomes, including shorter life expectancy, greater prevalence of chronic conditions, and higher infant mortality rates (The Commonwealth Fund, 2017).
17. The U.S.-based Joint Commission has an international component that has established the International Patient Safety Goals that are used worldwide.
18. The majority of hospitals in the United States (AHA, 2017) are required by the CMS to meet TJC accreditation requirements to be reimbursed for care received by Medicare and Medicaid beneficiaries, who represent the majority of hospitalized patients.
19. There are over 4,000 hospitals and approximately 77% of them are currently accredited by TJC (TJC, 2017).
20. The CEO of Merck Pharmaceuticals has an annual salary of $24.2 million.
21. The Baldrige Health Care Criteria for Performance Excellence has been used by many healthcare organizations to improve quality.
22. ANCC Magnet Recognition Program awards healthcare organizations that have achieved superior performance and is often referred to as the ultimate credential for high-quality nursing.

KEY TERMS

Adverse event	Sentinel events
Errors	Sharp end
Healthcare quality	Transparency
High-quality care	

REVIEW QUESTIONS

1. A group of emergency department nurses are asked to develop an action plan to improve the time before patients who present with chest pain receive an ECG. Which of the following would not be helpful when working on a QI effort like this?

   A. Identify an interprofessional group of individuals to help review current performance.

   B. Compare current hospital emergency department data results to benchmark comparison information reported on a national website.

   C. Post current hospital performance data results openly to staff in the nursing lounge.

   D. Identify whose fault it is that results are not very good.

2. As a staff nurse you are interested in making QIs in the overall care of patients with heart failure. Where would be most helpful to look for data and information to help you get started with these improvements?

   A. Explore the IHI website (www.IHI.org), which includes white papers, evidence-based protocols, blogs, and improvement stories that can be applied to patients with heart failure.

   B. Review the National Cancer Institute's website, which includes facts and statistics related to cancer care, resources, and latest research developments.

   C. Review drug companies' websites to see if there are any new medications available to treat heart failure.

   D. Google "heart failure" to see if you can get access to the latest treatment options for this patient population.

3. An 87-year-old patient was admitted to an acute care hospital. The patient was in a severe automobile vehicle accident. He is unconscious in intensive care and on a ventilator. On Day 3 of the patient's hospitalization, the patient experiences a cardiac arrest and a code blue is called. The code blue lasts for an hour. The patient's heart rhythm is restored. When the family is notified of the event, the wife is very upset. She states she had provided the hospital with the patient's advance directive, which clearly stated the patient should not be resuscitated. You are the nurse talking to the wife. What do you do?

   A. Apologize, but state that the patient was a full code, which means he must be resuscitated.

   B. Apologize, and assure the wife that you will be contacting the attending physician and your nurse manager that the problem occurred. The risk management department will probably review this case.

    C. Notify the wife that the advance directive is not legal or binding and that the wife needed to tell them specifically that the patient did not want to be resuscitated.

    D. Tell the wife to try to focus on the positive, that her 87-year-old husband is still alive.

4. A patient asks a nurse what it means to have a hospital accredited by TJC. Which one of the following is not a Joint Commission quality compliance requirement?

    A. Billing models

    B. Core measures

    C. Safe practice measures

    D. Process improvement efforts

5. A patient read that hospitals are not getting reimbursed by the CMS for certain never events and asks a nurse to explain. Which one of the following is an example of a never event?

    A. Absence of a hospice unit within the hospital

    B. Emergency department admissions of over 1,000 per month

    C. Nursing stations located at the end of the hall versus in the middle of the patient-care unit

    D. Stage IV hospital-acquired pressure ulcer

6. What is a common cause of errors within healthcare settings?

    A. Uncaring professionals

    B. Incompetent caregivers

    C. Communication problems between caregivers

    D. Phones not connecting to the nurse's station

7. QSEN has developed multiple quality and safety competencies to guide nursing practice. Identify which of these are considered a part of the six key competencies.

    A. QI, teamwork and collaboration, and EBP

    B. Fact finding, mission statements, and strategic planning

    C. Stakeholder feedback, budget reconciliation, and strategic planning

    D. Financial reporting, wait time measurements, and time delays in getting treatments

8. You are the nurse caring for a patient who was recently told he has heart failure. The patient will be relocating next week to a different state. The patient has a primary care provider in his new state and intends to follow up as instructed upon discharge. However, he would like to identify an acute care hospital in his new state that is adept in caring for heart failure patients, in the event that he needs to be admitted. The patient asks for your recommendation. All of the suggestions below may give him good information. What would be your *best* suggestion to the patient so that he may make a well-informed, objective decision?

    A. Tell the patient that hospitals publicly report their quality data associated with caring for heart failure patients on a website and instruct him where he can retrieve this information.

    B. Tell him to ask members in the community or family and friends where they have had good experiences.

    C. Tell him to ask his primary care provider for a recommendation.

    D. Tell him to visit the websites of hospitals in the community where he is moving.

9. You are an administrator working in an urban health system. You have been charged to lead the efforts of redesigning the patient-care delivery model. This model is intended to best represent patient expectations. As such, in developing the model, you recognize the importance of taking into account the patient's quality concerns. Which answer best represents the top patient quality concerns as described by the HFMA Value Project (2011)?

    A. Access: Make care available and affordable. Safety: Do not hurt me. Outcomes: Make me better. Respect: Respect me as a person, not a case.

    B. Access: Make care available and affordable. Safety: Do not hurt me. Quality: Provide high-quality care. Respect: Respect me as a person, not a case.

    C. Safety: Do not hurt me. Outcomes: Make me better. Value: Deliver care at a reasonable price. Inclusion: Include my loved ones in any care plans.

    D. Safety: Do not hurt me. Quality: Provide high-quality care. Value: Deliver care at a reasonable price. Respect: Respect me as a person, not a case.

QSEN ACTIVITIES

1. Go to the QSEN website (www.qsen.org) and search for Quality. Click on Quality Improvement (www.homehealthquality.org/Education/Best-Practices. aspx). Work on Cardiovascular Health Part 1 (www.homehealthquality.org/ Education/Best-Practices/BPIPs/Cardiovascular-Health-Part-1-BPIP.aspx). Can this information help improve patient safety?

2. Go to the QSEN website (www.qsen.org) and search for Quality. Click on Quality Improvement (www.homehealthquality.org/Education/Best-Practices.aspx). Work on Cardiovascular Health Part 2. Can this information help improve patient safety?

REVIEW ACTIVITIES

1. Go to the QSEN Institute website, qsen.org. Click on Competencies, Pre-Licensure. Also, click on Teaching Strategies. What did you find at these sites that apply to you as a student?

2. What patient safety challenges do you see in hospitals or in outpatient care sites?

3. Read through the summary of recommendations for two reports in the Quality Chasm series (go to www.nap.edu/catalog/21895/quality-chasm-series-health-care-quality-reports), and look at the list of recommendations. Of these recommendations, what surprised you?

CRITICAL DISCUSSION POINTS

1. Are all adverse events inevitable?

2. How is the FDA involved in improving patient safety?

3. Do sentinel events have to be reported to TJC?
4. Are there similarities in the measures of patient safety and the measures of quality of care (Table 1.3)?
5. Should only events that harm patients be reported to external quality and safety organizations?
6. Are patients safer if they stay in the hospital longer?
7. Name three of the QSEN competencies.
8. Does blaming a nurse for an error improve patient safety?
9. Name the six aims of the healthcare system from the IOM Crossing the Quality Chasm 2001 report.
10. Is improving quality and patient safety expensive?

EXPLORING THE WEB

1. AHRQ—www.ahrq.gov
2. ANCC—www.nurscredentialing.org
3. Baldrige Foundation—www.baldrigefoundation.org
4. CMS—www.cms.gov
5. FDA—www.fda.gov
6. IHI—www.ihi.org
7. NQF—www.qualityforum.org
8. QSEN Institute—qsen.org
9. Quality Chasm Series—www.nap.edu/catalog/21895/quality-chasm-series-health-care-quality-reports?gclid=EAIaIQobChMIjIeh35-31QIVBoNpCh2y0ASvEAAYASA AEgIhY_D_BwE
10. TJC—www.jointcommission.org
11. U.S. News and World Report ratings of hospitals—health.usnews.com/best-hospitals/rankings

EVIDENCE FROM THE LITERATURE

Citation: The Economist. (2018). Land of the free-for-all: America is a health-care outlier in the developed world. Retrieved from www.economist.com/news/special-report/21740871-only-large-rich-country-without-universal-health-care-america-health-care-outlier

DISCUSSION

America has some of the best hospitals in the world but it is also the only large rich country without universal healthcare coverage. About half of Americans have their health insurance provided by their employers. Healthcare costs can be financially ruinous for others. In 2016, America spent $10,348 per person on healthcare, roughly twice as much as the average for comparably rich countries. On average, both hospital cost and drug prices can be 60% higher than in Europe. The American Affordable Care Act expanded the health insurance system and cut the number of uninsured people from 44 million to 28 million but still left a gap among people not poor enough to qualify for Medicaid but not rich enough to buy private insurance.

In the United States, prices for the same service can vary enormously. Having your appendix removed, for example, can cost anywhere from $1,500 to $183,000 depending on the insurer. Add to this the fact that nine of the 10 best-paid occupations in the United States involve medicine and we see that doctors have little incentive to change the system.

Implication for practice: Nurses must participate in the discussion about the improvement of healthcare.

REFERENCES

Agency for Healthcare Research and Quality (AHRQ). (2011). *Health care quality still improving slowly, but disparities and gaps in access to care persist, according to new AHRQ reports*. Retrieved from https://archive.ahrq.gov/news/newsletters/patient-safety/66.html

Agency for Healthcare Research and Quality (AHRQ). (2015). *Efforts to improve patient safety result in 1.3 million fewer patient harms*. Rockville, MD: Agency for Healthcare Research and Quality. Retrieved from http://www.ahrq.gov/professionals/quality-patient-safety/pfp/interimhacrate2013.html

Agency for Healthcare Research and Quality (AHRQ). (2016). *Communication and optimal resolution toolkit (CANDOR)*. Retrieved from https://www.ahrq.gov/professionals/quality-patient-safety/patient-safety-resources/resources/candor/introduction.html

Agency for Healthcare Research and Quality (AHRQ). (2017a). *Patient safety indicators overview*. Retrieved from https://www.qualityindicators.ahrq.gov/modules/psi_resources.aspx

Agency for Healthcare Research and Quality (AHRQ). (2017b). *Inpatient quality indicators*. Retrieved from https://www.qualityindicators.ahrq.gov/modules/iqi_resources.aspx

Agency for Healthcare Research and Quality (AHRQ). (2017c). *Patient safety primer. Culture of safety*. Retrieved from https://psnet.ahrq.gov/primers/primer/5/safety-culture

American College of Physicians (ACP). (2010). *Healthcare transparency—Focus on price and clinical performance information*. Retrieved from https://www.acponline.org/system/files/documents/advocacy/current_policy_papers/assets/transparency.pdf

American Hospital Association (AHA). (2017). *AHA hospital statistics: A comprehensive reference for analysis and comparison of hospital trends*. Retrieved from http://www.aha.org/research/rc/stat-studies/fast-facts.shtml

American Nurses Association (ANA). (2010). *Nursing-sensitive indicators*. Retrieved from http://www.nursingworld.org

American Nurses Credentialing Center (ANCC). (2017). *Practice standards*. Retrieved from https://www.nursingworld.org/organizational-programs/pathway/

Aspden, P., Corrigan, J., Wolcott, J., & Erickson, S. M. (Eds.) (2004). *Patient safety: Achieving a new standard for care*. Washington, DC: National Academies Press.

ASQ. (2017). *Malcolm Baldrige national quality award (MBNQA)*. Retrieved from http://asq.org/learn-about-quality/malcolm-baldrige-award/overview/overview.html

Austin, J. M., McGlynn, E.A., & Pronovost, P.J. (2016). Fostering transparency in outcomes, quality, safety, and costs. JAMA, 316(16), 1661–1662.

Berwick, D. (2009, August 28). *In Bill Moyers" journal*. Retrieved from http://www.pbs.org/moyers/journal/08282009/transcript1.html

Berwick, D., James, B., & Coye, M. (2003). Connections between quality measurement and improvement. *Medical Care*, 41(1 Suppl), I30–I38.

Centers for Medicare and Medicaid Services. (2008). Medicare takes new steps to help make your hospital stay safer. Retrieved from https://www.cms.gov/Newsroom/MediaReleaseDatabase/Fact-sheets/2008-Fact-sheets-items/2008-08-045.html

Centers for Medicare and Medicaid Services (CMS). (2017a). Core measures. Retrieved from https://www.cms.gov/Medicare/Quality-Initiatives-Patient-Assessment-Instruments/QualityMeasures/Core-Measures.html

Centers for Medicare and Medicaid Services (CMS). (2017b). Hospital compare. Retrieved from https://www.cms.gov/medicare/quality-initiatives-patient-assessment-instruments/hospitalqualityinits/hospitalcompare.html

Committee on the Quality of Health Care in America. (2001). *Crossing the quality chasm: A new health system for the 21st century*. Washington, DC: National Academy Press.

The Commonwealth Fund. (2014). *Mirror, mirror on the wall, 2014 update: How the U.S. health care system compares internationally*. Retrieved from http://www.commonwealthfund.org/publications/fund-reports/2014/jun/mirror-mirror

The Commonwealth Fund. (2017). *U.S. health care from a global perspective*. Retrieved from http://www.commonwealthfund.org/publications/issue-briefs/2015/oct/us-health-care-from-a-global-perspective

Dolansky, M. A., & Moore, S. M. (2013). Quality and safety education for nurses (QSEN): The key is systems thinking. *The Online Journal of Issues in Nursing, 18*, 3. Retrieved from http://www.nursingworld.org/Quality-and-Safety-Education-for-Nurses.html

Food and Drug Administration (FDA), U.S. Department of Health and Human Services. (2016). *What is a serious adverse event?* Retrieved from https://www.fda.gov/safety/medwatch/howtoreport/ucm053087.htm

Food and Drug Administration (FDA), U.S. Department of Health and Human Services. (2017). *What we do*. Retrieved from https://www.fda.gov/aboutfda/whatwedo

Gawande, A. (2011). *The checklist manifesto: How to get things right*. New York, NY: Picador.

Glassdoor. (2017). Salary.com Salaries. Retrieved from https://www.glassdoor.com/Salary/Salary-com-Salaries-E35301.htm

The Health Foundation. (2015). *Focus on: International comparisons of healthcare quality*. Retrieved from http://www.qualitywatch.org.uk/content/focus-on-international-comparisons-health-care-quality#

Healthcare Financial Management Association (HFMA). (2015). *Value in health care: Current state and future directions*. Westchester, IL: Healthcare Financial Management Association. Retrieved from http://www.hfma.org/Content.aspx?id=1126

HIMSS. (2017). *2017 nursing informatics workforce survey executive summary*. Retrieved from http://www.himss.org/library/2017-nursing-informatics-workforce-survey-executive-summary

Institute for Healthcare Improvement. (2017a). Transforming care at the bedside. Accessed at http://www.ihi.org/Engage/Initiatives/Completed/TCAB/Pages/default.aspx

Institute of Medicine (IOM). (1999). In Kohn L. T., Corrigan J. M., and Donaldson M. S. (Eds.), *To err is human: Building a safer health system*. Washington, DC: National Academy Press. Retrieved from https://www.nap.edu/read/9728/chapter/1

Institute of Medicine (IOM). (2001). In Kohn L. T., Corrigan J. M., and Donaldson M. S. (Eds.), *To err is human: Building a safer health system*. Washington, DC: National Academy Press. Retrieved from https://www.nap.edu/read/9728/chapter/1

Institute of Medicine (IOM). (2010). *The future of nursing: Leading, changing, advancing health*. Retrieved from https://www.nursingworld.org/practice-policy/iom-future-of-nursing-report/

Institute of Medicine (IOM). (2015). *Assessing progress on the IOM report the future of nursing*. Washington, DC: National Academy Press. Retrieved from http://www.nationalacademies.org/hmd/Reports/2015/Assessing-Progress-on-the-IOM-Report-The-Future-of-Nursing.aspx

The Joint Commission (TJC). (2015). *The cost of Joint Commission Home Care Accreditation*. Retrieved from https://www.jointcommission.org/the_cost_for_joint_commission_home_care_accreditation/

The Joint Commission (TJC). (2017a). *Initiatives. Transforming care at the bedside*. Retrieved from http://www.ihi.org/Engage/Initiatives/Completed/TCAB/Pages/default.aspx

The Joint Commission (TJC). (2017b). *Facts about patient safety*. Retrieved from https://www.jointcommission.org/facts_about_patient_safety/

The Joint Commission (TJC). (2017c). *Facts about hospital accreditation*. Retrieved from https://www.jointcommission.org/facts_about_hospital_accreditation

Joint Commission International. (2017). *International patient safety goals*. Retrieved from http://www.jointcommissioninternational.org/improve/international-patient-safety-goals/

Leape, L. (2010). *Transparency and public reporting are essential for a safe health care system*. Perspectives on Health Reform. The Commonwealth Fund. Retrieved from http://

www.commonwealthfund.org/publications/perspectives-on-health-reform-briefs/2010/mar/transparency-and-public-reporting-are-essential-for-a-safe-health-care-system

The Leapfrog Group. (2017). *Never events*. Retrieved from http://www.leapfroggroup.org/influencing/never-events.

The Leapfrog Group. (2017). *Reports on hospital performance*. Retrieved from http://www.leapfroggroup.org/ratings-reports/reports-hospital-performance

Makary, M. A., & Daniel, M. (2016). Medical error—the third leading cause of death in the US. *BMJ, 353*, i2139. doi:10.1136/bmj.i2139

Marsa, L. (2017, September). *Take charge of your health care: How to research a surgeon* (p. 20) Retrieved from https://www.aarp.org/health/conditions-treatments/info-2017/choose-a-surgeon-doctor-surgeries.html

McCue, M. (2003). *Clamping down on variation. Managed Health Care Executive*. Retrieved from http://managedhealthcareexecutive.modernmedicine.com/managed-healthcare-executive/content/clamping-down-variation?page=full

McHugh, M. D., Hawkins, R. E., Mazmanian, P. E., Romano, P. S., Smith, H. L., & Spetz, J. (2014). *Challenges and opportunities in nurse credentialing research design*. Institute of Medicine of the National Academies. Retrieved from https://nam.edu/wp-content/uploads/2015/06/CredentialingResearchWashington, DCDesign.pdf,

Mello, M. M., Chandra, A., Gawande, A. A., & Studdert, D. M. (2010). National costs of the medical liability system. *Health Affairs, 29*(9), 1569–1577, doi:10.1377/hlthaff.2009.0807

Mello, M. M., Studdert, D. M., Thomas, E. J., Yoon, C. S., & Brennan, T. A. (2007). Who pays for medical errors? An analysis of adverse event costs, the medical liability system, and incentives for patient safety improvement. *Journal of Empirical Legal Studies, 4*(4), 835–860.

Modern Healthcare. *Technology price index*. Retrieved from http://www.modernhealthcare.com/section/technology-price-index

The Motley Fool. (2017). *5 drugs that are way cheaper in Canada*. Retrieved from https://www.fool.com/investing/2017/01/21/5-drugs-that-are-way-cheaper-in-canada.aspx

Mumford, V., Greenfield, D., Hogden, A., Forde, K., Westbrook, J., & Braithwaite, J. (2015). Counting the costs of accreditation in acute care: an activity-based costing approach. *BMJ Open, 5*(9), e008850. doi: 10.1136/bmjopen-2015-008850

National Committee for Quality Assurance (NCQA). (2017). *HEDIS® measures*. Retrieved from http://www.ncqa.org/hedis-quality-measurement/hedis-measures

National Institute of Standards and Technology (NIST). (2016). Baldrige performance excellence program. *Baldrige award process fees*. Retrieved from https://www.nist.gov/baldrige/baldrige-award/award-process-fees

National Quality Forum (NQF). (2004). *National voluntary consensus standards for nursing-sensitive care: An initial performance measure set*. Washington, DC: National Quality Forum. Retrieved from https://www.qualityforum.org/Publications/2004/10/National_Voluntary_Consensus_Standards_for_Nursing-Sensitive_Care__An_Initial_Performance_Measure_Set.aspx

National Quality Forum (NQF). (2017). *List of serious reportable events*. Retrieved from http://www.qualityforum.org/Topics/SREs/List_of_SREs.aspx

Needleman, J., Buerhaus, P., Pankratz, V. S., Leibson, C. L., Stevens, S. R., & Harris, M. (2011). Nurse staffing and inpatient mortality. *New England Journal of Medicine, 364*, 1037–1045, doi:10.1056/NEJMsa1001025 .

Nuckols, T. K., McGlynn, E. A., Adams, J., Julie Lai, J., Go, M. H., Keesey, J., & Aledort, J. E. (2011). Cost implications to health care payers of improving glucose management among adults with type 2 diabetes. *Health Services Research, 46*(4), 1158–1179, doi:10.1111/j.1475-6773.2011.01257.x.

Office of the Inspector General (OIG). (2010). *Adverse events in hospitals: National incidence among Medicare beneficiaries*. Washington, DC: U.S. Department of Health and Human Services. OIE-06-09-00090.

OECD. (2017). *OECD health statistics 2017*. Retrieved from http://www.oecd.org/els/health-systems/health-data.htm

Palmieri, P. A., DeLucia, P. R., Ott, T. E., Peterson, L. T., & Green, A. (2008). The anatomy and physiology of error in adverse healthcare events. In Savage T. & Ford E. W. (Eds.), *Patient safety and health care management, Advances in health care management* (Vol. 7, pp. 33–68), West Yorkshire, England: Emerald Publishing Limited.

Quality and Safety Education for Nurses (QSEN) Institute. (2014). *Graduate QSEN competencies.* Retrieved from http://qsen.org/competencies/graduate-ksas

Robert Wood Johnson Foundation (RWJF). (2014). *Becoming a Magnet hospital can increase revenue, offset costs of achieving Magnet status.* Retrieved from http://www.rwjf.org/en/library/articles-and-news/2014/05/becoming-a-magnet-hospital-can-increase-revenue--offset-costs-of.html

Van Den Bos, J., Rustagi, K., Gray, T., Halford, M., Ziemkiewicz, E., & Shreve, J. (2011). The $17.1 billion problem: The annual cost of measurable medical errors. *Health Affairs, 30*(4), 596–603, doi:10.1377/hlthaff.2011.0084.

Weingart, S. N., Wilson, R. M., Gibberd, R. W., & Harrison, B. (2000). Epidemiology of medical error. *Western Journal of Medicine, 172*(6), 390–393.

Wilson, R., Harrison, B., Gibberd, R., & Hamilton, J. (1999). An analysis of the causes of adverse events from the Quality in Australian Health Care. *Medical Journal of Australia, 170,* 411–415.

Wolf, Z. R., & Hughes, R. G. (2008). Error reporting and disclosure. In Hughes R. G. (Ed.). *Patient safety and quality: An evidence-based handbook for nurses.* AHRQ Publication No. 08–0043. Rockville, MD: Agency for Healthcare Research and Quality.

World Health Organization (WHO). (2009). Conceptual framework for the international classification for patient safety. Version 1.1. Final technical report. Retrieved from http://www.who.int/patientsafety/taxonomy/icps_full_report.pdf

▬▬ I SUGGESTED READINGS

Dekker, S. (2011). *Patient safety: A human factors approach.* Boca Raton, FL: CRC Press.

Gawande, A. (2011). *The checklist manifesto: How to get things right.* New York, NY: Picador.

Haviley, C., Anderson, A., & Currier, A. (2014). Overview of patient safety and quality of care. In Kelly, P., Vottero, B., & McAuliffe, C. (2014). *Introduction to quality and safety education for nurses: Core competencies.* New York, NY: Springer.

Hughes, R. G. (Ed.) (2008). *Patient safety and quality. An evidence-based handbook for nurses.* Rockville, MD: U.S. Agency for Healthcare Research and Quality (US).

Institute of Medicine (IOM). (2001). In Kohn L. T., Corrigan J. M., & Donaldson M. S. (Eds.), *To err Is Human: Building a safer health system.* Washington, DC: National Academy Press. Retrieved from https://www.nap.edu/read/9728/chapter/1

Institute of Medicine (IOM). (2001). *Crossing the quality chasm: A new health system for the 21st century.* Retrieved from https://www.nap.edu/catalog/10027/crossing-the-quality-chasm-a-new-health-system-for-the

Institute of Medicine (IOM). (2004). *Keeping patients safe: Transforming the work environment of nurses.* Washington, DC: National Academy Press. Retrieved from https://www.nap.edu/catalog/10851/keeping-patients-safe-transforming-the-work-environment-of-nurses

Institute of Medicine (IOM). (2010). *The future of nursing: Leading, changing, advancing health.* Retrieved from http://iom.edu/Reports/2010/The-Future-of-Nursing-Leading-Change-Advancing-Health.aspx

The Commonwealth Fund. (2015). *2015 international profiles of health care systems: Australia, Canada, China, Denmark, England, France, Germany, India, Israel, Italy, Japan, The Netherlands, New Zealand, Norway, Singapore, Sweden, Switzerland, and the United States.* Mossialos E., Wenzl M., Osborn R., & Sarnak D., D (Eds.), The Commonwealth Fund, Pub No. 1857.

The Joint Commission (TJC). (2017). *Initiatives. 5 million lives campaign.* Retrieved from http://www.ihi.org/Engage/Initiatives/Completed/5MillionLivesCampaign/Pages/default.aspx

The Joint Commission (TJC). (2017). *Initiatives. The IHI triple aim initiative.* Retrieved from http://www.ihi.org/Engage/Initiatives/TripleAim/Pages/default.aspx

The Joint Commission (TJC). (2017). *Sentinel event policy and procedures.* Retrieved from https://www.jointcommission.org/sentinel_event_policy_and_procedures/

Lee, D. S., & Mir, H. R. (2014, October). Global systems of health care and trauma. *Journal of Orthopedic Trauma, 28*(Suppl. 10), S8–S10, doi:10.1097/BOT.0000000000000213.

Wachter, R. M. (2012). *Understanding patient safety* (2nd ed.). New York, NY: McGraw-Hill.

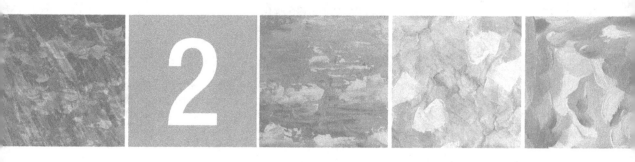

2

QUALITY AND SAFETY EDUCATION FOR NURSES

Catherine C. Alexander, Gail Armstrong, and Amy J. Barton

One goal of QSEN is to alter nursing's professional identity so that when we think of what it means to be a respected nurse, we think not only of caring, knowledge, honesty, and integrity. But also, that it means that we value, possess, and collectively support the development of quality and safety competencies. (Cronenwett, 2007)

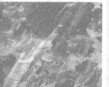

Upon completion of this chapter, the reader should be able to

1. Review a brief history of the Quality and Safety Education for Nurses (QSEN) initiative in the United States.

2. Discuss the various phases of development of the QSEN initiative.

3. Identify the six QSEN competencies, which are patient-centered care (PCC), quality improvement (QI), safety, teamwork and collaboration, evidence-based practice (EBP), and informatics.

4. Identify the knowledge, skills, and attitudes (KSAs) associated with each of the six QSEN competencies.

5. Identify QSEN competencies related to accreditation standards for nursing programs.

6. Recognize resources available for further learning about QSEN competencies.

7. Discuss special issues of nursing journals that have focused on QSEN.

An 86-year-old woman fell at home and suffered an intertrochanteric hip fracture. She will have a plate and screws surgically placed to stabilize the fracture. This patient has a past medical history of osteoporosis and atrial fibrillation. The patient takes Fosamax (alendronate sodium) 70 mg by mouth once a week and Coumadin (warfarin) 3 mg by mouth once a day. She proceeds to surgery without any member of the healthcare team checking her last dose of Coumadin or her international normalized ratio (INR) level. During surgery, the patient begins to bleed profusely and requires a transfusion of 5 units of packed red blood cells. The patient is transferred to the ICU for further monitoring. After this transfer, the interprofessional healthcare team gathers to review elements of this case (see Figure 2.1).

1. *Which members of the interprofessional healthcare team should be present to review this case?*
2. *How was patient safety and quality compromised in this case?*
3. *Which processes of patient care might be reviewed to ensure that this type of error does not occur again?*

The national nursing initiative, Quality and Safety Education for Nurses (QSEN), funded by the Robert Wood Johnson Foundation, has trained over 1,000 nursing faculty throughout the United States in how to build quality and safety content in prelicensure nursing curricula through education workshops sponsored by the American Association of Colleges of Nursing (AACN). In 2016, QSEN sponsored an international task force to guide the integration of the QSEN competencies in several countries across the globe (Canada, South Korea, Taiwan, Germany, and Sweden). The QSEN competencies are now translated into Spanish and can be found on the QSEN website (www.qsen.org). Plans are in place to translate the competencies into Chinese, Korean, and Swedish. Both faculty and students will find that the QSEN website (www.qsen.org) is a rich resource for ongoing education related to quality and safety.

This chapter outlines a brief history of QSEN, discusses the four phases of development of the QSEN initiative, and reviews the six QSEN competencies, that is, safety, informatics, patient-centered care (PCC), quality improvement (QI), teamwork and collaboration, and evidence-based practice (EBP). Built into each QSEN competency are the knowledge, skills and attitudes (KSAs) associated with each QSEN competency. The chapter then identifies how the QSEN KSAs are integrated into various phases of a nursing curriculum. The chapter also connects the QSEN competencies to accreditation standards for nursing programs. Finally, the chapter discusses nursing journals that have published QSEN-specific supplements and resources available for further learning about the QSEN competencies.

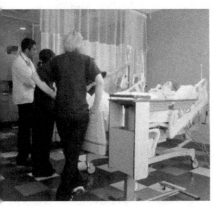

FIGURE 2.1 Interprofessional activities at the University of Colorado.

HISTORY OF QSEN INITIATIVES IN THE UNITED STATES

Educating the next generation of nurses in quality and safety is the overarching goal of the QSEN organization. To understand QSEN's history, one must go back to 1999. Since the Institute of Medicine (IOM, 1999) report, *To Err Is Human: Building a Safer Health Care System*, which estimated 98,000 lives were lost yearly in hospitals due to preventable medical error, a new era of consciousness about quality and safety in the U.S. healthcare system took root. Since the IOM report was published, healthcare leaders in both academia and practice have worked diligently to repair our fragmented healthcare system. However, progress has been slow since the report was issued. In 2015, The National Patient Safety Foundation (NPSF) convened an expert panel that concluded that despite advances in patient safety over the last 15 years, patients continue to experience harm that could be prevented (NPSF, 2015). In a report issued by Makary and Michael (2016), it was noted that medical errors are now the third leading cause of death, estimating 252,454 people lose their lives annually because of medical error.

Why are so many lives being lost to medical errors and what steps must be taken to fix the problem? Preventable deaths are linked to human factors including poor communication among providers, fatigue, time pressure, and systems breakdowns (Wachter, 2010). The NPSF acknowledges that our current healthcare system is far more complex than was previously understood and recommends that we rethink safety based on "systems thinking."

Dolansky and Moore (2013) define **systems thinking** as "the ability to recognize, understand and synthesize the interactions and interdependencies in a set of components designed for a specific purpose and understand how the components of a complex healthcare system influence the care of an individual patient" (p. 2). Healthcare leaders have a large role to play in providing safe, high-quality care. The NPSF report states "leaders must shift from a reactive approach to patient safety to one that consistently prioritizes a safety culture that includes the well-being and safety of the workforce" (NPSF executive summary, 2015). To accomplish this, leaders must be focused on patient safety at every level of an organization and, in particular, at the frontline of care. The *American Organization of Nurse Executives (AONE) Guiding Principles* document (2007) supports the following four patient safety goals: change from a culture of blame to one that is focused on teamwork, develop a leadership model that embraces shared decision making rather than the top down leadership style found in many hierarchical organizational structures, enhance collaboration within and external to the organization, and develop leadership competencies that are patient-centered and focused on patient safety.

Since the 1999 report, *To Err Is Human*, several subsequent reports have been published by the Institute of Health that address the causes of the startling number of preventable deaths in the acute care setting. The 2001 IOM report, *Crossing the Quality Chasm*, identified the need for safe, timely, efficient, equitable, effective, and patient-centered healthcare goals. The acronym STEEEP is often used as a mnemonic for these goals (IOM, 2001; Table 2.1).

In 2003, the IOM published *Health Professions Education: A Bridge to Quality* focused on the importance of all health professions students being educated in how to deliver care that exhibits qualities of patient-centeredness, QI, teamwork and collaboration, evidence-based practice (EBP), and **informatics**. The 2010 IOM report, *The Future of Nursing, Leading Change, Advancing Health*, called on nursing to lead the quality and safety movement. The report cited that nurses are in a unique position to impact the safety movement in the United States. However, there is a critical need to reassess nursing educational models that thread quality and safety throughout nursing curricula at the undergraduate, graduate, and doctoral levels. This reassessment is needed for nurses to lead QI initiatives at all levels of a healthcare organization. In 2015, a follow-up report by the IOM, *Assessing Progress on the Institute of Medicine Report—The Future of Nursing*, acknowledged that nursing had made significant strides in meeting many of the 2010 recommendations, but there is more work to do if nursing is going to lead collaborative improvement efforts through interprofessional teams. A pressing

TABLE 2.1 INSTITUTE OF MEDICINE'S (IOM) DEFINITIONS OF STEEEP

	IOM TERM	DEFINITION
S	Safe	Avoiding injuries to patients from the care that is intended to help them
T	Timely	Reducing waits and sometimes harmful delays for both those who receive and those who give care
E	Efficient	Avoiding waste, including waste of equipment, supplies, ideas, and energy
E	Equitable	Providing care that does not vary in quality because of personal characteristics such as gender, ethnicity, geographic location, and socioeconomic status
E	Effective	Providing services based on scientific knowledge to all who could benefit, and refraining from providing services to those not likely to benefit
P	Patient-centered	Providing care that is respectful of and responsive to individual patient preferences, needs, and values, and ensuring that patient values guide all clinical decisions

Source: STEEEP Healthcare Goals. Compiled with information from the report, IOM. (2001). *Crossing the quality chasm: A new health care system for the 21st century*. Washington, DC: National Academies Press.

question is how to engage healthcare professionals and frontline staff in QI "at the sharp end of the healthcare delivery system" where a patient's healthcare needs are met (Nelson, Batalden, & Godfry, 2007, p. 6).

The term "sharp end" has been used to identify the point in a healthcare system where providers, for example, nurses, physicians, aides, and so on, work and give care to patients. This point or sharp end of patient care is where errors may occur (Reason, 1990). Errors on the sharp end of patient care have often been considered to be the result of provider deficiencies such as careless behavior or lack of knowledge or skill. In fact, these sharp end errors have now been recognized to often be the result of organizational and extra-organizational issues, referred to as latent issues in a health-care system. These latent issues can be caused by healthcare system organization and management factors (Vincent, 2006), as well as by healthcare regulators, payers, insurance administrators, economic policymakers, and technology suppliers. All of these latent end issues affect the behavior of providers at the sharp end point of service with patients and may lead to patient-care errors.

PHASES OF DEVELOPMENT OF THE QSEN INITIATIVE

A group of nurse leaders, who had collaborated yearly since 1993 at an interprofessional conference with physicians and healthcare administrators, met to explore the impact of the 2003 IOM report, *Health Profession Education: A Bridge to Quality*, on health professions education. Engaging with other national thought leaders in nursing, this influential group asked the question: "What teaching strategies will prepare graduates in the health professions with the necessary skills to continuously improve the quality and safety of the healthcare system in which they work?" This question challenged this interprofessional group to outline a new curriculum that incorporates the principles of patient-centeredness, QI, teamwork and collaboration, EBP, and informatics outlined in the 2003 IOM report *Health Professions Education: A Bridge to Quality*. During the same period of time, the first phase of the Quality and Safety for Nurses (QSEN) initiative began with funding by the RWJF. The overall goal was to prepare nurses with the KSAs required to improve quality and safety in healthcare systems (Cronenwett et al., 2007). At the time, safety and high reliability consciousness were rising as critical components for the delivery of safe patient care. The QSEN Advisory Board decided to add safety apart from QI as the sixth competency. Cronenwett (2007) explains the QSEN Advisory Board's decision to add safety as a sixth competency this way: "The culture of nursing education was about preparing a competent, safe nurse and safety was viewed as a component of the individual professional rather than the system and we needed to make clear that preparation for future nurses needed to include that aspect of preparing for safety as well."

From 2005 to 2012 three phases of the QSEN initiatives were written that defined the quality and safety competencies that would be integrated into nursing programs throughout the United States. In Phase I, QSEN faculty outlined the KSAs appropriate for prelicensure education for each of the six competencies (Cronenwett et al., 2007). KSAs are defined as **knowledge**: the mental skills required to complete a task and the theoretical understanding of a subject; **skill**: the "hands on" or physical skills that one applies to his or her work, the proficiency or observable competence that is acquired or developed through education, and experience; and **attitude**: a behavior or point of view and the way a person views or responds to people or an experience. The KSAs for the six competencies can be found on the QSEN website (www.qsen.org). Phases II and III focused on faculty education and development and Phase IV, which began in 2012, expanded the competencies at the graduate level. Today, QSEN is a vibrant national initiative for nurses and nursing educators that offers resources for integrating the IOM's recommendations into models of nursing education both in prelicensure and graduate nursing education.

Phase I

Early QSEN data indicated that no nursing graduates were entering practice with updated knowledge about safe systems or knowledge from safety science. **Safety science** uses scientific methods and theoretical frameworks to achieve a trustworthy system of healthcare delivery. Safety science helps to describe how safety errors and near misses are recognized and reported, ways to manage human factors that impact safe healthcare delivery, and the competencies required for health professionals to provide safe care. Safety science has its roots in high-performance industries such as aviation and nuclear power and has now been adapted for use in healthcare. Safety science uses processes such as checklists and web-based reporting systems to improve care. Safety science has two important goals: It is the personal responsibility of all healthcare workers to both prevent errors and to continuously improve the delivery of healthcare services for both patients and staff.

Phase II

QSEN's Phase II work, also funded by the RWJF, occurred between 2007 and 2009 and focused on developing a QSEN Pilot School Learning Collaborative for faculty development. Fifteen nursing programs were selected to experiment with various pedagogical teaching strategies. The goal of this pilot program was to integrate the KASs, using the five competencies cited in the IOM 2003 report (i.e., PCC, QI, teamwork and collaboration, EBP, and informatics). Safety was added as the sixth competency given nursing's impact on patient outcomes at the frontline of care.

Phase III

QSEN's Phase III work occurred between 2009 and 2012, again funded by the RWJF. Phase III had three goals:

- Promote the ongoing development and evaluation of methods to assess student learning of KSAs of the six QSEN competencies and disseminate the new knowledge.
- Develop the faculty expertise necessary to assist the learning and assessment of achievement of quality and safety competencies in all types of nursing programs.
- Create a mechanism to sustain the will to change among all nursing education programs.

The focus of the Phase III work was to begin to change the content in nursing textbooks, accreditation certification standards, licensure exams, and continued competence requirements. Through the QSEN Phase III work, faculty from across the country were trained in how to integrate updated quality and safety concepts into their nursing education programs.

Phase IV

In 2012, the Tri-Council for Nursing, an alliance of four nursing organizations (i.e., the American Association of Colleges of Nursing [AACN], National League for Nursing [NLN], American Nurses Association [ANA], and American Association of Nurse Executives [AONE]) expanded the QSEN competencies at the graduate level. With support from the RWJF, the four nursing organizations led the $4.3 million effort to advance state and regional strategies to create a more highly educated workforce.

Integration of the KSAs Into Nursing Curricula

For practicing nurses, it is helpful to understand how nursing education is changing and to consider how QSEN KSAs are integrated into nursing curricula. Incorporating QSEN into a nursing curriculum requires an understanding of the six QSEN competency definitions of PCC, QI, teamwork and collaboration, EBP, informatics, and safety that are available on the QSEN website. Incorporating QSEN into a curriculum also requires a clear sense of how to effectively place the 162 KSA elements that operationalize those six QSEN competencies into a nursing curriculum. To provide guidance to faculty, a modified Delphi research strategy was used. The Delphi research strategy is an interactive forecasting method that allowed a panel of experts to gain consensus about where individual KSAs should be introduced in the nursing curriculum and where they should be emphasized (Barton, Armstrong, Preheim, Gelmon, & Andrus, 2009).

Each of the KSAs were identified as appropriate for introduction and emphasis either in a beginning-level nursing course, an intermediate-level nursing course, or an advanced-level nursing course. A beginning-level nursing course is one of a student's first nursing education courses. An intermediate-level nursing course is taken in the middle of a student's nursing education program. And an advanced-level nursing course is taken by a student just before graduation. The KSAs of the six QSEN competencies provide a strong foundation for quality and safety practices at the undergraduate level. The work of QSEN has only evolved over the last decade and many current nursing students will likely work with nurse preceptors who are not aware of the six competencies.

Table 2.2 provides a summary table of the Delphi results, indicating where KSAs from five of the six QSEN competencies should be introduced and where they should

TABLE 2.2 OVERVIEW OF DELPHI STUDY FINDINGS

QSEN COMPETENCY	BEGINNING INTRODUCTION	INTERMEDIATE INTRODUCTION	ADVANCED INTRODUCTION	BEGINNING EMPHASIS	INTERMEDIATE EMPHASIS	ADVANCED EMPHASIS
PCC	KSA competencies				KSA competencies	
Teamwork and collaboration	Skill and attitude competencies	Knowledge and skill competencies			Attitude competencies	Knowledge and skill competencies
EBP	Knowledge and attitude competencies	Skill competencies			Knowledge and attitude competencies	Skill and attitude competencies
Safety	KSA competencies			Attitude competencies	KSA competencies	Knowledge competencies
Informatics	Skill and attitude competencies	Knowledge competencies			Skills competencies	Knowledge and attitude competencies
QI	Attitude competencies	Skill and attitude competencies	Knowledge competencies		Attitude competencies	KSA competencies

EBP, evidence-based practice; KSA, knowledge, skill, and attitude; PCC, patient-centered care; QI, quality improvement; QSEN, Quality and Safety Education for Nurses.

Source: Compiled with information from Barton, A. J., Armstrong, G., Preheim, G., Gelmon, S. B., & Andrus, L. C. (2009). A national Delphi to determine developmental progression of quality and safety competencies in nursing education. Nursing Outlook, 57(6), 313–322.

be emphasized in a prelicensure nursing curriculum. Most interesting of these Delphi results is the clear message that all six quality and safety competencies need to be introduced and emphasized throughout a prelicensure nursing student's education program.

THE SIX QSEN COMPETENCIES

PCC

PCC emphasizes recognition of the patient or designee as the source of control and full partner in providing compassionate and coordinated care based on respect for the patient's preferences, values, and needs. For example, KSAs for this PCC competency are the following:

- K—Integrate understanding of the multiple dimensions of PCC: Patient/family/community preferences and values; coordination and integration of care; information, communication, and education; physical comfort and emotional support; involvement of family and friends; transition; and continuity.
- S—Elicit patient values, preferences, and expressed needs as part of clinical interview; implementation of the care plan; and evaluation of care.
- A—Value seeing healthcare situations through the patient's eyes (Cronenwett et al., 2007).

The KSAs for PCC allow for not only the basic needs of the patient to be met (bathing, feeding, toileting) but they also allow for the basic needs to be met in a way that considers patient preferences and values in the delivery of care. For example, when would the patient like to be bathed? How does he or she like to be fed? What aspects of the care is the patient able to carry out that they would prefer to do independently of the nurse? Do family members want to be active participants in their loved one's

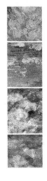

CASE STUDY 2.1

You are the charge nurse on a medical–surgical unit. A new graduate nurse is caring for a complex patient who has been hospitalized for over 2 weeks. The patient and the family have expressed frustration and mistrust in the healthcare team because of poor communication among members of the team. An individualized care plan was developed based on the unique needs of the patient. After report, you ask the new graduate nurse to read the plan of care for specific instructions related to the physical and psychosocial needs of the patient. The nurse states "I don't have time to read the plan of care, I have to pass my medications. I will read it later." Reading the plan of care later in the shift does not allow the nurse to consider the patient's preferences, values, or needs and may compromise the delivery of patient-centered care.

1. *Which (QSEN) competency would help you in expanding the nurse's practice?*
2. *Which resources for this QSEN competency might help you in working with this nurse?*
3. *Describe leadership attributes that would have helped this nurse provide PCC.*

TABLE 2.3 PATIENT-CENTERED CARE LEARNING ACTIVITIES

CURRICULUM LEVEL	LEARNING ACTIVITIES
Beginning level	Interview a patient about his or her diagnosis. What does the diagnosis mean to the patient? How does the patient's perspective of the diagnosis differ from that of the healthcare team? Write up your understanding of the patient's perspective and share it with the patient. Ask the patient for feedback about accuracy and interpretation.
Intermediate level	Are there barriers in your practice environment to actively involve families in patients' healthcare processes? Examine system barriers like limited visiting hours in the ICU or inability of family to be present in the perioperative setting. Are there policies that interfere with family involvement? What is the history of these policies? Do they still make sense?
Advanced level	Sometimes the nurse must initiate a conversation about patient-centered care. Use the following resource to identify effective strategies for such conversations: Toolkit: Conversations on Patient-Centered Care (https://www.orpca.org/files/Toolkit_Conversations_about_Pt_Ctrd_Care.pdf)

care? Physical comfort and emotional support are one knowledge aspect of the larger PCC competency. A report by the Picker Institute and the Commonwealth Fund titled *Patient-Centered Care: What Does It Take?* provides the contemporary context for PCC (Shaller, 2009). Table 2.3 offers learning activities for PCC at the beginning, intermediate, and advanced levels of nursing education.

CRITICAL THINKING 2.1

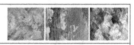

The video in which Donald Berwick shares his view of PCC: www.youtube.com/watch?v=SSauhroFTpk

1. Why is "indignity" promulgated and tolerated within healthcare institutions?
2. How can families be more authentically included in a patient-care experience?
3. Identify three concrete actions you can take to honor the concept of patient centeredness.

Teamwork and Collaboration

The QSEN competency of **teamwork and collaboration** emphasizes healthcare providers functioning effectively within nursing and interprofessional teams, fostering open communication, mutual respect, and shared decision making to achieve quality patient care. Examples of KSAs in this competency include the following:

- K—Describe scope of practice and roles of healthcare team members.
- S—Engage in appropriate handoff communication during shift report, patient-care rounds, discharge, or interfacility transfer.
- A—Value the personal contribution that team members make to achieve effective team functioning.

TABLE 2.4 TEAMWORK AND COLLABORATION LEARNING ACTIVITIES

CURRICULUM LEVEL	LEARNING ACTIVITIES
Beginning level	Explore the tools recommended for healthcare teams in the Team*STEPPS* program. These tools can be found at www.teamstepps.ahrq.gov. Which Team*STEPPS* communication strategies would be helpful for patient care on your unit?
Intermediate level	Teamwork and collaboration are core elements of surgical care processes. The IHI launched a national campaign to standardize aspects of perioperative teamwork and collaboration. Go to IHI's home page at www.ihi.org. Use the search box and type in SCIP. Look at the elements of the SCIP Project. What components of the SCIP Project are present in your perioperative services?
Advanced level	Review the article by Neily et al. (2010) and examine the implications of these authors' findings on training healthcare teams. Note the impact of teamwork training on patient outcomes. The first author on this research article is a nurse.

IHI, Institute for Healthcare Improvement; SCIP, Surgical Care Improvement Project.

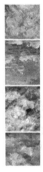

CASE STUDY 2.2

Emma, a new graduate, just completed her 3-month orientation. She is given a complex patient assignment without the assistance of a preceptor. After receiving a quick bedside report from the night nurse, Emma notices that her patient is restless and has an elevated respiratory rate. She is concerned, but realizes her patient is not wearing his oxygen. She puts the nasal cannula on the patient and tells him she will be back to check on him. Emma is starting to get behind in her work, but she wants to make a good impression with her colleagues and decides not to ask for help. One hour later, the nursing assistant tells Emma that her patient is in respiratory distress. Emma checks on her patient and decides to ask the charge nurse for help. After assessing the patient, the charge nurse calls the interprofessional rapid response team and tells Emma to bring the crash cart into the room. When the team arrives, they decide the patient is unstable and must be transferred to the ICU for close monitoring.

1. *What critical steps should Emma have taken to engage the interprofessional team sooner?*
2. *Describe the places where teamwork and communication could have been strengthened in this case.*
3. *Identify the quality and safety issues that emerged around teamwork and collaboration. What actions could have been taken to prevent a patient transfer to the ICU.*
4. *Describe one leadership concept that would have been beneficial for Emma to use to speak up and ask for help?*

Students begin to value the nurse's role in planning care and the nurse's impact on patient outcomes when the nursing scope of practice is learned within the context of interprofessional teams. Teamwork is one of the core competencies, along with communication, roles and responsibilities, and ethics, that all health professions students should achieve. The nurse is often at the center of communication for the healthcare team and frequently facilitates important patient-care transitions. For example, communication of the patient's changing status is vital to successful use of rapid response teams. **Rapid response teams** are a group of individuals from a variety of disciplines such as nursing, medicine, and respiratory therapy that use evidence-based interventions in the acute care setting to provide timely, focused care for patients experiencing rapid deterioration. The Institute for Healthcare Improvement's (IHI) *5 Million Lives Campaign* (2006) facilitated widespread adoption of this team-based intervention. Details about rapid response teams can be explored at IHI's website (go to www.ihi.org and search for rapid response teams). Table 2.4 offers learning activities that focus on the teamwork and collaboration competency at the beginning, intermediate, and advanced levels of nursing education.

Evidence-Based Practice

Nurses play a key role in protecting patients from harm by providing high-quality healthcare (Balakas & Smith, 2016). Research indicates that the implementation of EBP leads to higher quality of care, improved patient outcomes, and decreased healthcare costs (Melnyk, Fineout-Overholt, Gallagher, & Kaplan, 2012). The QSEN competency

TABLE 2.5 EVIDENCE-BASED PRACTICE LEARNING ACTIVITIES

CURRICULUM LEVEL	LEARNING ACTIVITIES
Beginning level	There is a body of research around barriers to utilizing EBP in nursing practice. Read the article titled "Evidence-Based Practice Barriers and Facilitators From a Continuous Quality Improvement Perspective: An Integrative Review," by Solomons and Spross (2011). Does the article resonate with what you are seeing in practice regarding the barriers for utilization of EBP? What did the authors identify as the barriers for continuous quality improvement in the clinical setting?
Intermediate level	Go to QSEN.org. On the search bar click the education tab. Both faculty and students will find competencies and teaching strategies related to evidence-based practice. Choose one to explore. Under the evidence-based practice tab there is a selection of articles for both students and faculty to read.
Advanced level	Nurses still struggle to get evidence into practice. The article, "Barriers and Facilitators to the Use of Evidence-Based Practice," by Scott and McSherry (2009) explains that, for evidence-based nursing to occur, nurses need to be aware of what evidence-based nursing means and what the process of EBP is to apply the evidence. This article examines the concept of evidence-based nursing and its application to clinical practice. Use the article as a basis for your discussion of nursing's struggle to get evidence into practice (Scott & McSherry, 2009).

EBP, evidence-based practice.

of **evidence-based practice** integrates the best current evidence with clinical expertise and patient/family preferences and values for the delivery of optimal patient care. Examples of this competency include the following:

- K—Describe EBP to include components of research evidence, clinical expertise, and patient/family values.
- S—Base individualized care plans on patient values, clinical expertise, and evidence.
- A—Value the concept of EBP as integral to determining best clinical practice (Cronenwett et al., 2007).

Traditional medical–surgical nursing skills are now often taught along with their bases in EBP. For example, nursing research highlights emerging best clinical practices related to fluid balance, peripheral intravenous insertion and maintenance, urinary catheter care, care of central lines, and nasogastric tube insertion. As confirmation of the core role of EBP in developing clinical practice, most nursing texts now include evidence-based support to explain rationales for clinical practice. Table 2.5 offers learning activities for this competency.

Quality Improvement

The QSEN competency of **quality improvement (QI)** is defined as the use of data to monitor the outcomes of care processes and using improvement methods to design and use changes to continuously improve the quality and safety of healthcare systems. Nursing programs have integrated QI methods and tools to help students engage in frontline improvement (IOM, 2003). Examples of KSAs for this competency include the following:

- K—Recognize that nursing and other health professions students are parts of systems of care and care processes that affect outcomes for patients and families.
- S—Use tools (such as control charts and run charts) that are helpful for understanding variation.
- A—Appreciate that continuous QI is an essential part of the daily work of all health professionals (Cronenwett et al., 2007).

Formal, systems-focused QI processes that engage a healthcare team, such as adverse events reporting, should be part of the early components of the nursing curriculum. Root cause analyses and resulting system changes are relevant to study in a clinical nursing course. As students progress through clinical courses, they will see many examples of nurses contributing to QI processes in the acute care setting. Nurses are well positioned to offer insights into how to improve patient-care processes to improve patient outcomes. Table 2.6 offers learning activities at the beginning, intermediate, and advanced levels of nursing education for this competency.

In addition to learning about QI from a nursing perspective, engaging with other health professional students is an effective learning strategy. Students can learn about QI together in classroom, simulation, and clinical settings (Headrick et al., 2012). In fact, the IHI has established an "open school" to distribute free online courses, provide experiential learning opportunities, as well as build community (available at www.ihi .org/offerings/ihiopenschool).

EVIDENCE FROM THE LITERATURE

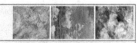

Citation

Hermann, C., Head, B., Black, K., & Singleton, K. (2016, January–February). Preparing nursing students for interprofessional practice: The interdisciplinary curriculum for oncology palliative care education. *Journal of Professional Nursing, 32*(1), 60–71.

Discussion

The Interprofessional Education Collaborative, a collaboration of key educational associations, including the American Association of Colleges of Nursing (AACN), established core competencies for interprofessional collaborative practice that apply to all students of the health professions. Evidence supports the collaboration of health professionals to improve patient outcomes, especially those related to quality and safety. This study identifies the development of an interprofessional Curriculum for Oncology Palliative Care Education (iCOPE) using team-based palliative oncology education as a framework for teaching students interprofessional practice skills.

Implications for Practice

The study concludes that health education can no longer be taught in separate silos, but must take an interprofessional approach to curriculum design. Nurse educators are ideally suited to lead these initiatives. The project serves as a model for ongoing efforts to develop and implement interprofessional education initiatives going forward.

TABLE 2.6 QUALITY IMPROVEMENT LEARNING ACTIVITIES

CURRICULUM LEVEL	LEARNING ACTIVITIES
Beginning level	Nurses are involved in QI work at every level of healthcare. A checklist, developed by Peter Pronovost, around central line insertion has standardized the practice of central line insertion and reduced central line-associated bloodstream infections. Read Atul Gawande's article on the development of this checklist, paying attention to the role of nurses in the checklist's implementation (Gawande, 2007)
Intermediate level	The article "Adverse Event Reporting and Quality Improvement in the Intensive Care Unit," by Heavner and Siner (2015) illustrates the process of QI and adverse event reporting. Form student teams to review an adverse event and propose system solutions.
Advanced level	Partner with someone who works in the QI department of your hospital. Shadow that person for 2 full days. Notice the focus of their work. Which patient outcomes is this department tracking? How are data gathered for these patient outcomes? What elements of nursing care are tracked for these patient outcomes? What insight can nurses provide about the patient-care processes to achieve these patient outcomes?

QI, quality improvement.

REAL-WORLD INTERVIEW

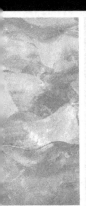

Quality and safety improvement is more than just a supplemental activity complementing core clinical education in the health professions. It directly impacts the health and lives of the people that healthcare professionals have pledged to help and directly affects the outcomes that we need to achieve in healthcare. Quality and safety, therefore, must be a personal commitment and part of the core professional role identity of every healthcare professional. To achieve this, health professions education must strive to integrate quality and safety into the core curriculum and prepare "clinician-leader-improvers" who are ready to lead and continuously improve the work they are doing in healthcare. QSEN is a key voice for quality and safety education in the nursing profession. QSEN also provides guidance and resources, which are essential in developing competence in quality and safety for health professions. It is critical that all health professions education programs integrate the QSEN competencies into their curricula and engage students in meaningful applied quality and safety education experiences at the beginning of their educational development and then onward into professional practice. To a great degree, the future of our health is in the hands of our students and in their efforts to improve healthcare quality and safety. As such, health profession educators have a critical obligation to help them to develop not only as clinicians, but as leaders and improvers

Brant J. Oliver, PhD, MS, MPH, APRN-BC
Assistant Professor, The Dartmouth Institute &
Geisel School of Medicine at Dartmouth
Adjunct Associate Professor, School of Nursing
MGH Institute of Health Professions
Faculty Senior Scholar
Veteran's Affairs National Quality Fellowship
in Healthcare Quality and Safety

Safety

The **safety** QSEN competency minimizes risk of harm to patients and providers through both system effectiveness and individual performance. Examples of KSAs for this competency include the following:

- K—Examine human factors and other basic safety design principles as well as commonly used unsafe practices, such as work-arounds and dangerous abbreviations.
- S—Demonstrate effective use of strategies to reduce the risk of harm to self or others.
- A—Value the contributions of standardization/reliability to safety (Cronenwett et al., 2007).

QSEN's definition of safety emphasizes team strategies to promote safe care in a healthcare system rather than focusing on blaming individuals for safety issues. For example, maintaining asepsis is a component of an individual nurse's practice and has multiple associated safety skills. Maintaining asepsis and reducing infections in

REAL-WORLD INTERVIEW

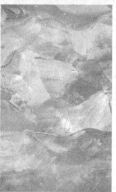
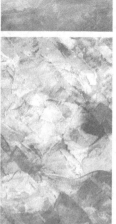

At the heart of our social identity as professionals is the ability to continually learn and improve our own work. No longer soloists, most of today's healthcare work is done with others. Interdependently, patients, families and people from multiple health professional disciplines work in complex, complicated and simple systems to cocreate and coproduce healthcare services. Changing and improving the coproductive work of relationships and actions requires diverse knowledge and skills (Batalden et al., 2016).

The European safety scholars, Charles Vincent and Rene Amalberti, remind us that, "we need to see safety through the patient's eyes, to consider how safety is managed in different contexts and to develop a wider strategic and practical vision in which patient safety is recast as the management of risk over time" (Vincent & Amalberti, 2016). This will involve moving from a focus on unusual events of failure and harm in hospital settings to a focus on the patient's journey over time. Attention to the coproduction and the coordination of services over time in diverse settings will open a new chapter in traditional safety efforts.

Paul Batalden, MD
Active Emeritus Professor
The Dartmouth Institute for Health Policy & Clinical Practice

Batalden, M., Batalden, P., Margolis, P., Seid, M., Armstrong, G., Opipari-Arrigan, L., & Hartung, H. (2016). Coproduction of healthcare service. *BMJ Quality & Safety, 25*, 509–517.

Vincent, C., & Amalberti, R. (2016). *Safer healthcare: Strategies for the real world.* Switzerland: Springer Open.

one's practice also has direct implications for supporting patient outcomes related to various national safety goals in a healthcare system. The *National Patient Safety Goals* (The Joint Commission, 2012), *5 Million Lives Campaign* (IHI, 2012), and *Safe Practices for Better Healthcare* (National Quality Forum, 2009) all state common goals around decreasing nosocomial infection rates in the acute care setting. Table 2.7 offers learning activities at the beginning, intermediate, and advanced level of nursing education for the competency.

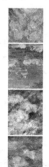

CASE STUDY 2.3

You are a new nurse working in a busy operating room. You notice that in the past month, three patients being transferred from the same adult patient-care unit in the hospital have not been given their preoperative antibiotics prior to transfer to the operating room.

1. *What patient-care processes might you address to attend to this recurring issue?*
2. *What data might you need?*
3. *Who would you invite to a meeting to address this patient-care issue?*

TABLE 2.7 SAFETY LEARNING ACTIVITIES

CURRICULUM LEVEL	LEARNING ACTIVITIES
Beginning level	Read and discuss the National Patient Safety Goals with colleagues. Describe how they apply in clinical practice. Go to www.jointcommission.org/2018_national_patient_safety_goals_presentation/ for a free 2018 National Patient Safety Goals slide presentation.
Intermediate level	The article "Lesson From Colorado: Beyond Blaming Individuals," by Smetzer (1998) summarizes the system failures that led to a sentinel event with a newborn.
Advanced level	Note the Nine Patient Safety Solutions identified by The Joint Commission and the World Health Organization: The purpose of the Nine Patient Safety Solutions is to guide the redesign of patient-care processes to prevent inevitable human errors from actually reaching patients. See www.who.int/mediacentre/news/releases/2007/pr22/en

Informatics

The QSEN competency of informatics calls for the use of information and technology to communicate, manage knowledge, mitigate (prevent) error, and support decision making. KSAs from this competency include the following:

- K—Explain why information and technology skills are essential for safe patient care.
- S—Apply technology and information management tools to support safe processes of care.
- A—Value technologies supporting decision making, error prevention, and care coordination (Cronenwett et al., 2007).

Documentation is an important skill in healthcare informatics. All members of a healthcare team contribute to an electronic health record that is used extensively to document shifting patient-care priorities. A broader view of informatics emphasizes not only documenting the patient care provided but also encourages the use of informatics in computerized clinical alerts and decision management. For example, a clinical alert signals to the provider that the patient is eligible to receive the pneumonia or flu vaccine. Decision management in healthcare focuses on having the appropriate data available at points in the decision making process to be able to make the best decision in a timely fashion. Data used in decision management may come from patient records, diagnostic results, providers' documentation, or EBPs. Table 2.8 offers learning activities at the beginning, intermediate, and advanced levels of nursing education regarding this competency.

QSEN COMPETENCIES RELATED TO NURSING EDUCATION ACCREDITATION STANDARDS

Nursing education accreditation standards are driven by rapid changes occurring in nursing practice. Several national reports have focused on the need for updated quality and safety content in nursing education. A 2010 report by the

TABLE 2.8 INFORMATICS LEARNING ACTIVITIES

CURRICULUM LEVEL	LEARNING ACTIVITIES
Beginning level	Many patients use Internet resources to become educated about their diagnosis. Use this QSEN learning activity to evaluate a health-related website that one of your patients may use. There is an evaluation form provided at qsen.org/website-evaluation-exercise.
Intermediate level	The Commission on Systematic Interoperability has been charged with developing a strategy to make healthcare information increasingly accessible at various care points in the healthcare process. Access the following website: www.endingthedocumentgame.gov. Click on the personal stories link and read the narratives provided by patients, healthcare professionals, and nurses about the importance of timely access to patient data.
Advanced level	Consider the number of electronic health records (EHRs) you have experienced during your nursing rotations. Answer the following questions: 1. How many EHR systems have you seen in your various clinical rotations? 2. What similarities have you seen among EHR systems? 3. Which EHR system seemed most "nurse friendly"? Identify what you mean by "nurse friendly." 4. What improvements do you think need to be made to existing EHR systems in the acute care setting to better support nursing care needs?

Carnegie Foundation for the Advancement of Teaching titled *Educating Nurses: A Call for Radical Transformation*, recommended several initiatives to address the practice–education gap (Benner, Sutphen, Leonard, & Day, 2010). The report's authors emphasize that both didactic academic classroom teaching and clinical practice teaching models need to more fully reflect the current healthcare emphasis on QI and patient safety. An interprofessional report published by the IOM in 2011, *The Future of Nursing: Leading Change, Advancing Health*, includes the key message that nurses need to be full partners with other healthcare team members to redesign healthcare in the United States. Quality and safety are two significant areas where interprofessional, collaborative efforts are needed to redesign U.S. healthcare systems. Accreditation standards for nursing programs have begun to clearly articulate the need for quality and safety content in prelicensure curricula. Standards from accrediting bodies for nursing programs, that is, the Accreditation Commission for Education in Nursing (ACEN), formerly the National League for Nursing Accrediting Commission (NLNAC), and the AACN are explicit about the necessity for the QSEN competencies in all nursing prelicensure curricula.

Table 2.9 connects each of the AACN Essentials of Baccalaureate Education to QSEN competencies. Many of the AACN Essentials of Baccalaureate Education contain several guidelines for prelicensure curricula, thus the connection to more than one QSEN competency in Table 2.9.

ACEN's accreditation standards similarly encourage the integration of QSEN competencies into prelicensure curricula. Table 2.10 connects several of the ACEN standards to QSEN competencies.

TABLE 2.9 SELECTED ACEN ESSENTIALS OF BACCALAUREATE EDUCATION AND QSEN COMPETENCIES

AACN ESSENTIALS OF BACCALAUREATE EDUCATION	QSEN COMPETENCY
II: Basic Organizational and Systems Leadership for Quality Care and Patient Safety	QI Safety
III: Scholarship for Evidence-Based Practice	Evidence-based practice
IV: Information Management and Application of Patient Care Technology	Informatics
V: Interprofessional Communication and Collaboration for Improving Patient Health Outcomes	Teamwork and collaboration QI

AACN, American Association of Colleges of Nursing.

Source: Developed with information from the American Association of Colleges of Nursing (AACN). (2008). *The essentials of baccalaureate education for professional nursing practice*. Retrieved from http://www.aacnnursing.org/Portals/42/Publications/BaccEssentials08.pdf

TABLE 2.10 SELECTED ACEN STANDARDS AND QSEN COMPETENCIES

ACEN STANDARD	QSEN COMPETENCY
4.5. The curriculum includes cultural, ethnic, and socially diverse concepts and may also include experiences from regional, national, or global perspectives.	PCC
4.6. The curriculum and instructional processes reflect educational theory, interprofessional collaboration, research, and current standards of practice.	Teamwork and collaboration Evidence-based practice QI
4.10. Students participate in clinical experiences that are evidence-based and reflect contemporary practice and nationally established patient health and safety goals.	Safety QI

ACEN, Accreditation Commission for Education in Nursing; PCC, patient-centered care; QI, quality improvement.

Source: Developed with information from the ACEN (2013).

QSEN RESOURCES

The QSEN website (www.qsen.org) has many resources for nurses, nursing students, and nursing faculty. Available on the website under the education tab are the competencies and KSAs for prelicensure nurses and graduate nurses. Here, students and faculty can read peer-reviewed articles on relevant teaching strategies and EBPs related to the QSEN competencies. Under the resource tab, faculty can access 18 learning modules that will assist them in integrating quality and safety competencies into their programs. The learning modules address topics such as appreciating and managing the complexity of nursing work, cognitive stacking (a process that assists students to more effectively manage the complexity of their work to promote safe, quality care), informatics, and other topics relevant for practicing nurses. Books, reports, toolkits, articles, and presentations can also be accessed under this tab. Under the publications tab, there are books and videos that highlight exemplar cases such as the Lewis Blackman story and the Josie King case. Both exemplar cases are potent tools that highlight the vital importance of quality and safety in nursing practice. Teaching strategies can be found in peer-reviewed articles at the site.

All of the relevant professional organizations that are making great strides in improving quality and safety in healthcare (e.g., IHI, www.ihi.org; Agency for Healthcare Research and Quality Patient Safety Network, psnet.ahrq.gov; National Association for Healthcare Quality, nahq.org/ and the NPSF, www.npsf.org) as well as many others can be found on the QSEN website. QSEN's well-designed website is an invaluable, updated resource for all nurses and nurse educators.

SPECIAL ISSUES OF NURSING JOURNALS THAT HAVE FOCUSED ON QSEN

Nurse Educator (2017) published a QSEN-dedicated issue in the September/October edition and included articles focused on QSEN'S impact on curriculum development in schools of nursing to date, as well as advancements in the integration of the QSEN competencies in the clinical setting. Earlier work in both *Nursing Outlook* (2009), November/December, *57* (6), and *Journal of Nursing Education* (2009), December, *48* (12) published QSEN-dedicated issues that are valuable resources and provide a substantive contribution to the literature about the importance and logistics of implementing QSEN competencies in nursing curricula.

CRITICAL THINKING 2.2

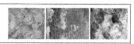

Go to this link at the IHI website: www.ihi.org/knowledge/Pages/HowtoImprove/ ScienceofImprovementHowtoImprove.aspx

Read about the Model for Improvement. Consider a unit-based project on an adult patient-care unit where a nurse wants to address decreasing the decubitus ulcer rate on her unit. Using the Model for Improvement with its three fundamental questions and its Plan-Do-Study-Act (PDSA) cycle as a model for such a project, answer the following questions:

1. What team members would have important input on this team?
2. Imagine yourself on the QI team. What change are you trying to accomplish?
3. What might be your goal?
4. What data will you collect that will show that your changes made a difference?

KEY CONCEPTS

- Historically, a major push for the six competencies of the QSEN initiative came from the 2003 IOM report, *Health Professions Education: A Bridge to Quality*, where competencies in quality and safety were recommended for all health professions students.
- All six of the QSEN competencies, that is, PCC, QI, safety, teamwork and collaboration, EBP, and informatics, are integral aspects of nursing clinical practice.

- Each of the six QSEN competencies has KSA elements that help operationalize each competency for practice.
- The QSEN competencies are fundamental components of accreditation standards for nursing programs and are integrated into beginning, intermediate, and advanced level nursing courses.
- There are a wide variety of quality and safety resources available for nurses at the QSEN website (www.qsen.org).
- There are several special issues of nursing journals that have focused on QSEN.

KEY TERMS

Attitudes
Evidence-based practice
Informatics
Knowledge
Patient-centered care
Quality improvement

Rapid response teams
Safety
Safety science
Skills
Teamwork and collaboration

REVIEW QUESTIONS

1. The nurse is caring for a newly admitted patient. She introduces herself using her first and last names and asks the patient what his values, needs, and preferences are for this hospital stay. The nurse is practicing which of the QSEN competencies?

   A. Evidence-based practice
   B. Safety
   C. Patient-centered care
   D. Teamwork and collaboration

2. The primary nurse is caring for a patient admitted to the unit from a nursing home with a Stage III decubitus ulcer. In looking at the electronic nursing notes, she notes a discrepancy in the patient's wound care procedures. The primary nurse calls the wound care nurse to consult and ensure a consistent plan of care. The wound care nurse assesses the patient and provides the necessary information reflecting the standard of care. The primary nurse is practicing which of the QSEN competencies? Select all that apply.

   A. QI
   B. Safety
   C. Teamwork and collaboration
   D. PCC
   E. Informatics

3. The nurse is transferring his patient to the Post Anesthesia Care Unit (PACU) from the surgical unit. He is calling the receiving nurse with a patient handoff report. Ensuring patient safety by using the handoff report, he is careful to describe the situation, background, assessment, and recommendation for the patient's continued care. Giving an accurate handoff report is an example of ensuring patient safety by using which QSEN competency?

   A. Teamwork and collaboration
   B. QI

C. PCC
D. Informatics

4. The nurse notices that there was an earlier medication error that resulted in an adverse patient outcome. She asks for assistance from her manager in analyzing the error. This is an example of using which QSEN competency?

   A. Safety
   B. QI
   C. PCC
   D. Teamwork and collaboration

5. A medical resident walks into a patient's room to complete a physical assessment. The nurse notices that the resident did not wash her hands before entering the room. The nurse gently reminds the resident to use the hand sanitizer before touching the patient. This reminder is an example of using which of the following QSEN competencies?

   A. Safety
   B. QI
   C. PCC
   D. Teamwork and collaboration
   E. Informatics

6. The nurse is using barcode administration technology to facilitate the administration of medications to her patients. This is an example of how barcode medication administration technology facilitates which of the following QSEN competencies?

   A. Teamwork and collaboration
   B. Safety
   C. Informatics
   D. EBP
   E. QI

7. The nurse is participating in a team meeting with her patient, the dietician, physician, and social worker. The nurse recalls that the patient had expressed that spirituality was important to her. A pastoral care representative is not present in the meeting. The nurse notices this and contacts pastoral care to be included in the meeting. This inclusion is an example of using which QSEN competency?

   A. Teamwork and collaboration
   B. Safety
   C. PCC
   D. Informatics

8. The nurse realizes that her patient's pain management is not effective. She has noticed this with other patients in the past and decides to analyze the unit-based pain control chart posted in the break room. She decides to explore additional pain management options for patients whose pain is not controlled with the usual pain management. Which QSEN competencies best describes her approach?

   A. Safety
   B. QI
   C. PCC
   D. Teamwork and collaboration

9. In administering medication to her patient, the nurse saw that the medication administration record indicated the dose amount to be 5 mg. She immediately double checked the order and confirmed that the dose was supposed to be 0.5 mg. The nurse remembered to always use a zero before a decimal when the dose is less than a whole unit and she updated the medication administration record accordingly. Which QSEN competency applies?

   A. Safety
   B. QI
   C. PCC
   D. Teamwork and collaboration

10. The nurse is concerned about his patient's lab values and medication regimen. The nurse uses the electronic health record to obtain information about medication doses, lab results, and notes that the patient's lab results are within normal limits. This use of the electronic health record is an example of using which QSEN competency?

   A. Teamwork and collaboration
   B. Safety
   C. PCC
   D. Informatics

REVIEW ACTIVITIES

1. Select one of the six QSEN competencies from the QSEN website (www.qsen.org) and create a 60-second video explaining the competency that was chosen and why it matters to professional nursing practice. Present the video in class and lead a discussion on the video's application to practice.
2. Interview three nurses on the unit where you are currently doing a clinical rotation. Ask each nurse, "What is the most pressing patient safety issue on this unit?" Take notes. Compare the nurses' answers. Discuss the results with your classmates and instructor in post conference. What did you find?

CRITICAL DISCUSSION POINTS

1. Discuss the importance of what QSEN has accomplished to date.
   • Defined quality and safety competencies for nursing and proposed targets for the KSAs to be developed in nursing prelicensure programs for each competency: patient-centered care, teamwork and collaboration, EBP, QI, safety, and informatics.
   • Completed a national survey of baccalaureate nursing program leaders and a state survey of associate degree nursing educators to assess beliefs about the extent to which the competencies are included in current curricula, the level of satisfaction with student competency achievement, and the level of faculty expertise in teaching the competencies.
   • Partnered with representatives of organizations that represent advanced practice nurses and drafted proposed KSA targets for graduate education.
   • Funded work with 15 pilot schools committed to active engagement in curricular change to incorporate quality and safety competencies
   • Discussed the goals of the QSEN competencies at the prelicensure level.

- Set the overall goal for QSEN to meet the challenge of preparing future nurses who will have the KSAs necessary to continuously improve the quality and safety of the healthcare systems in which they work.
2. Discuss one potential barrier for incorporating the QSEN competencies in a patient's plan of care. Are any of the following an issue in your clinical setting?
    - Lack of teamwork and collaboration among the interprofessional team members.
    - Developing a plan of care without consideration of the preferences/values of the patient/family.
    - Poor handoffs when a patient is being transferred from one unit to another.
3. Using the QSEN competency of *teamwork and collaboration,* discuss how you would apply those KSAs to a complex clinical situation.
4. Why it is essential that the QSEN competencies align with accreditation standards?
5. Select one article from *The Journal of Nursing Education,* September/October 2017, QSEN Supplement, and reflect on how the article is related to your practice. Discuss with colleagues what you have learned.
6. Discuss in class some of the most useful resources on the QSEN website.
    - Competencies
    - Teaching strategies
    - QSEN integration modules
    - Learning modules
    - Books, reports, toolkits
    - Evaluation tools
    - Videos
    - Conferences
7. What does the word "systems thinking" mean to you related to the QSEN competencies?

QSEN ACTIVITIES

1. Explore the teaching strategies published on the QSEN Website (www.qsen.org). These are peer-reviewed teaching strategies published on the site. Ask students to choose one of the strategies and apply it to a clinical situation. Discuss an implementation plan for the strategy chosen. Discuss which QSEN competencies apply.
2. Select one of the six QSEN competencies from the QSEN website (www.qsen.org) and create a 60-second video explaining the competency they chose and why it matters to professional nursing practice. Have students present the video in class and lead a discussion on the video's application to practice.

EXPLORING THE WEB

1. National Patient Safety Foundation—www.npsf.org
2. QSEN Institute—www.qsen.org
3. Institute for Healthcare Improvement—www.ihi.org
4. Team*STEPPS*—www.teamstepps.ahrq.gov
5. IHI Open School—www.ihi.org/offerings/ihiopenschool
6. Agency for Healthcare Research and Quality Patient Safety Network—psnet.ahrq .gov
7. National Association for Healthcare Quality. Q Essentials Info Session February 2016—www.youtube.com/watch?v=kP9-8V93s30

REFERENCES

Accreditation Commission for Education in Nursing (ACEN). Retrieved from www.acenursing .org/resources-acen-accreditation-manual/

American Association of Colleges of Nursing (AACN). (2008). *The essentials of baccalaureate education for professional nursing practice.* Retrieved from http://www.aacn.nche.edu/ education-resources/BaccEssentials08.pdf

American Organization of Nurse Executives (AONE). (2007). Guiding principles for nurse leaders. Retrieved from http://www.aone.org/resources/guiding-principles.shtml

Balakas, K., & Smith, J. (2016). Evidence based practice and quality improvement in nursing education. *The Journal of Perinatal & Neonatal Nursing, 30*(3), 191–194.

Barton, A. J., Armstrong, G., Preheim, G., Gelmon, S. B., & Andrus, L. C. (2009). A national Delphi to determine developmental progression of quality and safety competencies in nursing education. *Nursing Outlook, 57*(6), 313–322. doi:10.1016/j.outlook.2009.08.003

Benner, P., Sutphen, M., Leonard, V., & Day, L. (2010). *Educating nurses: A call for radical transformation.* San Francisco, CA: Jossey-Bass.

Cronenwett, L. (2007). *Emory Jowers lecture on "Quality and safety education for nurses."* Retrieved from http://qsen.org. Slide 10.

Cronenwett, L., Sherwood, G., Barnsteiner, J., Disch, J., Johnson, J., Mitchell, P., . . . Warren, J. (2007). Quality and safety education for nurses. *Nursing Outlook, 55*(3), 122–131.

Dolansky, M. A., & Moore, S. M. (2013). Quality and Safety Education for Nurses (QSEN): The key is systems thinking. *Online Journal of Issues in Nursing, 18*(3), 1–12.

Dolansky, M. A., Schexnayder, J., Patrician, P. A., & Sales, A. (2017, Septermber/October). Implementation science: A new approach to integrate QSEN competencies in nursing education. *Nurse Educator, QSEN Supplement, 42*(5), S12–S17. doi:10.1097/NNE.0000000000000422

Gawande, A. (2007, December 10). The checklist. *The New Yorker.* Retrieved from https://www .newyorker.com/magazine/2007/12/10/the-checklist

Headrick, L. A., Barton, A. J., Ogrinc, G., Strang, C., Aboumatar, H., Aud, M., & Patterson, J. (2012). Retooling for quality and safety: Integrating quality and safety into the required curriculum at twelve medical and nursing schools. *Health Affairs, 31*(12), 2669–2680. doi:10.1377/hlthaff.2011.012.1

Heavner, J. J., & Siner, J. M. (2015). Adverse event reporting and quality improvement in the Intensive care unit. *Clinical Chest Medicine, 36*(3), 461–467. doi:10.1016/j.ccm.2015.05.005

Hermann, C., Head, B., Black, K., & Singleton, K. (2016, January–February). Preparing nursing students for interprofessional practice: The interdisciplinary curriculum for oncology palliative care education. *Journal of Professional Nursing, 32*(1), 62–71.

Institute for Healthcare Improvement (IHI). (2012). *5 million lives campaign.* Retrieved from http:// www.ihi.org/offerings/Initiatives/PastStrategicInitiatives/5MillionLivesCampaign/ Pages/default.aspx

Institute of Medicine (IOM). (1999). *To err is human: Building a safer health system.* Washington, DC: National Academies Press. Retrieved from http://www.nationalacademies.org/hmd/~/ media/Files/Report%20Files/1999/To-Err-is-Human/To%20Err%20is%20Human% 201999%20%20report%20brief.pdf

Institute of Medicine (IOM). (2001). *Crossing the quality chasm: A new health care system for the 21st century.* Washington, DC: National Academies Press. Retrieved from http://www .nationalacademies.org/hmd/~/media/Files/Report%20Files/2001/Crossing-the-Quality-Chasm/Quality%20Chasm%202001%20%20report%20brief.pdf

Institute of Medicine (IOM). (2003). *Health professions education: A bridge to quality.* Washington, DC: National Academies Press. https://www.nap.edu/catalog/10681/health-professions-education-a-bridge-to-quality

Institute of Medicine (IOM). (2010). *Assessing progress on the institute of medicine report the future of nursing.* Washington, DC. National Academies Press. Retrieved from https://www.nap .edu/catalog/21838/assessing-progress-on-the-institute-of-medicine-report-the-future-of-nursing

Institute of Medicine (IOM). (2011). *The future of nursing: Leading change, advancing health.* Washington, DC: The National Academies Press. Retrieved from https://www.nap.edu/catalog/12956/the-future-of-nursing-leading-change-advancing-health

The Joint Commission. (2012). *National patient safety goals 2012.* Retrieved from http://www.jointcommission.org/standards information/npsgs.aspx

Makary, M. A., & Michael, D. (2016). Medical error-the third leading cause of death in the US. *BMJ: British Medical Journal (Online), 353,* i2139. doi:10.1136/bmj.i2139

Melnyk, B., Fineout-Overholt, E., Gallagher, L., & Kaplan, L. (2012). The state of evidence based practice in US nurses. *JONA, 42*(9), 410–417, doi:10.1097/NNA.0b013e3182664e0a

Mohn-Brown, E. (2017). Implementing quality and safety education for nurses in postclinical conferences: Transforming the design of clinical nursing education. *Nurse Educator, 42,* s18–s21. doi:10.1097/NNE.0000000000000410

National Patient Safety Foundation (NPSF). (2015). *Free from harm: Accelerating patient safety improvement 15 years after to Err is human.* Retrieved from http://www.npsf.org/page/freefromharm

National Quality Forum. (2009). *Safe practices for better healthcare.* Retrieved from http://www.qualityforum.org/Publications/2009/03/Safe_Practices_for_Better_Healthcare%E2%80%932009_Update.aspx

Neily, J., Mills, P. D., Young-Xu, Y., Carney, B. T., West, P., Berger, D. H., & Bagian, J. P. (2010). Association between implementation of a medical team training program and surgical mortality. *The Journal of the American Medical Association, 304*(15), 1693–1700.

Nelson, E. C., Batalden, P. B., & Godfry, M. M., 2007. *Quality by design: A clinical microsystems approach.* San Francisco, CA: Jossey Bass.

Reason, J. (1990). *Human error.* Boston, MA: Cambridge University Press.

Scott, K., & McSherry, R. (2009). Evidence-based nursing: Clarifying the concepts for nurses in practice. *Journal of Clinical Nursing, 18*(8), 1085–1095, doi:10.1111/j.1365-2702.2008.02588.x

Shaller, D. (2007). *Patient-centered care: What does it take?* The Commonwealth Fund. Retrieved from http://www.commonwealthfund.org/Publications/Fund-Reports/2007/Oct/Patient-Centered-Care–What-Does-It-Take.aspx

Smetzer, J. L. (1998). Lesson from Colorado: Beyond blaming individuals. *Nursing Management, 29*(6), 49–51.

Solomons, N. M., & Spross, J. A. (2011). Evidence-based practice barriers and facilitators from a continuous quality improvement perspective: An integrative review. *Journal of Nursing Management, 19,* 109–120. doi: 10.1111/j.1365-2834.2010.01144.x

The 5 Million Lives Campaign. (2006). Retrieved from http://www.ihi.org/about/Documents/5MillionLivesCampaignCaseStatement.pdf

Vincent, C. (2006). *Patient safety.* London, England: Elsevier.

Wachter, R. M. (2010). Patient safety at ten: Unmistakable progress troubling gaps. *Health Fairs, 29*(1), 165–173. doi:10.1377/hlthaff.2009.0785

SUGGESTED READING

Armstrong, G., Sherwood, G., & Tagliareni, M. E. (2009). Quality and Safety Education in Nursing (QSEN): Integrating recommendations from IOM into clinical nursing education. In *Clinical nursing education: Current reflections* (pp. 207–227). Washington, DC: National League of Nursing.

Altmiller, G., & Dolansky, M. A. (2017, September/October). Quality and safety education for nurses: Looking forward. *Nurse Educator, QSEN Supplement, 42*(5), S1–S2.

Avansino, J. R., Peters, L. M., Stockfish, S. L., & Walco, G. A. (2013). A paradigm shift to balance safety and quality in pediatric pain management. *Pediatrics, 131,* e921–e927. doi:10.1542/peds.2012-1378

Cohen, N. L. (2013). Using the ABCs of situational awareness for patient safety. *Nursing, 43,* 64–65. doi:10.1097/01.NURSE.0000428332.23978.82

Dekker, S. (2011). *Patient safety: A human factors approach.* Boca Raton, FL: CRC Press.

Dolansky, M. (2011). Teaching and measuring systems thinking in a quality and safety curriculum. In *Proceedings of the 2011 QSEN National Forum.* Milwaukee, WI (Available on QSEN website under 2011 National Forum Presentation Slides).

Finkelman, A., & Kenner, C. (2012). *Learning IOM. Implications of the institute of medicine reports for nursing education.* Silver Spring, MD: American Nurses' Association.

Gawande, A. (2001). *The checklist manifesto: How to get things right.* New York, NY: Henry Holt & Co.

Gawande, A. (2002). *Complications: A surgeon's notes on an imperfect science.* New York, NY: St. Martin's Press.

Gawande, A. (2008). *Better. A surgeon's notes on performance.* New York, NY: Henry Holt.

Hughes, R. G. (2008). *Patient safety and quality: An evidence-based handbook for nurses.* AHRQ Publication No. 08-0043. Rockville, MD: Agency for Healthcare Research and Quality.

Institute of Medicine (IOM). (2004). *Keeping patients safe: Transforming the work environment of nurses.* Washington, DC: National Academies Press.

Ko, H., Turner, T. J., & Finnigan, M. A. (2011). Systematic review of safety checklists for use by medical care teams in acute hospital settings—limited evidence of effectiveness. *BMC Health Services Research, 11,* 211.

Ogrinc, G. S., Headrick, L. A., Moore, S. M., Barton, A. J., Dolansky, M. A., & Madigosky, W. S. (2012). *Fundamentals of health care improvement: A guide to improving your patient's care* (2nd ed.). Oak Terrace, IL: Joint Commission Resources.

St. Onge, J., Hodges, T., McBride, M., & Parnell, R. (2013). An innovative tool for experiential learning of nursing quality and safety competencies. *Nurse Educator, 38,* 71–75. doi:10.1097/NNE.0b013e3182829c7d

Triola, N. (2006). Dialogue and discourse: Are we having the right conversation. *Critical Care Nurse, 26,* 60–66. AACN

Wachter, R. M. (2008). *Understanding patient safety.* New York, NY: McGraw-Hill.

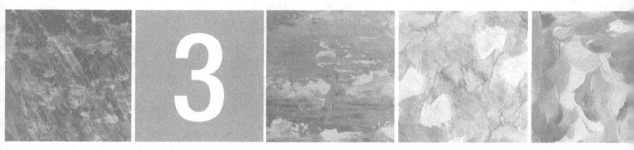

3

NURSES AS LEADERS AND MANAGERS FOR SAFE, HIGH-QUALITY PATIENT CARE

Carolyn A. Christie-McAuliffe

All truth passes through three stages: first it is ridiculed; second it is violently opposed; third it is accepted as being self-evident.

—Arthur Schopenhauer

Upon completion of this chapter, the reader should be able to

1. Explain major leadership theories in relation to the Quality and Safety Education for Nurses (QSEN).
2. Describe roles and responsibilities of leadership.
3. Define management as distinguished from leadership.
4. Discuss the importance of followership in relation to an organization's mission and vision.
5. Explain how the hospital's finances influence safety and quality of patient care.
6. Describe how a budget influences staffing.
7. Discuss the importance of the Code of Ethics for Nurses.
8. Discuss the importance of Emancipatory Knowing in relation to the call for every nurse to function as a leader.
9. Discuss the four key elements of the Future of Nursing (FON): Campaign for Action in the context of functioning as a leader at all levels of care.

S ally graduated from nursing school a year ago and is now working full time on a medical–surgical floor. Several novice nurses with no prior nursing experience have joined the staff and expressed feeling overwhelmed with all there is to know and be done. Sally is happy to have the additional help; however, she has noticed many patients are not being assisted out of bed or ambulated. She clearly remembers her first few months out of school and empathizes with the new nurses' feelings. However, she is also worried about the risk of pneumonia, bedsores, and other health complications in patients who remain in bed for extended periods of time.

- *What can Sally do to support her new colleagues?*
- *What are some things Sally can do to support her colleagues' patients?*
- *What could Sally do to prevent a similar situation the next time the floor hires new graduates?*

Leadership is frequently described in terms of personal attributes such as having confidence and being strong. Often, these leadership attributes have been assumed to be a quality one has been born with or cultivated by how the person has been raised. However, many experts now argue leadership can be taught, fostered, and refined. Many nurse leaders agree with this more contemporary viewpoint. Specifically, they are calling for nursing education that incorporates leadership content which encourages nurses to demonstrate leadership at all levels of nursing practice. The leadership they advocate would directly and indirectly impact the safety and quality of patient care.

This chapter provides the foundation for understanding leadership and this new call to action. Theories are presented as context for discussion as leadership is discussed in relation to management and followership. Similarities and differences of the qualities, roles, and responsibilities of leadership, managers, and followers are described within the framework of economic and financial constraints. The impact of economics and finance will be discussed in relation to the ability to deliver safe, quality care. However, the emphasis of this chapter is substantiating the need to shift the focus of care from individual patients to now include care of the healthcare system as well. This substantiation comes from many influences, including Nursing's Social Contract as well as the Code of Ethics for Nurses, the Quality and Safety Education for Nurses (QSEN), the Future of Nursing (FON) Campaign for Action, and the understanding of Emancipatory Knowing.

Nursing has a rich history of leading change. Florence Nightingale, Clara Barton, Margaret Sanger, and Hazel Johnson-Brown are but a few nurses who have advanced nursing and healthcare through their efforts to facilitate change. More recently, leadership has been demonstrated by nursing in response to the Institute of Medicine's (IOM) reports, *To Err Is Human: Building a Safer Health System* (2000) and *Crossing the Quality Chasm* (2001), which documented the need to restructure the healthcare system. These reports revealed issues of both safety and quality of care, specifically in the context of increased complexity within the healthcare system. The IOM reports identified many causes of this complexity, including the health status of patients, technology, as well as economics, politics, and social factors. National organizations such as The Joint Commission (TJC) and the Institute for Healthcare Improvement (IHI) launched programs in response to the IOM findings. Similarly, nurse leaders responded to the same IOM findings at local, state, and national levels with many initiatives; however, two of these initiatives stand out: The QSEN Initiative and the FON: Campaign for Action.

In 2005, QSEN was formed to develop competencies of knowledge, attitude, and skill related to safety of patient care and as a means to ensure continuous quality improvement in healthcare organizations and institutions. Six core competencies were developed with measures differentiated at prelicensure and graduate levels as follows:

1. Patient-Centered Care
2. Teamwork and Collaboration
3. Evidence-Based Practice (EBP)
4. Quality Improvement (QI)
5. Safety
6. Informatics (QSEN, 2017)

The aim of the QSEN competencies was and is to provide relevant materials and resources to nurse educators that can be incorporated into existing curricula. In addition, QSEN wanted to provide objective measures of knowledge, attitude, and skill that nurse faculty could use to determine if students understood and could apply interventions aimed at increasing safety and quality of care. Since its formation, QSEN has funded and/or supported innovative programs in specific schools, the Veterans Administration, the American Association of Colleges of Nursing, and more.

The FON: Campaign for Action is another powerful initiative within nursing. In 2008, the Robert Wood Johnson Foundation (RWJF) partnered with the IOM to launch a specific study investigating the role of nursing in transforming healthcare. Their research discovered much diversity of educational preparation, underutilization of nursing knowledge and skill, and fragmentation of purpose within the nursing profession. However, they also found great potential. In 2011, the IOM published *The Future of Nursing: Leading Change, Advancing Health*. In this report, eight recommendations were offered to policymakers, educators, healthcare organizations, and businesses, as follows:

1. Remove scope-of-practice barriers.
2. Expand opportunities for nurses to lead and diffuse collaborative improvement efforts.
3. Implement nurse residency programs.
4. Increase the proportion of nurses with a baccalaureate degree to 80% by 2020.
5. Double the number of nurses with a doctorate by 2020.
6. Ensure that nurses engage in lifelong learning.
7. Prepare and enable nurses to lead change to advance health.
8. Build an infrastructure for the collection and analysis of interprofessional healthcare workforce data (IOM, 2011, pp. 9–15).

As a result of this report, the RWJF joined forces with AARP (formerly known as the American Association of Retired Persons) to create the FON: Campaign for Action. All 50 states now have an Action Coalition Committee aimed at meeting the eight recommendations of the IOM report.

Despite these initiatives, little improvement in safety and quality of care has been demonstrated. The call to action has never been more ardent or urgent. Nurses at all levels, from the patient bedside to the boardroom, are now asked to step into their authentic power with moral courage to be leaders for change. No longer can responsibility for leading change sit solely with nurse administrators or academicians; nurses at every level of educational preparation and position are now called to improve patient safety and quality of care within the healthcare system in which they work, as well as with individual patients. As a profession, nursing now realizes all nurses should function as leaders to heal patients as well as the healthcare system.

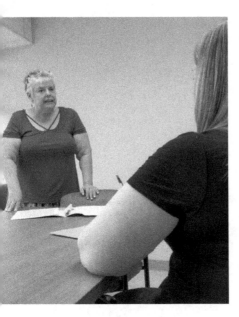

FIGURE 3.1 Leadership as mentor.

Cultivating leadership in nursing has not been studied extensively. However, residency programs for new graduate nurses have provided some valuable insight. Curtis, de Vries, and Sheerin (2011) discuss factors that contribute to leadership in nursing including the offering of educational activities and role modeling as well as the opportunity to practice leadership skills. They discuss being open to new ideas and being extroverted as traits likely to foster leadership. Likewise, the role of age and experiences are positive influences. Interestingly, they found the most important skill necessary for leadership involved fostering effective relationships. They describe this specific skill as more important than knowledge surrounding management skill or technical abilities (Figure 3.1). They found that the most important qualities of effective relationships include effective communication, approachability, and emotional intelligence. Wagner, Cummings, Smith, Olson, Anderson, and Warren (2010), as cited in Curtis et al. (2011), discovered the organizations that promoted nurse empowerment resulted in increased "positive work behaviors and attitudes, including leadership behavior" (p. 308).

LEADERSHIP THEORY

Historical review of how leadership has been perceived provides insight into how and why nursing gravitates to some leadership theories over others. During the Industrial Revolution, leadership was focused almost exclusively on how to manage productivity. Success was measured by precise, scientific measurements and standards, which was appropriate and beneficial for institutions primarily focused on manufacturing. During the mid-20th century, organizations identified the need for clearer structure and standardization. Max Weber (1864–1920) offered a theoretical framework based on establishing a hierarchy of authority and power that clearly delineated policies and procedures as a way of standardizing work. As institutions grew focused mainly on efficiency and growth, a dehumanizing quality to administration and leadership developed. In response, government organizations enacted regulations to protect workers. With this national shift, unions formed to further ensure safe and fair working conditions. The focus of leadership then evolved further to the individual within an organization, specifically looking at maximizing their efforts and strengths. With this new focus, a movement toward "human relations" emerged that continues today. Many, if not most, contemporary leadership theories are based on the behavioral sciences, which aim to explain human behavior. This perspective of leadership provides organizations with a better understanding of what influences behavior. Having a clear understanding of what an organization wants allows its leaders improved ability to manage those influences.

Dinh et al. (2014) conducted a comprehensive literature review of established and emerging leadership theories that revealed 23 thematic categories and 66 domains or areas of foci. Nursing does not espouse a single theory of leadership but, rather, most often views leadership through the lens of nursing theory, incorporating and applying relevant leadership theory as appropriate. Three commonly referred to theories of leadership that nursing utilizes include Chaos, Quantum, and Systems Theories. Each of these theories relates and interrelates to each other.

Chaos Theory

Chaos theory is based on the belief that underneath the seemingly unpredictable nature of life and/or business, a pattern or order exists. While many leadership styles and strategies are based on the belief that events are predictable and can be controlled, Chaos Theory calls for leaders to be vigilant to the dynamic changing nature of economic, political, and social cues. This awareness allows leaders to guide their organization through disorder. By seeking insight from these cues, the leader finds a new pattern of understanding. Through this pattern of understanding, leaders accept the reality of complexity as well as unpredictability in order to learn to anticipate needed change and flexibility (Porter-O'Grady & Malloch, 2011). The leader then translates this understanding for the need for change and flexibility to the organization in a way that provides relevance, importance, and direction.

Quantum Theory

Quantum Theory acknowledges the complexity and chaotic nature of life. This theory is based on quantum physics, which states particles or matter can exist simultaneously in two different states of being. Quantum Theory asks leaders to simultaneously consider the reality of a situation and the potential or ideal. Porter-O'Grady and Malloch (2011) explain that in order to achieve this requirement, leaders must adopt a whole systems approach versus an approach of individual parts. They explain that every part of a system is part of one comprehensive system and smaller systems are linked to form larger, more complex systems. This explanation provides the need and benefit of interdependence (Box 3.1). They continue their explanation that Quantum Theory requires leaders to focus on outcomes, not the process; in other words, what a job or

---

BOX 3.1 INTERDEPENDENCE

In nature, everything is interdependent. There is an ebb and flow among all elements of life. Leaders must see their role from this perspective. Most of the work of leadership will be managing the interactions and connections between people and processes. Leaders must keep aware of the following truths:
- Action in one place has an effect in other places.
- Fluctuation of mutuality means authority moves between people (followers can be leaders and leaders can be followers in a dynamic relationship).
- Interacting properties in systems make outcomes mobile and fluid (function in the present but work toward the future).
- Relationship building is the primary work of leadership.
- Trusting feeling is as important as valuing thinking.
- Acknowledging in others what is unique in their contribution is vital.
- Supporting, stretching, challenging, pushing, and helping are part of being present to the process, to the players, and to the outcome (Porter-O'Grady & Malloch, 2011, p. 22).

work *results in* rather than just that someone preformed the work for work's sake. It asks leaders to emerge from all levels of nursing, independent of educational preparation or position, learning to adapt to dynamic, unpredictable change in order to see *what is* alongside *what could be*. In this way, the leader functions for the present but works toward the future.

Systems Theory

Systems Theory espouses the same belief as Quantum Theory that all parts of a system are vital and interdependent of the whole. Based on General Systems Theory developed by biologist von Bertalanffy, Systems Theory addresses seven fundamental elements: input (resources), output (product or service), throughput (planning), feedback (data on service or product that allow for self-correction), control (evaluation), environment (milieu), and goals (vision, mission). Ultimately, to be viable or sustainable, an organization as a system, must have a clear vision and mission that is substantiated by feedback and able to adapt to changing economic, political, and social conditions. Dolansky and Moore (2013) argue Systems Theory or thinking allows nurses to move from a specific focus on individual patient care to a perspective that sees patient care in the context of the care of the "system." In this broadened and more global view, the nurse is able to appreciate and impact safety and quality of care on multiple levels. With this viewpoint, nurses are able to see how various actions benefit the patient directly and indirectly. Their example (Figure 3.2) of how this occurs on a continuum is poignantly illustrative.

Leadership Defined

Leadership can be explained or described in many ways; however, simply put, **leadership** is the ability to lead or command a person or group of people (Figure 3.3). In this simplistic perspective, anyone who leads and facilitates change by speaking up, providing education, role modeling, and/or coaching resulting in changed behavior of an individual or group is a leader. As mentioned earlier, historically, leadership has been viewed as something a person is born with that demonstrates a list of specific characteristics. That viewpoint is no longer considered accurate. More contemporary views of leadership consider the possibility of success to be a cocreation of a group that allows for creativity and innovation. Grossman and Valiga (2016) explain this cocreation and shared responsibility for success occurs when a group can appreciate and foster one another's strengths and attributes and commit to inspiring each other, as well as to be self-aware, insightful, and accountable. The qualities of responsibility and accountability share a sense of fidelity or dependability to others. Both of these qualities are components of being a leader; however, each quality is slightly different from the another.

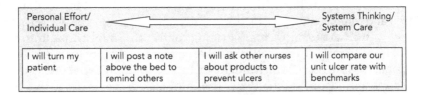

FIGURE 3.2 Example of continuum of systems thinking for quality and safety in healthcare.

Source: From Dolansky, M. A., & Moore, S. M. (2013). Quality and safety education for nurses (QSEN): The key is systems thinking. *The Online Journal of Issues in Nursing, 18*(3), Manuscript 1. Retrieved from https://www.nursingworld.org/Quality-and-Safety-Education-for-Nurses.html

Responsibility is typically a requirement of assigned tasks, roles, and/or a position (i.e., a staff nurse on a medical surgical floor is responsible for monitoring vital signs of her assigned patients), whereas **accountability** speaks to one's willingness to accept responsibility for an assignment (i.e., the nurse accepts accountability for all assignments related to her job).

Nursing leaders such as Porter-O'Grady and Malloch (2011) distinguish leadership that simply facilitates change from that which transforms, explaining, "A transformational leader creates a new and improved system that allows individuals to contribute to their fullest potential

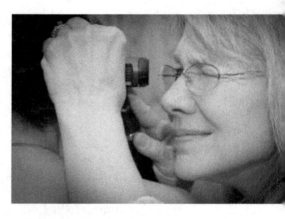

FIGURE 3.3 Direct patient care; leadership at the front line.

to deliver the most effective healthcare possible" (p. 375). As described earlier, this model of leadership abdicates sole "control" by the individual or individuals holding formal, authorized power in exchange for shared ownership. In this new model, everyone involved owns responsibility to identify strengths, weaknesses, and opportunities.

ROLES AND RESPONSIBILITIES OF LEADERS

Distinct roles and responsibilities are associated with the various positions within an organization. These are typically outlined in a job description. A **role** is a position or the part the position fulfills within an organization, such as a CEO or Vice President (VP) of Nursing. Depending on the formal position, appropriate responsibilities will be delegated or assigned. For a leader, these roles typically involve developing a vision and facilitating change on a large scale, such as for a department or institution. John Gardner (1993), considered one of the experts in the field of leadership, distinguishes leaders from managers in six respects. Leaders:

1. Think long term.
2. Influence the organization/unit they lead.
3. Reach out to those impacted by, as well as those impacting their organization.
4. Focus on facilitating a vision by actualizing values through motivation and guidance.
5. Exhibit political skill in managing conflict related to multiple and potentially differing and/or competing priorities.
6. Include measures to always improve how an organization or institution functions to meet their stated mission and vision.

Gardner (1993) further distinguishes the tasks or responsibility of the leader to include, first and foremost, that of creating a vision for the group. This vision includes a detailed plan as well as directions for managing conflict that might arise from competing goals. The second task of the leader involves affirming the organization or group's values, vision, and mission, which might include facilitating agreement between people or groups with opposing thoughts. The third task of the leader is to motivate the group by fostering ownership, positivity, and excitement for what has been committed to by the group. Managing priorities and work in order to actualize the group's vision and mission is the fourth task of the leader, whereas the fifth task is to facilitate cohesion of mind and purpose. This fifth task is accomplished by establishing trust and loyalty among the members of the group. Gardner further states, the sixth task is to accept responsibility for ensuring understanding of the vision and mission, specifically as it relates to individual roles and responsibilities of group members. The seventh task of the leader is to serve as a role model. Gardner explains, the leader serves as the risk taker, the group's voice as well as the force that brings the group together and provides positivity that they can accomplish their goal. The eighth task of the leader involves serving as the advocate for the group and their vision; the leader speaks as well as acts on behalf of the group. The last task of leadership that Gardner speaks to is the responsibility for ensuring the renewing or sustainability of the group's mission; this task is accomplished by balancing continuity with change so that group members do not become complacent or satisfied with the status quo. The leader helps to maintain momentum and movement toward accomplishing their goal.

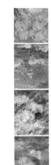

CASE STUDY 3.1

A new graduate nurse is eager to be a valuable member of the Dialysis Unit he has just been hired to work on. He quickly realizes patient safety is a concern because of short staffing.

1. *What is the most pressing concern related to short staffing?*
2. *What course of action could the nurse pursue to help this situation?*
3. *What aspects of leadership could he employ to facilitate change?*

REAL-WORLD INTERVIEW

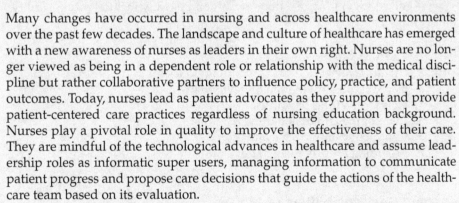

Many changes have occurred in nursing and across healthcare environments over the past few decades. The landscape and culture of healthcare has emerged with a new awareness of nurses as leaders in their own right. Nurses are no longer viewed as being in a dependent role or relationship with the medical discipline but rather collaborative partners to influence policy, practice, and patient outcomes. Today, nurses lead as patient advocates as they support and provide patient-centered care practices regardless of nursing education background. Nurses play a pivotal role in quality to improve the effectiveness of their care. They are mindful of the technological advances in healthcare and assume leadership roles as informatic super users, managing information to communicate patient progress and propose care decisions that guide the actions of the healthcare team based on its evaluation.

Nurses lead in promoting a culture of best practices for their patients and mutually share in organizational goals to justify their services through empirical, ethical, theoretical, and seminal works across disciplines. Nurses are influencers as they collaborate with peers in best evidence and care practices, promote professional practice environments, and adhere to national parameters that ensure safety and quality outcomes. Today's nurses at every level are leaders as they assume their role and responsibility to influence others and continue to transform the landscape of healthcare for future generations.

Esther Bankert, PhD, RN
Board Member, St. Elizabeth's Hospital, Utica, NY

Formal and Informal Leadership

Leadership within an organization can occur both formally and informally. Formal leadership involves specific role responsibility and authority related to the position one holds. This type of leadership is typically based on certain skill, knowledge, and experience. A variety of formal leadership positions exist within healthcare organizations including nurse executives that might hold positions such as Chief Nursing Officer or VP of Nursing. Other positions of leadership include a head nurse or charge leader. Effective leadership exemplifies the qualities of trustworthiness, courage, commitment, and perseverance.

In contrast, informal leadership is not explicit or official. It is based on personal power or credibility in the eyes of others. This credibility can come from many sources but typically evolves from education and/or experience as well as from personal characteristics such as charisma, certainty, and/or courage to speak up or take action. Nurses at all levels, even newly graduated nurses have the potential for informal leadership and facilitating positive change by asking question, speaking up when something doesn't appear right, and engaging in continuous quality improvement.

MANAGEMENT

Clearly, managers can also be leaders, inspiring and motivating their subordinates. However, the roles and responsibilities of a manager are distinct and different from that of formal leaders within an organization. A **manager** is someone who is responsible for controlling all or parts of an organization. The focus of a manager is getting the work of the designated group or unit done effectively. As a nurse manager of a patient care unit, the role and tasks or responsibilities associated with this position involve the running of a floor or unit and usually include responsibilities such as the following:

1. The hiring of nursing staff.
2. Creating, reviewing, and amending policies and procedures.
3. Coordinating orientation of new nurses.
4. Creating staffing schedules.
5. Developing and maintaining a budget.
6. Conducting employee evaluations.
7. Providing for professional development.

Roles and Responsibilities of Managers

While the ultimate goal of nurse managers is safe and high-quality patient care, most often they do not provide direct patient care themselves. Rather, they manage nurses giving the care, coordinate quality improvement of that care, and help resolve any patient care concerns. In this role, nurse managers work closely with nursing and other inter-professional team members including ancillary staff and managers from other units, departments and disciplines. This list could include individuals from any department or discipline within the organization, such as pharmacy, physicians and other providers, as well as administration. Meetings, emails, safety huddles, and other forms of interaction help the nurse manager to coordinate communication and efforts of the interprofessional team.

The list of tasks a nurse manager is responsible for directly and indirectly help ensure that patient care is both safe and of high quality. They aim to hire qualified staff, provide adequate staffing to meet their unit's needs, allow for sufficient resources, and foster continuous quality improvement. Policies and procedures help to provide clear expectations to relevant staff. Policies and procedures also provide measures of performance, knowledge, and skill. As a working document, periodic review and modifications of policies should occur. This review provides additional opportunity for continuous improvement.

FOLLOWERSHIP

Not everyone in an organization can be a leader at the same time. And good followers are just as important as good leaders. Neither exists without each other. A **follower** is an individual who supports and is guided by another person who usually functions as a leader. However, a good follower is not blindly led but rather exhibits traits of discernment, commitment, and trustworthiness; that is, exhibits similar traits of a leader. A relationship must exist between the leader and the follower that, to be effective, must be based on mutual trust and shared goals. As with effective leadership, effective followership approaches this relationship as equally responsible partners in accomplishing the vision and mission at hand. Ideally, followers know their own strengths and weaknesses as they critically appraise the leader and group's ideas, thus providing support and intelligent advocacy.

Shared Responsibility

To be effective leaders, managers, and followers, effective communication is required. QSEN emphasizes this importance throughout its competencies with specific interventions/tools such as SBAR and Team*STEPPS*, which are topics discussed in depth in subsequent chapters.

Chain of Command

Considering the importance of communication to the effective running of any organization, understanding chain of command is important. **Chain of command** is the order or hierarchy of authority within an organization typically delineates flow of communication and delegation. For example, using a chain of command, a staff nurse reports to a charge nurse who reports to the head nurse, who in turn might report to a Department Supervisor. That person might then report to a senior manager who reports to the VP of Nursing. That VP then typically reports to the CEO who heads the organization. The chain of command is important for communication and direction of power. In most institutions and organizations, to initiate or suggest change, following the chain of command is a well-established process. For staff nurses, typically the chain of command starts with their head nurse.

Strategic Planning

Strategic planning and goal setting are based on an organization's vision and mission. Many resources exist to aid organizations in developing a strategic plan. One such resource is the Society for Human Resource Management (SHRM). These resources or associations help organizations distinguish between similar but different terms. Access to resources sometimes requires a membership to an organization. SHRM is one of those associations; however, membership is free and comes with many advantages. According to SHRM, the vision of an organization is a statement that describes its ideal or future state, whereas the mission describes why an organization or institution exists. Based on the vision and mission of an organization, goals are set. Based on the set goals, the organization will then develop a strategic plan to accomplish them. This strategic plan typically includes very specific steps, clearly stating who will do what with exact timelines. Specific units within a hospital will set goals and a strategic plan that flows from the executive level to them. That is, the unit's strategic plan helps them to meet the unit's goals which support the institution's goals and strategic plan. QSEN as well as the FON call nurses to participate in this strategic planning on all levels of an organization to affect change. This includes sitting on relevant committees and boards within the healthcare organization as well as within the community in order to partici-pate equally alongside other interprofessional team members.

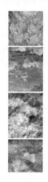

CASE STUDY 3.2

Samantha is a nurse manager of a busy neuro floor. She has noticed a steady decline in patient satisfaction rates.

1. *Should she ignore this situation?*
2. *How should Samantha approach this matter with her staff?*
3. *How could Samantha's supervisor help her with this matter?*

FINANCIAL AND ECONOMIC INFLUENCES

Though nursing is in the business of caring, healthcare is clearly a business that must be financially solvent to exist. As a business, revenue is generated by the care given to patients. This revenue pays for the expenditures incurred. A **budget** is an estimate of anticipated earnings and expenses that allows organizations to plan and function with forethought. A budget stems from the organization's mission and goals. While a variety of budgets exist, most hospitals employ both a capital and an operating budget. A capital budget focuses on fixed costs such as land and buildings, whereas an operating budget focuses on day-to-day expenses such as linen and clerical items. An operating budget typically involves the allocation of resources including those resources involving staff and needed supplies. Nursing units normally function with an operating budget that focuses on salaries and supplies required for the care the unit provides (Sherman, 2012).

Incoming Revenue

The revenue of an organization comes from reimbursement paid for patient care. Reimbursements come from insurance companies, governmental agencies, and out-of-pocket payments made by the patient. If a hospital is fortunate to conduct research and/or allow for auxiliary boards, unique and separate sources of funding or money can augment what is received in reimbursements.

Up until more recently, healthcare reimbursement has been tied to patient care provided in a fee-for-service model. A fee-for-service model of reimbursement pays a provider or institution for each individual or separate component of care, independent of quality or patient satisfaction. However, healthcare reimbursement is now based on additional factors such as patient outcomes (how well did the patient respond to the care provided?) as well as patient satisfaction measures. These additional performance measures alongside decreased reimbursements from many private and public insurers have tightened hospital's and organization's budgets significantly.

Staffing

Misuse of finances within the healthcare setting can have dramatic consequences on individual patients as well as on the institution. As professionals responsible for patient care, nurses have a moral obligation to understand how finances impact their ability to do their jobs safely, including how budgets affect staffing, which in turn affects patient care. In fact, studies show that patient mortality and morbidity is directly affected by the number of patients assigned to a nurse in a given shift. The number of patients assigned to a nurse depends on staffing of the unit. Staffing can be centralized where one unit or department is responsible for determining the needs for all units. Staffing can also be decentralized where the individual unit or department determines its specific staffing needs. Typically, staffing needs are expressed in a ratio of nurses to patients, which can be determined by one or more factors including budget allocation, beds filled, and patient acuity (Mensik, 2014). An example of this ratio on a medical–surgical floor might be one nurse to 24 patients or a 1:3 ratio. Adequate staffing helps to ensure nurses are able to provide safe and high-quality care. Organizations like the Agency for Healthcare Research and Quality: Advancing Excellence in Healthcare and Planetree.org provide valuable tools to nurses and healthcare organizations to use for many aspects of healthcare, including safe staffing.

In 2004, California became the first state to mandate minimum nurse–patient ratios. The legal mandate was limited to the following ratios:

- 6:1 patient-to-nurse workload in psychiatrics
- 5:1 patient-to-nurse in medical–surgical units, telemetry, and oncology
- 4:1 in pediatrics
- 3:1 in labor and delivery
- 2:1 in ICUs

Aiken et al. (2010) studied the impact of this mandate on patient outcomes and found it significantly improved patient outcomes and nurse retention.

Ensuring that the competencies of QSEN are implemented has been shown to save hospitals money. For example, cost savings have been demonstrated with the provision of patient-centered care. See the Evidence From the Literature for one such study.

CRITICAL THINKING 3.1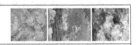

A nurse has been working on an oncology floor for 1 year. At times she feels frustrated that concerns regarding patient safety are not being taken seriously. She cares deeply for her patients as well as the floor itself and believes she could make a difference as a more formal leader. When an opening for a nurse manager position opens up, she applies for and gets the position.

(continued)

CRITICAL THINKING 3.1 *(continued)*

1. How could her understanding of Quantum Leadership Theory guide her in her new role?
2. How might she ensure staff feel heard?
3. In what other ways can she help staff be effective leaders?
4. In what ways can she help staff be effective followers?

EVIDENCE FROM THE LITERATURE

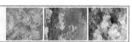

Citation

Wong, C. A., Cummings, G. G., & Ducharme, L. (2013). The relationship between nursing leadership and patient outcomes: A systematic review update. *Journal of Nursing Management, 21*(5), 709–724.

Discussion

A systematic review of existing studies was undertaken to examine the relationship between the practice of nursing leadership and patient outcomes. The authors identified 20 articles documenting the study of this relationship. They found a distinct correlation between positive, effective leadership and better patient outcomes. The specific leadership qualities found to most effective were positive, relationship based, and transformational, and reflected organizational goals and missions. Patient outcomes of this positive leadership included improved patient satisfaction and decreased mortality, medication errors, nosocomial infections, and use of patient restraints.

Implications for Nursing: Patient safety and quality of care is affected by leadership. Therefore, efforts to encourage leadership of nurses at all levels of practice are warranted.

CASE STUDY 3.3

Maria works as a staff nurse on a medical–surgical floor. She is asked to join a new committee focused on improving communication between the various departments providing care on her floor. The committee is led by a dynamic and inspiring pharmacist.

1. *How is Maria a leader in this scenario?*
2. *How is she a follower?*
3. *How could her understanding of Chaos Theory helps her in this scenario?*

NURSING'S SOCIAL CONTRACT AND CODE OF ETHICS

Nurses' right and authority to practice as nurses are based on an ethical social contract with society that explicates specific rights and responsibilities based on education and licensure. Within this contract, nursing describes and agrees to the essence of the profession with clear guidelines for behavior and intention. Documented as Nursing's Social Policy Statement, the relationship between nursing (and individual nurses within the profession) and society is explained and spelled out. The behaviors expected of nurses are based on autonomy to function and perform within the scope of nursing practice. The autonomy of nurses is in turn based on nursing's acknowledgment of public trust as well as nursing's agreement to self-regulate and accept legal parameters and regulations.

Within the social contract is a Code of Ethics for Nurses that lists nine provisions. These provisions allow nurses to fulfill the commitment made to their patients. However, it also guides nurses to effectively serve as leaders in any and all positions. The nine provisions are the following:

- The nurse practices with compassion and respect for the inherent dignity, worth, and unique attributes of every person.
- The nurse's primary commitment is to the patient, whether an individual, family group, community, or population.
- The nurse promotes, advocates for, and protects the rights, health, and safety of the patient.
- The nurse has authority, accountability, and responsibility for nursing practice; the nurse makes decisions and takes action consistent with the obligation to promote health and to provide optimal care.
- The nurse owes the same duties to self as to others, including the responsibility to promote health and safety, preserve wholeness of character and integrity, maintain competence, and continue personal and professional growth.
- The nurse, through individual and collective effort, establishes, maintains, and improves the ethical environment of the work settings and conditions of employment that are conducive to safe, quality healthcare.
- The nurse, in all roles and settings, advances the profession through research and scholarly inquiry, professional standards development, and the generation of both nursing and health policy.
- The nurse collaborates with other health professionals and the public to protect human rights, promote health diplomacy, and reduce health disparities.
- The profession of nursing collectively through its professional organizations must articulate nursing values, maintain the integrity of the profession, and integrate principles of social justice into nursing and health policy (American Nurses Association, 2015).

CRITICAL THINKING 3.2

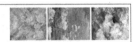

Your hospital is hosting the next FON: Campaign for Action in your area. You express interest in attending the meeting; however, your nurse manager denies your request because the floor will be short staffed.

1. What options do you have in response to this decision?
2. In this scenario, how can you be an effective informal leader?
3. In this scenario, how can you be an effective follower?

To Be a Profession

In the mid-1980s, reimbursement for patient care moved from a retrospective reimbursement system or fee-for-service to one of prospective payment. Reimbursing for care prospectively meant providers and hospitals were paid based on standardized care related to a patient diagnosis. Diagnostic-related group formulas (DRGs) were created as a way to control hospital costs, which represented a way to "capitate" or control costs. At the time, some nurse leaders believed it provided an opportunity for nursing to become more visible. Because patients are admitted to the hospital for nursing care, it was hoped DRGs would emphasize the centrality of nursing. Along with this realization, it was thought nursing would also move into a position of more authority. At the time, a revered nurse leader Donna Diers (1986) addressed District Four of the New York State Nurses Association. The title of her speech was "To Profess—To Be a Professional." She began by explaining the meaning of "to profess," which infers a dishonesty or insincerity of beliefs. She argued nurses were and are professional; however, she also stated nurses had not yet obtained the authority for the responsibility they had been delegated. Like others, she spoke of the social contract nurses have with their patients and society. She also spoke of nursing's primacy of caring. Diers believed the DRGs were the start of a revolution that offered nurses the opportunity to step into a place of authentic and deserved authority. Nurse's moral imperative is to care. But simply providing care or exerting compassion and concern are not enough. Diers and many others throughout nursing's history have argued caring must be intelligent and intentional. She states:

> Nursing is not just comfort, care, coordination, collaboration, or just applied psychology, physiology, sociology, anthropology or diluted medical science. Nursing is all of those things and more. It requires an effort of considerable intellectual acuity—which looks to an outsider like intuition—to thread one's way through all the knowledge, technique, and tenderness one has and to come out with the right action to serve the patient's particular need. (Diers, 1986, p. 27)

Like many of her contemporary counterparts, Diers acknowledged that the application of caring must extend from individual patient care to the creation of budgets, committees, curricula, community efforts, and legislative work. However, what she argued most ardently was nurses' legitimacy as professionals would not come from advanced degrees or credentialing. Rather, Dier's proposed, nursing's professionalism and authority would be established when nursing's practice was professional. She argued this would only happen if and when nurses took ownership of the work performed once education occurred.

This argument has been made by many others over time, both within as well as outside the nursing profession. Suzanne Gordon is another powerful and ardent champion of nursing and nurses' need to "own the knowledge of their work." Ms. Gordon is a journalist who has become a nationally recognized expert in healthcare systems but specifically on teamwork, nursing, and patient safety. She is a prolific author, speaker, and advocate/activist. Like Diers, Gordon argues nurses are solely responsible for how they are viewed in her 2006 landmark book authored with Bernice Buresch, *From Silence to Voice:*

> If nurses aren't willing to talk about their work, the results will be catastrophic for nursing. Nursing, like every other profession in today's work, must justify its existence and compete for resources. If nursing is misunderstood by the public and those with influence, it will continue to be disproportionately vulnerable to

the budget ax, and new resources for nursing education and practice will not be forthcoming at sufficient levels.

If nursing's script continues to emphasize the virtues of the nurse as a person to the detriment of the knowledge work that nurses do, then nurses themselves offer a rationale for limiting resources for nursing. Focusing on who the nurse is rather than what the nurses does can be an invitation to seek not the best and the brightest recruits, but the most virtuous, meekest and self-sacrificing who will try to do more and more with less and less. (p. 4)

CRITICAL THINKING 3.3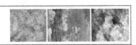

You work on a busy pediatric floor. During casual conversation with colleagues, you realize medication errors are increasing significantly.

1. How could you proactively respond to this realization?
2. With whom should you first begin discussing this realization?
3. Who else should be involved in assessing and addressing this situation?

EMANCIPATORY KNOWING

Acknowledging and accepting responsibility for the knowledge required to do the work of nursing is an important start. But knowledge is based on *knowing,* which speaks to subjective perception and a dynamic ontology or way of being. When knowing is expressed in a way that can be shared, it is considered to be knowledge. Knowledge of a discipline, such as nursing, encompasses the body of shared knowledge. This process of sharing knowledge within a discipline is vital to the creation of a community. According to Chinn and Kramer (2013), once knowledge moves beyond the individual to the discipline as a group, "social purposes form, and knowledge development and shared purposes form a cyclical interrelationship that moves us toward perspective, value-grounded change or praxis" (p. 4). For Chinn and Kramer, praxis is the outcome of critical thought and reflection of the art and science of nursing. Change occurs with the inclusion of ethics and the therapeutic use of self that ultimately results in some type of action. This process of thinking and reflection that leads to action is called Emancipatory Knowing.

As with Chaos and Quantum Theories, Emancipatory Knowing stems from critical evaluation of economic, social, and political influences of a reality or status quo simultaneously looking at its potential for positive change. For Chinn and Kramer, this positive change must involve alleviating injustice in order to ensure equitable conditions for individual and groups. In doing so, individuals and groups are provided the opportunity to fulfill their potential.

FON: CAMPAIGN FOR ACTION

As discussed earlier, the IOM reports of 2000 and 2001 have led to many initiatives, including the formation of the FON: Campaign for Action. Within this initiative, several organizations joined forces to support nurses in a unique way. The RWJF, AARP, and the AARP Foundation pledged their support and resources to aid the nursing

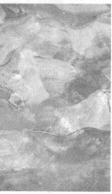

REAL-WORLD INTERVIEW

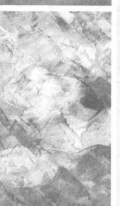

Nurses entering the profession often voice their reason for choosing nursing as a desire to "make a difference" by impacting or facilitating another's physical and mental well-being. Through helping others, a challenge develops that offers the nurse an opportunity to grow morally, ethically, and spiritually. The challenge is the quest for "doing the right thing" for the patient. This implies that the nurse must be responsible for developing therapeutic alliances, monitoring and evaluating patient needs, as well as ensuring interventions have produced the intended results and outcomes. This further implies that nurses must be successful in critically questioning and then identifying necessary changes, within their own nursing practice, as well as using their leadership skills in the development of teams that promote evidence-based practice with patient-focused care and goals.

Nurses' growth and experience in providing quality care happens over time. Quality is achievement, refinement, and satisfaction in and of practice, but the quest to become "REAL" requires a continuous commitment to the very process that is often infused with the challenges that we ethically, morally, and spiritually need to address in order to "become." Rising to the challenge requires developing leadership skills in defining and critically analyzing what is inherent in quality nursing practice; for example, doing a nursing intervention because it is the "right thing to do" and not because that "is how it has always been done." Essential to achieving best outcomes requires that:

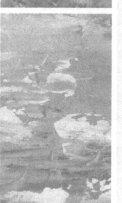

- Quality, the quest for best practice, becomes the way we do business.
- Mentors for quality who are respected clinicians and knowledgeable role models with moral courage will step forward when necessary to serve as patient advocates and to promote quality care endeavors, such as critically questioning, investigating, and promoting nursing practice in the ever-changing healthcare arena.
- Academic nursing programs support clinical experiences with practicing nurses that routinely incorporate quality behaviors on the front line and embrace quality endeavors as the main approach to promoting best outcomes.
- Reinforcement of quality and change theory principles in continuing education for all healthcare professionals and the expectation that these principles be used by all in the patient-centered setting.

If we choose to make a committed difference individually, what follows is the collective commitment to quality and safe nursing practice that offers the nurse, patient, team, and health administrative staff the best care.

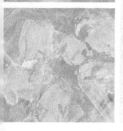

Judy Kilpatrick, RN, MS, CCNS, ANP
Syracuse, NY
Denise A. Karsten RN, MS, DC, Adult/Gero Nurse Practitioner
Primary Spine Practitioner
Upstate Brain and Spine Center
Syracuse, NY

profession in addressing the eight recommendations listed earlier. While the FON acknowledges the importance of all recommendations, they identified four specific or key elements to ensuring all nurses will be prepared to assume a leadership role within institutions and healthcare as a whole (Box 3.2).

BOX 3.2 KEY ELEMENTS

1. Nurses should practice to the full extent of their education and training.
2. Nurses should achieve higher levels of education and training through an improved education system that promotes seamless academic progression.
3. Nurses should be full partners with physicians and other health professionals in redesigning healthcare in the United States.
4. Effective workforce planning and policy making require better data collection and an improved information infrastructure (IOM, 2011, p. 58).

The call to action by multiple nurse leaders and organizations is clear: Nurses must step into leadership positions at all levels of practice. From advocating for the primary prevention of nosocomial infections to safer staffing to working on committees to refine policies ensuring safer and higher quality patient care on units, in institutions, and on more global levels, nursing can have a powerful and important role to play. Nursing's social contract requires nursing to engage in a more global systems thinking that embraces moral courage and the knowing of its profession. By doing so, nursing will step into leadership that influences the safety and quality of care of patients individually and as a whole.

KEY CONCEPTS

1. Nursing education must prepare nurses to demonstrate leadership at all levels of nursing practice, directly and indirectly impacting the safety and quality of patient care.
2. Three theories of leadership that guide nursing practice are Chaos Theory, Quantum Theory, and Systems Theory.
3. Leadership is the ability to lead or command a person or a group of people.
4. The roles of a leader typically involve developing a vision and facilitating change on a large scale, such as for a department or institution.
5. A manager is someone responsible for controlling all or part(s) of an organization, and for getting a designated group or unit's work done effectively.
6. A follower is an individual who supports and is guided by a leader, who shares mutual trust and goals with the leader, and who is an equally responsible partner in accomplishing the vision and mission at hand.
7. Nursing care must be provided within the context of the business of healthcare. It must generate revenue and operate within the constraints of the budget.
8. Nursing practice is based on an ethical social contract with society that explicates specific rights and responsibilities of nurses, such as those embodied in the Nursing Code of Ethics.
9. Nursing practice should be guided by emancipatory knowing, which is a process of thinking and reflection that leads to action.

10. The FON: Campaign for Action is an initiative in which several organizations have joined forces to support nurses and prepare them to assume leadership roles with institutions and healthcare as a whole.

KEY TERMS

Accountability	Manager
Follower	Responsibility
Leadership	Roles

REVIEW QUESTIONS

1. The nurse is working on a busy medical–surgical floor caring for oncology patients. One of the patients with a poor prognosis is asking for a glass of wine with dinner. The floor policy states that patients are not allowed to consume alcohol while admitted to their floor. The nurse believes the policy as stated does not take into consideration the circumstances this patient is experiencing. The nurse approaches the manager with a request to review and potentially modify the current policy. The manager agrees a review of the policy is warranted but would like the nurse to invite several other interdisciplinary team members to the meeting in order to consider their perspective. The manager specifically invites them to this discussion because they understand the impact allowing alcohol could have on departments such as Dietary, Pharmacy, and Physical Therapy. What leadership theory explains the manager's perspective most accurately:

A. Chaos
B. Quantum
C. Change
D. Systems

2. A nurse decides to apply for a hospital leadership position after receiving a glowing performance review at her fifth year anniversary as a floor manager. The nurse is aware that a formal leadership position will include unique roles and responsibilities. Which of the following apply to leadership (distinguished from management)? Select all that apply.

___ Improve on ways an organization functions to meet its goals and objectives.
___ Conducts periodic review of unit policies and procedures.
___ Develop skills in managing conflicts of different groups with differing priorities.
___ Enforce policies such as continuing education requirements for nursing staff.
___ Focus on the long term.
___ Identify areas for marketing campaigns to increase income, thus increasing staffing.
___ Create the staffing schedule for the medical–surgical unit.
___ Actualize and demonstrate the organization's mission by motivating others.
___ Lead by displaying your education and professional certifications to inspire others.

3. A nurse applies for a position as a unit manager. In the interview process, the nurse is asked to list responsibilities they assume will come with the position. List three tasks that could be included in this list:

   A. _____

   B. _____

   C. _____

4. A nurse has just taken a new position on an orthopedic floor as a staff nurse. Before this new position, the nurse had been a Team Leader on the Telemetry Unit for almost 5 years. In this new position and role, the nurse is aware that being a follower is a vital piece of demonstrating an organization's mission and values. The nurse also understands that all nurses are followers and leaders, often at the same time. How can the nurse best demonstrate followership in this new role? Select all that apply:

   ___ Demonstrate the organization's missions and values in patient care.
   ___ Know the strengths and weaknesses that you bring to both roles.
   ___ Challenge every suggestion the group leader makes.
   ___ Build relationships with those you follow.
   ___ Only accept tasks that are of personal interest.
   ___ Recognize that followers always support their leaders.

5. The nurse works for a hospital that is experiencing budget cuts and layoffs due to decreased reimbursements. The nurse is concerned about how this might affect patient care. What potential ramifications should the nurse be concerned about? Select all that apply.

   ___ Poor staffing ratios
   ___ Use of unqualified staff
   ___ Increased patient satisfaction
   ___ Fewer supplies on the unit
   ___ Hiring freezes
   ___ Poor patient outcomes

6. The nurse is asked to work overtime because replacements have not been hired yet to fill recent vacancies. The nurse is very concerned about agreeing to this overtime, because the shift is already down two nurses. The nurse is also concerned because the hospital is freezing budgets and most likely will not fill these vacant positions for a while. What outcome is the nurse concerned about relative to safety and quality of care? What factor in a hospital budget has the most direct effect on patient morbidity and mortality?

   _____

7. The nurse is attending general orientation with a group of new graduates. A clinical nurse specialist (CNS) presents a 1-hour talk on professionalism and responsibility to function as leaders in the new positions the nurses will assume. Within this presentation, the CNS states all nurses practice within a Code of Ethics and agree to a social contract with society. What are the components of Nursing's Code of Ethics? Select all that apply.

   ___ Compassion
   ___ Patient dignity
   ___ Commitment to the patient

___ Protecting patient rights
___ Health and safety
___ Promotion of health
___ Participating in improving ethical environment in care setting and/or larger community
___ Collaborating with others to establish/maintain standards, articulate values, and generate policy

8. Jim, a nurse, has volunteered to sit on a professional development committee as a representative from the floor he works on. In one of the first committee meetings, Jim is asked what he would be interested in knowing more about. Jim explains he is confused about the meaning of autonomy. Which of the following is false?

   A. Autonomy refers to delegating responsibility to others.
   B. Autonomy refers to the right to self-regulate or govern.
   C. Autonomy in nursing has been earned by society's trust.
   D. Autonomy in nursing includes legal parameters delineating scope of practice.

9. Mary works as a nurse in an NICU with a few unhappy colleagues. Unfortunately, the demeanor of these few nurses affects many people, including the parents of the neonates. Mary knows the impact of stress on these vulnerable families and infants so she begins to explore how to change the situation. In researching ideas, Mary discovers an intervention that might help and reflects on the interpersonal dynamics of the unit alongside the complexity of the health of its patients. Mary considers each person's right to self-determination and autonomy and also considers how best to approach proposing change. Ultimately, the thought, reflection, and therapeutic use of self leads to deliberate action by Mary, facilitating effective change. What is this process called?

   _____

10. A nurse is orienting to a new position on a transplant floor. Part of the job expectations includes serving on committees. The nurse is interested in promoting the nursing profession, particularly as it relates directly and indirectly to ensuring safe and high-quality patient care. As such, the nurse is interested in joining the local Action Coalition of the FON: Campaign for Action. Because this activity will require quite a bit of time off the unit, the nurse will need to provide a brief explanation of this initiative. As a foundation, the nurse lists the four key elements of the FON. Please list two of the four elements:

    A. _____
    B. _____

REVIEW ACTIVITIES

1. Consider how the Key Elements of the FON, Campaign for Action could help you as a nurse leader in your first position as a staff nurse.
2. How does the Nursing Code of Ethics impact how you will practice as a new nurse?
3. What characteristics of leadership do you bring to the frontline of patient care?

CRITICAL DISCUSSION POINTS

1. Leadership theories provide effective guidance in understanding how best to facilitate change.
2. The roles and responsibilities of leaders directly and indirectly affect the safety as well as the quality of patient care.
3. Management incorporates aspects of leadership but is primarily focused on getting the work of an assigned group accomplished.
4. Being an effective follower includes critical thinking, commitment to the group's goals, and mutual trust.
5. The FON: Campaign for Action is a national initiative that provides a forum for collaborative effort aimed at empowering the nursing profession.
6. Staffing directly affects patient satisfaction surveys but more importantly, patient outcomes.
7. Staffing adequacy is based on a sufficient budget.
8. Nursing's Code of Ethics provides guidance for practice and action.
9. Emancipatory Knowing requires one to integrate critical thought, reflection, ethics, and therapeutic use of self within a community created by shared knowledge. This integration leads nurses to take action and facilitate change at all levels of practice.

EXPLORING THE WEB

1. Visit QSEN.org and review the various Graduate QSEN Competencies, specifically noting the knowledge, attitude, and skill for each of them. Reflect on which of these competencies you feel comfortable with at this time. Consider which you feel are essential to have acquired before you start as a graduate nurse.
2. Visit the following websites to compare and contrast resources: Agency for Healthcare Research and Quality: Advancing Excellence in Healthcare and Planetree.org.
3. Search the Internet for how the FON is referenced and incorporated into action plans within nursing and as an interprofessional approach to change.
4. Conduct an Internet search for the terms "leadership" and "nursing." Describe what your search reveals.

REFERENCES

Aiken, L. H., Sloane, D. M., Cimiotti, J. P., Clarke, S. P., Flynn, L., Seago, J. A., … Smith, H. L. (2010). Implications of the California nurse staffing mandate for other states. *Health Services Research*, 45(4), 905.

American Nurses Association. (2015). *Code of ethics for nurses with interpretive statements*. Silver Spring, MD: American Nurses Association.

Buresh, B., & Gordon, S. (2006). From silence to voice: What nurses know and must communicate to the public (2nd ed). Ithaca, NY: ILR Press/Cornell University Press.

Chinn, P. L., & Kramer, M. K. (2013). *Integrated theory and knowledge development in nursing* (7th ed.). St. Louis, MO: Mosby Elsevier.

Curtis, E. A., de Vries, J., & Sheerin, F. K. (2011). Developing leadership in nursing: Exploring core factors. *British Journal of Nursing*, 20(5), 306–309.

Diers, D. (1986). To profess—To be a professional. *Journal of Nurse Administration*, 16(3), 25–30.

Dinh, J., Lord, R. G., Gardner, W. L., Meuser, J. D., Liden, R. C., & Hu, J. (2014). Leadership theory and research in the new millennium: Current theoretical trends and changing perspectives. *The Leadership Quarterly*, 25(1), 36–62.

Dolansky, M. A., & Moore, S. M. (2013). Quality and safety education for nurses (QSEN): The key is systems thinking. The *Online Journal of Issues in Nursing*, *18*(3), 1–10. Retrieved from www.nursingworld.org/Quality-and-Safety-Education-for-Nurses.html

Gardner, J. (1993). *On leadership*. New York, NY: The Free Press.

Grossman, S. C., & Valiga, T. M. (2016). *The new leadership challenge: Creating the future of nursing* (5th ed.). Philadelphia, PA: F.A. Davis.

Institute of Medicine (IOM). (2011). *The future of nursing: Leading change, advancing health*. Washington, DC: The National Academies Press.

Mensik, J. (2014). What every nurse should know about staffing. *American Nurse Today*. Retrieved from www.americannursetoday.com/what-every-nurse-should-know-about-staffing

Oxford Dictionary. (2017). Integrity. Retrieved from https://en.oxforddictionaries.com/definition/integrity

Porter-O'Grady, T., & Malloch, K. (2011). *Quantum leadership: Advancing innovation, transforming health care* (3rd ed.). Sudbury, MA: Jones & Bartlett Learning.

QSEN. (2017). QSEN institute: Quality and safety education for nurses. Retrieved from www.qsen.org

Sherman, R. (2012). The business of caring: What every nurse should know about cutting costs. *American Nurse Today*. Retrieved from www.americannursetoday.com.

Society for Human Resource Management (SHRM). (2017). Mission & vision statements: What is the difference between mission, vision and values statements? Retrieved from https://www.shrm.org/

SUGGESTED READINGS

AHRQ. (2016). *AHRQ patient safety tools and resources*. Retrieved from http://www.ahrq.gov/professionals/quality-patient-safety/patient-safety-resources/resources/pstools/index.html

American Nurses Association. (2010). *Nursing's social policy statement: The essence of the profession*. Silver Spring, MD: American Nurses Association.

Anderson, C. L., & Agarwal, R. (2011). The digitalization of health care: Boundary risk, emotion, and consumer willingness to disclose personal health information. *Information Systems Research*, *22*(3), 469–490.

Bertakis, K. A., & Azari, R. (2011). Patient-centered care is associated with decreased health care utilization. *Journal of the American Board of Family Medicine*, *24*, 229–239.

Chinn, P. L. (2013). *Peace and power: New directions for building community*. Burlington, MA: Jones and Bartlett Learning.

Fischer, S. A. (2016). Transformational leadership in nursing: A concept analysis. *Journal of Advanced Nursing*, *72*(11), 2644–2653.

Hughes, R. G. (2008). *Patient safety and quality*. Rockville, MD: Agency for Health Care Research and Quality.

Kreidler, M. L. (2015). *Quality improvement in health care*. Research Starters: Business (Online Edition).

Nadeem, E., Olin, S., Hill, L., Hoagwood, K., & Horwitz, S. (2013). Understanding the components of quality improvement collaboratives: A systematic literature review. *Milbank Quarterly*, *91*, 354–394.

National Committee for Quality Assurance. (2007). *About NCQA*. Retrieved from http://www.ncqa.org/AboutNCQA.aspx

The National Academies of Press. (2011). The future of nursing: Leading change, advancing health. Retrieved from http://www.nap.edu/read/12956/chapter/10#235

Wong, C. A., Cummings, G. G., & Ducharme, L. (2013). The relationship between nursing Leadership and patient outcomes: A systematic review update. *Journal of Nursing Management*, *21*(5), 709–724.

Wong, C. A., Lashchinger, H. K., & Cummings, G. G. (2010). Authentic leadership and Nurses' voice, behavior, and perceptions of care quality. *Journal of Nursing Management*, *18*, 889–900.

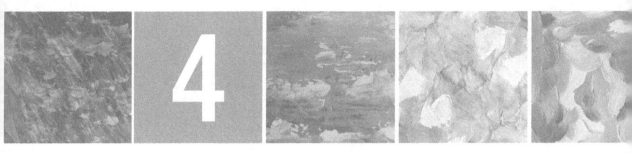

4

QUALITY AND SAFETY IN HIGH-RELIABILITY ORGANIZATIONS

Patti Ludwig-Beymer

Every system is perfectly designed to get the results it gets. (Attribution disputed)

Upon completion of this chapter, the reader should be able to

1. Define high-reliability organizations (HROs).
2. Evaluate the characteristics of HROs.
3. Describe how high reliability affects all aspects of an organization.
4. Identify how healthcare can learn about high reliability from other industries.
5. Analyze healthcare system changes essential for HRO.
6. Discuss nursing responsibilities and interprofessional team functions required for achieving high reliability.
7. Compare and contrast methods for assessing a culture of high reliability.
8. Discuss barriers to achieving high reliability.
9. Identify internal and external resources helpful in an organization's journey to high reliability.

A patient who was discharged postabdominal surgery at General Hospital returned a week later with sepsis from a surgical site infection. During her rehospitalization, x-rays revealed that a sponge was retained in her abdomen during the initial surgical procedure. By definition, this is a sentinel event, and it is thoroughly investigated by a team that includes nurses, physicians, surgical technicians, anesthesiologists, and staff from risk management and quality. The team conducts a root cause analysis to determine the underlying cause of the retained sponge and to create a corrective action plan. The sentinel event is reviewed and the corrective action plan is approved by hospital leadership and governance. Everyone at the hospital expresses confidence that the processes put into place will prevent this event from happening again. Unfortunately, within a few months, a sponge is retained in another patient's abdomen after a gynecological surgical procedure.

- *How could this sentinel event error happen again?*
- *What unit or organizational characteristics may have contributed to this sentinel event?*
- *What can the interprofessional healthcare team do to prevent future errors?*

In *To Err Is Human*, the Institute of Medicine (IOM;1999) described the safety of healthcare in the United States and suggested that up to 98,000 people die in hospitals each year as a result of medical errors that could have been prevented. *To Err Is Human* provided a roadmap to safety, including strategies to enhance knowledge about safety; identifying and learning from errors; raising expectations for improving safety; and implementing safety systems in healthcare organizations to ensure safe practices at the patient care delivery level. Unfortunately, errors that cause harm to patients continue to occur.

More recently, Makary and Daniel (2016) estimated medical errors cause 251,000 deaths each year, making it the third leading cause of death in the United States, after heart disease and cancer. Yet medical error is not even recorded on U.S. death certificates. Most medical errors do not result from individual recklessness or the actions of a particular group but are instead caused by faulty healthcare systems, processes, and conditions that lead people to make mistakes or fail to prevent them. As a result, mistakes can best be prevented by designing the health system to make it easier to do the right thing and harder to do the wrong thing.

Makary and Daniel propose a three-part model for reducing harm from individual and system errors: (a) transparency to make errors more visible, (b) rapid response to errors, and (c) decrease the frequency of errors. **Transparency** is defined as openly sharing and making errors and other aspects of performance visible so that everyone can learn from the errors and improve quality. Within the model, the responsibility for reducing harm lies with both the organization and the individual.

The Joint Commission (TJC, 2017), an independent, not-for-profit group in the United States that administers voluntary accreditation programs for hospitals and other healthcare organizations, adopted a formal Sentinel Event Policy in 1996 to help hospitals that experience serious adverse sentinel events improve safety and learn from those sentinel events. A **sentinel event** is a healthcare error that reaches a patient and results in death, permanent harm, or severe temporary harm and requires healthcare interventions to sustain life. A sentinel event requires immediate investigation and response by the interprofessional healthcare team to prevent it from happening again.

Each year, TJC publishes a list of the most frequent sentinel events that occurred nationally (Box 4.1). TJC recommends, but does not require reporting of sentinel events. As a result, this published sentinel events list represents only a fraction of the actual number of sentinel events. Careful investigation and analysis of sentinel events and other patient safety events and creation of corrective actions are essential to reducing risk and preventing patient harm.

BOX 4.1 TOP 10 SENTINEL EVENTS IN THE UNITED STATES, 2017

1. Unintended retention of a foreign body—116 reported
2. Wrong patient, wrong site, wrong procedure—95 reported
3. Falls—114 reported
4. Suicide—89 reported
5. Unassigned (category unassigned at time of report)—54 reported
6. Delay in treatment—66 reported
7. Other unanticipated event (including asphyxiation, burn, choked on food, drowned, or found unresponsive)—60 reported
8. Operative/postoperative complication—19 reported
9. Medication error—32 reported
10. Criminal event—37 reported

Source: The Joint Commission (TJC). (2018). Summary data of sentinel events reviewed by The Joint Commission. https://www.jointcommission.org/assets/1/18/Summary_4Q_2017.pdf

This chapter focuses on building a high-reliability organization (HRO), a cultural transformation designed to ensure safe practices and reduce errors and sentinel events in healthcare. The chapter begins by defining HROs and presenting the characteristics of HROs. The effect of high reliability on all aspects of an organization is described. Healthcare changes essential for creating HROs are discussed, and the nurse's responsibilities required for achieving high reliability are described. The importance of interprofessional team function is addressed. Finally, barriers to achieving high-reliability and internal and external resources helpful in a journey to high reliability are summarized.

HIGH-RELIABILITY ORGANIZATIONS

HROs, such as commercial aviation and nuclear power plants, operate under very trying conditions all the time and yet manage to have fewer than their fair share of accidents. HROs in healthcare establish and maintain high quality and safety expectations for patient care and keep quality and safety error rates near zero (Weick & Sutcliffe, 2007). HROs have the ability to provide consistent healthcare at a high level of excellence over a long period of time. **Reliability** is defined as the probability of failure-free performance over a specified timeframe. It is also called quality over time (www.businessdictionary.com/definition/reliability.html). Morrow (2016) describes reliability as "getting the expected outcome throughout the expected time" (p. 9). The risk of healthcare error is a function of both probability and consequence.

Healthcare can be dangerous and errors can have devastating consequences. For example, administering IV fluids safely is an important aspect of treating a dehydrated patient who has heart failure. Administering fluids too slowly can result in prolonged hypotension. Administering fluids too rapidly can result in worsening of the heart failure. An IV pump is used to assist the nurse in providing accurate amounts of fluid. The IV pump decreases the probability of error. However, if the pump fails, the consequences can still be catastrophic. By decreasing the probability of an error, HROs operate to make healthcare systems safer. In an HRO, a culture of safety permeates the organization, and everyone is expected to ensure safety.

To improve safety, HROs maintain a focus on reducing errors. An **error** is a deviation from generally acceptable performance standards. Generally acceptable performance standards are found internally within a healthcare organization and externally outside of an organization. Internal standards include policies, procedures, protocols, and order sets. External standards include healthcare industry and accreditation imposed practice requirements and professional practice standards. For example, a hospital may establish a protocol that requires a nurse to assess an IV infusion site in pediatric patients every 2 hours. This is an internal standard. On the other hand, the American Association of Critical-Care Nurses (2015, p. 14) requires that the nurse "intervenes to prevent and minimize complications and alleviate suffering." If the nurse fails to assess a patient on a ventilator and provide sedation and pain medication as needed, the nurse has deviated from generally acceptable external performance standards.

A deviation from performance standards may cause varying levels of harm to a patient. A **near miss safety event** occurs when the safety event does not reach the patient because it is caught by chance or because the process was engineered with a detection barrier. For example, the medication reconciliation process in hospitals is often designed with purposeful redundancies. On admission, a nurse or pharmacist meets with a patient to obtain an accurate list of current medications. The physician then reviews the list, verifies it with the patient, and places the medication orders. A pharmacist reviews the medications, and the nurse administers the medications. Despite these steps, sometimes an incorrect medication is ordered. If this is discovered before the medication is administered, it is considered a near miss event. Nurses and other clinicians may fail to report near misses, rationalizing that no one was hurt. However, near miss safety events serve as an early warning system of something that could go wrong. By reporting near miss safety events, healthcare organizations can work on improving processes so that no one else makes the same error.

Precursor safety events occur when the healthcare error reaches the patient and results in no harm or minimal detectable harm. **Adverse events** or **serious safety events** occur when the error reaches the patient and results in moderate-to-severe harm or even death. They are an undesired or unintended consequence of the care provided, such as a significant decrease in blood pressure after a wrong dose of medication is given.

To differentiate a precursor safety event from a serious safety event, consider this example. A nurse assesses Mr. Z and determines that he is a high fall risk. The nurse puts fall prevention precautions in place, including placing the bed in its lowest position, activating the bed alarm, and using floor mats to cushion the floor around the bed. However, Mr. Z gets out of bed and falls before anyone can respond to his bed alarm. If Mr. Z suffers no harm, the event is considered a precursor safety event. Like near miss safety events, the nurse should report this precursor event and the care team should investigate what could have been done differently to keep Mr. Z safe from falls. After all, Mr. Z's lack of injury was due to luck rather than healthcare system design. On the other hand, if Mr. Z suffers a fall and fractures his hip, the injury is a serious safety event. In addition to providing immediate patient care and reporting the serious safety event, the nurse should participate in an in-depth analysis called a **root cause analysis** (RCA). An RCA allows a healthcare team to determine the primary cause of the safety event and put together an action plan to prevent it from happening again. See Chapter 10 for further discussion of RCAs.

The healthcare team often becomes aware of errors at the point of care, where nurses and other clinicians interact with patients. According to Cook and Woods (1994), this is the "sharp end" of a triangle, where clinicians interface with patients. Clinicians experience remorse and blame themselves when errors happen. However, their work with patients is influenced by many factors and decisions made by individuals prior to an actual error event. These factors and decisions are the "blunt end" of the triangle. For example, policies and procedures put in place to ensure consistent healthcare processes may be inaccurate, difficult to interpret, or hard to access. Work processes might be convoluted and patient handoffs can be inadequate. The environment may be cramped and noisy, making it difficult to concentrate. Technology can be cumbersome or may fail completely. The culture of the hospital might hinder a nurse's ability to speak up about safety concerns. Groups and individuals may blame others rather than taking responsibility for their actions. All of these "blunt end" factors can contribute to an error at the "sharp end," where the consequences of all healthcare activities reach the patient.

James Reason (1997) proposed the Swiss cheese model to illustrate how errors occur. The model suggests that every step in a process has the potential for error. The holes in the Swiss cheese represent opportunities for a process to fail, and each slice is a defensive layer to prevent an error in the process. An error may pass through a hole in one layer but in the next layer, the hole is in a different spot and catches the error before it reaches the patient. More layers of cheese and smaller holes allow more errors to be stopped or caught. When the holes in the Swiss cheese line up, the defenses are defeated and an error occurs.

For example, a nurse may be caring for a female patient who requires the insertion of an indwelling urinary catheter. The intent is to place the catheter into the correct patient using aseptic technique. A variety of protective layers are in place to prevent errors as the nurse performs this procedure. The nurse is educated on the policy, procedure, and equipment. The nurse verifies the order and checks the patient's identification using two patient identifiers. The nurse explains the procedure to the patient and obtains an assistant to help with proper patient positioning. The nurse ensures the environment is appropriate, with privacy and sufficient lighting. If one or more of these protective layers are circumvented, an insertion error may occur, resulting in patient harm.

CHARACTERISTICS OF HIGH-RELIABILITY ORGANIZATIONS

Weick and Sutcliffe (2007) identified five key principles of high reliability organizations: preoccupation with failure, reluctance to simplify, sensitivity to operations, commitment to resilience, and deference to expertise (Table 4.1). These characteristics, when present, help an organization to achieve high reliability.

Preoccupation With Failure

Preoccupation with failure requires the nurse and other healthcare providers to be aware that the risk of error is always present. An HRO acknowledges that failures can occur and puts healthcare processes in place to diminish harm. An HRO proactively identifies high-risk activities and analyzes all the potential error points in the process. Conducting a failure modes and effect analysis (FMEA) is one way of accomplishing

TABLE 4.1 HIGH-RELIABILITY ORGANIZATION CHARACTERISTICS

CHARACTERISTIC	ELEMENTS
Preoccupation with failure	• Be alert to near-miss events • Recognize weaknesses in healthcare systems early
Reluctance to simplify	• Recognize the complexity of work • Do not focus on superficial causes of failure
Sensitivity to operations	• Acknowledge the complexity of healthcare processes • Have situational awareness of the environment, distractions, availability of resources and supplies • Be aware of relationships
Resilience	• Anticipate and mitigate failure • Determine how to diminish risk of harm to patients • Identify strategies to recover when an adverse event occurs
Deference to expertise	• Use teamwork that recognizes each member's knowledge, skill, and expertise • Facilitate active participation from healthcare professionals • Be comfortable in sharing information • De-emphasize hierarchy

Source: Adapted from Weick K. E., & Sutcliffe, K. M. (2007). *Managing the unexpected: Resilient performance in an age of uncertainty* (2nd ed.). San Francisco, CA: Jossey-Bass.

this analysis. **FMEA** is a rigorous process in which a team of clinicians identify and eliminate known and potential failures, errors, or problems before they actually occur (Hughes, 2008). "Failure modes" refer to the ways in which something might fail and cause potential or actual harm. "Effect analysis" examines the consequences of those failures. Failures are prioritized according to the seriousness of the consequences, how frequently they occur, and how easily they can be detected. The purpose of an FMEA is to take actions to eliminate or reduce failures, starting with the highest priority ones.

For example, during an acute bleeding episode, a nurse may need to administer multiple units of blood during a very short time period. This requires cooperation among physicians, nurses, the blood bank staff, transportation staff, and many others. A hospital might examine the process used for massive blood transfusion by convening an interprofessional team. The team identifies each step in the process, from ordering of the blood to administration and determines where failures might occur. Through the FMEA, the hospital might learn that the greatest risk of error occurs in small units with a limited number of nurses. As a result, they may create a code transfusion team to bring additional resources to the bedside during acute bleeding episodes.

Preoccupation with failure also requires that critical information is communicated across time, across the healthcare team, and across sites of care. For example, the day shift nurse communicates her concerns about the patient and what should be monitored with the oncoming night shift nurse. Last, preoccupation with failure requires the nurse to pay attention to near miss safety events and precursor safety events as an early warning that something is wrong. This requires that nurses and others report questionable or unsafe practices. Nurses need to recognize when an error can or has occurred, feel confident in stopping unsafe practices, and assume the responsibility for reporting errors or near misses. HROs then use those reports to correct unsafe processes through rigorous process improvement activities.

Reluctance to Simplify

Reluctance to simplify drives an organization's search to understand the cause of errors. Staff members in HRO healthcare facilities focus on drilling down to determine the true cause of error. They take nothing for granted and challenge the status quo to make healthcare processes and structures safer. For example, a nurse may fail to change a dressing. Upon questioning to determine why this event occurred, the easy answer is "I forgot." However, probing further for contributing factors to this failure encourages the organization to find real, sustainable solutions. In the case of the dressing change, the information may not have been shared at change of shift, or a prompt in the electronic health record (EHR) may have been missing, or the necessary supplies may not have been available at the time the nurse had planned to change the dressing. An examination of each of these factors allows an HRO to determine ways to improve the healthcare process.

Reluctance to simplify also addresses work arounds, a common phenomenon in healthcare. **Work arounds** occur when nurses and other clinicians use shortcuts in an effort to streamline care without realizing the potential impact on safety. For example, healthcare organizations require dual (two person) verification for high-risk medications. Letty, a nurse in critical care, generally abides by this policy. However, she has been administering a propofol infusion to her patient for several days and has begun to adjust the dose without seeking an independent double check. Letty uses this work around to save time. Unfortunately, it also increases risk to her patient. Leaders in HROs identify and extinguish these types of workarounds.

Sensitivity to Operations

Sensitivity to operations creates an awareness of the many factors that influence the care environment. Healthcare workflows are complex and factors such as fatigue, distractions, and workload can contribute to unsafe conditions. Sensitivity to operations requires healthcare leaders to make rounds and talk to staff to look for weaknesses in the care delivery system that allow errors to occur. Once weaknesses are identified, leaders provide guidance and feedback and allocate resources to prevent harm. For example, in an attempt to create an open-floor plan on a medical–surgical unit, the automated medication dispensing system was placed in an alcove in the hallway. With no barrier in place, the nurse was frequently interrupted by physicians, patients, visitors, and other staff while obtaining medications from the dispensing system. Nurses expressed concern about this process, which interfered with their ability to concentrate on the task at hand. Nursing leaders observed this when making rounds and resolved the problem by creating a small medication room to house the automated medication dispensing system and minimize distractions for the nurse while preparing medications.

Commitment to Resilience

Commitment to resilience addresses the need to talk about and learn from mistakes. Rather than blaming others, clinicians in HRO healthcare settings discuss how the error occurred and what can be done to prevent such an error in the future. Because we are human, mistakes will happen. Resilience describes the ability to recover when something bad happens. For an HRO, resilience is the ability to overcome problems, learn from mistakes, and move forward. Transparency is paramount. An HRO openly discusses errors and uses them to improve healthcare processes. Nurses and other clinicians in an HRO are taught to perform quick situation assessments when an error occurs, work as a team to contain or manage the error, and then take steps to reduce the harm.

HROs ensure that clinicians are offered support when they are involved in a safety event. When a nurse or other clinician makes an error that harms a patient, she or he feels guilty. The term "second victim" has been coined to label the pain and anguish experienced by the clinician (Wu, 2000). Programs have been developed to assist clinicians to build resilience and recover from these safety events. The forYOU program (Scott, 2015) is an evidence-based second victim intervention that provides immediate emotional and social support. Members of the forYOU team provide emotional support using a three-tiered methodology. In tier one, local support is provided by colleagues. In tier two, specially trained peers provide support. In tier three, support is provided by a referral network of chaplains, social workers, and employee assistance programs.

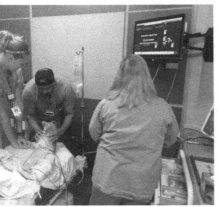

FIGURE 4.1 An interprofessional team responds to a code in a simulation center.

Last, simulation learning is a tool used in HROs to practice responses to errors or safety events. Drills for rapid responses, cardiopulmonary resuscitation, active threats, and environmental disasters help nurses and other clinicians to work as an interprofessional team and build resilience for emergency situations (Figure 4.1).

Deference to Expertise

Deference to expertise acknowledges that collective expertise is better than any individual's expertise. This deference allows an HRO to take advantage of the unique skills of everyone involved. In an HRO, teams recognize that each member has knowledge and skills unique to his or her profession and role. HROs minimize the authority gradient and hierarchy so that everyone feels comfortable to speak up. **Authority gradient** refers to positions within a group or profession, such as a direct care nurse and the nurse manager or a medical resident and the attending physician. The term was defined first in aviation when it was noted that pilots and copilots did not always communicate effectively in stressful situations if there was a significant difference in their perceived authority. A number of unintentional aviation, aerospace, and industrial incidents have been attributed to authority gradients. The concept of authority gradient was introduced to medicine in the IOM's(1999) report *To Err Is Human*. **Hierarchy** refers to perceived level of power across groups, such as a housekeeper and a direct care nurse, or a direct care nurse and a physician. Healthcare has been and remains hierarchical. Physicians are viewed as the "captain of the ship," with nurses and other clinicians viewed as less powerful.

Regardless of authority gradient or hierarchy, deference to expertise specifies that team members with the most expertise about the issue have the authority to make decisions. For example, in an HRO, decisions about nursing practice are informed by and driven by practicing nurses rather than by the chief nursing officer (CNO) or by physicians. Ignoring a team member's expertise can generate anger, indifference, or a failure to respond, which create opportunities for error to occur. Open communication with information flowing in all directions among all team members is essential for the delivery of consistently safe care.

THE EFFECT OF HIGH RELIABILITY

A culture of reliability affects all aspects of an organization. HRO improves safety, which was identified as one of the six elements of quality healthcare in the IOM's (2001) report *Crossing the Quality Chasm*. Patient safety is recognized as an important element of an effective, efficient healthcare system. **Safety** has to do with lack of harm and focuses on avoiding bad events. Safety makes it less likely that mistakes and errors will happen. When care processes are performed as intended over long periods of time, the result is no harm. For example, an interprofessional team may focus on reducing harm to patients caused by catheter-associated urinary tract infections (CAUTIs). Using evidence from the literature and standards from professional organizations, the team constructs a CAUTI bundle, a standard set of procedures to be used consistently to prevent CAUTIs. If the procedures are consistently applied by every clinician providing care to the patient, the likelihood of harming the patient with a hospital-acquired CAUTIs usually drops exponentially. Functioning in a culture of reliability prevents harm and enhances safety.

Similarly, a culture of high reliability enhances quality. **Quality** has to do with efficient, effective, and purposeful care that gets the job done at the right time for the right cost. It focuses on doing things well and employs quality improvement techniques so that the overall care continues to improve. CAUTI rates are widely measured and reported as a quality measure for healthcare systems. At the individual level, preventing CAUTI simproves quality for that patient.

In addition, a culture of reliability enhances the **patient experience**. The patient experience is more than patient satisfaction. It is "the sum of all interaction, shaped by an organization's culture, that influences patient perceptions, across the continuum of care" (The Beryl Institute, 2017). Most clinicians strive to provide patient-centered care in a kind and compassionate manner. Yet all too often, patients receive mixed messages and inconsistent information. This occurs because care is provided by humans, and humans are fallible and variable in their approaches. However, in a culture of high reliability, enhanced communication among staff results in more consistent communication with patients. Clinicians are educated to be competent, compassionate, and consistent. Patient satisfaction scores, one measure of the patient experience, tend to rise in such an environment. Patients and their family members are unhappy when their care is unsafe or of poor quality. Returning to the earlier CAUTI example, no patient wants to develop a urinary tract infection, with the corresponding symptoms and required treatment. Patients who have this experience often evaluate their overall care less positively when they complete patient satisfaction surveys. They may also express their dissatisfaction when talking with friends and families, thus eroding the reputation of the hospital.

Last, a culture of reliability also improves **financial performance**, which reflects the income and the expenses of a healthcare organization. A culture of reliability helps to increase income and decrease expense. Hospitals and ambulatory care settings are increasingly being reimbursed based on safety, quality, and patient experience outcomes. The Centers for Medicare and Medicaid Services (CMS) oversees three hospital-based pay-for-performance programs that tie reimbursement to reliability: Value-Based Purchasing (VBP) Program, Readmission Reduction Penalty Program, and Hospital-Acquired Conditions (HAC) Reduction Program. In VBP, hospitals earn scores based on achievement or improvement of their safety, quality, patient experience, and financial scores. VBP scores a hospital on five domains as follows:

- Patient- and caregiver-centered experience of care/care coordination (contributing 25% of the score)
- Clinical care outcomes (contributing 25% of the score)

- Efficiency and cost reductions (contributing 25% of the score)
- Safety (contributing 20% of the score)
- Clinical care processes (contributing 5% of the score)

The Readmission Reduction Penalty Program focuses on patients being readmitted to hospitals for specific conditions, including acute myocardial infarction, coronary artery bypass graft surgery, chronic obstructive pulmonary disease, heart failure, pneumonia, and total hip and knee arthroplasty. The hospital's actual readmission rate is compared to the expected rate of readmissions given the patient's comorbidities. **Comorbidities** are two or more coexisting medical conditions or disease processes that are additional to an initial diagnosis. For example, a patient may be admitted for a total knee arthroplasty. If the patient has diabetes and heart failure, these coexisting conditions must be documented because they make patient care more complex.

The HAC Reduction Program examines the hospital's performance on coded data derived from the documentation of physicians and advanced practice clinicians. The coded data are then analyzed as part of the Agency for Healthcare Research and Quality (AHRQ, 2013a) Patient Safety Indicators (PSI-90) and the Centers for Disease Control and Prevention (CDC) National Healthcare Safety Network (NHSN) databases. In 2017, 6% of Medicare reimbursement to hospitals was tied to these three pay-for-performance programs, representing billions of dollars. Hospitals with better than expected outcomes received higher reimbursement for patients insured under Medicare, whereas those with worse than expected outcomes received lower reimbursements.

Additionally, healthcare organizations may experience less waste and lower cost when care is provided in a consistent manner. Returning to CAUTI prevention as an example, an important first step in preventing the infection is to clearly identify which patients truly require the insertion of an indwelling urinary catheter. By providing evidence-based care and inserting indwelling urinary catheters only when needed for care, the number of indwelling catheters can be reduced, with a corresponding decrease in the CAUTI rate and the cost of urinary catheter supplies. According to the Association for Professionals in Infection Control and Epidemiology (2017), each urinary tract infection adds on average $5,904 to the cost of the hospital stay. Simply put, hospitals and patients can save money by preventing CAUTIs.

LEARNING FROM OTHER INDUSTRIES

Commercial Aviation

Commercial aviation has worked diligently to change the culture in airplane cockpits to advance airline safety. Their work began after research conducted by the National Aeronautics and Space Administration in the 1970s suggested that the majority of commercial airplane crashes were caused by failure of communication among pilots and crew, not by mechanical failures. As a result, crew resource management (CRM) training programs were developed and implemented. Teams make fewer errors than individuals, especially when each team member knows his or her own responsibilities along with those of other team members. The CRM program is widely credited with the dramatic safety improvements in the airline industry (Helmreich, Merritt, & Wilhelm, 1999) and has tremendous applicability in healthcare.

Nuclear Power

Similarly, the nuclear power industry has worked for many years to improve safety. The Institute of Nuclear Power Operations defines seven safety culture characteristics that are adaptable to the healthcare environment as follows:

1. Leaders demonstrate commitment to safety in their decisions and behaviors.
2. Decisions that support or affect safety are systematic, rigorous, and thorough.
3. Trust and respect permeate the organization.
4. Opportunities to learn about ways to ensure safety are sought out and implemented.
5. Issues potentially impacting safety are promptly identified, fully evaluated, and promptly addressed and corrected, commensurate with their significance.
6. A safety-conscious work environment is maintained where personnel feel free to raise safety concerns without intimidation, harassment, discrimination, or fear of retaliation.
7. The process of planning and controlling work activities is implemented so that safety is maintained.

CRITICAL THINKING 4.1 APPLYING NUCLEAR POWER SAFETY CHARACTERISTICS TO HEALTHCARE

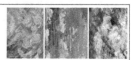

Review the seven nuclear power safety characteristics outlined in the chapter.

1. Which characteristics can be applied to healthcare?
2. How might a nurse leader demonstrate commitment to safety in decisions and behaviors?
3. How have you seen nurses demonstrate trust and respect in your clinical setting?
4. What experiences have you had at school to learn about ways to ensure safety? What experience have you had in your clinical setting?
5. How might you raise safety concerns during your clinical rotations?

Science of Human Error: How Humans Function

Humans function primarily in three modes: skill-based performance, rule-based performance, and knowledge-based performance. Each mode is described in the following along with the errors that can occur when functioning in that mode.

When individuals are using skill-based performance, they are essentially on auto-pilot. **Skill-based performance** is used for routine, familiar tasks that can be done without thinking about them. For example, the drive to work or school may be so familiar that the driver arrives without knowing how he or she got there. Nurses often function in this mode because of the repetitive nature of some nursing tasks. Consider, for example, Jim, a nurse completing his documentation in the EHR. Jim logs onto the EHR many times each day. He does not need to think about his user identification or his password. He is on auto-pilot. He pulls up his assigned patients in the EHR and begins to document.

In general, skill-based performance is accurate. But even though these repetitive tasks may be simple, there is still a risk for error. Slips occur when, without intending to, the individual does the wrong thing. Jim could pull up the wrong patient and document care that was delivered to a different patient. Lapses occur when, without intending to, the individual fails to do what he meant to do. Jim could document on his patient but forget to save or file his work before closing the record. Fumbles occur when, without intending to, an individual mishandles a word or action. Jim may be documenting using a hand-held device. If he drops the device, he has experienced a fumble.

Skill-based errors may be prevented by stopping and thinking before acting. Double checking one's own work helps to prevent these errors. This is why nurses learn to check, recheck, and recheck again before administering medications. Determining that the right drug in the right dose is being given by the right route, at the right time, and to the right patient involves checking the medication label against the medication order or medication administration record three times. In addition, two unique patient identifies need to be used prior to administering the medication. Healthcare facilities typically define which two patient identifiers are to be used, most often full name and date of birth. High-risk medications, such as insulin, require independent verification by another nurse. The independence of this double check helps to prevent skill-based errors.

In **rule-based performance**, the clinician has learned a rule and applies it in appropriate situations. The delivery of healthcare is largely based on rules, often called protocols. Rules may be learned in nursing school or through continuing education, clinical experience, or life experiences. Errors may also occur when functioning in a rule-based performance mode. Sometimes, clinicians use the wrong rule. They may have been taught or somehow learned the wrong response for a situation. For example, Susan learned many years ago in nursing school to treat patients with hypoglycemia if glucose was 60 mg/dL or less. If Susan has not kept current with more recent diabetes and hypoglycemia guidelines, she will fail to treat a patient with glucose of 70. The solution to this type of error is to educate clinicians with the right rule.

A rule-based error may also occur if the clinician misapplies the rule. The nurse may know the right response but select another response instead. For example, Susan may know that a blood sugar of 68 should be treated with 15 g of glucose. However, she may misapply the rule, and give 30 g of carbohydrates instead. This could over-correct the low blood sugar, causing the blood sugar to spike and creating another patient safety event. This can be prevented by pausing and thinking a second time.

Noncompliance can also cause a rule-based performance error. The clinician may know the rule but choose not to follow it. For example, Susan knows that she should recheck her patient's glucose level 15 to 30 minutes after treating hypoglycemia. Susan's patient has a hypoglycemic event and she treats it appropriately. Susan sees that the patient looks fine, is alert, and oriented. She assumes the patient will put on her call light if she runs into any problems, so Susan decides not to recheck the blood sugar. Noncompliance with rules can be prevented in several ways. First, Susan needs to understand the risks involved in not following the rules. In addition, organizations need to reduce the burden or difficulty of following the rules. For example, are there an adequate number of bedside glucose monitors so that a glucose recheck is easy? Is staffing sufficient to allow time for the glucose recheck? Susan also may need to be coached by her supervisor to make better decisions. If this is a repeated behavior, Susan needs to be counseled.

In **knowledge-based performance**, a clinician is solving problems in a new and unfamiliar situation. The clinician tries to figure out how to perform based on what they already know. They may use trial and error or even guess at a solution. This is very dangerous. Up to 60% of all knowledge-based decisions may be made in error. For example, consider Cathy, an experienced nurse who has been working in critical care for 15 years. When she arrives on her shift, her patient is receiving continuous renal replacement therapy. Cathy has not previously managed this therapy and is not familiar with the supplies and fluids used. Rather than proceeding independently, Cathy needs to stop and consult an expert. The expert may be a colleague or another member of the healthcare team. Or the expert may be a written resource, such as an evidence-based protocol.

The concepts of skill-, rule-, and knowledge-based performance are essential when investigating errors. Clinicians involved in the error should focus on how they made the decision they did. Did they develop a shortcut or work-around to save time? Did they fail to do a double check of their own work? Did they proceed even though they were not familiar with the procedure? Each type of error requires a different solution. The three performance modes are critical to keep in mind when designing error prevention strategies.

THE ROLE OF LEADERSHIP IN CREATING A HIGH-RELIABILITY ORGANIZATION

For the purposes of this chapter, leadership is defined as the governing body of an organization, typically the board of directors or trustees, senior health system management, and nursing, physician, and other clinical leadership. To build an HRO, all of these leaders must share the vision of eliminating harm to patients (Chassin & Loeb, 2013). The governing body plays a critical role in setting goals and priorities for healthcare organizations and in overseeing patient safety. Ganghi and Yates (2017) identify the following eight questions board members should ask to ensure that the healthcare organization is focused on safety:

- Is safety positioned as an uncompromising core value?
- Is there a comprehensive plan for improving patient and workforce safety and for monitoring progress?
- Is transparency embraced for sharing adverse patient safety events and lessons learned across the system?
- Do we have a healthy reporting environment and a fair and just culture?
- Do we expect respect for patients, coworkers, and physicians within the organization?
- Are patient stories heard regularly?
- Are quality and safety implications considered for every major organizational decision?
- Does the board devote sufficient time to safety, quality, and the patient experience of care?

REAL-WORLD INTERVIEW

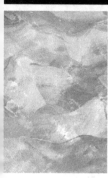

What is the role of the board of directors in our journey toward high reliability? We begin with the philosophy that "good isn't good enough." We need to be sensitive to our systems and processes to identify where things may not work or can be improved upon. And we must build a culture of open communication and reporting by all, for the good of all, to inspire and achieve greater results.

Joseph DePaulo
Board Member, Edward-Elmhurst Health; and Chair, Edward Hospital Quality
Committee of the Board

Creating a Culture of Safety

Leadership is accountable for the provision of effective and efficient care while protecting the safety of patients, employees, and visitors. Competent leaders understand that every step of the care process has the potential for failure simply because humans make mistakes. TJC's Sentinel Event Database suggests that leadership's failure to create an effective safety culture is a contributing factor for many types of adverse events (TJC, 2017, February 17). Understanding and shaping an organization's culture is essential for enhancing safety.

A culture of safety is what an organization is and does in the pursuit of safety (TJC, 2017). Leaders in HRO healthcare facilities realize their role in creating a culture of safety. As such, leaders need to show their commitment to safety and eliminate fear of reporting. Leaders must make their commitment to safety clear. This is accomplished in a variety of ways: telling safety stories at each meeting; expecting, encouraging, and rewarding the reporting of safety events; and expecting and supporting staff to speak up for safety. The focus of a safety story can be on an event of harm, an explanation of why safety is important, a review of an error prevention tool, a thank you for being committed to patient or employee safety, or an example of using a safety tool at home or at work. Many hospitals use these techniques to keep safety at the top of everyone's mind.

Leaders in HRO organizations know they must eliminate the fear of reporting in order to encourage and reward the reporting of safety events. This may be accomplished by thanking staff for reporting errors, mistakes, events, and near misses. The Good Catch award is one way to recognize staff who report near misses or close calls (Figure 4.2). Many hospitals across the nation have implemented the Good Catch award program. Edward Hospital in Naperville, Illinois, implemented the Good Catch award in 2008. Each month, risk managers identify safety events that have been identified by staff and have not reached the patient to cause harm. They summarize the top safety events and ask members of the senior leadership team to vote on the most important event. The person or team responsible for submitting the top safety event is recognized at a management team meeting and receives a certificate, a lapel pin, and a Good Catch traveling trophy, which rotates monthly. The Good Catch program recognizes those who speak up about near miss safety events, and fosters a culture of transparency and safety.

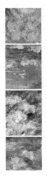

CASE STUDY 4.1

During handoff report from the emergency department, Colleen Erhardt, RN, learned that her patient had become increasingly confused. Upon arrival to the floor, her patient remained disoriented, had garbled speech, and was lethargic. No family was present and the patient's spouse could not be reached. Physician's orders included a neurology consult, stat head CT scan, and NPO status. While the patient was receiving his CT scan, Colleen reviewed the patient's morning lab work and noted his blood sugar was 70 mg/dL. Realizing there had not been a repeat blood sugar obtained since that time, Colleen proceeded to the radiology department to check the patient's blood sugar and found it had decreased to 31 mg/dL. Colleen administered 50 mL of D50. The patient immediately responded and was able to answer all orientation questions appropriately. The neurologist was notified of the blood sugar and CT results, which revealed no acute neurological problem. The neurologist noted the source of the patient's confusion appeared to be hypoglycemia and after this was resolved, the patient returned to normal.

1. *What type of error is a Good Catch?*
2. *What factors allowed Colleen to make this Good Catch?*
3. *What are the typical signs and symptoms of hypoglycemia?*
4. *Why might this patient have experienced this episode of hypoglycemia?*
5. *Why is it important to identify and discuss Good Catches?*

HRO leaders support investigations into how errors occur. This encourages reporting and learning. HRO leaders make errors visible in a way that has meaning to the audience. For example, hospitals tend to report injuries as percentages, rates, or raw numbers. However, putting a face to that number is essential for understanding the impact of the error. For example, consider this communication, which demonstrates transparency and paints a vivid picture of the event: "We had one fall with injury reported this week. The patient was a grandmother who required surgery to repair her fractured hip and experienced a prolonged separation from her family because of her stay in a skilled nursing facility."

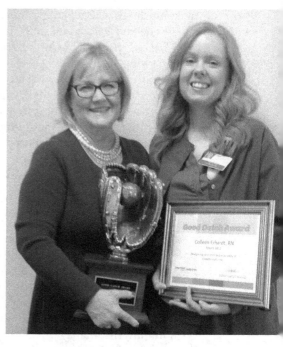

FIGURE 4.2 Colleen Erhardt, RN (right), receiving the Good Catch Award with her manager, Deb Kocsis, RN.

Correcting System Problems

Consistent with sensitivity toward operations, leaders must identify and correct system problems. HRO leaders are always on the lookout for system problems and work diligently to fix those problems. A helpful tool to accomplish this is a **daily safety huddle**. This brief huddle includes senior and operational leaders who meet at the start of each day to discuss safety concerns and resolve problems. Operational leaders prepare for the daily safety huddle by reviewing the past 24 hours and anticipating the next 24 hours. They summarize safety issues that have already occurred and identify if those safety issues impact other departments. They discuss any barriers to providing safe care, such as inadequate supplies, staffing, or technology. They describe any high-risk or nonroutine situations, such as two patients with the same first and last names on the same unit. At the daily safety huddle, issues critical to the safety of patients or staff can be addressed quickly and efficiently. Appropriate experts are mobilized and empowered to solve the problem. For example, safety huddles may reveal an increase in work place injuries inflicted by patients. This information may be used to launch a system-wide task force designed to decrease violence in the workplace, including early identification of potential problems, environmental modifications, and employee training. Workplace injuries will begin to decrease if the interventions are effective.

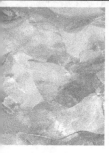

REAL-WORLD INTERVIEW

"The single best thing we've implemented here as part of our 'Road to Zero Harm' is the daily Safety Huddle. While it only lasts 10 to 15 minutes, we all attend or call in to hear 49 operational leaders report on the safety issues in their areas. The Safety Huddle allows us to quickly identify and act on safety trends. It's helping to make our care safer."

Bill Kottmann
President and CEO, Edward Hospital

Building and Reinforcing Accountability

HRO leaders are also responsible for building and reinforcing accountability. They reinforce sound safety habits, console those who make honest mistakes, and counsel those who make risky choices. To build a culture of accountability, leaders must set clear expectations, educate and build skills within the staff, and build and reinforce accountability. The behavioral expectations should be consistent with the organization's mission, vision, goals, and standards for performance. Edward Hospital uses the phrase "Road to Zero Harm" to connote their journey toward high reliability. Individuals at all levels of the organization must be educated on these expectations. In addition, leaders need to create a system that allows nurses and other staff members to convert all their behaviors into safe work habits.

Individuals experience three sources of accountability: vertical, horizontal, and intrinsic. Vertical accountability is applied by leaders, that is, the sense that managers are watching. Peers account for horizontal accountability, the sense of teamwork and the desire to function as effectively as others. Intrinsic accountability exists within the individual. All three types of accountability are important in creating a culture of safety and accountability. Leaders need to expect accountability and build the intrinsic motivation of the individual to meet performance expectations. HRO leaders take every opportunity to build and reinforce accountability by making regular rounds and creating a just culture.

Leaders who visit and make rounds to clinical practice areas are essential for building a culture of high reliability. "Management by walking around" allows leaders to see firsthand the conditions that exist at the front line, where care is being delivered. Making rounds demonstrate leadership's commitment to safety and allow leaders to talk with staff about safety concerns for themselves and their patients. It also provides an opportunity for leaders to provide quick feedback and reinforcement to staff. The science of human performance suggests that providing both positive and constructive feedback is needed to decrease human errors, and that the overwhelming majority of feedback should be positive. Instant feedback helps to reinforce positive behaviors and should be immediate and based on facts. A verbal thank you for practicing safely is very effective in reinforcing safe behaviors. During rounds, leaders may observe unsafe behaviors and should immediately correct the behavior and offer a practice tip to extinguish the unsafe behavior.

For example, nurses and clinicians in many hospitals and healthcare settings are inconsistent in performing hand hygiene before and after patient contact (see Figure 4.3). Edward Hospital is no exception. As a result, leaders decided to focus on hand hygiene during rounds. To prepare leaders, a rounding tool was created by Mary Anderson, an infection preventionist at Edward Hospital. The rounding tool allowed leaders to relate hand hygiene to the core value of safety. Clinicians were then asked how they perform hand hygiene and expectations were clarified if necessary. Clinicians were asked what barriers exist for performing hand hygiene and how hand hygiene can be better met in the future. Last, clinicians were asked to commit to performing hand hygiene and helping others to do the same. This effective rounding tool provided actionable feedback to leaders (for more information, go to www.eehealth.org). For example, leaders received input on the need for structural modifications, and they are working to increase the number of sinks and hand gel stations.

Creating a Fair and Just Culture

Leaders are also responsible for creating a fair and just culture. A fair and just culture minimizes blame and punishment and creates an environment that encourages individuals to report errors so that the system problems can be corrected. Traditionally, healthcare's

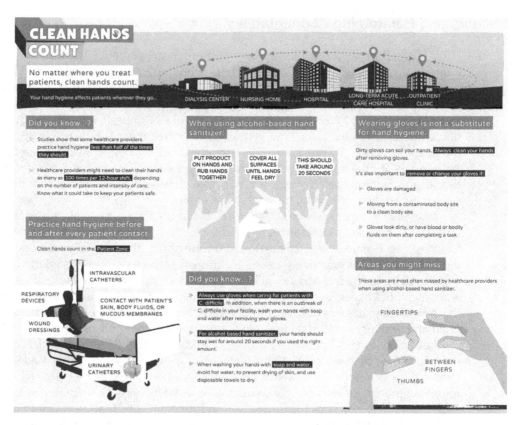

FIGURE 4.3 Clean Hands Count for Healthcare Providers.
Source: Centers for Disease Control and Prevention. Retrieved from http://cdc.gov/handhygiene

culture has held individuals accountable for all errors that occur with patients under their care. This punitive approach toward errors views those who make errors as "bad apples" (IOM, 1999). This approach has served as a disincentive to reporting errors and mistakes. After all, who would report an error if it meant they would get in trouble? As a result, organizations missed opportunities to uncover and correct problems that impacted performance and outcomes. The pendulum then swung to the opposite extreme, to a nonpunitive culture. This was interpreted by some to mean the individual was always blameless when an error occurred, which allowed intentional disregard for work rules. Most recently, the concept of a just culture has been embraced within healthcare.

James Reason (1997) wrote that a just culture creates an atmosphere of trust, encouraging and rewarding people for providing essential safety-related information. A just culture also clearly identifies what constitutes acceptable and unacceptable behavior. Marx David (2001) wrote that individual practitioners should not be held accountable for system failings over which they have no control. He held that discipline should be tied to the behavior of individuals and the potential risks of their behavior rather than only to the actual outcome of their actions. A just culture recognizes that many errors represent predictable interactions between human operators and the systems in which they work. In a 2010 position paper, the American Nurses Association (2010) endorsed the just culture model, noting its wide use in the aviation industry.

Ultimately, the just culture model is about creating a learning culture that is open and fair; managing behavioral choices; and designing safe healthcare systems. The model acknowledges that humans make mistakes and because of this no system can be designed to produce perfect results. A just culture views errors as opportunities to improve the understanding of both healthcare system risk and individual behavioral risk. It changes staff expectations and behaviors so that everyone looks for risks in the environment; reports errors; helps to design safe healthcare systems; and makes safe choices, such as following procedures, policies, and protocols.

The just culture model requires leadership competencies that appropriately hold individuals accountable for their behaviors and investigates the behavior that led to the error. James Reason (1997) developed a Performance Management Decision Guide that is used across the world to guide management decisions when human error occurs. It starts with a deliberate act test. If the individual acted with malicious intent, disciplinary action and a report to a professional group, regulatory body, and/or law enforcement is warranted. If there is confirmed ill health and the individual was unaware, a leave of absence and physician referral are appropriate. If substance abuse is suspected, testing and disciplinary action are warranted. If the individual chose to take an unacceptable risk based on policies, procedures, and protocols commonly used within the organization, disciplinary action may be warranted. However, if the individual adhered to generally accepted performance expectations and simply made an unintended error, the individual needs to be consoled and coached. In every case, leadership is also responsible for correcting all safety problems that contributed to the error.

Fostering a Learning Environment

The learning organization was first described by Peter Senge (1990) as an organization where people continuously learn and enhance their capabilities to create. An HRO cannot exist in the absence of learning. A learning organization views each failure as an opportunity to learn from mistakes. An HRO readily admits its weaknesses and commits to learning from its mistakes (Hughes, 2008). Key tenets of improving patient safety at the organizational level include taking a systems approach to safety and improving the culture of safety. Healthcare systems that embody this approach are considered learning organizations. Leaders in these organizations support learning and create a supportive learning environment. They put specific processes in place to facilitate learning and encourage creativity among employees. Such a learning environment requires a level of transparency related to safety, so that everyone is aware of opportunities for improvement. Reporting errors and near miss safety events can assist in understanding a problem rather than hiding that a problem exists.

Enhancing Process Improvements

An HRO has a strong commitment to healthcare process improvement. Becoming an HRO requires a systematic look at the complexity of the healthcare process, identification of the root causes of failures in the healthcare process, implementation of solutions, measuring and monitoring outcomes from the implemented solutions, and then building ways to sustain the improvement. In some cases, an entirely new process may be required to enhance safety. Increasingly, patients and their families are being engaged to assist in healthcare process improvements. The use of systematic process improvement methodologies and tools such as Six Sigma and Lean are discussed in Chapter 13.

Identifying and Reporting Events

In an HRO, all healthcare providers are responsible for reporting safety events, including near misses, adverse events, and sentinel events. This type of reporting has its limitations, as it depends on both the recognition of the safety event and the completion of a safety event report. When using voluntary reporting and error tracking, only around 10% to 20% of all errors are reported in healthcare organizations (Classen, Lloyd, Provost, Griffin, & Resar, 2008). Hospitals need a more effective way to identify events that cause harm to patients in order to select and test changes to reduce harm.

In an HRO, a multifaceted reporting approach is needed that is comprehensive and provides accurate measurements of errors and near misses. The Institute for Healthcare Improvement (IHI) Global Trigger Tool (GTT; IHI, 2017c) helps healthcare organizations get a clearer understanding of the safety of care by measuring risk and harm at the hospital level. The GTT uses specific patient care triggers as indicators that an adverse event (AE) may have occurred. Using GGT to identify AEs is an effective method for measuring the overall level of harm from patient care in a healthcare organization. The GTT provides an easy-to-use method for accurately identifying AEs (harm) and measuring the rate of AEs over time. Tracking AEs over time is a useful way to tell if changes being made are improving the safety of the patient care processes.

For example, transfer to a higher level of care is one of the Global Triggers. A patient is transferred to the ICU from a medical–surgical unit due to a rapid drop in blood pressure and decreased level of consciousness. This would cause activation of the trigger and a review of the patient's EHR to determine what happened to the patient, when it happened, and if it could have been avoided. There are more than 50 triggers that are consolidated into categories on the GTT related to the provision of surgical, ICU, perinatal, medication, and emergency department care. The categories and triggers can be viewed at the IHI website (www.ihi.org/resources/Pages/Tools/IHIGlobalTriggerToolforMeasuringAEs.aspx). In an HRO, investigation results and the GTT results are shared with healthcare providers and process improvement changes are put into protocols, policies, and procedures to reduce the chance of future safety problems occurring.

Deploying Technology

In an HRO, health technologies help facilitate and sustain quality improvement efforts to improve patient safety. For example, the use of IV pumps with built in limits for high and low medication doses helps to reduce medication errors. Elaine is caring for a patient with a pulmonary emboli. She reviews the medication orders to administer 80 units of heparin per kilogram by IV bolus, followed by 18 units per kilogram as an hourly infusion. Elaine knows her patient weighs 150 pounds, or 68 kg. She correctly calculates and administers the initial dose of 5,540 units. Elaine calculates the continuous infusion rate at 1,224 units per hour. When programming the pump, however, her finger slips and she enters 12,244. Because that dose is beyond the normal range for heparin, the pump does not administer the drug, and Elaine receives an error message. She quickly identifies and corrects the programming. A double check from a peer for this high-risk medication would also catch this programming error before it reaches the patient.

All too often, however, hospital leaders apply technology to faulty healthcare processes and hope to prevent errors with technology. Technology can only help improve healthcare processes when applied appropriately. A focus on a safe and efficient healthcare process design using technology to support and sustain any improvement is critical.

Committed leaders are needed to implement system changes that are essential for becoming an HRO. However, leadership is not sufficient. Every individual within an organization needs to be committed to high reliability. The next section addresses the individual responsibilities for nurses and other members of the interprofessional healthcare team on a journey toward high reliability.

INDIVIDUAL RESPONSIBILITIES: SAFETY BEHAVIORS FOR NURSES

While many contributing factors lead to errors, an actual error occurs when the clinician interacts with the patient, at the "sharp end" of care. The nurse is often the last line of defense against healthcare errors. As such, the nurse must be cognizant of both internal behaviors to enhance safety and communication techniques that can be helpful in preventing errors and patient harm.

Internal Behaviors to Enhance Safety and High Reliability

Nurses and other members of the interprofessional healthcare team must always strive to focus their attention and to think before they act. This is effective in preventing many task-based errors, especially in stressful, noisy, and pressured situations. A tool used to focus and think in these situations is Pause-Act-Review (PAR). Nurses and other clinicians are asked to pause for 1 or 2 seconds to focus their attention on the task; act by concentrating and performing the task; and review their actions to check for the desired result. This self-checking takes only a few seconds but greatly reduces the probability of making an error.

For example, Karly, a nurse on the telemetry unit, uses the PAR technique when pulling medications from the automated medication dispensing system (Figure 4.4). She pauses, acts, and reviews her action. The automated medication dispensing system is located in the supply room; the area gets considerable traffic and can become noisy. Karly recognizes that noise and congestion can increase the risk of errors. She takes her concern to the Practice Council, and a decision is made to post a sign by the automated medication dispensing system. The sign serves two purposes. It reminds other staff to be quiet and avoid interrupting the nurse who is preparing medications, and it reminds the nurse to use PAR.

Another internal behavior helpful in enhancing safety is maintaining a questioning attitude when providing patient care. The nurse must carefully consider the patient care situation and ask questions of herself. Is this what I expected to see? Does this fit with what I know? Does this make sense to me? If a question or concern remains, the nurse confirms by checking with independent, expert sources, either competent people or written materials that can help in resolving the question.

As an example of a questioning attitude, Chris is caring for a 3-month-old with a history of supraventricular tachycardia who is admitted to the pediatric ICU with a cough and congestion. Chris reviews the medication orders and finds orders for propranolol 20 mg TID. As an experienced pediatric nurse, Chris realizes that this dose is high. He knows pediatric doses are weight-based and consults a drug reference book (an external expert) to determine the appropriate dose. Chris also talks with the mother

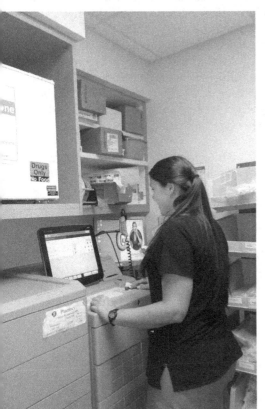

FIGURE 4.4 Karly Blaschak, RN, focuses on retrieving medications from an automated medication dispensing system.

(an expert in her child's care) and finds that the infant was taking 2 mg of propranolol TID at home. Chris questioned what he saw and investigated appropriately. He then spoke to the physician, who changed the medication order and thanked Chris for his diligence.

Communication Techniques

In the fast-paced healthcare arena, clear communication is essential, both within nursing and with other members of the interprofessional team. Communication ensures that messages are heard correctly and accurately and prevents incorrect assumptions and misunderstandings that could lead to wrong decisions. One of the National Patient Safety Goals (NPSGs) is to improve the effectiveness of communication among caregivers (TJC, 2016). TeamSTEPPS® (AHRQ, 2013b) provides a variety of tools that can be helpful in improving communication, including callout and closed loop (or three-way) communication. Callout is a tool used to communicate important information. It informs all team members simultaneously during an emergency and helps team members anticipate next steps. For example, during a code, the nurse uses a callout to report "I've administered 1 mg epinephrine IV."

Closed-loop communication ensures that the message received is the same as the message sent. The sender initiates communication with a receiver by providing an order, request, or information. The receiver acknowledges the communication with a repeat-back of the order, request, or information. The sender then confirms the accuracy of the acknowledgment by saying "that's correct." If communication is not clear, the nurse must clear up the confusion. "Let me ask a clarifying question" is a helpful and nonthreatening phrase to use when attempting to clarify communication. As an example, Pam is a nurse on a medical–surgical unit. When she receives a telephone order from a physician, she enters it into the EHR and reads it back to the physician. Pam waits for the physician to verify the order before terminating the conversation. Pam also uses closed-loop communication when communicating with or delegating to a patient care tech (PCT).

Communication also includes the transfer of information during transitions of care, for example, during shift changes, transfer to another unit, or discharge from the hospital. These communication handoffs provide an opportunity to ask questions, clarify information, and confirm understanding. The tools I PASS the BATON and SBAR can be used effectively in handoffs. The I PASS the BATON acronym for remembering the key components of the handoff is presented in Box 4.2.

The acronym, SBAR, stands for Situation, Background, Assessment, and Recommendation. It was originally adapted by Kaiser Permanente from a U.S. Navy tool to enhance collaboration between nurses and physicians (IHI, 2017b). In the structured SBAR communication, Situation refers to a concise statement of the immediate problem. Background includes brief and pertinent information related to the situation. Assessment refers to analysis and consideration of action options. Recommendation addresses the actions requested.

Jean uses SBAR as a nurse in labor and delivery. When caring for Mrs. Jones, she calls the obstetrician to report, "Here's the situation. I'm concerned about the decelerations that Mrs. Jones is experiencing. Mrs. Jones is 34 years old, gravida 2, para 1. My assessment finds baseline fetal heart tones are 120 with minimal variability and repetitive late decelerations. I've initiated all intrauterine resuscitation measures without improvement. I need you to come assess Mrs. Jones as quickly as possible. When can I expect to see you?"

BOX 4.2 I PASS THE BATON

I—Introduction—Introduce self and role
P—Patient—Name, identifiers, and basic demographic information
A—Assessment—Present chief complaint, vital signs, and diagnoses
S—Situation—Current status, including code status, recent changes, and response to therapy
S—Safety Concerns—Critical lab values, allergies, alerts such as high fall risk and isolation
B—Background—Comorbidities, previous issues, current medications, family history
A—Actions—Actions taken or provided with rationale
T—Timing—Level of urgency and prioritization
O—Ownership—Identify who is responsible, including patient and family members
N—Next—Plan of care, anticipated changes, contingency plan

Source: Adapted from Agency for Healthcare Research and Quality (AHRQ). (2013). *TeamSTEPPS® pocket guide.* Retrieved from https://www.ahrq.gov/sites/default/files/wysiwyg/professionals/education/curriculum-tools/teamstepps/instructor/essentials/pocketguide.pdf

Initially, it appears that speaking up for safety is an easy behavior. After all, healthcare providers come into healthcare to do the right thing, help patients, and cause no harm. However, speaking up for safety requires a change in culture. Leadership must clearly communicate that everyone has the authority to stop for a safety concern at any time. Nurses are expected to voice their concern and "stop the line" if they sense or discover a safety issue. The acronym CUS may be used, representing "I am **C**oncerned"; "I am **U**ncomfortable"; and "This is a **S**afety Issue." A phrase like "I have a safety concern" is useful to help staff feel comfortable with speaking up.

Consider this example of a culture where nurses feel empowered to speak up for safety, regardless of authority gradient. Mary Ann was caring for an infant in the NICU. At the request of the infant's parents, the hospital's CEO, COO, and CNO arrived in the private NICU room. Mary Ann calmly and professionally asked, "Did you scrub in?" All three retreated to the sink, scrubbed in, and thanked Mary Ann for speaking up. In fact, Mary Ann received recognition for her actions at a management team meeting. Mary Ann's action ensured safety for a vulnerable infant. The story of the positive response of the CEO, COO, and CNO spread widely throughout the hospital, helping to promulgate the understanding that everyone is rewarded for speaking up for safety.

The Interprofessional Team

The delivery of healthcare requires strong and supportive healthcare teams. Team members monitor team function, share the workload, and support each other. TeamSTEPPS (AHRQ, 2013) provides team strategies and tools to enhance performance and patient safety. CRM, described earlier in this chapter, has been adopted from aviation into healthcare to promote and reinforce team behaviors such as cooperation, coordination, and sharing regardless of formal position. It has been used to improve patient care in obstetrics, the operating room, emergency department, and other settings (Kreiser, 2012).

Providing feedback to team members is important for fostering high performance. HROs foster a culture where nurses and other staff members are expected to provide and are comfortable providing both positive and constructive feedback to team members. Positive feedback is essential for reinforcing safe behavior. Clinicians perform many safe actions every day and should be recognized for that. Constructive feedback is needed to discourage and change unsafe behaviors. People tend to avoid constructive feedback because they are uncomfortable providing it. However, as in the speaking up example earlier in this chapter, Mary Ann reminded others to wash their hands before entering the patient's room. This simple reminder is often all that is needed to correct behavior. Constructive feedback should always be met with a thank you and a change in behavior.

Cross-monitoring is tool to assist in error reduction during team functioning. Cross-monitoring allows team members to take advantage of working together and monitor unusual situations or hazards, identify safety slips

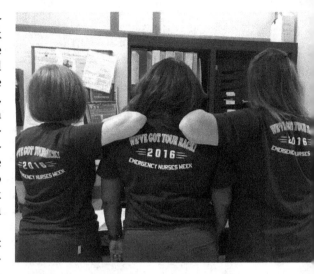

FIGURE 4.5 Three Edward Hospital emergency department nurses have each other's backs.

or lapses, and provide impromptu consultation and feedback. For example, TJC (2017, March 1) has set an NPSG to improve the accuracy of patient identification. Because of the negative outcomes that could occur if incorrect blood were administered to a patient, the NPSG requires a two-person identification process if automated identification technology is not available. The two-person process with a peer is an essential safety step and reinforces teamwork when providing care. Some hospitals adopt a phrase such as "I've got your back" to connote a supportive team environment (Figure 4.5). In this way, staff support each other and feel comfortable asking each other for help.

Providing **mutual support** to team members builds a strong team and helps members avoid work overload situations. Mutual support is the ability to anticipate team members' needs and provide assistance as needed through accurate knowledge about their workloads and responsibilities. By providing mutual support and feedback to a team member, team function is enhanced. Feedback should be timely, respectful, specific, considerate, and directed toward quality improvement. Team members are expected to advocate for the patient, particularly when a team member's view doesn't coincide with that of the main decision maker on the team. If conflict erupts on the team, the DESC tool can be used to manage and resolve the conflict: First, describe the specific situation or behavior you are concerned about and provide concrete data about it. Next, express how the situation makes you feel and what your concerns are. Third, suggest alternative actions and seek agreement. Last, state possible consequences in terms of impact on established team goals and strive for team consensus. Try using this tool the next time you have a safety concern.

ASSESSING THE CULTURE OF A HIGH-RELIABILITY ORGANIZATION

Organizational culture is the shared values and beliefs of individuals in a group or organization. Schein (2004) describes organizational culture at three levels: observable artifacts, values, and basic underlying assumptions. Observable artifacts are visible manifestations of values and may include signage, décor, dress code, traffic flow, medical equipment, and visible interactions. Values are explicitly stated norms and social principles and are manifestations of an organization's assumptions. Basic underlying assumptions are the shared beliefs and expectations that influence perceptions, thoughts, and feelings about an organization. They are the core of an organization's culture. These assumptions define the culture of the organization, but because they are invisible, they may not be recognized. At times, the assumptions of an organization are unclear and self-contradictory, especially when an organizational merger or acquisition has occurred.

Essentially, culture is how we act when no one is looking. Take for example, Elizabeth, a patient care technician caring for a patient in isolation. Elizabeth entered the patient's room without donning appropriate personal protective equipment. She deviated from policy and may have put herself, her family, patients, staff, and everyone she encountered at risk of infection. When asked about her behavior, she admitted that she knew the patient was in isolation and that she should put on a gown and gloves. Elizabeth stated, however, that she did not think anyone was watching. This illustrates an employee who has not yet internalized a culture of safety.

On the other hand, consider Tom, a housekeeper who informed his supervisor that he found a piece of metal that came off the door handle in a restroom on the Adolescent Behavioral Health Unit. Tom was concerned that there were sharp edges and that someone could get hurt. The supervisor asked facilities to fix the handle as quickly as possible. The facilities manager noted that two screws were missing and asked Tom if he had found them. When Tom said no, the manager of the Adolescent Unit was notified of the situation and staff members searched each patient's room. After a long and exhaustive search, the missing screws were located in a patient's orthodontic retainer case. Because of Tom's attention to detail and willingness to speak up, the patient was kept safe from harming himself. This scenario exemplifies an employee who is living a culture of safety.

Many organizations use a culture of safety survey tool to capture the perspectives of healthcare providers. Two commonly used tools are the survey on patient safety culture (AHRQ, 2017) and the safety attitudes questionnaire (Sexton et al., 2006). Organizations may also choose to assess their stage of organizational maturity toward becoming an HRO using a model proposed by Chassin and Loeb (2013).

To support a culture of patient safety and quality improvement, AHRQ sponsored the development of separate patient safety culture surveys for hospitals, nursing homes, medical offices, community pharmacies, and ambulatory surgery centers. Each survey measures various dimensions of the safety culture. For example, the hospital survey measures teamwork within units; supervisor/manager expectations and actions promoting patient safety; organizational learning; management support for patient safety; overall perceptions of patient safety; feedback and communication about error; communication openness; frequency of event reporting; teamwork across units; staffing; handoffs and transitions; nonpunitive response to errors; and number of events reported; and asks the participant to assign a patient safety grade to the organization. The patient safety culture surveys are available in English and Spanish and are publicly available at no cost on the AHRQ website (https://www.ahrq.gov/sops/quality-patient-safety/patientsafetyculture/index.html).

AHRQ has established comparative databases for patient safety culture survey data from organizations that administer the surveys. The databases allow healthcare organizations to compare their patient safety culture survey results to similar sites in support of patient safety culture improvement. AHRQ provides an action-planning tool to assist an organization in analyzing and improving its patient safety culture. Survey results are used by organizations to:

- Raise staff awareness about patient safety
- Diagnose and assess the current status of the patient safety culture

- Identify strengths and areas of opportunity for patient safety culture improvement
- Examine trends in patient safety culture changes over time
- Evaluate the cultural impact of patient safety initiatives and interventions
- Conduct internal and external evaluations of the culture of safety

The safety attitudes questionnaire was developed with funding from the Robert Wood Johnson Foundation and AHRQ (med.uth.edu/chqs/surveys/safety-attitudes-and-safety-climate-questionnaire/). The 36-item survey is designed to obtain frontline staff perspectives about specific patient care areas. The key factors that are measured on the survey are teamwork climate, safety climate, perceptions of management, job satisfaction, working conditions, and stress recognition. The survey is known to be accurate in measuring these factors and is used by healthcare organizations to compare themselves to other organizations, identify interventions needed to improve safety attitudes, and measure the effectiveness of the interventions.

Chassin and Loeb (2013) developed a grid to allow healthcare organizations to assess their stage of organizational maturity toward becoming an HRO: beginning, developing, advancing, and approaching. Chassin and Loeb identified performance based on position in the organization (board member, CEO/management, physicians); initiatives (quality strategy, quality measures, information technology); safety culture (trust, accountability, identifying unsafe conditions, strengthening systems, and assessment); and robust process improvement (methods, training, and spread). Their grid may be used by leaders to assess their journey toward becoming an HRO.

IDENTIFYING AND OVERCOMING BARRIERS TO HIGH RELIABILITY

Achieving high reliability in an organization is an ongoing journey, with many barriers along the way. The culture, history, and traditions of a healthcare organization can pose a barrier to becoming an HRO. Workplace intimidation and disruptive behaviors can oppose the creation of an HRO. Blending various professional healthcare subcultures into a common professional culture creates challenges for leaders. In addition, the lack of robust health technology and information systems can undermine the ability to achieve high reliability and safety. Regardless of the challenges, organizations can overcome each barrier.

Culture, History, and Traditions

The overall culture of an organization is a reflection of past learning experiences. Revising the cultural patterns of basic assumptions and beliefs is difficult, time consuming, and anxiety provoking. If a past experience with reporting an error resulted in punishment, it may deter future reporting of errors. The fear of punishment can be a significant barrier to error reporting. Changing the culture requires a significant leadership commitment to focus on healthcare processes and systems that lead to errors rather than on individual blame. Considerable effort is required to change a long-standing tradition of blame and punishment.

The history and traditions of a healthcare organization set the stage for becoming an HRO. Some healthcare organizations assume that high reliability is not achievable in healthcare. The amount of change needed to address the complexity of the work needed to achieve HRO status may overwhelm the organization. The past history of how quality improvements were made in the healthcare organization can limit future improvements.

For instance, a nurse is preparing an insulin injection at the medication station. When reaching for an insulin syringe, the nurse discovers that insulin and tuberculin syringes are mixed together in the same container. Using the wrong syringe would result in a medication error. The last time a medication error was made on the unit, the nurse was suspended for 3 days. Due to the punishment associated with the last medication error, the nurse decides to separate the insulin and tuberculin syringes into two containers rather than reporting the near miss. In this example, the organization does not have the opportunity to examine why the two syringes were mixed together in the same container since the nurse fixed the problem. Without knowledge of the near miss, no actions can be taken to prevent the problem from occurring again.

Workplace Intimidation and Disruptive Behavior

Workplace intimidation and making others feel fearful, timid, orinferior destroys the trust environment that is essential for a culture of high reliability. Workplace intimidation is created by disruptive behaviors or behaviors that do not support a culture that makes safety a priority. A culture of safety is a necessary element of an HRO. Workplace intimidation behaviors such as refusing to answer a question, not answering a page, using nonverbal gestures of disapproval, and raising one's voice need to be eliminated in an HRO to build the critical component of trust. Accepting disrespectful or disruptive behavior from any interprofessional team member is a potential threat to quality and safety for an organization. Committed leaders must recognize and manage this unwanted behavior to create a culture or safety.

Interprofessional Complexity

The complexity of the healthcare environment creates challenges for the HRO. The safety of patient care relies on effective coordination and communication among the diverse interprofessional staff who provide healthcare. Different members of the interprofessional team come from very diverse educational preparation and may use different terminology. This diversity creates a challenge in making decisions required for safe care. The complex dependency of healthcare processes requires coordination of efforts across the healthcare continuum. For example, the coordination of interprofessional healthcare processes is essential for a safe patient transition when preparing a patient to be discharged from the acute care setting to the home environment. Extensive coordination and clear communication among the entire healthcare team facilitates the provision of posthospital services the patient may require, the prescriptions needed, follow-up appointments, patient and family understanding of care instructions, and appropriate transportation.

Hierarchies

Challenges inherent in healthcare hierarchies was discussed earlier in this chapter. Traditionally, the physician was the leader in the provision of healthcare, and the hierarchical roles of physicians, nurses, and organizational leadership create a challenge to implementing the HRO principles. In contrast, the HRO values the perspective of all healthcare team members. In doing so, the HRO works toward eliminating power hierarchies and allowing for open communication among the interprofessional healthcare team to ensure safety.

Information Systems

The use of health information systems for the documentation of care and the gathering of quality and safety information is essential. Additionally, healthcare information systems provide a means for reporting errors and near misses. The lack of health information systems can impede progress to an HRO. Healthcare organizations may be challenged with devoting scarce resources to implement information systems that require significant capital expense and ongoing maintenance costs.

INTERNAL STRUCTURES AND ROLES TO SUPPORT AN HRO

A strong infrastructure is needed to support the goals and strategies of the organization's quest toward becoming an HRO. The governing body, typically the board of directors, must set the priority for quality and safety. Implementing quality and safety initiatives requires an executive team that is committed to leading an organization on the journey to high reliability. Nurses, physicians, and all members of the interprofessional team must be engaged at all levels of the quality and safety infrastructure.

The CEO sets the tone when creating an HRO. The CEO oversees safety and quality efforts within the organization. Often, the CEO chairs an interprofessional safety and quality committee. Committee membership includes a patient safety officer; physicians; nurses; pharmacists; staff from risk management, quality, patient experience, and infection control; and a community member. Multiple committees, defined in Table 4.2, exist to support the overall work of the board of directors and the safety and quality committee.

In addition to the committees discussed, certain departments and key positions in an organization support the infrastructure of an HRO. Supporting departments can perform multiple functions. They may ensure public reporting of quality and safety data, identify external benchmarks, facilitate process improvements, participate in external learning collaboratives, improve clinical documentation, detect and prevent infections, expedite peer review, oversee regulatory and accreditation compliance, provide risk management, and improve the customer experience.

Key positions in an organization also support the journey to high reliability. Not all healthcare organizations will have every position described in the following, but most will have a majority of the positions. A patient safety officer is the quality and safety leader at the executive level. The patient safety officer provides leadership for error prevention, error identification and reporting, and reduction of the severity of harm. The role of the patient safety officer closely aligns to the role of risk manager. The risk manager is responsible for protecting the assets of the organization by undertaking activities to identify, evaluate, and reduce the likelihood of patient injury and the risk of loss to the organization.

In the journey to high reliability, several new roles have emerged or expanded in healthcare organizations. A human factors engineer (HFE) may be engaged in an HRO as a support professional. Human factor engineering is an interprofessional approach that looks at the safety and efficiency of work systems. The HFE examines how people, policies, technology, and work structures interact to improve quality, safety, efficiency, and reliability of healthcare provision. The HFE can also function as educator and project consultant for clinical effectiveness and quality improvement teams. A quality analyst can also function as an expert in the process

TABLE 4.2 COMMITTEES THAT SUPPORT A JOURNEY TOWARD HIGH RELIABILITY

Board Quality Committee	Provides oversight for patient safety and quality of care, including physicians and other professional credentialing and privileging. In some hospitals, the board of trustees may perform these functions.
Medical Staff Executive Committee	Supports medical staff processes and clinical quality improvement.
Credentials Committee	Ensures that qualified, competent providers practice in the organization.
Hospital Safety and Quality Committee	Provides leadership to implement the safety and quality plan.
Infection Control Committee	Provides leadership for the infection prevention and control program.
Utilization Review Committee	Oversees appropriate utilization of care and services provided by the hospital; ensures the management of the appropriate admission status of the patient (inpatient, outpatient, or observation) based on the severity of the patient's illness.
Medical Staff Quality Committee	Conducts retrospective reviews of patient care (peer review), focused professional practice evaluation, and ongoing professional practice evaluation to identify opportunities for improvement and to share what was learned with other physicians, licensed independent practitioners, and advanced practice clinicians.
Safety Event Review Committee	Reviews and classifies safety events and commissions root cause analyses.
Nursing Quality Committee	Fosters nursing and interprofessional performance improvement activities.
Nursing Peer Review Committee	Conducts retrospective reviews of nursing patient care, focused professional practice evaluation, and ongoing professional practice evaluation to identify opportunities for improvement and to share what was learned with other clinicians.
Pharmacy and Therapeutics Committee	Provides leadership for safe medication processes. May include a subcommittee focused on antibiotic stewardship.
Environment of Care Committee	Provides leadership for the ongoing evaluation and improvement of the environment of care safety management program.
Ethics Committee	Provides support for ethical dilemmas that present themselves in clinical care.
Institutional Review Board Committee	Responsible for ensuring that all research practices are safe and follow standard guidelines for the conduct of research.
Workplace Safety Committee	Reviews workplace injuries and sets goals and strategies for improving workplace safety.

improvement methodologies and tools. A clinical documentation expert assesses and supports documentation processes to ensure that they accurately reflect the patient's condition and the level of service required to meet the patient's care need.

A patient experience expert provides leadership to ensure that the patient receives respectful and coordinated care and to facilitate a process to address complaints that may arise when failure to meet patient's healthcare expectations occur.

As healthcare increases its focus on coordinated healthcare across multiple providers and settings, many organizations are expanding care management and social services to encompass transitional care for patients. This community case management role focuses on ensuring safe patient transitions to home or to another healthcare service. An initial primary focus is on the transition from hospital to home for patients with chronic disease and end-of-life issues to ensure that healthcare is provided seamlessly. Transitional care nurses help coordinate care between transitions to different care settings such as hospital to home healthcare and assist patients to navigate the complex healthcare system. A well-defined organization infrastructure that promotes teamwork and communication supports the transition to an HRO.

EXTERNAL INFLUENCES FOR CHANGE AND HRO RESOURCES

Increasingly, the government is mandating that hospitals publicly report safety, quality, and financial indicators. This transparency is designed to help the consumer make informed choices about selecting healthcare providers. Transparency holds healthcare providers and organizations accountable for quality care. In other purchase transactions, consumers can easily obtain information about cost and value to make informed purchases. Healthcare is now being asked to follow the same practice of transparency. Public awareness of medical errors, poor quality outcomes, and perceived low value are driving changes in healthcare.

Centers for Medicare and Medicaid Services

Healthcare costs have escalated along with poor quality of care and patient outcomes, healthcare errors, and waste. Historically, organizations were rewarded for the volume of healthcare services delivered instead of for their achievement of high-quality and safety outcomes. For example, a hospital used to be reimbursed for the number of appendectomies performed regardless of the outcome. As previously described, safety, quality, and experience outcomes now affect hospital reimbursement. In addition, safety, quality, and patient experience data are posted on the CMS website (www. medicare.gov/hospitalcompare/search.html). Last, the Centers for Medicare and Medicaid Innovation was created as part of the Affordable Care Act to enhance the quality of healthcare and reduce costs through innovative approaches to healthcare delivery.

Leapfrog

Leapfrog, a business consortium, is a voluntary reporting agency that collects and publishes quality information. The Leapfrog website allows insurance companies and the public to access hospital ratings and use the information to make informed healthcare decisions. The Leapfrog consortium works on behalf of the public and employers to inform Americans about the performance of hospitals on quality measures. The Leapfrog group promotes full disclosure of hospital performance information and helps provide employers with information to provide the best healthcare benefits to employees.

Accreditation Agencies

Several accrediting agencies for hospitals address patient safety. These agencies include TJC, Healthcare Facilities Accreditation Program (HFAP), and Det Norske Veritas Healthcare, Inc. (DNV, n.d.; Meldi, Rhoades, & Gippe, 2009).

The mission of **TJC** is to continuously improve healthcare for the public, in collaboration with other stakeholders, by evaluating healthcare organizations and inspiring them to excel in providing safe and effective care of the highest quality and value (TJC, 2017). TJC uses the Donabedian conceptual framework of structure, process, and outcomes to assess an organization. Using this framework, TJC (2017, March 1) set 11 expectations for leadership in developing a safety culture as follows:

1. Create a transparent, nonpunitive approach to reporting and learning from adverse events, close calls, and unsafe conditions.
2. Establish clear, just, and transparent risk-based processes for recognizing and separating human error and error arising from poorly designed systems from unsafe or reckless actions that are blameworthy.
3. Adopt and model appropriate behaviors and champion efforts to eradicate intimidating behaviors.
4. Establish, enforce, and communicate to all team members the policies that support safety culture and the reporting of adverse events, close calls, and unsafe conditions.
5. Recognize team members who report adverse events and close calls, who identify unsafe conditions, or have good suggestions for safety improvements.
6. Establish an organizational baseline measure on safety culture performance using the AHRQ hospital survey on patient safety culture or another tool, such as the safety attitudes questionnaire.
7. Analyze safety culture survey results from across the organization to find opportunities for quality and safety improvement.
8. Develop and implement unit-based quality and safety improvement initiatives designed to improve the culture of safety.
9. Embed safety culture team training into quality improvement projects and organizational processes to strengthen safety systems.
10. Proactively assess system strength and vulnerabilities and prioritize them for enhancement or improvement.
11. Repeat organizational assessment of safety culture every 18 to 24 months to review progress and sustain improvement.

HFAP was originally created in 1945 to conduct an objective review of services provided by osteopathic hospitals. In 1965, HFAP received authority from the CMS to provide accreditation to hospitals, ambulatory care/surgical facilities, mental health facilities, physical rehabilitation facilities, clinical laboratories, and critical access hospitals. HFAP has adopted the 34 Safe Practices set forth by the National Quality Forum (NQF) in 2009 (HFAP, 2017).

DNV is dedicated to empowering quality and patient safety through an efficient and outcomes-based accreditation program. DNV received authority from the CMS to provide accreditation to hospitals in 2008, and has accredited nearly 500 hospitals of all sizes and in every region of the United States. They integrate the CMS Conditions of Participation with the ISO 9001 Quality Management Program. The ISO 9001 quality system is a structured way of delivering a better service or product, supported by detailed procedures such as work instructions, quality manuals, and written quality policies to provide all employees with detailed, understandable, and workable instructions that define both expectations and actions to achieve the stated quality goals. DNV's goal is to enable a broader culture change toward high performance and continual improvement by combining the mandatory CMS evaluation with a quality management system into one seamless program.

State Requirements

Along with the quality and safety measures publicly reported by the CMS, many states are now requiring some form of mandatory reporting of safety and quality indicators and specific adverse events.

Public Recognition of Quality Achievements

In the race to achieve competitive advantages for patient safety and quality, healthcare organizations are seeking recognitions that set them apart from other healthcare organizations. The **Baldrige Award** recognizes organizations that have improved and sustained quality results. The purpose of the Baldrige Award in healthcare is to challenge organizations to improve their effectiveness of care and healthcare outcomes to pursue excellence, which moves organizations toward becoming an HRO. The Baldrige framework embraces integration among leadership, strategy, customers, workforce, operations, and results. The Baldrige framework is built on core values and concepts and requires measurement, analysis, and knowledge management (NIST, 2016).

Designation by the American Nurse's Credentialing Center (ANCC) as a **Magnet®** organization denotes nursing excellence and is factored into payer reimbursement and recognition (ANCC, 2013). The components of the Magnet Recognition Program®, discussed in Chapter 1, are congruent with the HRO concepts. The Magnet® components include Transformational Leadership; Structural Empowerment; Exemplary Professional Practice; New Knowledge, Innovations, and Improvements; and Empirical Outcomes. The original forces of Magnetism emphasized structure and process. The current Magnet Model recognizes that an excellent infrastructure must result in positive outcomes in order to create a culture of excellence and innovation. Safety is a main component of a culture of excellence.

The Transformational Leadership component of the Magnet Model requires strong advocacy and support for staff and patients by all nursing leaders. In a Magnet-designated hospital, the CNO is an active leader in creating an HRO by establishing strategic goals for quality and safety in conjunction with the hospital's executive team. These strategic goals support the organization's commitment to zero major quality failures. For example, one source of evidence related to Transformational Leadership calls for nurse leaders and clinical nurses to advocate for resources to support nursing unit and organizational goals. The Structural Empowerment component of Magnet addresses the need to create structures and processes that allow nurses to practice safely and effectively. For example, one source of evidence related to Structural Empowerment calls for clinical nurse involvement in interprofessional decision-making groups at the organizational level. In total, five of the 11 Structural Empowerment sources of evidence address the culture of safety for patients and nurses. Both the Transformational Leadership and Structural Empowerment components of Magnet require the active engagement of nurses.

The Exemplary Professional Practice component of Magnet indicates that "achievement of exemplary professional practice is grounded in a culture of safety, quality monitoring, and quality improvement" (ANCC, 2013, p. 42). Many of the Exemplary Professional Practice sources of evidence require documentation of safe nursing practices. For example, Magnet acute care organizations with ambulatory services are required to report on these six nurse-sensitive clinical indicators: patient falls with injury, hospital-acquired pressure ulcers, central line-associated bloodstream infection, CAUTI, one indicator from the Core Measures Set, and one indicator from primary or specialty outpatient services. The performance on each of these indicators must exceed the mean or median value on the majority of units the majority of the time to meet Magnet standards. The New Knowledge, Innovations, and Improvements component of Magnet requires nurses to use evidence and innovation for safe, high quality care. Last, the Empirical Outcomes component of Magnet requires the organization to continually assess and monitor a variety of indicators for nursing leadership and clinical practice. Sustained quality performance on empirical outcomes will move an organization on the journey to becoming an HRO.

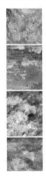

CASE STUDY 4.2

A nurse works for an organization that has achieved Magnet designation. The nurse is a member of the Quality and Safety Unit Practice Council. As a member of the Council, the nurse is assigned the task of educating nursing and other peers on how the Magnet designation supports and helps the organization become an HRO. Complete a web literature search on the Magnet components and correlate the key Magnet principles to the HRO concepts.

1. *How do the Magnet components support the organizational requirements for high reliability?*
2. *How do the Magnet components align with the HRO process concepts?*
3. *How do the Magnet components support a culture of safety?*

Additional Resources for Organizations Striving for High Reliability

A **patient safety organization (PSO)** is a group, institution or association that improves patient care by reducing errors. PSOs exist to allow organizations to learn from their own safety events and the safety events of others. The Patient Safety and Quality Improvement Act of 2005 (Public Law 109–41), signed into law on July 29, 2005, was enacted in response to growing concern about patient safety in the United States and the IOM's (1999) report *To Err Is Human*. A healthcare provider can obtain the confidentiality and privilege protections of the act by working with a federally listed PSO.

The law provides confidentiality protections and privilege protections, which means the information cannot be included in a law suit. A complete list of federally approved PSOs may be found on the AHRQ website (www.pso.ahrq.gov/listed).

The **AHRQ**'s mission is to produce evidence to make healthcare safer, higher in quality, more accessible, equitable, and affordable, and to work with the U.S. Department of Health and Human Services and with other partners to make sure that research findings are understood and used. AHRQ creates materials to teach and train healthcare systems and professionals to put the results of research into practice and funds a variety of initiatives. In addition to the AHRQ initiatives already discussed in this chapter, successful initiatives include the following:

- Re-Engineered Discharge (RED)—a structured protocol and suite of implementation tools that help hospitals rework their discharge processes to reduce readmissions by determining patients' needs and carefully designing and communicating discharge plans.
- The Comprehensive Unit-based Safety Program (CUSP)—a highly effective method of preventing healthcare-associated infections (HAIs) by combining improvement in safety culture, teamwork, and communication.
- EvidenceNOW, an initiative aligned with Million Hearts®—provides clinical practice support to over 5,000 primary care physicians with the goal of improving the heart health of millions of patients and improving the capacity of the practices to incorporate new research findings and information into practice.
- AHRQ's Healthcare Cost and Utilization Project—helps highlight the opioid overdose epidemic and contributed to the Department of Health and Human Services' launch of a major multipronged initiative to reduce opioid abuse.

The work of the **IHI** began in the late 1980s as part of the National Demonstration Project on Quality Improvement in Health Care to redesign healthcare into a system without errors, waste, delay, and unsustainable costs. IHI uses the science of improvement approach to work with health systems, countries, and other organizations on improving quality, safety, and value in healthcare. The approach is characterized by the combination of expert subject knowledge with improvement methods and tools. It is interprofessional, drawing on clinical science, systems theory, psychology, statistics, and other fields.

IHI's methodology traces back to W. Edwards Deming (1900–1993), who taught that by adhering to certain principles of management, organizations can increase quality and simultaneously reduce costs. Based on Deming's work, the IHI Model for Improvement asks three questions as follows:

1. What are we trying to accomplish?
2. How will we know that a change is an improvement?
3. What changes can we make that will result in improvement?

The Model then employs Plan-Do-Study-Act (PDSA) cycles for small, rapid-cycle tests of change. IHI uses the Model for Improvement in all of its improvement efforts (IHI, 2017a).

The vision of the **National Patient Safety Foundation (NPSF, 2017)** is to create a world where patients and those who care for them are free from harm. A central voice for patient safety since 1997, NPSF partners with patients and families, the healthcare community, and key stakeholders to advance patient safety and healthcare workforce safety and disseminate strategies to prevent harm. Committed to a collaborative approach in all that it does, the NPSF offers a portfolio of programs targeted to diverse stakeholders across the healthcare industry. The American Society of Professionals in

Patient Safety (ASPPS) is part of NPSF. It provides education and oversees professional certification (ASPPS, 2017).

The Institute for Safe Medication Practices (ISMP) is the nation's only nonprofit organization devoted entirely to medication error prevention and safe medication use. It is respected worldwide as a resource for impartial, timely, and accurate medication safety information. ISMP's medication error prevention efforts began in 1975. ISMP began a voluntary practitioner error-reporting program to learn about errors happening across the nation, understand their causes, and share "lessons learned" with the healthcare community. Today, ISMP's initiatives, which are built upon a nonpunitive approach and system-based solutions, fall into five key areas: knowledge, analysis, education, cooperation, and communication (ISMP, 2017).

ISMP is also responsible for reviewing all medication error reports submitted by healthcare facilities to the Commonwealth of Pennsylvania Patient Safety Authority. Each year, ISMP's national Medication Errors Reporting Program (MERP) receives hundreds of error reports from healthcare professionals. In addition, ISMP's wholly owned corporate subsidiary, Med-ERRS (Medical Error Recognition and Revision Strategies), works directly and confidentially with the pharmaceutical industry to prevent errors that stem from confusing or misleading naming, labeling, packaging, and device design.

The mission of **NQF** is to improve the quality of healthcare. Patient safety is central to achieving this mission. Of the over 600 NQF-endorsed quality measures, approximately 100 are patient-safety focused. NQF has also endorsed 34 Safe Practices for Better Healthcare and 28 Serious Reportable Events (NQF, 2017). Despite these achievements, there are still significant gaps in the measurement of patient safety. By convening panels and other educational forums, NQF works with quality measure developers and others in healthcare to help understand measurement gaps and encourage strategies to fill them. A list of 28 adverse events, also called never events because they should never occur in healthcare, is grouped into six categories: surgical, product or device related, patient protection, care management, environmental, radiologic, and potential criminal events (www.qualityforum.org/topics/sres/serious_reportable_events.aspx).

Medical Product Safety Network (MedSun)

The Medical Product Safety Network (MedSun) is an adverse event reporting program launched in 2002 by the U.S. Food and Drug Administration's Center for Devices and Radiological Health (FDA, 2017). The primary goal for MedSun is to work collaboratively with the clinical community to identify, understand, and solve problems with the use of medical devices. Once a problem is identified, MedSun clarifies the problem and shares lessons learned with the clinical community and the public, without facility and patient identification, so that clinicians nationwide may take necessary preventive actions.

The Safe Medical Devices Act defines device user facilities as hospitals, nursing homes, and outpatient treatment and diagnostic centers, and requires them to report medical device problems that result in serious illness, injury, or death. MedSun participants are also highly encouraged to voluntarily report problems with devices, such as "close-calls," potential for harm, and other safety concerns. By monitoring reports about problems and concerns before a more serious event occurs, the FDA, manufacturers, and clinicians work together proactively to prevent serious injuries and death. Human Factor Engineers can play a key role here, as they examine how clinicians, products, policies, and the work environment interact to affect safety.

Healthcare organizations are recognized for reporting events that result in manufacturing changes. For example, Nancy is a nurse in the ICU. She received a patient from surgery who was wearing a purple armband, which designates a Do Not Resuscitate (DNR) status in Nancy's hospital. There was no indication of a DNR order for this patient, so Nancy asked the patient about the purple band. The patient explained that she received the purple band at an outpatient surgical center when her port was implanted. It was part of the port kit provided by the manufacturer, and staff suggested that the patient wear the band to remind healthcare providers of her port. Nancy then explained the meaning of the band at most hospitals. When the patient heard this, she stated her desire to be resuscitated, Nancy asked permission to remove the band. The patient granted this permission and Nancy reported the event as a near miss. Nancy received a Good Catch award for averting harm. In addition, the organization reported the event to MedSun. MedSun worked with the manufacturing company to change their practices and the company stopped including the purple band in their port kits. This is an example of high reliability at its finest—focusing on improving patient safety internally and nationally.

The journey toward high reliability is complex and involves every aspect of an organization. Errors in healthcare cause harm to patients. Healthcare organizations can apply what has been learned in other safety-focused industries to improve patient safety. Nurses are in a strong position to advocate for patient safety and lead interprofessional efforts to achieve high reliability. While barriers to HRO exist, they can be overcome with the use of internal and external resources.

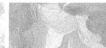

KEY CONCEPTS

- An HRO targets near-zero rates of failure.
- Characteristics that differentiate healthcare HROs from other healthcare organizations are preoccupation with failure, reluctance to simplify, sensitivity to operations, commitment to resilience, and deference to expertise.
- Being a HRO affects a healthcare organization's safety, quality, patient experience, and financial performance.
- Healthcare has learned a great deal about high reliability from other industries, such as commercial aviation and nuclear power.
- To achieve high reliability, an organization must have strong leadership commitment, an established culture of safety, and a well-developed quality improvement program.
- A fair and just culture minimizes blame and punishment and creates a learning environment where errors are reported so that system problems can be corrected.
- The nurse is responsible for implementing internal behaviors and communication techniques and working effectively in an interprofessional team in a healthcare HRO.
- Organizational culture can be assessed with valid and reliable tools to support a journey toward becoming an HRO.
- Barriers to achieving high reliability may include culture, history and traditions, workplace intimidation and disruptive behavior, interprofessional complexity, hierarchies, and information systems.
- A healthcare organization's infrastructure must provide support to achieve high reliability.

- Many organizations influence a healthcare organization's decision to become an HRO and provide support for the journey toward high reliability.
- The components of the Magnet Recognition Program are congruent with HRO concepts.

KEY TERMS

Adverse event or serious safety event
AHRQ
Authority gradient
Baldrige Award
Comorbidities
Cross-monitoring
Culture of safety
Daily safety huddle
Error
Fair and just culture
Financial performance
FMEA
Hierarchy
HRO
IHI
ISMP
Knowledge-based performance

Magnet
Mutual support
Near miss safety event
NQF
Organizational culture
Patient experience
Precursor safety event
PSO
Quality
RCA
Reliability
Rule-based performance
Safety
Sentinel event
Skill-based performance
Transparency
Work arounds

REVIEW QUESTIONS

1. Which of the following recommendations was not made by the Institute of Medicine's publication *To Err Is Human*?

   A. Identify and learn from errors.
   B. Avoid talking about errors.
   C. Improve safety.
   D. Ensure safe practices at the delivery level.

2. Which statements about an HRO are false? Select all that apply.

   A. HROs avoid discussing failures.
   B. HROs explore a variety of reasons for errors and are reluctant to simplify explanations.
   C. HROs are aware of the many factors that influence the care environment.
   D. HROs understand that decisions should be made by the highest ranking official.
   E. HROs know that when small things go wrong it is often a sign of a larger problem.

3. Errors occur when there is a deviation from generally acceptable performance standards. Which of the following is not an example of a generally acceptable performance standard?

   A. Professional practice standard.
   B. Article published in the *Wall Street Journal*.

C. Evidence-based policy.

D. Evidence-based order set.

4. High reliability affects the entire organization. Which of the following statements is false?

   A. Quality often improves in HRO organizations.

   B. An HRO improves patient and staff safety.

   C. Enhanced communication and reliability helps to increase patient satisfaction in HROs.

   D. Financial performance is negatively impacted in HROs.

5. Healthcare can learn about high reliability from a variety of other industries. Which of the following statements is false?

   A. Commercial aviation found that the most common cause of error was mechanical failures.

   B. The Institute of Nuclear Power Operations believes that trust and respect are needed in an HRO.

   C. Human beings can make skill-based, rule-based, and knowledge-based errors.

   D. Commercial Aviation embraced CRM training programs in an effort to enhance communication in the cockpit.

6. Leadership plays an important role in creating an HRO. Which of the following statements demonstrates the best understanding of the role of leadership?

   A. Leaders are accountable for the provision of effective and efficient care while protecting the safety of patients, employees, and visitors.

   B. Leaders must identify system problems and ask employees to fix them.

   C. While fostering a learning environment, leaders must never discipline employees for their behaviors.

   D. Leaders may rely solely on technology to build and reinforce accountability.

7. A nurse is asked how quality, safety, and performance improvement are addressed in an HRO. Which response demonstrates the best understanding?

   A. "We have an interprofessional committee on our unit that looks at patient outcomes, practice issues, and most recently, the number of falls on our unit. Together, we figure out the best way to fix the problem and suggest changes."

   B. "A couple of nurses got together last night to look at the number of falls on our unit. We are concerned about the problem and think there is a better way to do it."

   C. "I saw an article about falls on a unit like ours. I took the article to work to show my unit director but she said the solution isn't feasible on our unit."

   D. "Our fall rates are so high that the physical therapist formed a committee to address the issue and came back to the nursing staff with some recommendations for changes in our care delivery."

8. Which of the following methods are helpful for assessing the culture of an HRO? Select all that apply.

   A. Observe the behaviors of employees when they think no one is watching to determine if they are adhering to the policies and expectations of the organization.

   B. Review safety event reports, including near miss, precursor, and serious safety events.

C. Use a standard tool to assess the patient safety of the organization.

D. Assume the culture exists if process improvement activities are underway.

9. Many barriers keep healthcare organizations from becoming HROs. Which of the following statements is false?

   A. Culture, history, and tradition may be a barrier to becoming an HRO.

   B. Information systems always serve as a barrier to creating an HRO.

   C. Workplace intimidation and disruptive behavior cannot be tolerated in an HRO.

   D. The hierarchical roles of physicians, nurses, and organizational leadership create a challenge to implementing HRO principles.

10. Which of the following external organizations strongly influence hospitals to change to become HROs? Select all that apply.

   A. CMS

   B. Magnet recognition by the American Nurses Credentialing Center

   C. The National Labor Relations Board and Office of Human Subjects Protection

   D. Accreditation agencies, such as TJC and DNV

   E. Consumer groups, such as Leapfrog

   F. Vendors of EHRs

REVIEW ACTIVITIES

1. During one of your clinical days, ask nurses to describe the process in place to report an error in their hospital and what happens when an error is reported. Ask the nurses if they have ever reported an error. Based on what you have learned, is the reporting method focused on blame or learning?

2. Leaders are responsible for creating a culture of high reliability. Review the roles of the leader as outlined in this chapter. During your next clinical rotation, assess the culture of the healthcare organization. Is it obvious that the leaders are committed to safety? Are the leaders visible? Does the healthcare organization provide a learning environment? Are process improvements underway? Is technology used to enhance safety?

3. Review the chapter content related to Safety Stories. Why is it important to share Safety Stories? How does it strengthen the HRO culture and a healthcare organization? During your next clinical day, identify a Safety Story and share it with your classmates.

4. Review the chapter content related to the Science of Human Error. Why is it important to know if the error is skill-based, rule-based, or knowledge-based? What types of errors have you made in your personal or professional life? What types of tools would be helpful in preventing these errors?

5. Review the chapter content related to the SBAR and I PASS the BATON communication tools. The next time you are providing care, try using one of these tools in your handoff to another provider. How effective was the tool? Did the tool help you to organize your thoughts more concisely? Did it prompt you to share the most pertinent information?

6. Review the external forces that influence the need for change in quality and safety. How does transparency influence quality and safety? What resources are available to assist a healthcare organization on the road to high reliability?

CRITICAL DISCUSSION POINTS

1. Consider a recent clinical experience. What characteristics of an HRO were visible? Describe what you felt met the explanation in the text of characteristics of HROs.
2. Interview a nurse about the error reporting process in his or her current practice setting. Is it anonymous? Does it include reporting near misses or just errors? Ask if the nurse feels comfortable reporting his or her own or other's errors. Why or why not?
3. What would you consider a priority for an organization that is working towards a culture of safety? Explain why you selected the priority.

EXPLORING THE WEB

1. Go to the website for the AHRQ (www.ahrq.gov). Review one of the patient safety survey tools. How would you complete the survey for the site of your most recent clinical rotation?
2. Go to the website for the CMS Hospital Compare at www.medicare.gov/hospital compare/search.html. Review the ratings for several hospitals close to your zip code.
3. Go to TJC website at www.jointcommission.org. Review their vision for healthcare. Review the most recent NPSGs.

REFERENCES

Agency for Healthcare Research and Quality (AHRQ). (2013a). *Agency for Healthcare Research and Quality (AHRQ)*. Retrieved from https://www.ahrq.gov

Agency for Healthcare Research and Quality (AHRQ). (2013). *TeamSTEPPS pocket guide*. Retrieved from https://www.ahrq.gov/teamstepps/instructor/essentials/pocketguide.html

Agency for Healthcare Research and Quality (AHRQ). (2017). *Surveys on patient safety culture™*. Retrieved from https://www.ahrq.gov/sops/quality-patient-safety/patientsafetyculture/index.html

American Association of Critical-Care Nurses (2015). AACN Scope and Standards for Acute and Critical Care Nursing Practice. Aliso Viejo, California: AACN.

American Nurses Credentialing Center (ANCC). (2013). *2014 Magnet application manual*. Silver Spring, MD: American Nurses Credentialing Center.

American Nurses Association. (2010). *Position statement: Just culture*. Retrieved from http://www.nursingworld.org/practice-policy/nursing-excellence/

ASPPS. (2017). *American Society of Professionals in Patient Safety*. Retrieved from http://www.npsf.org/default.asp?page=aspps&DGPCrPg=1&DGPCrSrt=7A

Association for Professionals in Infection Control and Epidemiology. (2017). *Health care-associated infection cost calculators*. Retrieved from https://apic.org/Resources/Cost-calculators

The Beryl Institute. (2017). Retrieved from http://www.theberylinstitute.org/

Business Dictionary. (2017). Retrieved from http://www.businessdictionary.com/definition/reliability.html

Chassin, M. R., & Loeb, J. M. (2013). High-reliability health care: Getting there from here. *The Milbank Quarterly, 91*(3), 459–490.

Classen, D. C., Lloyd, R. C., Provost, L., Griffin, F. A., & Resar, R. (2008). Development and evaluation of the Institute for Health care Improvement Global Trigger Tool. *Journal of Patient Safety, 4*(3), 169–177.

Cook, R., & Woods, D. (1994). Operating at the sharp end: The complexity of human error. In M. S. Bogner (Ed.), *Human error in medicine* (pp. 255–310). Hillsdale, NJ: Erlbaum and Associates.

DNV (n.d.). *Hospital Accreditation*. Retrieved from http://dnvglhealthcare.com/accreditations/hospital-accreditation

Ganghi, T. K., & Yates, G. (2017). Safety champions. *Trustee, 70*(5), 17–19.

Helmreich, R. L., Merritt, A. C., & Wilhelm, J. A. (1999). The evolution of crew resource management training in commercial aviation. *International Journal of Aviation Psychology, 9*(1), 19–32.

HFAP (2017). *Overview*. Retrieved from http://www.hfap.org/about/overview.aspx

Hughes, R. G. (2008). *Tools and strategies for quality improvement and patient safety*. In R. G. Hughes (Ed.), *Patient safety and quality: An evidence-based handbook for nurses*. Rockville, MD: Agency for Healthcare Research and Quality.

Institute for Healthcare Improvement (IHI). (2017a). *Institute for Healthcare Improvement*. Retrieved from http://www.ihi.org/Pages/default.aspx

Institute for Healthcare Improvement (IHI). (2017b). SBAR Toolkit. Retrieved from http://www.ihi.org/resources/Pages/Tools/sbartoolkit.aspx

Institute for Healthcare Improvement (IHI). (2017c). Trigger Tools. Retrieved from http://www.ihi.org/Topics/TriggerTools/Pages/default.aspx

Institute for Safe Medication Practices (ISMP). (2017). *Institute for Safe Medication Practices*. Retrieved from http://www.ismp.org/about/default.aspx

Institute of Medicine. (2001). *Crossing the quality chasm*. Washington, DC: National Academy of Sciences.

Institute of Medicine. (1999). *To err is human*. Washington, DC: National Academy of Sciences.

The Joint Commission (TJC). (2017). *About The Joint Commission*. Retrieved from https://www.jointcommission.org/about_us/about_the_joint_commission_main.aspx

The Joint Commission (TJC). (2016, December 2). *National patient safety goals effective January 2017*. Retrieved from https://www.jointcommission.org/assets/1/6/NPSG_Chapter_HAP_Jan2017.pdf

The Joint Commission (TJC). (2017, February 17). *Sentinel event policy and procedure*. Retrieved from https://www.jointcommission.org/sentinel_event_policy_and_procedures/

The Joint Commission (TJC). (2017, March 1). *Sentinel event alert*. Retrieved from https://www.jointcommission.org/assets/1/18/SEA_57_Safety_Culture_Leadership_0317.pdf

Kreiser, S. (2012). High reliability healthcare: Applying CRM to high-performing teams, Part 5. *PSQH—Patient Safety and Quality Healthcare*. Retrieved from https://www.psqh.com/news/high-reliability-healthcare-applying-crm-to-high-performing-teams-part-5

Makary, M. A., & Daniel, M. (2016, May 3). Medical error—The third leading cause of death in the U.S. *British Medical Journal, 353*, i2139.

Marx, David (2001). Patient Safety and the "Just Culture": A Primer for Health Care Executives. New York City: Columbia University.

Morrow, R. (2016). *Leading high reliability organizations in health care*. Boca Raton, FL: CRC Press.

National Institute of Standards and Technology (NIST). (2016). *Baldrige performance excellence program*. Retrieved from https://www.nist.gov/baldrige/publications/baldrige-excellence-framework/businessnonprofit

National Patient Safety Foundation (NPSF). (2017). *National Patient Safety Foundation*. http://www.npsf.org

National Quality Forum (NQF). (2017). *Patient Safety*. Retrieved from https://www.qualityforum.org/Topics/Safety_pages/Patient_Safety.aspx

Reason, James (1997). Managing the risks of organizational accidents. Aldershot, England: Ashgate.

Reason, J. (1997). *Managing the risks of organizational accidents*. Burlington, VT: Ashgate Publishing.

Schein, Edgar H. (2004). Organizational Culture and Leadership, 3rd ed. San Fransisco, CA: Jossey-Bass.

Scott S. D. (2015, September/October). Second victim support: Implications for patient safety attitudes and perceptions. *PSQH, 12*, 26–31.

Senge, P. (1990). *The fifth discipline. The art and practice of the learning organization*. New York City, NY: Doubleday.

Sexton, J. B., Helmreich, R. L., Neilands, T. B., Rowan, K., Vella, K., Boyden, J., Roberts, P. R., & Thomas, E. J. (2006, April 3). The Safety Attitudes Questionnaire: Psychometric properties, benchmarking data, and emerging research. *BMC Health Services Research, 6*, 44.

U.S. Food and Drug Administration (FDA). (2017). *MedSun: Medical Product Safety*. Retrieved from https://www.fda.gov/medicaldevices/safety/medsunmedicalproductsafetynetwork/

Weick K. E., & Sutcliffe, K. M. (2007). *Managing the unexpected: Resilient performance in an age of uncertainty* (2nd ed.). San Francisco, CA: Jossey-Bass.

Wu, A. (2000). The second victim: The doctor who makes the mistake needs help too. *British Medical Journal*, 320, 726–727.

SUGGESTED READINGS

Conner, M., Duncombe, D., Barclay, E., Bartel, S., Borden, C., Gross, E., . . . Ponte, P. R. (2007). Creating a fair and just culture: One institution's path toward organizational change. *The Joint Commission Journal on Quality and Patient Safety*, 33(10), 617–624.

Dekker, S. (2011). *Patient safety: A human factors approach*. Boca Raton, FL: CRC Press Taylor and Francis Group.

Graban, M. (2008). *Lean hospitals: Improving quality, patient safety and employee satisfaction*. Boca Raton, FL: CRC Press Taylor and Francis Group.

Henriksen, K., Dayton, E., Keyes, M. A., Carayon, P., & Hughes, R. G. (2008). Understanding adverse events: A human factors framework. In R. Hughes (Ed.), *Patient safety and quality: An evidence-based handbook for nurses* (pp. 67–85). AHRQ Publication No. 08–0043. Rockville, MD: Agency for Healthcare Research and Quality.

Marx, D. (2009). *Whack a mole; the price we pay for expecting perfection*. Plano, TX: By Your Side Studios.

Pepe, J., & Cataldo P. J. (2011). *Manage risk: Build a just culture*. Retrieved from https://www.researchgate.net/publication/51568049_Manage_risk_build_a_just_culture

Spath, P. L. (2011). *Error reduction in healthcare: A systems approach to improving patient safety* (2nd ed.). San Francisco, CA: Jossey-Bass.

Stolzer, A. J., Halford, C. D., & Goglia, J. J. (2011). *Implementing safety management systems in aviation*. Burlington, VT: Ashgate Publishing.

Studer, Q. (2013). *A culture of high performance*. Gulf Breeze, FL: Fire Starter Publishing.

Wakefield, M. K. (2008). The quality chasm series: Implications for nursing. In R. Hughes (Ed.), *Patient safety and quality: An evidence-based handbook for nurses* (chap. 4). AHRQ Publication No. 08–0043. Rockville, MD: Agency for Healthcare Research and Quality.

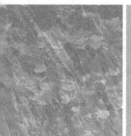

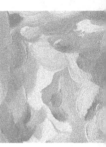

5

LEGAL AND ETHICAL ASPECTS OF NURSING

Theodore M. McGinn

As a nurse, we have the opportunity to heal the heart, mind, soul and body of our patients, their families and ourselves. They may not remember your name but they will never forget the way you made them feel.

—Maya Angelou

Upon completion of this chapter, the reader should be able to

1. Identify the three branches of the U.S. Government.
2. Define the role of Administrative Agencies.
3. Review the role of law in shaping nursing practice.
4. Identify the four elements of negligence.
5. Discuss negligence and malpractice.
6. Review the Health Insurance Portability and Accountability Act of 1996 (HIPAA).
7. Discuss Medicare.
8. Discuss the Anti-Kickback Law.
9. Discuss the Stark Law.
10. Review the International Council of Nurses' Code of Ethics and the American Nurses Association's Code of Ethics.
11. Describe common ethical principles that influence the practice of nursing.

Y ou are a nurse with 15 years of experience and have always been proud of the care you provide and the rapport you create with your patients and their families. Late one evening, the ED calls with handoff report for an admission to your unit. During report, you learn that while in the ED for the past 14 hours, the patient has been uncooperative, difficult to manage, and lashing out at staff and other patients. The patient was in a motor vehicle accident and tested positive for both alcohol and drugs. Upon arrival to the ED, the examination of the patient revealed two broken ribs, bruising on his chest, and multiple facial lacerations. The ED nurse states that the patient is currently stable and must be moved immediately because they are expecting multiple patients with critical injuries to arrive in the ED shortly. Currently, your medical–surgical unit is short-staffed because of nurse call-offs. The patient arrives on the unit and is quiet and withdrawn. His initial vital signs include a pulse rate of 110 and blood pressure of 90/50. These assessment findings concern you, so you make a note of rechecking the patient's vitals after you assess your other patients. Within an hour of admission, before you have an opportunity to reassess the patient, the patient experiences a cardiac arrest and dies. Three weeks after the incident you are informed of a lawsuit that has been filed and that you are named as a defendant.

1. *Will you be arrested and have to go to jail?*
2. *Should you call the patient's family and apologize?*
3. *Will you lose your nursing license?*
4. *Should you hire a lawyer?*

The law provides guidance for the way we live our lives and, in many instances, for the manner in which we conduct our work. The healthcare system is highly regulated with laws and regulations that guide the way nurses interact with patients and identify the rights that patients can legally expect during healthcare delivery. These laws and regulations derive from federal statutes, state statutes, state common law, and administrative rules and codes. Simply put, nurses are bombarded with laws.

The expanding role of the nurse in direct patient care and the expanding roles that nurses occupy in our healthcare system make it imperative that nurses understand our current legal system and nurses' role in complying with the laws governing nursing practice. Advances in technology, healthcare, and pharmacology are also constantly changing the care that is reasonably expected to be provided to the patient. As an integral part of the healthcare system with significant interaction with patients and families, nurses must not only stay current with emerging risks and trends, but must also assume leadership and management in designing healthcare systems and processes to minimize those risks.

This chapter describes the three branches of the U.S. government system and defines the role of administrative agencies. It reviews the role of law in shaping nursing practice and discusses negligence and malpractice. The chapter reviews the Health Insurance Portability and Accountability Act of 1996 (HIPAA) and discusses Medicare. It also discusses the Anti-Kickback Law and the Stark Law. Finally, the chapter reviews the International Council of Nurses' Code of Ethics and the American Nurses' Association Code of Ethics and describes common ethical principles that influence the practice of nursing.

THE U.S. GOVERNMENT SYSTEM

Following the American Revolution, the nation floundered under the Articles of Confederation. The Founding Fathers, Benjamin Franklin, George Washington, Thomas Jefferson, and Alexander Hamilton, understood that the Articles of Confederation failed miserably in that too much power was left to the individual states. Without an effective central government, the United States lacked a cohesive economic and political structure. As more states became interested in changing the Articles of Confederation, a meeting was set in Philadelphia on May 25, 1787. This became the Constitutional Convention. It was quickly realized that changes would not work and instead the entire Articles needed to be replaced (Kelley, 2017). On March 4, 1789, the government under the Articles of Confederation was replaced with the federal government under the Constitution (Rodgers, 2011). The new Constitution provided for a much stronger federal government by establishing a chief executive (the President), courts, and taxing powers.

In drafting the U.S. Constitution, the Founding Fathers set forth three branches of federal government, each with specific and occasionally overlapping roles and duties. They devised this federal government with a **separation of powers**, a government system with checks and balances that allow one branch of government to limit another and that ensure that no one single branch of government can ever have total control or power. For example, the U.S. Supreme Court may declare a law passed by Congress and signed into law by the President as unconstitutional. The three branches of the federal government are the executive branch, the legislative branch, and the judicial branch.

Branches of Government

The **executive branch** of the federal government consists of the office of the president of the United States. The executive branch of the government shapes the agenda for the country. This agenda is theoretically based on promises made during elections and is often based on how the president's party seeks to advance its agenda. The president has a significant role in making law. Although the president does not write legislation, the president can approve a bill passed by Congress, thus making it a law. The president may also veto a bill, preventing it from becoming a law. This veto may be overturned by Congress. The president is responsible for the execution and implementation of federal laws, often through the members of the Cabinet and through numerous governmental agencies. The president is also the Commander in Chief, responsible for defending the country and leading the U.S. Armed Forces. The president can sign treaties, issue executive orders, declare states of emergency, make appointments to the judiciary, and grant pardons.

The **legislative branch** of the federal government has the responsibility under the U.S. Constitution to make laws. This branch of government is also known as Congress. It is composed of the House of Representatives and the Senate. The Founding Fathers were very intentional when they defined the duties of the legislative branch and when they set the terms for holding office. The members of the House of Representatives are elected to 2-year terms. Currently, there are 435 members of the House of Representatives. The number of representatives each state has is based on the respective state's population. The members of the Senate are elected to 6-year terms. Each state has two senators.

The legislative branch also has the power to tax and spend. It may regulate interstate commerce, borrow money, and ratify treaties signed by the president. The legislative branch has the sole power to approve members appointed by the president to the judiciary. Finally, the legislative branch has the sole power of impeachment of the president, judges, and members of Congress.

The **judicial branch** of the federal government has the responsibility of interpreting federal laws and ensuring that the laws are in compliance with the U.S. Constitution. The Supreme Court judges who comprise the judicial branch are appointed by the president and approved by Congress. Justices of the Supreme Court are appointed for lifetime terms. This is intended to ensure that Supreme Court justices are not subject to the whims of the electorate who may seek to have a federal or Supreme Court justice removed from his or her position because he or she rendered a decision in a manner that might have been contrary to other political beliefs. Judges are expected to base their decisions only on the facts of the case at hand and their interpretation of the law relevant to the case.

CRITICAL THINKING 5.1

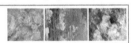

President Jones was elected in 2022 on a campaign promoting tax code reform. Unfortunately for President Jones, the other party has control of Congress. After several months of inaction, President Jones becomes impatient and orders the Internal Revenue Service to reduce the effective tax rates across the board.

1. Is that constitutional?
2. Will President Jones be able to reduce the tax code?

Administrative Agencies

The legislative branch and the executive branch of the federal government often delegate authority to governmental administrative agencies. These governmental administrative agencies may arise under the cabinets of various presidents. Other agencies are created by Congress by statute. The 50 states also have a web of state governmental agencies in existence. Regardless of the source, such agencies permeate the landscape of America.

One of the most influential agencies in the healthcare industry is the U.S. Department of Health and Human Services (HHS). This agency consists of 11 operating units that influence laws surrounding many aspects of our healthcare delivery system, including payment of healthcare services, regulation of medical drugs and devices, vaccine programs, healthcare research, and patient safety. HHS agencies can also write regulations but often run into difficulties with some of the branches of government, for example, when Congress refuses to allocate dollars to enact laws. Table 5.1 lists the agencies under HHS and briefly describes its most important functions. Many of these HHS agencies are familiar to nurses working both in direct patient care and in administration.

TABLE 5.1 U.S. DEPARTMENT OF HEALTH AND HUMAN SERVICES (HHS) AGENCIES AND FUNCTIONS

U.S. DEPARTMENT OF HEALTH AND HUMAN SERVICES AGENCY	MOST IMPORTANT FUNCTIONS
The Administration for Children and Families	Promotes the economic and social well-being of families, children, individuals, and communities through a range of educational and supportive programs in partnership with states, tribes, and community organizations.
The Administration for Community Living	Increases access to community support and resources for the unique needs of older Americans and people with disabilities.
The Agency for Healthcare Research and Quality	Produces evidence to make healthcare safer, higher quality, more accessible, equitable, and affordable, and to work within the HHS and with other partners to make sure that the evidence is understood and used.
The Agency for Toxic Substances and Disease Registry	Prevents exposure to toxic substances and the adverse health effects and diminished quality of life associated with exposure to hazardous substances from waste sites, unplanned releases, and other sources of environmental pollution.
The Centers for Disease Control and Prevention	Part of the Public Health Service; it protects the public health of the nation by providing leadership and direction in the prevention and control of diseases and other preventable conditions and responding to public health emergencies.
The Centers for Medicare & Medicaid Services	Combines the oversight of the Medicare program, the federal portion of the Medicaid program and State Children's Health Insurance Program, the Health Insurance Marketplace, and related quality assurance activities.
The Food and Drug Administration	Part of the Public Health Service; it ensures that food is safe, pure, and wholesome; human and animal drugs, biological products, and medical devices are safe and effective; and electronic products that emit radiation are safe.
The Health Resources and Services Administration	Part of the Public Health Service; it provides healthcare to people who are geographically isolated or economically or medically vulnerable.
The Indian Health Service	Part of the Public Health Service; it provides American Indians and Alaska Natives with comprehensive health services by developing and managing programs to meet their health needs.
The National Institutes of Health	Part of the Public Health Service; it supports biomedical and behavioral research with the United States and abroad, conducts research in its own laboratories and clinics, trains promising young researchers, and promotes collecting and sharing medical knowledge.
Substance Abuse and Mental Health Services Administration (SAMHSA)	Part of the Public Health Service and improves access and reduces barriers to high-quality, effective programs and services for individuals who suffer from or are at risk for addictive and mental disorders, as well as for their families and communities.

THE ROLE OF THE LAW IN SHAPING NURSING PRACTICE

The federal government is generally responsible for carrying out those powers specifically delegated to it in the U.S. Constitution. All other powers are reserved to the states. The U.S. Constitution does not directly address the regulation of nursing. Therefore, the states are the bodies that have created most of the nursing regulations. Moreover, the law that governs individual practice is dependent upon the particular state where the practice in question takes place. There are many state and federal laws that govern the healthcare industry and influence the practice of nursing. Nurses are regulated by both criminal law and civil law as well as by both common law and statutory law.

Criminal Law Versus Civil Law

Generally, law is divided into two distinct categories: criminal law and civil law. The primary distinction between the two categories relates to the particular goal of the law in question. Is the law designed to punish the wrongdoer? If so, then it is criminal law. On the other hand, civil law aims to provide for compensation to a victim. Examples of criminal law would include traffic violations, assault or battery, burglary, and/or murder. Examples of civil law would include negligence, breach of contract, and/or infringement of trade secrets. There are many differences in purposes and objectives for these two law categories.

One of the most significant differences is the burden of proof required in any legal proceeding. In a criminal law matter, the prosecution must prove its case beyond a reasonable doubt. For a civil law matter, the plaintiff must prove its case by a preponderance or greater amount of evidence. Another important distinction is that in a criminal law matter, the case is initiated by the prosecution who is working on behalf of the government. Criminal law proceedings are referred to as criminal prosecutions. In a civil law matter, the legal case is initiated by private individuals or corporations.

Another difference between criminal law and civil law relates to the resolution of the case. In a criminal law matter, if the prosecution is successful, the defendant is required to spend time incarcerated in jail or are assessed a fine. In a civil law matter, if the plaintiff or the person who brings a case against another in a court of law is successful, the defendant, that is, an individual, company, or institution sued or accused in a court of law, has to reimburse the plaintiff for the amount of damages determined by the court.

Statutory Law Versus Common Law

Within the category of civil law, law is further divided into two additional categories: statutory law and common law. **Statutory laws** are written laws that derive from a legislative body; for example, written laws from the U.S. Congress, a state legislative body, or a municipal board of trustees of a city or town. Members of these legislative bodies are elected by the citizens of their respective communities. An example of statutory law would be the applicable state Nurse Practice Act that is enacted by the various states that govern the licensure process for nurses.

Common law is the body of law that has been created through the application of prior court decisions, that is, precedents, to a unique set of facts; it has been developed by judges, courts, and other special courts or tribunals appointed to deal with a particular problem. If a similar matter has been heard by a court in the past, a court will generally follow the prior court decision and apply the reasoning given in the earlier precedent case to the matter that is pending before the court at that time. There are times, however, where the set of facts in the pending case are different from all prior cases and there are no statutes that are applicable, whereupon the court is required to render a decision. This is known as a matter of first impression. There are other situations where a statute may be applicable, but the statute does not expressly address the facts in question. In that situation, the court is required to interpret the statute using prior decisions and/or legislative history. Examples of common law would be negligence or malpractice matters.

Nurse Practice Acts

The nursing industry is regulated by **nurse practice acts** (NPAs), which are laws that have been enacted by state governments to protect the public's health, safety, and welfare by overseeing and ensuring the safe practice of nursing. As with state laws, NPAs also vary by state but generally include a definition of the scope of nursing practice allowed in the state, the types of licenses and the requirements for each, grounds for disciplinary action and remediation, education standards for nursing programs, and the authority and power of the state Board of Nursing.

NPAs generally are designed to protect the public's health, safety, and welfare. NPAs are designed to shield the public from nurses who lack the minimum qualifications to preform competent nursing services. In addition, the NPAs also contain protections to punish and/or suspend any nurses who fail to follow proper protocol or otherwise unsafe practices. NPAs also define the minimum requirements in order to obtain a license within a particular state. NPAs are designed to ensure that nurses have a minimum level of competency. Finally, NPAs usually set forth any minimum ongoing continuing education that is required in order to maintain a license within a state.

In addition to NPAs, state legislatures and agencies also enact certain administrative codes and rules that regulate the nursing industry. Such administrative codes and rules contain more of the minimum requirements for nurses in practice and define different disciplinary structures for misconduct. The administrative codes and rules typically will allow a state governing body the right to suspend or revoke a license for the following acts:

1. Engaging in conduct likely to defraud or harm the public or demonstrating a willful disregard for the health, welfare, or safety of a patient.
2. Departing from or failing to conform to standards of practice.
3. Engaging in behavior that crosses professional boundaries (such as signing wills or other legal documents) not related to healthcare.
4. Engaging in sexual conduct with a patient.
5. Demonstrating actual or potential inability to practice nursing with reasonable skill, safety, or judgement by reason of illness, use of alcohol, drugs, chemicals, or any other material, or as a result of any mental or physical condition (Illinois Administrative Code, Title 68, Section 1300.90).

Administrative codes also will set forth the number of hours of continuing education required in order to maintain current status of the state licensure. For example, in the state of Illinois, licensed nurses are required to complete 20 hours of approved continuing education per 2-year license cycle (Illinois Administrative Code, Title 68, Section 1300.130).

All individuals entering into nursing practice must become familiar with their particular state's NPA. Failure to understand and comply can jeopardize a nursing license and the ability to legally practice nursing within a state. Moreover, such failure may also subject an individual to discipline including fines and license revocation.

The policies and procedures of an organization that define the manner in which nurses are to practice in a specific work setting should always be aligned with a state's NPA. It is important that these policies and procedures are not only descriptive of the work nurses are performing in an organization but also are compliant with the state's NPA. Because these documents may be used in court to both determine the standard of care for nurses and to assess whether a nurse was in compliance with the standard of care, clarity and specificity of these documents are important. Periodic review and revision of hospital policies and procedures are essential to ensure that they are current with the NPAs, as well as evidence based and related to the ever-expanding role of nurses.

NURSE LEADER AND MANAGER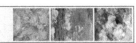

Imogene King, EdD, MSN, RN, FAAN, is recognized as an international pioneering nurse theorist and educator. She is known for her Theory of Goal Attainment. Read more about her at www.nursingworld.org/halloffame.

NEGLIGENCE

Negligence is a failure to exercise the care that a reasonably prudent person would exercise in like circumstances. **Malpractice** is one form of negligence and is improper, illegal, or negligent professional activity or treatment by a healthcare practitioner, lawyer, or public official. In today's litigious environment, all professionals must take care to ensure that they do not make mistakes. Malpractice claims against nurses are increasing, with more than $90 million paid in nurses' malpractice claims over a 5-year period (AHC Media LLC, 2016). Table 5.2 identifies common causes of nursing malpractice (McGuire & Mroczek, 2017). All nurses must understand their responsibilities in order to avoid common causes of nursing malpractice

A suit for negligence or malpractice is a civil suit brought by a person to recover damages from the person who caused such damages. A party bringing a malpractice suit must prove, by a preponderance or a large amount of evidence, the following:

- That a duty of care was owed to the patient;
- That there was a breach in that duty;
- That any injury was proximately caused by the breach in duty; and
- That there were damages.

TABLE 5.2 COMMON CAUSES OF NURSING MALPRACTICE

NURSING MALPRACTICE	EXAMPLE
Negligent infliction of emotional distress	In *Spangler v. Bechtel* (958 N.E.2d 458 [2011]), the Supreme Court found that the defendants, which included a nurse-midwife, could be liable for negligent infliction of emotional distress following the death of the plaintiffs' stillborn child.
Burns	In *Pillers v. Finley Hospital* (2003 Iowa App. LEXIS 792), the Court concluded that a nurse was liable along with the physician when the nurse applied a tourniquet to the plaintiff, as ordered, prior to surgery. Prep solution leaked around the tourniquet resulting in chemical burns to the plaintiff's thigh.
Falls	The California Third Circuit Court in *Massey v. Mercy Medical Center Redding* (180 Cal. App. 4th 690 [2009]) concluded that expert testimony was not necessary to prove a nurse's negligence in preventing a 65-year old, who had recently had surgery, from falling.
Failure to properly diagnose	The Supreme Court of Kansas held that the defendant's advance practice nurse and physician failed to diagnose the decedent's urinary tract infection, which later caused the decedent's death *Puckett v. Mt. Carmel Reg'l Med. Ctr.*, 290 Kan. 406 (2010).
Assault and battery	The Illinois Fifth Circuit Court of Appeals found a nurse and hospital guilty of battery, alleging that the nurse attending the plaintiff-patient observed and touched her without her permission, citing religious standards and beliefs (*Cohen v. Smith*, 269 Ill. App. 3d 1087 5th Cir. 1995).
HIPAA violations	In *Guardo v. Univ. Hosps., Geneva Medical Center* (2015-Ohio-1492), Eleventh District Court of Appeals in Ohio upheld the defendant-hospital's decision to terminate the plaintiff-nurse due to an unwarranted disclosure of HIPAA-protected information.
Breach of privilege	The Fourth District Ohio Court of Appeals found that the defendant-nurse and physician breached the physician-patient privilege by revealing the plaintiff's pregnancy to the plaintiff's parents. The liability extended to the nurse as well as to the physician because she contacted the plaintiff's parents at the supervising physician's direction (*Hobbs v. Lopez*, 96 Ohio App. 3d 670 [4th Dist. 1994]).
Failure to observe/ report	Reviewing a decision of the Nevada State Board of Nursing, the Supreme Court of Nevada upheld the Board's determination that the plaintiff-nurse had, among other things, failed to "observe the conditions, signs and symptoms of a patient, to record the information or to report significant changes to the appropriate persons" in treating one of the nurse's patients. The nurse did not timely deliver medication to a patient, and the patient subsequently passed away. Additionally, the nurse back-timed the order for the medication in his report (*Nevada State Bd. of Nursing v. Merkley*, 113 Nev. 659 [1997]).
False imprisonment	The Supreme Court of Mississippi held in *Lee v. Alexander* (607 So. 2d 30 [1992]) that "all who united in the illegal commitment are equally liable" in a false imprisonment case. This would extend to nurses who take part in a patient's involuntary confinement.
Medication errors	The Fourth Circuit Court of Appeals in Louisiana affirmed the district court's failure to instruct the jury to consider intervening cause. In that case, the patient suffered an adverse reaction to a drug administered and not monitored by the attending nurse (*Cagnolatti v. Hightower*, 692 So. 2d 1104 [La.App. 4 Cir. 1996]).

HIPAA, Health Insurance Portability and Accountability Act.

Duty of Care

The element of duty of care is generally the easiest of the four elements to prove in a healthcare negligence or malpractice case. **Duty of care** is the legal obligation of professionals to deliver a certain standard of care when performing acts that could directly or indirectly harm others. A duty of care is often viewed as a social contract that requires members of a society to behave responsibly toward one another.

Because negligence or malpractice is a state common law, the applicable law depends on the state where the conduct took place. Each state may have a slightly different legal interpretation. In many states, the test for duty of care is whether the harm to the patient due to the nurse's actions was foreseeable. Many states consider the following factors that are weighed to determine if a duty of care exists:

- Foreseeability of harm
- Degree of likelihood of harm
- Relationship of the parties
- Policy of preventing harm
- Available alternative conduct (how could the nurse have handled the situation differently)

Once a duty of care has been established, a nurse is expected to use the degree of skill, knowledge, and care that would be offered by a similarly trained nurse in a similar situation. It is important to note that a nurse is not expected to guarantee a perfect result or outcome, but a nurse is expected to conform to specific standards of care.

In some unique situations, it may appear that a duty of care may be owed. For example, a nurse while exercising at a local health club may encounter someone having a heart attack. In such a situation, public policy eliminates the duty of care. The nurse is not obligated to assist the person having the heart attack. Contrast that situation with a Good Samaritan case, where a nurse or other well-meaning citizen comes to the aid of a person who has sustained a physical injury or is in physical peril or harm. Courts want to encourage people to render aid to those in need. If the law of negligence were not modified in the case of the Good Samaritan, it could discourage people from getting involved in rendering aid to those in need. Although Good Samaritan laws vary by state, there are a few principles that are universally accepted. Good Samaritan laws generally apply when someone renders aid to an individual in an emergency on a voluntary basis without the expectation of remuneration or compensation. In most states, it is acknowledged that a person, even a person with medical or nursing training, does not need to come to the aid of someone who has been injured, but if they elect to do so, they must act in a manner that is reasonable. For example, they cannot come to the scene and offer assistance and then decide they need to leave and abandon the patient. In many states, the reasonable person standard is used to judge the conduct of the nurse rather than the standard of the reasonable nurse professional. This is due to the fact that when rendering care or assistance as a Good Samaritan, a nurse would not have access to the tools and support he or she might have when practicing in a formal healthcare environment.

Breach in Duty

A **breach in duty** occurs when a nurse or other healthcare professional has a duty of care toward another person but fails to live up to the accepted standard of care. Nursing standards of care are established by external and internal sources. Expert

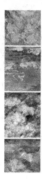

CASE STUDY 5.1

Mary, RN, is busy with four patients. She receives a new intravenous piggyback medication (IVPB) order from the healthcare provider and orders it from the pharmacy for her patient. When the unit clerk tells Mary that her patient's IVPB has arrived from the pharmacy, Mary quickly grabs the medication and hangs it. A few minutes later, the patient becomes short of breath. As Mary checks her patient over, she notes to her horror that she hung another patient's IVPB for this patient.

1. *What action should Mary take immediately?*
2. *What should she do next?*
3. *What should the hospital pharmacy and the nursing unit do to prevent future errors like this?*
4. *Is a problem like this the fault of the healthcare system, the fault of the nurse, or both?*

testimony and scholarly, evidence-based articles and practice guidelines can be used to establish whether the nurse acted in accordance with best and acceptable standards of care or whether he or she did not. Hospitals, home health agencies, and physician and nursing practices adopt policies and procedures on how to treat patients. Such policies are always evolving based on technology and medication.

A breach in duty can be either an act of commission (doing something but doing it incorrectly) or an act of omission (not doing what was expected or ordered). Often hospital policies and procedures are used to determine if a nurse breached a duty of care. A failure to conform to hospital policies and procedures is evidence of a breach in duty. The policies and procedures and the nurse's adherence to them are then supported or refuted and disproved by a nurse expert, who is credible in light of experience and background. Determining the applicable standard of care is the crux of the legal debate on whether a duty in care was breached. Generally, the standard of care is how a reasonable nurse would treat a patient under the same circumstances. Note that the standard of care in one community may be different in another community and may change and evolve based on research and technology.

Injury, Proximately Caused by a Breach in Duty of Care

The third element of negligence or malpractice is Injury, Proximately Caused by a Breach in Duty of Care. Proximate cause is often very difficult to prove or to get a jury to understand. Proximate cause of injury consists of successfully proving that a patient was indeed injured and that a breach in the duty of care was the cause of the injury sustained. Often nurses care for patients who are already very vulnerable and might be subject to exacerbations of their condition or further injury by the very nature of their condition. Thus, it can be difficult to prove that an injury was not part of the natural progression of the patient's illness or that the injury would not have occurred except for the breach in duty of care. Lawyers who seek to prove this element of negligence or malpractice again use experts for this. In addition, many times a patient may have contributed toward the injury. This is known as contributory negligence. If a lawyer can prove contributory negligence, the amount of a patient's monetary award is reduced.

Damages

Finally, the fourth element of negligence or malpractice is that the plaintiff's attorney must present evidence that, as a result of the conduct of the nurse, the plaintiff (patient) suffered some type of economic or physical damage. The goal of civil litigation is to award compensation and/or make the patient whole. Typical components of damages include the following:

1. Actual cost of reversing the injury
2. Future anticipated economic losses because of the injury
3. Pain and suffering
4. Emotional distress that those close to the injured person might have sustained while witnessing the harm to a loved one
5. Punitive damages, where the plaintiff seeks an amount to punish the nurse or the organization for particularly egregious bad conduct

The monetary amount of damages that can be awarded varies from state to state and in rare cases, there may be partial or limited immunity from liability. The damages award is generally covered under the malpractice insurance program that has been set up by the organization employing the nurse. That program generally covers attorney's fees and any money paid to the plaintiff to compensate for the injuries. Information about damage caps on a state-by-state basis can be found at www.alllaw.com/resources/personal-injury/personal-injury-state-law. A table that lists the limits to punitive damages in each of the 50 states and the District of Columbia is available at www.legalmatch.com/law-library/article/limits-on-punitive-damages.html.

HEALTH INSURANCE PORTABILITY AND ACCOUNTABILITY ACT (HIPAA) OF 1996

Advances in technology have impacted the healthcare profession in many ways. One significant impact is the advent of electronic patient information. On one hand, technology has made it easier for patient information to be shared among healthcare professionals, which in turn has made it easier to diagnose and treat patients. On the other hand, patient information may fall into the wrong hands or otherwise be misused, potentially causing damages or harm to the rights of patients. Organizations, individuals, or other entities could discriminate against patients based upon their medical condition.

To address this issue, the **Health Insurance Portability and Accountability Act (HIPAA)** was passed in 1996 to set national standards for the protection of patient information. The HHS published final rules implementing HIPAA in 2000 and 2002. These rules are applicable to health plans, healthcare clearinghouses, and healthcare providers who electronically transmit health information in connection with transactions for which HHS has adopted standards. Generally, these transactions concern billing for services or insurance coverage by hospitals, academic medical centers, physicians, and other healthcare providers who electronically transmit claims to a health plan. The major goal of HIPAA is to ensure individuals that their patient information will be protected, while at the same time promoting the free flow of information that is needed to provide the best care for patients' health and well-being. HIPAA attempts to strike a balance that enables professionals to use patient information but it also protects patient privacy.

Patient Information

HIPAA regulates the use and maintenance of patient information. Patient information is information including demographic data that relates to an individual's past, present, or future physical or mental health or condition; the provision of healthcare to that individual; or the past present, or future payment for the provision of healthcare to that individual. In order for the information to constitute protected health information, the information must include identifier information that identifies the individual with a reasonable basis of belief that it could be used to identify the individual. Identifiable health information may include the name, address, birthdate, or Social Security number of the patient. There are ways to deidentify health information where the specified identifiers have been removed.

Permitted Uses of Patient information

HIPAA defines when patient information may be used and disclosed. HIPPA rules provide that a healthcare provider may not use or disclose protected patient info except (a) as the rule permits, for example, for treatment or payment, and so on, and (b) as the individual who is the subject of the information has authorized in writing. Healthcare providers must rely on professional ethics and best judgments in deciding which of the permitted uses and disclosures to make. Providers must also disclose protected health information to patients when they specifically request access to it or to the HHS when it is undertaking a compliance investigation.

Authorized Disclosure

A healthcare provider is required to turn over patient information to the patient upon request. Many times a nurse may be faced with a request for patient information by a family member or another person other than the patient in question or another healthcare professional. HIPAA allows healthcare providers to treat a legally appointed personal representative the same as the individual with respect to information uses and disclosures. A **personal representative** is a person that is legally authorized to make healthcare decisions on an individual's behalf or to act for a deceased individual or an estate (such as under a power of attorney or guardianship). However, a healthcare provider is not permitted to disclose patient information to others who are not a patient's personal representative. In the situations of minors, the parents are considered to be personal representatives of the patient.

Penalties

The HHS Office for Civil Rights may impose a penalty on a healthcare provider for a failure to comply with HIPAA. These penalties may vary and it depends on many factors that are relevant to the violation in question. The penalty ranges from $100 to $50,000 or more per HIPAA violation depending on the severity of the violation. Moreover, a criminal penalty may be involved and assessed against a person who knowingly obtains or discloses protected patient information. Such fines could be up to $50,000 as well as up to 1-year imprisonment. Furthermore, if the violation includes false pretenses, such as an effort to defraud the patient, the fine cap rises from $200 to $50,000 and up to 10-years imprisonment.

MEDICARE COMPLIANCE

The exploding baby boomer population has impacted many facets of American society including the healthcare industry. In addition, medical technology has contributed to the longer lifespan of individuals. Within nursing, one area that has gained additional popularity is the home healthcare arena. **Home healthcare** is the provision of limited healthcare services by a nurse or other healthcare professional in the home of the patient. Although not exclusively, much of the care is funded through the U.S. Centers for Medicare & Medicaid Services (Medicare), which covers individuals 65 years of age and older. Many nurses today provide services through a home healthcare agency. Within that industry, there are certain regulatory requirements that must be understood.

Certification Compliance

In order for an individual to be eligible for reimbursement for home healthcare services, an individual must meet certain requirements. The requirements are summarized as follows:

1. Patient must have medical necessity
2. Patient must be homebound
3. A physician must certify and/or prescribe the need for home healthcare services

If any person, nurse, and/or agency attempts to submit claims to Medicare for reimbursement for the provision of healthcare services to a patient that does not meet these three requirements, they may be subject to penalties and/or criminal prosecution.

Federal Anti-Kickback Statute

The **Federal Anti-Kickback Statute** is a law that prohibits the payment or receipt of any gift or remuneration in exchange for federal healthcare referrals to Medicare patients. Congress has determined that a compensation structure that rewards referring patients for the receipt of Medicare reimbursement is potentially abusive and would lead to fraud and waste within the Medicare program. The term, remuneration, is broad and includes anything of value, transferred either directly or indirectly, in cash or gifts. In other words, remuneration can include trips, meals, and tickets to sporting events or other shows or concerts. Accordingly, the Anti-Kickback Statute cannot be avoided merely by using gifts or goods or services in exchange for healthcare referrals.

Although the Federal Anti-Kickback Statute concerns any individual, the Stark Law relates strictly to a physician. The **Stark Law** prohibits a physician from making a Medicare or Medicaid referral to a healthcare provider or organization with whom the physician or his or her family member has a financial relationship. Similar to the Federal Anti-Kickback Statute, the Stark Law seeks to prevent potentially abusive circumstances whereby Medicare may be defrauded due to corrupt physicians.

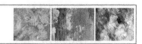

CRITICAL THINKING 5.2

Dr. Thompson operates a thriving patient practice in Chicago. Many of his patients are over 65 years of age. Many of them suffer from various healthcare conditions but do not require hospitalization. Dr. Thompson's wife is a nurse who started a home healthcare agency that is eligible to seek reimbursements from Medicare.

1. Can Dr. Thompson refer a patient to his wife's agency?
2. Does the Stark Law apply to this situation?

Civil Monetary Penalty Law

In addition to the Federal Anti-Kickback Statute and the Stark Law, there are also other penalties relating to certain misconduct within the Medicare program. A civil monetary penalty may be assessed against a person if the person provides remuneration to a Medicare or Medicaid beneficiary when the person knows or should know that such action is likely to influence the beneficiary's selection of a particular provider, practitioner, or supplier. When evaluating whether a civil monetary penalty should be assessed, there is a three-prong test:

- Was there remuneration of an item or service to a Medicare or Medicaid beneficiary?
- Was it likely that the item or service influenced the beneficiary to select the providers?
- Did the provider know that the item or service was likely to influence the beneficiary's selection of the provider?

It is generally held that items of value of $10 or less are considered to be not subject to the Civil Monetary Penalty Law. Those guilty of a Federal Anti-Kickback Statute violation may be convicted of a felony, assessed a $25,000 fine, or potentially given a 5-year prison sentence. For the Civil Monetary Penalty Law violation, there may be a penalty of up to $10,000 for each violation.

Exclusions

The Office of the Inspector General has the authority to exclude certain individuals and entities from participation in the Medicare, Medicaid, or other federal healthcare programs. Excluding an individual or entity is a severe penalty. Organizations employing or contracting with an excluded individual are not eligible to be paid directly or indirectly by a federal healthcare program for any items or services such excluded individual provides. Those found guilty of violating the Federal Anti-Kickback Statute or the Civil Monetary Penalty Law may be excluded from the Medicare program. In addition, any provider who employs an excluded individual may be required to return to Medicare any revenue received that is attributable, directly or indirectly, to the excluded individual.

ETHICAL CODES AND PRINCIPLES

In addition to the laws that govern the practice of nursing, there are also ethical codes and principles that nurses must observe in the performance of their duties. The International Council of Nurses' Code of Ethics (2012) groups ethics under four fundamental nursing responsibilities:

- Promote health
- Prevent illness
- Restore health
- Alleviate suffering

Ethical codes and principles guide the practice of nursing (Table 5.3). The American Nurses Association's (ANA) Code of Ethics (ANA, 2015) has been developed to provide an ethical framework for nurses. The Code of Ethics make it clear that inherent in nursing is respect for human rights, including the right to life, to dignity, and to be treated with respect.

The ANA's Code of Ethics provides a succinct statement of the ethical values, obligations, and duties of every individual who enters the nursing profession. It is available at www.nursingworld.org/practice-policy/nursing-excellence/ethics/code-of-ethics-for-nurses/. A short list of ANA Definitions of Ethical Principles is available at www.happynclex.com/wp-content/uploads/2016/04/ANA-ethics-definitions-and-examples.pdf.

TABLE 5.3 ETHICAL PRINCIPLES THAT GUIDE THE PRACTICE OF NURSING

ETHICAL PRINCIPLES	DEFINITION	APPLICATION
Benef-icence	Compassion; taking positive action to help others; desire to do good; core principle of patient advocacy	• Provide all patients, including the terminally ill, with caring attention and information • Become familiar with state laws regarding organ donations • Treat every patient with respect and courtesy • Give pain medication as quickly as possible
Nonma-leficence	Avoidance of harm or hurt; core of medical oath and nursing ethics	• Always work within your scope of practice • Never give information or perform duties when you are not qualified to do so • Check that patient is oriented when signing consents • Keep areas safe from hazards • Perform procedures according to facility protocols; never take shortcuts • Ask an appropriate person about anything you are unsure of • Keep your skills and education up to date

(continued)

TABLE 5.3 ETHICAL PRINCIPLES THAT GUIDE THE PRACTICE OF NURSING (*continued*)

ETHICAL PRINCIPLES	DEFINITION	APPLICATION
Justice	This principle refers to an equal and fair distribution of resources, based on analysis of benefits and burdens of decision. Justice implies that all citizens have an equal right to the goods distributed, regardless of what they have contributed or who they are. For example, in the United States, we all have rights to services from the postal service, firefighters, police, and access to public schools, safe water, and sanitation.	• Treat all patients equally, regardless of economic or social background • Learn the laws and your facility's policies and procedures for reporting suspected abuse
Autonomy	Agreement to respect another's right to self-determine a course of action; support of independent decision making	• Respect all patient choices and rights to decision making • Become familiar with federal and state laws and facility policies dealing with autonomy and privacy, e.g., HIPAA legislation, Patient Self-Determination Act • Never release patient information of any kind unless there is a signed patient release • Do not discuss patients with anyone who is not professionally involved in their care
Fidelity	This principle requires loyalty, fairness, truthfulness, advocacy, and dedication to patients. It involves an agreement to keep our promises. Fidelity refers to the concept of keeping a commitment and is based upon the virtue of caring	• Be sure that contracts have been completed • Be careful what you say to patients. They may only hear the "good news" • Keep promises to patients
Respect for others	The right of people to make their own decisions regarding diagnosis, therapy, and prognosis. This principle is heavily laden as an application of power over the patient	• Do not make paternal decisions for patient based on what you think is best for them • Let patients choose what is best for them • Provide all persons with information for decision making

(*continued*)

TABLE 5.3 ETHICAL PRINCIPLES THAT GUIDE THE PRACTICE OF NURSING (*continued*)

ETHICAL PRINCIPLES	DEFINITION	APPLICATION
Veracity	The obligation to tell the truth	• Admit mistakes promptly. Offer to do whatever is necessary to correct them • Refuse to participate in any form of fraud
Advocacy	The obligation to look out or speak up for the rights of others	• Provide patients with high-quality, evidence-based care • Participate in community actions to improve patient care • Participate in professional nursing actions to improve patient care

Sources: Little, C.B., Dorman, J. Ethical Aspects of Health Care. (2012). In Kelly, P. Nursing Leadership and Management. Third Edition. Clifton Park, New York: Cengage Learning.

American Nurses Association. Short definitions of ethical principles' and theories' familiar words, what do they mean? Retrieved from https://www.coursehero.com/file/11324675/ANA-defined-ethical-principles/

KEY CONCEPTS

- The three branches of government are the executive branch, the legislative branch, and the judicial branch.
- The U.S. Department of Health and Human Services (HHS) has 11 operating units that influence laws surrounding many aspects of our healthcare delivery system, including payment of healthcare services, regulation of medical drugs and devices, vaccine programs, healthcare research, and patient safety.
- There are many state and federal laws that govern the healthcare industry and influence the practice of nursing. Nurses are affected by both civil and criminal law.
- Nurse practice acts vary by state but generally include a definition of the scope of nursing practice allowed in the state.
- A person bringing a malpractice or negligence suit must prove, by a preponderance of the evidence, that a duty of care was owed to the patient; that there was a breach in that duty; that any injury was proximately caused by the breach; and that there were damages.
- The Health Insurance Portability and Accountability Act (HIPAA) was passed in 1996 to set national standards for the protection of patient information.
- The International Council of Nurses' Code of Ethics (2012) identifies four fundamental responsibilities for nurses. These responsibilities are promoting health, preventing illness, restoring health, and alleviating suffering.

- The American Nurses Association's Code of Ethics (2015) identifies distinct provisions.
- Ethical principles guide the practice of nursing.
- Nurses take action in order to improve the environment of patients, themselves, other nurses, and members of the interprofessional team.
- Nurses should participate in their professional organizations to assist in the advancement of quality healthcare policies, civic values, professional standards, and clinical practice protocols.
- Nurses should also take action to collaborate with the public and promote community, national, and international efforts to meet the healthcare needs of the community.

KEY TERMS

Breach in duty
Common law
Duty of care
Executive branch
Federal Anti-Kickback Statute
Health Insurance Portability and
   Accountability Act (HIPAA)
Home healthcare
Judicial branch

Legislative branch
Malpractice
Negligence
Nurse practice acts
Personal representative
Separation of powers
Stark Law
Statutory laws

REVIEW QUESTIONS

1. A healthcare provider has ordered you to discharge Mr. Jones from the hospital despite a new temperature of 102°F (38.8°C). The provider refuses to talk with you about the patient. In this situation, which of the following is an appropriate nursing action?

   A. Administer an antipyretic medication and discharge the patient.
   B. Discharge the patient with instructions to call 911 if he has any problems.
   C. Do not discharge the patient until you have discussed the matter with your nursing manager and are satisfied regarding patient safety.
   D. Discharge the patient and tell the patient to take acetaminophen (Tylenol) when he gets home.

2. A healthcare provider has issued a Do Not Attempt to Resuscitate (DNAR) order for your patient, a 55-year-old man with cancer. You spoke with the patient this morning and he clearly wishes to be resuscitated in the event that he stops breathing. What is the most appropriate course of action?

   A. Ignore the patient's wishes because the healthcare provider ordered the DNAR.
   B. Consult your hospital's policies and procedures, speak to the healthcare provider, and discuss the matter with your nurse manager.
   C. Attempt to talk the patient into agreeing to the DNAR.
   D. Contact the medical licensing board to complain about the healthcare provider.

3. The Health Insurance Portability and Accountability Act (HIPAA) protects which of the following?

    A. A patient's right to be insured regardless of employment status or ability to pay.
    B. The confidentiality of certain protected health information.
    C. The nurse's right to health insurance.
    D. The hospital's right to disclose protected health information.

4. Which of the following elements is not necessary for a nurse to be found negligent in a court of law?

    A. A duty or obligation for the nurse to act in a particular way.
    B. A breach of that duty or obligation.
    C. The nurse's intention to be negligent.
    D. Physical, emotional, or financial harm to the patient.

5. Inez, RN, did not put the bed-side rails up on a confused patient. The patient fell and was injured. When there is a connection between the nurse omitting a duty and the damages occurring to a patient, it is an example of which of the following?

    A. Breach of duty
    B. Duty
    C. Causation
    D. Damages

6. Select the most appropriate documentation example in the following.

    A. Patient found covered in stool. The night nurses were too busy to change the bed.
    B. The patient fell because we are short of staff.
    C. The patient's family is difficult and argumentative.
    D. Dr. M. Bresley notified through the medical exchange at 0610 of patient's complaints of difficulty breathing. Orders received for oxygen and arterial blood gases (ABGs).

7. You call the surgeon for your new postoperative patient who is bleeding excessively. The patient's blood pressure has decreased 20 mmHg, and his pulse rate has increased by 20 beats over the past hour. The surgeon's response to this information is "Why did you wake me up at 2 a.m. for this? I am hanging up as I expect a postoperative patient to be oozing from the operative site and these changes are not significant. Just watch him." You are quite concerned about your patient. What will you do next?

    A. Go to the nursing station and complain to the other nurses about how rude the surgeon was on the phone.
    B. Document and quote the surgeon's response in your nurse's notes.
    C. Inform the surgeon that you do not agree with continuing to just observe this patient and that you are going to initiate the chain of command.
    D. Tell the family what the surgeon said.

8. An 80-year-old man who lives with his son is brought to your unit because "he just isn't acting right." On physical examination, you note that the patient is malnourished, noncommunicative, and has poor hygiene. When you ask the patient some questions, he avoids eye contact and does not respond. The son is answering questions for the patient and refuses to leave the room. You suspect elder abuse. Choose the most appropriate documentation of the situation.

   A. The patient is very thin and does not make eye contact with the nursing or medical staff. It is obvious that he has been abused and neglected by his family.
   B. The patient is a thin elderly male who presents to the unit wearing clothing that is soiled. He does not make eye contact with the staff or answer our questions. Social services notified.
   C. It appears that the patient's son manipulates his father by refusing to let his father answer any questions. We suspect elder abuse.
   D. The patient's son states that the patient "isn't acting right." The patient does not answer questions from the staff due to his abuse.

9. The nurse is given a written order by a healthcare provider to administer an unusually large dose of pain medicine to a patient. In this situation, which of the following is an appropriate nursing action?

   A. Administer the medication because it was ordered by a healthcare provider.
   B. Refuse to administer the medication, and move on to another patient.
   C. Speak with the healthcare provider about your concerns, and clarify whether the medication dose is accurate.
   D. Select a dose that you feel comfortable with, and administer that dose.

REVIEW ACTIVITIES

1. Identify the ways in which nurses you observe in your clinical rotations discuss orders and treatments with healthcare providers. How do nurses address incorrect or questionable medication orders? Talk with nurses you see about how they handle these situations.
2. Go to the website and search for your state's Nurse Practice Act. Discuss what you find there.

CRITICAL DISCUSSION POINTS

1. What are the three branches of the American legal system?
2. How does the law play a role in shaping nursing practice?
3. How can nurses protect themselves against a negligence lawsuit?

QSEN ACTIVITIES

1. Go to qsen.org/faculty-resources/patient-centered-care-resources/. Review the information about the Patient Safety Movement. How can nurses help prevent the more than 200,000 preventable patient deaths each year?

2. Review the "Guide to Patient and Family Engagement in Hospital Safety and Quality" at www.ahrq.gov/professionals/systems/hospital/engagingfamilies/index.html. Review how this guide helps patients, families, and health professionals work together as partners to promote improvements in care.

EXPLORING THE WEB

1. www.nso.com/risk-education/individuals/legal-case-studies
2. www.rmf.harvard.edu/Clinician-Resources/Article/2008/Medical-Malpractice-Cases-Involving-Nurses
3. listverse.com/2013/05/29/10-horrible-cases-of-medical-malpractice/
4. www.dprnesq.com/pages/news/malpractice-suits-against-nurses-on-the-rise
5. www.nursingworld.org/practice-policy/nursing-excellence/ethics/code-of-ethics-for-nurses/
6. www.nursingworld.org/practice-policy/nursing-excellence/ethics/

REFERENCES

AHC Media LLC. (2016). *More nurses, hospitalists being sued for malpractice, studies say*. Retrieved from https://www.ahcmedia.com/articles/137567-more-nurses-hospitalists-being-sued-for-malpractice-studies-say

American Nurses Association. (2015). *Short definitions of ethical principles and theories familiar words, what do they mean?* Retrieved from http://www.nursingworld.org/MainMenuCategories/Ethics-Standards/Resources/Ethics-Definitions.pdf

American Nurses Association Code of Ethics (ANA). (2015). The Code of Ethics for Nurses with Interpretive Statements. Retrieved from http://www.nursingworld.org/MainMenuCategories/EthicsStandards/CodeofEthicsforNurses/Code-of-Ethics-For-Nurses.html

Beauchamp, T. L., & Childress, J. F. (2009). *Principles of biomedical ethics* (6th ed., pp. 38–39, 152–153). New York, NY: Oxford University Press.

Butts, J. B., & Rich, K. L. (2008). *Nursing ethics across the curriculum and into practice* (2nd ed., pp. 48, 263). Sunbury, MA: Jones and Bartlett.

Ethics Advisory Board. (2011). Retrieved from http://www.addpriv.eu/uploads/public%20_deliverables/1.1%2089–ADDPRIV_20110424_WP1_ULANCS_EthicsAB_R2.pdf

Ethics Resource Center. (2009, May 29). *Definition of values*. Retrieved from http://www.ethics.org/resources/free-toolkit/definition-values

The International Council of Nurses (ICN) Code of Ethics (2012). Retrieved from http://www.icn.ch/images/stories/documents/about/icncode_english.pdf

Kelley, M. (2018, March 2). Why did the Articles of Confederation fail? *About Education*. Retrieved from https://www.thoughtco.com/why-articles-of-confederation-failed-104674

McGuire, C., & Mroczek, J. (2017). *Nurse malpractice*. National Center of Continuing Education, Inc., Retrieved from https://www.nursece.com/courses/99

Rodgers, P. (2011). *United States constitutional law: An introduction* (p. 109). McFarland.

SUGGESTED READINGS

Andersson, Å., Frank, C., Willman, A. M., Sandman, P. O., & Hansebo, G. (2015). Adverse events in nursing: A retrospective study of reports of patient and relative experiences. *International Nursing Review, 62*(3), 377–385. doi:10.1111/inr.12192

Ferrell, K. (2015). *Nurse's legal handbook* (6th ed.). Philadelphia, PA: Lippincott Williams & Wilkins.

Gostin, L. O. (2017). Five ethical values to guide health system reform: The JAMA forum. *JAMA*, 318(22), 2171–2172. doi:10.1001/jama.2017.18804

Guido, G. W. (2014). *Legal and ethical issues in nursing* (6th ed.). London, England: Pearson.

Hinno, S., Partanen, P., & Vehviläinen-Julkunen, K. (2012). Nursing activities, nurse staffing and adverse patient outcomes as perceived by hospital nurses. *Journal of Clinical Nursing*, 21(11–12), 1584–1593. doi:10.1111/j.1365-2702.2011.03956.x

Lucero, R. J., Lake, E. T., & Aiken, L. H. (2009). Variations in nursing care quality across hospitals. *Journal of Advanced Nursing*, 65(11), 2299–2310. doi:10.1111/j.1365-2648.2009.05090.x

Lucero, R. J., Lake, E. T., & Aiken, L. H. (2010). Nursing care quality and adverse events in US hospitals. *Journal of Clinical Nursing*, 19(15–16), 2185–2195. doi:10.1111/j.1365-2702.2010.03250.x

Van Bogaert, P., Timmermans, O., Weeks, S. M., van Heusden, D., Wouters, K., & Franck, E. (2014). Nursing unit teams matter: Impact of unit-level nurse practice environment, nurse work characteristics, and burnout on nurse reported job outcomes, and quality of care, and patient adverse events—A cross-sectional survey. *International Journal of Nursing Study*, 51(8), 1123–1134. doi:10.1016/j.ijnurstu.2013.12.009

Watts, A. (2017). Limits on punitive damages. LegalMatch. Retrieved from https://www.legalmatch.com/law-library/article/limits-on-punitive-damages.html

Westrick, S. (2013). *Essentials of nursing law and ethics*. Burlington, Massachusetts: Jones and Bartlett.

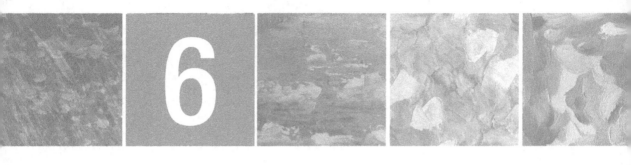

6

DELEGATION AND SETTING PRIORITIES FOR SAFE, HIGH-QUALITY NURSING CARE

Maureen T. Marthaler

Embraced for their wisdom and ability to provide outstanding patient-centered care, nurses are now optimally positioned to influence and help lead our national and global health care systems in the future.

Michele Mittelman, RN MPH. Founder and Editor, *Global Advances in Health and Medicine* (2014).

Upon completion of this chapter, the reader should be able to

1. Define delegation, responsibility, delegated responsibility, assignment, accountability, authority, and supervision.
2. Discuss the National Guidelines for Nursing Delegation developed by the National Council of State Boards of Nursing.
3. Describe the Five Rights of Delegation.
4. Discuss delegation related to the healthcare organization and members of the healthcare team.
5. Review communication factors influencing the delegation process.
6. Utilize the Scope of Nursing Practice Decision-Making Framework.

M orning report was given to an RN and one unlicensed assistive personnel (UAP) for five patients on a busy medical-surgical unit. One of the patients was to receive one unit of packed red blood cells (PRBC) if the patient's hemoglobin (Hgb) was less than 8.0 gm/dL. Later that morning, the patient's Hgb results came back as 7.1 gm/dL. The nurse went to the blood bank and picked up the unit of PRBC. The policy and procedure for administering blood includes two RNs to check the blood at the bedside and identify the patient, the patient's wristband, the unit of blood, the patient's blood bank wristband, the blood type and unit number, and the blood expiration date. Prior to the start of the blood transfusion and during and after the blood transfusion, the patient's vital signs are to be obtained and recorded by the nurse.

The policy and procedure was followed by the nurse. Fifteen minutes after the unit of blood was started, another set of vital signs was obtained by the Unlicensed Assistive Personnel (UAP). At this time, the patient complained of difficulty breathing and lower back pain. The UAP rubbed the patient's back and assured the patient these complaints were nothing to worry about. The UAP documented the vital signs and went on a break for lunch. Forty-five minutes later, the nurse was making rounds and found the patient gasping for air and covered in a raised rash all over the face and arms.

1. How could this patient's symptoms have been prevented?
2. Was the policy and procedure for blood administration followed? If not, what part was not followed?
3. Were the Five Rights of Delegation employed or not?

Delegation is a complex nursing skill requiring nursing leadership and management skills, setting priorities, using good clinical judgment, and assuming accountability for patient care. Delegation is guided by one's state Nurse Practice Act (NPA)

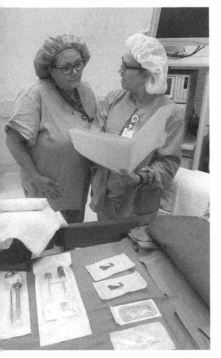

and requires nursing assumption of authority for the decisions and outcomes associated with patient care, sharing the process of patient care with other responsible members of the nursing team, and holding all members of the nursing team accountable for their responsibilities. Delegation requires nurses to use critical thinking, good communication skills, and leadership and management to build good relationships with staff and the interprofessional team to meet patient needs.

The National Council of State Boards of Nursing (NCSBN) convened two groups of experts representing education, research, and practice in 2015. They developed a set of National Guidelines for Nursing Delegation that standardized the nursing delegation process in 2016. The guidelines are meant for licensed nurses. A large piece of the National Guidelines for Nursing Delegation addresses UAP advanced roles. Skills that were once exclusive to licensed practical nurses/licensed vocational nurses (LPNs/LVNs) are now taught in advanced UAP programs. The NCSBN and other professional nursing organizations will continue to explore delegation as healthcare advancements and the roles and responsibilities of providers in a variety of state settings continuously change over time.

The roles of the nurse vary by geographic location and/or institution. The state NPA and the National Guidelines for Nursing Delegation guide the nurse in nursing delegation to UAP. The number one priority for nurses is to deliver safe patient care. The nurse is responsible and accountable for determining the appropriate delegation of responsibilities to UAP consistent with state NPAs, the policies and procedures of the healthcare organization, and the nurse's obligation to deliver safe, high-quality patient care. To ensure that this obligation is met, nurses are accountable for patient care delivered by both themselves and other personnel under their supervision.

This chapter discusses the concept of delegation with an emphasis on quality and safety. It discusses responsibility, delegated responsibility, assignment, accountability, authority, and supervision. NCSBN, National Guidelines for Nursing Delegation, and the Five Rights of Delegation are discussed. Delegation related to the healthcare organization and members of the healthcare team is discussed and communication factors influencing the delegation process are reviewed. The Scope of Nursing Practice Decision-Making Framework is also explored with applications throughout the chapter.

DELEGATION

Delegation is allowing a delegatee to perform a specific nursing activity, skill, or procedure that is beyond the delegatee's traditional role and not routinely performed (NCSBN, 2016). The National Guidelines for Nursing Delegation were created in 2016 by the NCSBN. The states have different NPAs and rules and regulations. This is information all licensed nurses must review prior to delegating. It is the nurses' responsibility to know what is permitted in their state's NPA and rules and regulations, along with the policies of their employer.

Delegation has been a source of significant debate for many years and there have been many philosophical discussions over the differences between assignment and delegation. Much of the literature surrounding nursing delegation has focused on the nursing home setting (NCSBN, 2016). Delegation is needed because of the advent of cost containment, the nursing shortage, increases in patient acuity levels, an elderly chronic patient population, and advances in healthcare technology.

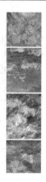

CASE STUDY 6.1

An armed services member returned home after a 13-month deployment to Afghanistan. He has come to the clinic where you work with his wife. The nurse delegates to the UAP to complete the assessment form with him. This is the first time the UAP has been delegated to complete this task. The UAP opens the computer and starts asking the patient the questions from the form. Under the history section on the form, a question reads "Have you ever experienced post-traumatic stress disorder (PTSD)?" The UAP then asks the patient if he had ever experienced a sexually transmitted disease. The patient questioned the UAP as to what was meant by "experienced"? The UAP responded by saying, "I am just reading the form, sir. I do not write the questions."

1. *What steps should the nurse have taken prior to delegating the completion of the computerized assessment form to the UAP?*
2. *What guides the process of delegation in an organization?*
3. *Should completing the assessment form be delegated to an UAP? Why or why not?*

EVIDENCE FROM THE LITERATURE

Citation

Shannon, R. A., & Kubelka, S. (2013). Reducing the risks of delegation use of procedure skills checklist for unlicensed assistive personnel in schools, Part 1. *NASN School Nurse, 28* (4), 178–181. doi:10.1177/1942602X13489886

Discussion

The school nurse will adhere to the state's NPA with many state boards of nursing allowing for some degree of delegation appropriate to the circumstance. School administrators are responsible for the assignment of specific employees to carry out the delegated tasks. Administration of medicines for asthma, anaphylaxis, diabetes, and seizures can be delegated. The decision to delegate is based on guidance by the state's NPA, state board of nursing, an organization's administration, policies, and procedures, and the Five Rights of Delegation.

Implications for Practice

Delegation of tasks in a school setting is no different than in a hospital setting. The same considerations are employed.

RESPONSIBILITY

Responsibility is the obligation involved when a person accepts an assignment. The delegation process is not complete until the person who receives the assignment accepts the responsibility for the assignment. Without this acceptance of responsibility, assignments cannot be delegated. Further, if a person does not have the knowledge, skill, experience, or willingness needed to complete an assignment, it is inappropriate to accept responsibility for the assignment. Once a person accepts responsibility for an assignment, this responsibility is retained.

NATIONAL GUIDELINES FOR NURSING DELEGATION

All decisions related to delegation are based on the fundamental principles of health, safety, and welfare of the public. The nursing profession takes responsibility and accountability for the provision of nursing practice (American Nurses Association [ANA], 2016). The **National Guidelines for Nursing Delegation** (NCSBN, 2016; Figure 6.1) identifies responsibilities of the employer/nurse leader, the licensed nurse, and the delegatee for public protection. In addition, the National Guidelines for Nursing Delegation highlight the need to communicate information about the delegation process and the delegatee competence level; the need for two-way communication; and the need for training and education.

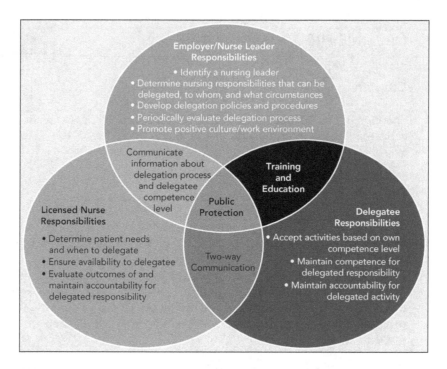

FIGURE 6.1 National Guidelines for Nursing Delegation.

Source: National Council of State Boards of Nursing. (2016). National Guidelines for Nursing Delegation. *Journal of Nursing Regulation, 7*(1), 5–12.

Each person in the National Guidelines for Nursing Delegation has specific responsibilities that he or she is expected to exercise for public protection. For example, the employer will identify a nurse leader who will determine nursing responsibilities that can be delegated, to whom, and under what circumstances; develop delegation policies and procedures; periodically evaluate the delegation process; and promote a positive culture and work environment. The nurse leader will also communicate information about the delegation process and delegatee competence level to the licensed nurse and provide training and education.

The Licensed Nurse Responsibilities include to determine patient needs and when to delegate, ensure availability to delegatee, evaluate outcomes of and maintain accountability for delegated responsibility. The Licensed Nurse will communicate information about the delegation process and delegatee competence level to the Employer/Nurse Leader. The Licensed Nurse will also maintain two-way communication with the Delegatee. The Delegatee responsibilities are to accept activities based on his or her own competence level and to maintain competence and accountability for delegated responsibility.

DELEGATED RESPONSIBILITY

A **delegated responsibility** is a nursing activity, skill, or procedure that is transferred from a licensed nurse to a delegatee; according to the National Guidelines for Nursing Delegation (NCSBN, 2016), "Any decision to delegate a nursing responsibility must be based on the needs of the patient or population, the stability and predictability of the patient's condition, the documented training and competence of the delegatee, and the ability of the licensed nurse to supervise the delegated responsibility and its outcome, with special consideration to the available staff mix and patient acuity." The responsibilities considered for delegation must be in accordance to the state's/jurisdiction's laws and rules and organizational policies and procedures prior to the licensed nurse making a final decision to delegate. If at any point, the nurse does not feel delegation of a responsibility is appropriate, the nurse must complete the responsibility himself or herself. The licensed nurse will maintain accountability for the patient at all times. The UAP is responsible for the delegated responsibility.

ASSIGNMENT

Assignment is the routine care, activities, and procedures that are within the authorized scope of practice of the RN or LPN/LVN or part of the routine functions of the UAP (NCSBN, 2016). An example of an assignment is the LPN/LVN caring for a patient with Crohn's disease. The nurse expects the LPN/LVN to assess the patient, monitor intake and output (I and O), administer medications, and take vital signs. As an assignment, these skills were taught in the LPN/LVN education program and thus are part of the LPN/LVN scope of practice.

There are exceptions when speaking to the basic educational preparation of a UAP. The skills once believed to be performed only by a licensed nurse are now taught to UAPs in certain advanced UAP education programs. Such roles of the UAP include administering injections and medications. For example, certified medication assistants (CMAs) are given special training to pass oral medications and give injections. Since there is a significant level of skill needed when administering medications or injections, employers and nurses will validate CMA competency. To validate competency, employers and nurses give skill tests or make observations as needed. Once employers and nurses are comfortable with a UAP's competence, procedures can be routinely delegated to him or her (NCSBN, 2016).

ACCOUNTABILITY

According to the ANA, **accountability** is defined as "to be answerable to oneself and others for one's own choices, decisions and actions as measure against a standard such as that established by the *Code of Ethics for Nurses with Interpretive Statements*" (ANA, 2015). The licensed nurse is accountable for the performance of the responsibilities delegated to others, for responsibilities the nurse personally performs, and for the act of delegating responsibilities to others. The nurse is ultimately accountable for the overall care provided to a patient. The delegatee shares the responsibility for the patient and is fully responsible for the delegated responsibilities. Licensed nurse accountability involves compliance with legal requirements as set forth in states/jurisdictions laws and rules governing nursing. The nurse is also accountable for the quality of nursing care provided and for recognizing limits, knowledge, competency, and experience of delegatees (ANA, 2015). Furthermore, the ANA (2015) states, nurses are accountable even in the event of system and/or technology failure.

UAPs and LPN/LVNs are also accountable to the licensed nurse. Accountability for the act of delegating involves the appropriate choice of delegatee and responsibility. For example, a nurse might delegate to the UAP a certain responsibility. If the nurse has not determined in advance that the UAP understands the delegated responsibility and has the skills, knowledge, and judgment to complete the responsibility, or the nurse does not supervise the completion of the responsibility and the UAP does not carry out the responsibility adequately, the nurse would be accountable for this act of improper delegation.

AUTHORITY

Authority is the right to act or to command the action of others. Authority comes with the job and is required for a nurse to take action. The person with authority must be free to make decisions regarding the activities involved. Without authority, the nurse will be unable to provide quality and safe patient-centered care (PCC). Authority is based on the state's/jurisdiction's NPA and guides the development of an organization's job description. If the nurse is in charge of a group of patients, the nurse must have the authority to act or command the action of others.

EVIDENCE FROM THE LITERATURE

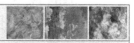

Citation

Buppert, C. (2016, December 8). Can a patient-care tech perform this task? *Medscape*. Retrieved from https://www.medscape.com/viewarticle/873589

Discussion

A nursing educator recently hired at a community hospital in New York observed a patient-care tech (PCT) removing a peripheral intravenous (IV) line. The nursing educator looked for a policy and procedure for this task to be completed by a PCT but was unsuccessful. The nursing educator asks the nursing administrator about it. The nursing administrator stated she wanted a policy to be written for this particular procedure. The nurse educator contacted the state board of nursing for New York and was told PCTs are not allowed to perform this task as stated in the NPA for the state of New York.

Implications for Practice

Some states specify, in the form of a regulation or policy, the tasks UAPs, such as a PCT, may perform. Some states specify what they may not do and some states are silent on this issue.

The state NPA trumps the community hospital's decision to allow PCTs to remove peripheral IV lines. The hospital's decisions must refer to their particular state's NPA prior to determining a policy and procedure related to nursing care.

SUPERVISION

Supervision is the provision of guidance or direction, evaluation, and follow-up by the licensed nurse for accomplishment of a nursing task delegated to the UAP (NCSBN, 1995). Supervision is generally categorized as on site (the licensed nurse being physically present or immediately available while the activity is performed) or off site (the licensed nurse has the ability to provide direction through various means of written and verbal communication).

A licensed nurse supervising care will provide clear directions to the interprofessional team. The supervising nurse must identify when and how a task is to be done and what information must be collected as well as any patient-specific information.

The licensed nurse must identify what outcomes are expected and the time frame for reporting results. The organization will monitor staff performance to ensure compliance with established standards of practice, policy, and procedure.

CRITICAL THINKING 6.1

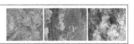

A nurse working in the emergency department asks a UAP if he wants to try to start an IV line. The nurse knows the UAP is graduating from nursing school in May. Without hesitation, the UAP agreed to start the IV.

1. Can this task be delegated to a UAP?
2. Who is responsible in the event the IV insertion site becomes infected?
3. What are the implications for the UAP if he declined the opportunity to start the IV?

FIVE RIGHTS OF DELEGATION

When the needs of the patient coincide with the skills, knowledge, and competency of UAP and can be performed safely, the licensed nurse will decide that delegation of a responsibility can occur. This decision is guided by the NCSBN Five Rights of Delegation (1995, 1996) (Table 6.1).

TABLE 6.1 FIVE RIGHTS OF DELEGATION

Right task	• The activity falls within the delegatee's job description or is included as part of the established written policies and procedures of the nursing practice setting. The facility needs to ensure the policies and procedures describe the expectations and limits of the activity and provide any necessary competency training.
Right circumstance	• The health condition of the patient must be stable. If the patient's condition changes, the delegatee must communicate this to the licensed nurse, and the licensed nurse must reassess the situation and the appropriateness of the delegation.
Right person	• The licensed nurse, along with the employer and the delegatee, is responsible for ensuring that the delegatee possesses the appropriate skills and knowledge to perform the activity.
Right direction and communication	• Each delegation situation should be specific to the patient, the licensed nurse, and the delegatee. • The licensed nurse is expected to communicate specific instructions for the delegated activity to the delegatee; the delegatee, as part of two-way communication, should ask any clarifying questions. This communication includes any data that need to be collected, the method for collecting the data, the time frame for reporting the results to the licensed nurse, and additional information pertinent to the situation. • The delegatee must understand the terms of the delegation and must agree to accept the delegated activity. • The licensed nurse should ensure that the delegatee understands that she or he cannot make any decisions or modifications in carrying out the activity without first consulting the licensed nurse.

(continued)

TABLE 6.1 FIVE RIGHTS OF DELEGATION (*continued*)

Right supervision and evaluation	• The licensed nurse is responsible for monitoring the delegated activity, following up with the delegatee at the completion of the activity, and evaluating patient outcomes. The delegatee is responsible for communicating patient information to the licensed nurse during the delegation situation. The licensed nurse should be ready and available to intervene as necessary. • The licensed nurse should ensure appropriate documentation of the activity is completed.

Source: National Council of State Boards of Nursing (NCSBN). (1995). *Delegation: Concepts and decision-making process*. National Council of State Boards of Nursing 1995 Annual Meeting Business Book; National Council of State Boards of Nursing (NCSBN). (1996). *Delegation: Concepts and decision-making process*. National Council of State Boards of Nursing.

REAL-WORLD INTERVIEW

I am a veteran labor and delivery travel nurse. We had a patient develop an amniotic fluid embolism in labor on my unit. This is a phenomenon that occurs in about one in 20,000 births. Therefore, it is not widely recognized nor easily diagnosed until autopsy. Not only was this patient mine, but I was in charge of a busy unit and it was 4 o'clock in the morning, when only skeleton crews are available. Due to quick thinking, 10 years of experience, and a lot of divine intervention, we were able to save this mother and her unborn baby. I remained at the bedside, prepping the patient for an emergency cesarean section. I delegated to another RN to obtain blood that we had on hold from the laboratory, so the patient could be transfused stat, as we knew disseminated intravascular coagulation (DIC) was looming. I was able to delegate to two other RNs at the same time to set the operating room up and call the house supervisor to alert the main operating room on-call staff. My final act of delegation was to have another RN call in our own on-call staff and our management team. This was all done while at the bedside. Granted, I had an amazing staff that evening, but being able to "hold it together" and think quickly and clearly to delegate within seconds in a crisis lent a glimmer of hope to a potentially fatal outcome. That outcome, thanks to skill and prayer, was a mother and her infant walking out of the hospital 5 days later, going home alive and well.

Sharon Murphy, RNC, BSN
Silver Spring, Maryland

The UAP's knowledge and level of competence impacts effective delegation. This knowledge and competency can be obtained from a formal educational program or from on the job training. For example, a licensed nurse in some states can delegate to UAPs such as secretaries, teachers, or other individuals in a school setting when certain medications need to be administered. The Five Rights of Delegation must be followed and the knowledge the UAP has gained from such things as an inservice followed by a return demonstration for competency testing is tested.

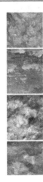

CASE STUDY 6.2

The hospital was preparing to initiate the use of high-flow nasal oxygen therapy (HFNOT). A committee was charged with writing the policy and procedure for this new form of oxygen therapy. The policy and procedure for the HFNOT was not completed prior to the initial use on a patient in the NICU. An anesthesiologist was present during the time of the administration of HFNOT. The nurse started to feed the neonatal patient a bottle of formula once the oxygen saturation was over 97%. The anesthesiologist told the nurse to stop feeding the patient, as it was contraindicated when HFNOT was being administered.

1. *How should the nurse respond to the directive by the anesthesiologist?*
2. *What is the hospital's responsibility to ensure new equipment such as HFNOT is implemented correctly?*

NURSE LEADER AND MANAGER

In 1854, Florence Nightingale and her staff of 38 female volunteer nurses were sent to the Crimean War, where they improved the unsanitary conditions at a British base hospital and reduced the death count by two thirds. In 1859, Nightingale wrote *Notes on Nursing* and in 1860, she funded the establishment of St. Thomas' Hospital and the Nightingale Training School for Nurses. *Notes on Nursing* served as the cornerstone of the curriculum at the Nightingale School and other nursing schools. Read more about her at www.victorianweb.org/history/crimea/florrie.html.

DELEGATION RELATED TO THE HEALTHCARE ORGANIZATION AND HEALTHCARE TEAM

The process of delegation begins with the states/jurisdictions NPA. From there, the healthcare organization selects a nurse leader to oversee the process of nursing delegation. It is imperative this nurse leader is familiar with the NPA, the policies and procedures of the organization, the National Guidelines for Nursing Delegation, and the Five Rights of Delegation. Organizational accountability for delegation also includes the need to provide sufficient staffing, an appropriate staffing mix, and ongoing education and competency support for all those involved in the delegation process. Requiring ongoing education and regular competency assessment will keep everyone involved in the delegation process up to date.

A nursing committee is usually established to create the policies and procedures for delegation. The nursing committee is often led by the nurse leader. Appropriate nurse and UAP staffing, the roles of the nurse and UAP, appropriate lines of communication, and the procedure for delegation are developed. The nursing committee will consider various factors as they write the delegation policy and procedure. These factors include but are not limited to:

- The nursing responsibilities that can be delegated
- The standards of nursing practice to maintain patient-centered, high quality, safe care

- Job descriptions of all healthcare team members that are part of the delegation process, for example, RN, LPN/LVN, UAP

Licensed nurses throughout the organization are then given the responsibility to delegate, oversee the delegation process, and evaluate the effectiveness of delegation. A systematic approach to the delegation process fosters communication and consistency of the process throughout the facility.

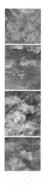

CASE STUDY 6.3

The nurse is caring for a patient who is on day 2 post-op gastric bypass surgery. The patient has been using oxygen periodically. The order is written for oxygen per nasal cannula at 2 L/min whenever necessary. The respiratory therapist explains to the patient that it is necessary for the oxygen to be worn at all times. The patient replies that the doctor said to use the oxygen only when needed. The nurse entered the room just as the patient made the statement and the nurse concurred. The respiratory therapist then said she had been taking care of gastric bypass patients longer than the surgeon has performed them. She said to trust her, it is best to wear the oxygen all the time.

1. *How does the nurse know when the patient should wear the oxygen? On what basis did you determine your answer?*
2. *Who is responsible for the care of the patient's respiratory status? Why?*

EVIDENCE FROM THE LITERATURE

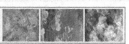

Citation

Buchwach, D. (2017). Helping new nurses with the fine art of delegation. Adapted from *Quick-E! Pro Time Management: A Guide for Nurses.* Retrieved from http://www.strategiesfornursemanagers.com/content.cfm?content_id=233639&oc_id=602#

Discussion

Delegation is a five-step process. First, as the nurse, determine how, where, and when assistance can be provided. Next, select an appropriate person. A discussion occurs wherein authority to complete the task is given from one person to another. The task is carried out under supervision. Finally, the delegation process is evaluated and feedback is given. Some questions to consider when matching a delegated task with skill level are: Is the person licensed or unlicensed? Is the person in orientation or off orientation? How long has the person worked in the role? Has the person been checked off on this particular skill? Does the person feel confident that he or she can complete the task? Does the person need additional training or practice prior to completing the

(continued)

> ### EVIDENCE FROM THE LITERATURE (*continued*)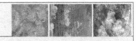
>
> skill independently? Use the Five Rights of Delegation to reflect on each step of the delegation process as you do the exercises in the article to examine how to delegate. Implications for nursing. It is useful to think through various scenarios prior to being faced with the decision to delegate as a new nurse.

CHAIN OF COMMAND

The licensed staff nurse, including the new graduate nurse, is accountable to the charge nurse of the unit where they are working. The charge nurse is accountable to the nurse manager. The nurse manager is accountable to the Chief Nursing Executive. The Chief Nursing Executive is accountable to the hospital's Chief Executive Officer. The hospital's Chief Executive Officer is accountable to the Board of Directors. The Board of Directors is accountable to the community it serves and often to another larger healthcare organization, as well as being accountable to state nursing and medical licensing boards and accreditation agencies, for example, The Joint Commission (TJC), Det Norske Veritas Healthcare, Inc. (DNV), Healthcare Facilities Accreditation Program (HFAP), or American Osteopathic Association. All of the aforementioned are accountable for their actions to the patients and the communities that they serve. See the organizational chain of command in Figure 6.2.

COMMUNICATION FACTORS INFLUENCING DELEGATION

Communication is a cornerstone to achieving success when delegating patient care. The Quality and Safety in Educating Nurses (QSEN) Patient-Centered Care (PCC) competency is defined as, "Recognize the patient or designee as the source of control and full partner in providing compassionate and coordinated care based on respect for patient's preferences, values, and needs" (www.qsen.org). The knowledge, skills, and attitudes of PCC include communication; the Five Rights of Delegation identify the necessity for communication; and the National Guidelines for Nursing Delegation has communication in the center of the Guidelines.

An excellent guide for communication with coworkers is the golden rule, "Do unto others as you would have them do unto you." Communication between nurses and coworkers often involves nursing delegation. Offering positive feedback to a UAP such as, "I appreciate the way you spoke with the patient in room 2345 to get him to ambulate twice this shift," goes a long way toward team building. "I will help you as soon as I can," is a statement that acknowledges that all team members' responsibilities are important.

The licensed nurse also ensures that all communication is culturally appropriate and respectful. Evidence shows that the better the communication and collaborative relationship between the licensed nurse and the delegatee, the better the chance a positive outcome of the delegation process will ensue (Corazzini et al., 2013; Damgaard & Young, 2014; Young & Damgaard, 2015). Reviewing the delegated responsibility with the delegatee and allowing for questions for clarification should be welcomed by the nurse. The licensed nurse should be available to the UAP for assistance and guidance in an ongoing manner. Under no circumstance is

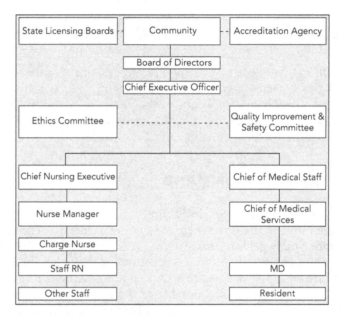

FIGURE 6.2 Organizational chain of command.

the nurse permitted to delegate a responsibility that requires any form of clinical reasoning, nursing judgment, or critical decision making. For example, a licensed nurse delegates the responsibility of checking a patient's blood sugar every 2 hours and reporting the results to the licensed nurse. The delegation cannot include having the delegatee make a nursing judgment of what action to take when the patient's blood sugar is low.

Communication on a patient-care unit often begins with a handoff report from one nurse to another to ensure continuity of patient care. The receiving nurse then completes an assignment sheet (Figure 6.3), a written or computerized plan that identifies the patient-care assignments on the unit to team members and the priorities for the shift. Assignments should consider several factors (Table 6.2) and include specific reporting guidelines, times for interventions, and deadlines for accomplishment of tasks.

SCOPE OF NURSING PRACTICE DECISION-MAKING FRAMEWORK

In early 2015, the Tri-Council for Nursing, consisting of the American Association of Colleges of Nursing (AACN), the ANA, the American Organization of Nurse Executives (AONE), and the National League for Nursing (NLN), in collaboration with NCSBN developed a Scope of Nursing Practice Decision-Making Framework to assist nurses and their employers in determining the responsibilities a nurse can safely perform. While decisions to delegate patient-care responsibilities are unique to different situations, the Scope of Nursing Practice Decision-Making Framework (Ballard et al., 2016) in Figure 6.4 can be applied to most situations. This Framework is for all nurses with various types of education and roles in different settings.

Nurse Manager: _____   House Supervisor: _____

Charge Nurse:_____Day_____SHIFT_____

Census	Isolations	Discharges	Planned Transfers

Patient Care Communication	Special Assignments
	CODE PAGER: _____

RNs:			UAP:		
Room	RN	UAP	Room	RN	UAP
401			405		
402			406		
403			407		
404			408		

FIGURE 6.3 Unit nursing assignment sheet.

TABLE 6.2 FACTORS CONSIDERED IN MAKING ASSIGNMENTS

- Number and acuity of patients
- Priority patient needs
- Number and type of staff
- State laws
- Organizational policies and procedures
- Patient-care standards
- Accreditation regulations
- Unit routines
- Geography of nursing unit
- Complexity of patient needs
- Staff responsibilities
- Attitude and dependability of staff
- Need for continuity of care by same staff

(continued)

TABLE 6.2 FACTORS CONSIDERED IN MAKING ASSIGNMENTS (*continued*)

- Need for fair work distribution among staff
- Need of patient for isolation and/or protection
- Skill, education, and competency of staff, i.e., RN, LPN/LVN, UAP
- Need to protect patient and staff from injury
- Environmental concerns
- Lunch/break times
- All delegation policies

LPN, licensed practical nurses; LVN, licensed vocational nurses, UAP, unlicensed assistive personnel.

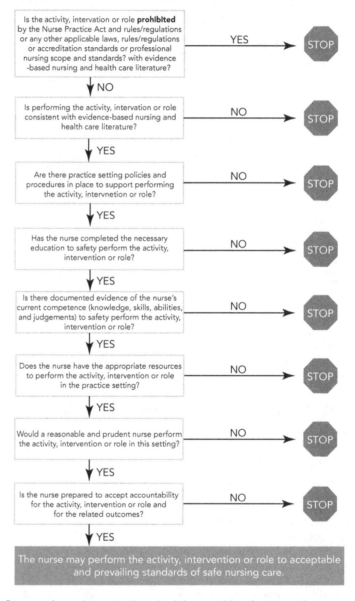

FIGURE 6.4 Scope of nursing practice decision-making framework.

Source: Ballard, K., Haagenson, D., Christiansen, L., Damgaard, G., Halstead, J. A, Jason, R. R., ... Alexander, M. (2016). Scope of nursing practice decision-making framework. *Journal of Nursing Regulation*, 7(3), 19–21.

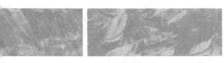

KEY CONCEPTS

- **Delegation** is allowing a delegatee to perform a specific nursing activity, skill, or procedure that is beyond the delegatee's traditional role and not routinely performed (NCSBN, 2016).
- The National Guidelines for Nursing Delegation were created in 2016 by the NCSBN.
- Different states have different NPAs and rules and regulations.
- **Responsibility** is the obligation involved when a person accepts an assignment. The delegation process is not complete until the person who receives the assignment accepts the responsibility for the assignment. Without this acceptance of responsibility, assignments cannot be delegated.
- If a person does not have the knowledge, skill, experience, or willingness needed to complete an assignment, it is inappropriate to accept responsibility for the assignment.
- Once a person accepts responsibility for an assignment, this responsibility is retained.
- A **delegated responsibility** is a nursing activity, skill, or procedure that is transferred from a licensed nurse to a delegatee. According to the National Guidelines for Nursing Delegation (NCSBN, 2016), "Any decision to delegate a nursing responsibility must be based on the needs of the patient or population, the stability and predictability of the patient's condition, the documented training and competence of the delegatee, and the ability of the licensed nurse to supervise the delegated responsibility and its outcome."
- **Assignment** is the routine care, activities, and procedures that are within the authorized scope of practice of the RN or LPN/VN or part of the routine functions of the UAP (NCSBN, 2016).
- Accountability is defined as "to be answerable to oneself and others for one's own choices, decisions, and actions as measured against a standard such as that established by the *Code of Ethics for Nurses with Interpretive Statements*" (ANA, 2015).
- **Authority** is the right to act or to command the action of others. Authority comes with the job and is required for a nurse to take action. The person with authority must be free to make decisions regarding the activities involved.
- Authority is based on the states/jurisdiction NPA and guides the development of an organization's job description with special consideration to the available staff mix and patient acuity.
- **Supervision** is the provision of guidance or direction, evaluation, and follow-up by the licensed nurse for accomplishment of a nursing task delegated to the UAP (NCSBN, 1995).
- When the needs of the patient coincide with the skills, knowledge, and competency of a UAP and can be performed safely, the licensed nurse will decide that delegation of a responsibility can occur. This decision is guided by the NCSBN Five Rights of Delegation (1995, 1996).
- The licensed staff nurse, including the new graduate nurse, is accountable to the charge nurse of the unit where they are working. The charge nurse is accountable to the nurse manager. The nurse manager is accountable to the Chief Nursing Executive. The Chief Nursing Executive is accountable to the hospital's Chief Executive Officer. The hospital's Chief Executive Officer is accountable to the Board of Directors. The Board of Directors is accountable to the community it serves and

often to another larger healthcare organization, as well as being accountable to state nursing and medical licensing boards and accreditation agencies, for example, TJC, DNV, HFAP, or American Osteopathic Association. All of the aforementioned are accountable for their actions to the patients and the communities that they serve.

• Communication on a patient-care unit often begins with a handoff report from one nurse to another to ensure continuity of patient care. The receiving nurse then completes an assignment sheet, a written or computerized plan that identifies the patient-care assignments on the unit to team members and the priorities for the shift. Assignments should consider several factors and include specific reporting guidelines, times for interventions, and deadlines for accomplishment of tasks.

• The Tri-Council for Nursing, consisting of AACN, ANA, AONE, and NLN, in collaboration with the NCSBN developed a Scope of Nursing Practice Decision-Making Framework to assist nurses and their employers in determining the responsibilities a nurse can safely perform.

KEY TERMS

Accountability
Assignment
Authority
Delegated responsibility

Delegation
Responsibility
Supervision

REVIEW QUESTIONS

1. The nurse is performing an assessment on a patient who is taking 400 mg of naproxen for abdominal pain. Which assessment can be delegated to the unlicensed nursing personnel?

   A. Review the results of the patient's Hgb and hematocrit.
   B. Collect and send a stool sample to the laboratory for guaiac testing.
   C. Auscultate the abdomen for bowel sounds.
   D. Ask the patient what other medications they are taking.

2. Which of the following is a responsibility of the employer and/or nurse leader when delegating nursing responsibilities to the UAP?

   A. Assigning the UAP responsibilities.
   B. Establishing licensure guidelines for UAP.
   C. Making certain that appropriate policies and procedures for delegation are in place.
   D. Encouraging staff to create a delegation sheet at the beginning of every shift.

3. The licensed nurse delegated to the UAP to ambulate the patient to the bathroom. The UAP is having difficulties completing this delegated task. What is the proper action the UAP must take?

   A. Delegate the task to another UAP.
   B. Notify the employer of the UAP's inability to complete this particular task.
   C. Notify the licensed nurse of the UAP's difficulties with completing this task.
   D. Document that the patient was unable to ambulate to the bathroom.

4. The patient assigned to a new graduate nurse has an order to have a nasogastric tube inserted. The nurse has never completed this type of procedure. How should the new graduate nurse proceed?

   A. Request assistance from an experienced nurse.
   B. Delegate the procedure to a UAP.
   C. Notify the physician of the new graduate nurse's inexperience.
   D. Look-up the policy and procedure, then insert the tube.

5. The nurse delegated to another nurse to disconnect an IV line from a patient once the infusion is complete. Which factors should the nurse consider prior to delegating this to another nurse? Select all that apply.

   A. Right person
   B. Right supervision and evaluation
   C. Right direction and communication
   D. Right task
   E. Right circumstance

6. A new graduate nurse is caring for two patients during the fifth week of new employee orientation. The new graduate nurse asks one of the unit nurses to see the policy and procedure for delegation. The unit nurse looks at the new graduate nurse with a puzzled look and says, "I don't know if we have one." What is the best reason for the unit nurse's reply?

   A. There probably is not a delegation policy or procedure.
   B. The new graduate nurse should not be asking this question when caring for only two patients.
   C. The unit nurse is not aware of a policy or procedure for delegation.
   D. Delegation is something taught in nursing school, but is not practiced in the real world.

7. Who is legally responsible for nursing care provided to patients?

   A. Physician
   B. Nurse manager
   C. RN assigned to patient
   D. UAP providing care to patient

8. QSEN has developed multiple quality and safety elements to guide nursing practice. Identify which of these are considered a part of the six key elements.

   A. Quality improvement (QI), teamwork and collaboration, and evidence-based practice
   B. Fact finding, mission statements, and strategic planning
   C. Stakeholder feedback, budget reconciliation, and strategic planning
   D. Financial reporting, wait time measurements, and time delays in getting treatments.

9. The nurse is preparing to review discharge instructions with a patient. The nurse instructs the patient regarding medications and wound care for her foot. What indicates to the nurse the level of understanding the patient has regarding discharge instructions?

    A. The patient signs the discharge instruction sheet.
    B. When asked by the nurse, the patient denies any questions or concerns.
    C. The patient asks for new prescriptions for the pharmacy.
    D. The nurse observes the patient changing the dressing on her foot wound.

10. The nurse is transferring a patient from the ICU to the step-down patient-care unit. When the ICU nurse calls report to the receiving unit, what is the best way for the nurse to provide the handoff information?

    A. Situation, background, assessment, requirements
    B. Situation, background, assessment, recommendations
    C. Systems, background, activities, recommendations
    D. Systems, background, activities, requirements

REVIEW ACTIVITIES

1. Click on the link from QSEN to watch the Lewis Blackman story: qsen.org/qsen-videos-lewis-blackman-story-released/. What responsibilities should the nurse have delegated to allow more time to focus on the patient?
2. Interview three nurses on the unit where you are currently doing a clinical rotation. Ask each nurse, "What responsibility is delegated to Unlicensed Assistive Personnel (UAP) most often on this unit?" Make a list. Compare their answers. Review the policy and procedure for the delegated responsibilities to UAPs. What did you find?
3. Show two nursing instructors the Scope of Nursing Practice Decision-Making Framework in Figure 6.4. Ask each instructor how they implement the Framework in their practice. What were their responses?

CRITICAL DISCUSSION POINTS

1. What references should a licensed nurse refer to when considering delegating to a UAP in a state other than his or her own?
2. During your clinical, what examples of delegation did you observe? Were the delegated responsibilities in the delegatee's job description? How was it decided what could be delegated and what could not?

QSEN ACTIVITY

1. Go to the QSEN website (www.qsen.org) and search for Delegation. Click on Delegation: A Collaborative, Patient-Centered Approach (qsen.org/delegation-a-collaborative-patient-centered-approach/). Click on one of the Case Studies and work through it to improve your Delegation skills.
2. Go to the QSEN website (www.qsen.org) and search for Delegation. Click on Learning Module 1 (qsen.org/faculty-resources/courses/learning-modules/module-one/). Use the module to improve your nursing delegation skills.

EXPLORING THE WEB

1. Visit www.youtube.com and search for "Delegating effectively NCSBN." Select some of the Popular Videos on Delegation & Nursing and begin viewing some of them.
2. Visit the Indiana Center for Evidence Based Nursing Practice at www.ebnp.org. Hover over "About Us" then click on "Evidence into Practice."
3. Login and register your name at www.nursingcenter.com to receive articles, continuing education, and information on topics such as quality and safety and delegation.

REFERENCES

American Nurses Association (ANA). (2015). *Code of ethics for nurses with interpretive statements.* Retrieved from http://nursingworld.org/DocumentVault/Ethics-1/Code-of-Ethics-for-Nurses.html

American Nurses Association (ANA). (2016). *Code of ethics for nurses.* Silver Spring, MD: Author.

American Nurses Association and National Council of State Boards of Nursing. (2006). *Joint statement on delegation.* Retrieved from https://www.NCSBN.org/Delegation_joint_statement_NCSBN-ANA.pdf

Ballard, K., Haagenson, D., Christiansen, L., Damgaard, G., Halstead, J. A., Jason, R. R., … Alexander, M. (2016). Scope of nursing practice decision-making framework. *Journal of Nursing Regulation, 7*(3), 19–21.

Buppert, C. (2016, December 28). Can a patient care tech perform this task? Medscape.

Corazzini, K. N., Anderson, R. A., Mueller, C., Hunt-McKinney, S., Day, L., … Porter, K. (2013). Understanding RN and LPN patterns of practice in nursing homes. *Journal of Nursing Regulation, 4*(1), 14–18.

Damgaard, G., & Young, L. (2014). Virtual nursing care for school children with diabetes. *Journal of Nursing Regulation, 4*(4), 15–24.

National Council of State Boards of Nursing (NCSBN). (1995). *Delegation: Concepts and decision-making process.* National Council of State Boards of Nursing 1995 Annual Meeting Business Book.

National Council of State Boards of Nursing (NCSBN). (1996). *Delegation: Concepts and decision-making process.* National Council of State Boards of Nursing 1996 Annual Meeting Business Book.

National Council of State Boards of Nursing (NCSBN). (2016). Nursing guidelines for nursing delegation. *Journal of Nursing Regulation, 7*(1), 5–12.

Shannon, R. A., & Kubelka, S. (2013). Reducing the risks of delegation use of procedure skills checklist for unlicensed assistive personnel in schools, part 1. *NASN School Nurse, 28*(4), 178–181. doi:10.1177/1942602X13489886

Young, L., & Damgaard, G. (2015). Transitioning the virtual nursing care for school children with diabetes study to a sustainable model of nursing care. *Journal of Nursing Regulation, 6*(2), 4–9. doi:10.1016/S2155-8256(15)30380-X

SUGGESTED READINGS

Agency for Healthcare Research and Quality. (2016). *Patient safety primer: Handoffs and signouts*. Retrieved from https://psnet.ahrq.gov/primers/primer/9/handoffs-and-signout

Anthony, M. K., & Vidal, K. (2010). Mindful communication: A novel approach to improving delegation and increasing patient safety. *The Online Journal of Issues in Nursing, 15(2)*. doi:10.3912/OJIN.Vol15No2Man02

Barra, M. (2011). Nurse delegation of medication pass in assisted living facilities: Not all medication assistant technicians are equal. *Journal of Nursing Law, 14(1)*, 3–10.

Flicek, C. L. (2012, November/December). Communication: A dynamic between nurses and physicians. *Medsurg Nursing: Pitman, 21(6)*, 385–387.

Hansen, F., McKenna, H. P., & Keeney, S. (2013). Delegating and supervising unregistered professionals: The student nurse experience. *Nurse Education Today, 33(3)*, 229–235. doi:10.1016/j.nedt.2012.02.008.

Kalisch, B. J. (2011). The impact of RN-UAP relationships on quality and safety. *Nursing Management, 42(9)*, 16–22.

Kreitzer, M. J., & Koithan, M. (2014). *Integrative nursing*. Oxford, England: Oxford University Press.

Lloyd, J. (2014). Still trying to do it all yourself? Tips for effective delegation. *Health Care Collector, 28(7)*, 8.

McCloskey, R., Donovan, C., Stewart, C., & Donovon, A. (2015). How registered nurses, licensed practical nurses and resident assistants spend time in nursing homes: An observational study. (2015). *International Journal of Nursing Studies, 52(9)*, 1475–1483.

McMullen, T. L. Resnick, B., Chin-Hansen, J., Geiger-Brown, J. M., Miller, N., & Rubenstein, R. (2015). Certified nurse aide scope of practice: State-by-state differences in allowable delegated activities. *Journal of the American Medical Directors Association, 16(1)*, 20–24.

Mueller, C., & Vogelsmeier, A. (2013). Effective delegation: Understanding responsibility, authority, and accountability. *Journal of Nursing Regulation, 4(3)*, 20–27.

Quality and Safety Education for Nurses. (2017). *QSEN*. Retrieved from www.qsen.org

Saccomano, S. J., & Pinto-Zipp, G. (2011). Registered nurse leadership style and confidence in delegation. *Journal of Nursing Management, 19*, 522–533.

Twigg, D. E., Myers, H., Duffield, C., Pugh, J. D., Gelder, L., & Roche, M. (2016). The impact of adding assistants in nursing to acute care hospital ward nurse staffing on adverse patient outcomes: An analysis of administrative health data. *International Journal of Nursing Studies, 63*, 189–200.

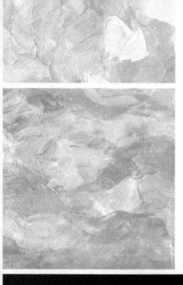

UNIT II.

**THE USE OF QUALITY AND SAFETY
EDUCATION CONCEPTS BY NURSING
LEADERS AND MANAGERS**

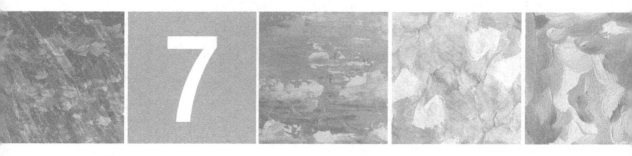

PATIENT-CENTERED CARE

Carolyn A. Christie-McAuliffe

Transforming Health Care One Nurse, One Caregiver, One Organization, At a Time.

(Dr. Jean Watson, 2012, World Caring Science Institute, watsoncaringscience.org)

Upon completion of this chapter, the reader should be able to

1. Describe characteristics of patient-centered care (PCC).
2. Identify basic components of empathetic communication and describe its importance to PCC.
3. Discuss the psychosocial factors associated with the impact of physical illness and injury.
4. List strategies to support patient-centered healthcare.
5. Describe the impact of legislation such as the Patient Protection and Affordable Care Act (ACA) in facilitating PCC.
6. Discuss discharge planning as a means of ensuring continuity of care.
7. List information technologies that facilitate PCC.
8. Explain the significance of patient-centered measures and monitors of quality healthcare.
9. Describe the importance of patient satisfaction relative to measuring the accomplishment of PCC.

Y ou are a nurse on a very busy medical–surgical unit. Mrs. Rodriguez is a 76-year-old patient who suffered a stroke and is being discharged within the next few days. She is a widow whose children live an hour away and her most frequent visitor is the priest from her church.

Each day, the interprofessional team completes rounds on the unit. As the contact point for Mrs. Jones and her family, you have been directed by the charge nurse to communicate the discharge plan to the patient and family/designee.

- *Before you can effectively participate in the interprofessional team rounds, what must you understand about your patient?*
- *What are some interventions that will support an effective care transition for this patient?*
- *Who will be key contact points in the family to ensure patient continuity of care posthospitalization?*

Decades ago a paradigm shift to caring within healthcare settings was introduced that emphasized moving from a technocratic focus to establishing caring relationships, identifying the patient as a consumer of care to recognizing the patient as a partner in care, and providing service from the perspective of the expert provider for healthcare services to the perspective of the collaborative partnership between patient and provider for healthcare services. This new paradigm embraces values, relationships, and preferences, recognizing the patient as a participant in his or her own care. Although this paradigm shift has taken time to be accepted within a highly technological and authoritative healthcare system, it has awakened the need for nursing and healthcare providers to support the patient's role in control of his or her own healthcare decisions.

Currently, many federal initiatives are being implemented to address the need for quality care and patient safety and are transforming healthcare settings into accountable, safe, patient-centered environments that respect the unique needs and values of the patient. This process of transformation within healthcare has evolved into providing compassionate care that recognizes the patient as an integral member of the interprofessional team. With patients central to all services, nurses and healthcare providers are establishing true, collaborative relationships as partners in healthcare service to address healthcare needs through the lens of the patient.

Thus, this chapter focuses on strategies and practices that support patient-centered care (PCC) that aim to improve patient safety and quality patient care. Characteristics of PCC are discussed as are the components of communication that help to ensure it is actualized. Psychosocial factors associated with the realities of disease and illness are described within the context of how the interprofessional team can implement strategies that support patient-centered healthcare. Legislation impacting the ability to deliver PCC is presented. Innovations that foster PCC are discussed including how continuity of care is augmented with effective discharge planning and use of novel technologies empowering patients to function as integral members of the interprofessional healthcare team. Finally, patient-centered measures and monitors of quality healthcare and measurements of patient satisfaction are presented in relation to PCC.

PATIENT-CENTERED CARE

PCC "recognizes the patient or designee as the source of control and full partner in providing compassionate and coordinated care based on respect for patient's preferences, values, and needs" (Quality and Safety Education for Nurses [QSEN], 2012, p. 1). Nurses and healthcare providers coordinate patient-care services with compassion and respect through a collaborative partnership between the patient and interprofessional team.

Today, with nurse leaders in the forefront of healthcare services, the Institute of Medicine (IOM) as well as other national campaigns for quality care have drawn attention to the necessity of maintaining safety, providing quality care, and keeping the patient at the center and in control of his or her care to meet his or her health needs. This attention is intended to ensure that all healthcare providers are accountable for quality care through PCC services, careful monitoring of patient outcomes, and validation of improvement in the patient's health. It is paramount that nurses and healthcare providers recognize that the patient is a full partner within the interprofessional team and that the patient is in control of his or her care. PCC is a new way of practicing and providing care through the lens of the patient with respect for his or her values, meaning of health, and preferences. To achieve true PCC, healthcare practice must include the characteristics of PCC that ensure patient engagement via effective communication, education, and coordination of services. Within this goal, Pettetier and Stickler (2014) address the need for nurse leaders to accept the responsibility for the achievement of PCC by specifically ensuring patients are fully engaged in all aspects of their care. They begin this argument by stating the absolute need and commitment to PCC by healthcare facilities based on respect for patient self-determination (or right to make decisions for oneself) and autonomy (right to self-govern based on values). To effectively implement PCC within an organization, they delineate competencies of the healthcare providers from those of the patient in order to ensure patient engagement. For providers, Pettetier and Stickler (2014) echo the competencies outlined by QSEN (2012), which include the need for effective communication that allows the patient to articulate their values, needs, and desires for care. For nurses, once this information is obtained, it is expected they will communicate the patient's preferences to the rest of the care team. Within this process of integrating the patient's wishes, the healthcare professional will also assess for any barriers that might impede their actualization, including the potential need for patient education not to sway the individual's choice but rather to ensure full informed decision making. In contrast, the authors explain, patients need only to be "empowered" through the provision of knowledge as well as know how to "negotiate" with healthcare providers. While these are important characteristics, it is important to note that many patients will have difficulty with either or both of these competencies. However, nurses are in a unique and effective position to provide education, support, and advocacy that facilitate engagement.

It is vital to understand PCC is based on the unique values held by *the patient*. These values can be based on many aspects of the person including physical condition, culture, generation or age, socioeconomic factors, as well as religion and/or spirituality (see Table 7.1). Soliciting these values becomes a cornerstone of ensuring PCC. Miles and Mezzich (2011) substantiate the need to consider all aspects of the patient's value system within the context of evidence-based medicine in order to allow the clinician and patient the opportunity to establish a relationship based on respect, trust, equality, and shared responsibility. They contend this ensures the successful intersection of science, compassion, and quality.

TABLE 7.1 INDIVIDUAL FACTORS THAT INFLUENCE PATIENTS' VALUE SYSTEMS

Ethnicity and cultural background
Religion and/or spirituality
Gender identification
Age or generational difference
Educational level
Socioeconomic status
Moral development

REAL-WORLD INTERVIEW

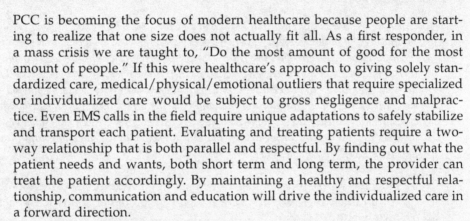

PCC is becoming the focus of modern healthcare because people are starting to realize that one size does not actually fit all. As a first responder, in a mass crisis we are taught to, "Do the most amount of good for the most amount of people." If this were healthcare's approach to giving solely standardized care, medical/physical/emotional outliers that require specialized or individualized care would be subject to gross negligence and malpractice. Even EMS calls in the field require unique adaptations to safely stabilize and transport each patient. Evaluating and treating patients require a two-way relationship that is both parallel and respectful. By finding out what the patient needs and wants, both short term and long term, the provider can treat the patient accordingly. By maintaining a healthy and respectful relationship, communication and education will drive the individualized care in a forward direction.

I work in an urban ED with a high daily patient volume. When patients come into the ED in a tense situation where emotion and stress are high, I find that it is essential to communicate PCC in short and simple ways. When moving together, the patient can get the highest quality care and the provider can ensure no harm is done. The nurse may be the first person to sense what a patient may need, as nurses are often the first to interact with the patient. The nurse also knows the medical staff and can anticipate the dynamics of a patient-care team. This demonstrates how important it is for nurses to identify the patient's needs as sometimes the nurse is the only person that the patient has to advocate for them.

Cara Carpenter, BSN, RN, CEN
St. Joseph's Hospital and Health Center
Syracuse, New York

Advocacy

Serving as an advocate to patients is another key hallmark of PCC and is an essential component of nursing and leadership within the interprofessional healthcare team. Advocacy refers to any activity that ultimately assists a patient in receiving the "best" care depending on the patient's needs and wishes. Florence Nightingale emphasized nurses must keep the patient central to nursing care, an obligation that remains embodied in nursing's application of values such as beneficence and fidelity (Bradshaw, 1999; Hoyt, 2010). Patient empowerment reflects a form of self-directed advocacy that enables and motivates patients to bring about changes and make decisions to manage and improve their health (Bann, Sirois, & Walsh, 2010). Through a patient-centered approach to advocacy and empowerment, a partnership between the caregiver and the patient can increase the patient's autonomy and involvement in his or her own care, especially in chronic illnesses such as diabetes (Asimakopoulou, Gilbert, Newton, & Scambler, 2012; Figure 7.1).

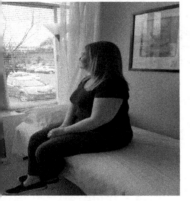

FIGURE 7.1 A patient waiting for test results.

CRITICAL THINKING 7.1

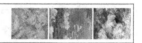

Consider the following situation and identify the nurse's behaviors associated with promoting the patient's sense of control over her care. Mrs. Dawes is in a subacute rehabilitation facility recovering from a knee replacement. Sue Jones is her primary nurse. Nurse Jones approaches Mrs. Dawes, introduces herself, and asks Mrs. Dawes how she would like to be addressed. She also reviews with Mrs. Dawes what she might expect from the rehabilitation program and how she might deal with the discomfort that could result from her therapy. Nurse Jones also gives Mrs. Dawes her choices of times for therapy and menus for meal selection. She answers all her questions and provides her with the list of her therapies.

1. How has Nurse Jones engaged the patient in a number of behaviors that would likely increase Mrs. Dawes's perception of her ability to impact her own health?
2. What are strategies Nurse Jones could have implemented to include others on the interprofessional team at the onset of her meeting with Mrs. Dawes to ensure advocacy and PCC?

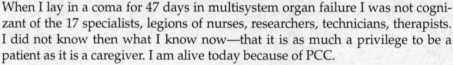

REAL-WORLD INTERVIEW

When I lay in a coma for 47 days in multisystem organ failure I was not cognizant of the 17 specialists, legions of nurses, researchers, technicians, therapists. I did not know then what I know now—that it is as much a privilege to be a patient as it is a caregiver. I am alive today because of PCC.

My continuity of care has spanned several decades so much so that my professional and personal life in the field often feel like one and the same. I take my responsibility as a patient and caregiver seriously. It is not simply a right but a privilege to be included in conversation about an individual's well-being and safety—be it my own or someone else's. I hold practitioners to an extremely high standard, not only for what they already know, but what they want to know and take the time to learn. In this field, it is time we often seem to be racing rather than respecting.

We are, in American healthcare, surrounded by resources, research, and genius. Yet we are all too often lacking in relationship and communication with patients. The challenges are many: a fractured socioeconomy; a somewhat unknowable future as it relates to funding and access; and all the nuances of care for varying populations and needs. Add to that quotas, liability, and privacy restrictions along with other elements of industry invading the patient experience, it is a wonder the Hippocratic Oath has not been rewritten to include bylaws with a daily reminder of the regulations and a mandate of self-care for the provider.

Quality and quantity of service look different with every individual be it in an office or at the bedside. Triaging patients for myocardial infarctions, GSWs, and nausea may be your skill set. Triaging mind, body, and spirit is far trickier and no less important. For every cell in the body of a patient that needs specific

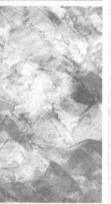

(continued)

REAL-WORLD INTERVIEW (*continued*)

treatment there is a unique corresponding memory or experience in those cells that makes the patient a person, a human being, just like you. And you matter! The next time you begin your shift, or rounds, or class, remember that everyone has a story beyond their symptoms that will inform their care. It might be the one that changes your life. It certainly changed mine.

Kate D. Mahoney
International Speaker, Actorvist, Ambassador to Patients and Caregivers
Author, The Misfit Miracle Girl: Candid Reflections

EMPATHETIC COMMUNICATION

As discussed earlier, effective communication is essential for patient engagement and PCC. To effectively communicate information, consideration for clarity and readiness to learn must be made. However, to elicit subjective beliefs and values, healthcare professionals must employ strategies that convey respect and facilitate trust. Strategies or types of communication that encourage this level of sharing are based on communication that is based on empathy. **Empathetic communication** is simply the act of communicating with someone else from the vantage point of that person's feelings, values, and perspective, and is the foundation of establishing relationships that are consistent with PCC. When using empathetic communication, the nurse and patient enter into a relationship characterized by both empathy and a genuine sense of respect for the patient's opinions and decisions. To better understand the nature of empathetic communication, the nurse and healthcare provider must first recognize the difference between empathy and sympathy, be proficient in the basic elements of communication, and appreciate the major psychosocial factors associated with the role of patient.

While empathy and sympathy are highly related concepts as well as integral to the provision of PCC, they are distinct and different (Decety & Michalska, 2010). Empathy involves the ability to understand and share the emotional experience observed in another person. Sympathy by contrast is defined as emotional concern for another (Kunzmann, 2011). Empathetic communication has three essential components: the ability to take the perspective of another, the ability to appreciate the emotions of another even when they are different from your own, and the ability to communicate that understanding to the patient (Burks & Kobus, 2012). There are a number of behaviors that facilitate empathetic communication and thus promote PCC. Likewise, there are nonempathetic communication behaviors that hinder communication and thereby impede PCC. Table 7.2 lists a representative sample of empathetic and nonempathetic communication behaviors.

TABLE 7.2 EMPATHETIC AND NONEMPATHETIC COMMUNICATION BEHAVIORS

EMPATHETIC COMMUNICATION	NONEMPATHETIC COMMUNICATION
Listens carefully and reflects back a summary of the patient's concerns	Interrupts patient with irrelevant information
Uses terms and vocabulary that are appropriate for the patient	Uses vocabulary that is either beneath the level of the patient or not understandable to the patient

(*continued*)

TABLE 7.2 EMPATHETIC AND NONEMPATHETIC COMMUNICATION BEHAVIORS (*continued*)

EMPATHETIC COMMUNICATION	NONEMPATHETIC COMMUNICATION
Calls patient by patient's preferred name	Uses language that may be perceived as cajoling, patronizing, or demeaning, for example, "honey"
Uses respectful and professional language	Uses nonprofessional language
Asks patient what they need and responds promptly to those needs	Chastises patient
Provides helpful and informative information	Provides patient with inappropriate information
Solicits feedback from the patient	Asks questions at inappropriate times and gives patient advice inappropriately
Uses self-disclosure appropriately	Self-discloses inappropriately
Employs humor as appropriate	Preaches to the patient
Provides words of comfort when appropriate	Scolds the patient

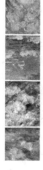

CASE STUDY 7.1

On morning rounds, a doctor and nurse enter a patient's room to assess him in preparation for his cardiac catheterization scheduled later in the day. The nurse introduces herself to the patient, "Good morning, Mr. Potter, I am Jane Smith, the nurse, and I will be assisting Dr. Turk with the procedure today." Mr. Potter replies, "Okay, I hope you know what you are doing. I am already in pain and I don't need you to add to it." Mr. Potter's emotional undertones are obviously hostile and offensive.

1. *How do you think Jane Smith, the nurse, felt when listening to hostile tones in the patient's voice and remarks toward her competency?*
2. *How would you respond, maintaining a respectful and open dialogue between you and the patient?*
3. *How would you respond if the doctor or another member of the interprofessional team was criticizing your skills and competency in caring for a patient?*
4. *How would you respond, maintaining a respectful relationship with the healthcare team?*

Elements of Communication

Communication simultaneously takes place verbally and nonverbally. Verbal communication has a cognitive (what we say) and affective (emotional) component, while nonverbal communication has a behavioral (what we do) and affective (emotional) component. To communicate effectively, the listener must attend to all elements of the communication process. This is not always easy to do although particularly important to remember in terms of providing PCC.

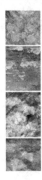

CASE STUDY 7.2

As a senior nursing student, you are under much pressure to follow PowerPoint slides, listen to the lecture, and take notes, all at the same time! You ask a friend if you can borrow her notes from class so you can be sure you have everything you need for the next test. Your friend verbally agrees but places her notes in her book bag and immediately leaves the room. You try to contact her later that day, but she does not respond to your calls, texts, or emails.

1. *What are major factors underlying the communication process?*
2. *What conflict in values or beliefs might exist to explain what happened?*

Nonverbal Communication

Sometimes the verbal and nonverbal components of a patient's communication are incongruent and provide conflicting messages. For example, a patient might verbally indicate that nothing is bothering him or her but his or her nonverbal body language is communicating something quite different (Table 7.3). The empathetic communicator must discern the real meaning behind the patient's verbal and nonverbal behavior. It is the nonverbal aspect of the communication that provides nurses and healthcare providers with the most important clues about inner feelings. For example, if your patient states he or she is not afraid to have surgery but looks away from you and/or begins wringing his or her hands as you discuss the upcoming operation, you would probably think to yourself that your patient's words do not match his or her nonverbal communication.

Cultural Influences and Beliefs on Communication

Smiles, warm gestures, and welcoming words are universal signs of caring in many cultures. Nurses and other interprofessional members of the healthcare team, however, must also realize that expressions of caring can be perceived differently across cultures. In addition, there are many factors that can affect the quality and clarity of communications and healthcare providers must be proactive to address any potential barriers. For

TABLE 7.3 EXAMPLES OF NONVERBAL BEHAVIOR

NONVERBAL BEHAVIOR	EXAMPLES
Eye movement and features	Either steady eye contact or inability to make eye contact, blinking, teary eyes opened or closed
Body position, movement, behavior, and stance	Tense, relaxed, jerky, fidgety, legs crossed, arms crossed, agitated, calm, use of hands, gestures
Facial expression	Grimaces, smiles, frowns, no expression or flat affect, exaggerated expression
Tone of voice	Mumbles, whispers, high pitched, quiet; rate of speech either speedy or slowed
Skin	Blushes, sweats, general pallor
General appearance	Appropriateness of dress for weather and/or event, neatness, accessories, stature

example, language barriers may be present. The use of interpreters can provide a safe space where patients can freely express their concerns and be understood through the interpreter, calming their fears and apprehensions in an unfamiliar situation and setting. While bilingual family members can be appropriately used for basic exchanges of information, communication of complex healthcare information may require the help of other interpreters. When bilingual family member interpreters are not available in person, healthcare providers can access trained interpreters through various certified telephone services, for example, CTS Language Link, which can be accessed through its website at www.ctslanguagelink.com. Certified healthcare interpreters can help all parties understand the strengths and needs of the patient and family.

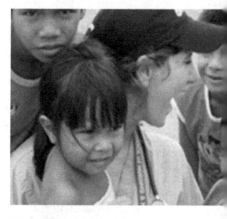

FIGURE 7.2 Nonverbal communication.

Effective patient-centered communication, even when done through an interpreter, provides an opportunity for a personal exchange between patient and provider that fosters clarity and understanding of what is needed to continue the patient's care and include the patient as an active partner in the recovery process. Patience and fortitude in understanding the patient's cultural norms and healthcare practices that are unique to the patient's culture must be respected (Figure 7.2).

CRITICAL THINKING 7.2

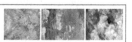

Nurse Johnson is caring for a patient newly diagnosed with diabetes. The patient speaks English as a second language and is a recent immigrant to the United States. The patient is able to make her basic needs known but does not ask questions or speak unless prompted to do so. Nurse Johnson has been unable to determine if this patient can self-inject her insulin. The patient nods and smiles as Nurse Johnson begins teaching her about insulin and her diagnosis.

1. What strategies can Nurse Johnson employ to facilitate self-management in this patient?
2. What resources and/or services can the nurse use to ensure that the patient has understood the instruction?

PSYCHOSOCIAL FACTORS ASSOCIATED WITH THE ROLE OF THE PATIENT

Understanding how a person's life is affected by illness is essential in understanding patient reactions and emotions. This level of understanding leads to the ability to take another's perspective and is a precursor to empathetic communication, the cornerstone of PCC (Burks & Kobus, 2012). Being a patient is a role that most people find challenging. This is because illness can greatly impact a person's self-concept (Taylor, 2011). For a better understanding of the impact of illness on the patient, nurses and healthcare providers need to understand self-concept and the impact illness has on how one perceives oneself. **Self-concept** is the conception an individual holds about his or her own particular traits, aptitudes, and unique characteristics; it typically includes physical, social, and personal components (Taylor, 2011).

Physical self refers to the conception a person has of his or her physical body and physical capacities. Illness and chronic illness impact a person's physical self because it changes how an individual evaluates his or her body. Consider, for example, a newly diagnosed breast cancer patient facing a mastectomy. The mastectomy has the potential of challenging the patient's perception of herself as a woman. The mastectomy might also change the patient's conception of how she sees herself sexually. Social self involves the roles the individual holds in a social environment. In the case of the breast cancer patient, the mastectomy might affect the patient's social self as a wife and member of the community. A serious illness may change the social self the patient has in his or her family or work situation. Serious illness and injury may change the patient's role from being the family breadwinner to role of the dependent person requiring care and assistance. Personal self embodies all the goals and dreams we have for ourselves now and in the future. Illness or injury sometimes prohibits the realization of those goals and dreams. For example, the young high school football star may have had aspirations of becoming a professional football player. A serious injury on the field may thwart those plans forever.

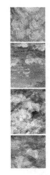

CASE STUDY 7.3

Mary is a 28-year-old female in the prime of her life. Mary has completed her master's degree in education and is employed as a kindergarten teacher, which she absolutely loves. She has always been independent and enjoyed being single. Mary developed generalized pain that progressively worsened over the course of 2 years. Mary also found that her general energy level was low and she could no longer concentrate for any length of time. Mary sought medical care and was diagnosed with fibromyalgia. She was forced to give up her kindergarten job and found herself not only in pain but frustrated professionally. She believes the fibromyalgia has impacted her physically and professionally.

1. *How can chronic illness impact Mary's perspective on her personal life?*
2. *Explore the web for support services that are available to her at home. What might a few services be?*

STRATEGIES TO SUPPORT PATIENT-CENTERED PRACTICE

As discussed earlier, the IOM's (2001) report identified specific aims to improve the quality and safety of healthcare. Among these aims, the patient-centered model of care has become a core component that ensures patient values and guides clinical decisions. Through this patient-centered model of care, the healthcare industry is called upon to develop innovative strategies to support patients and caregivers in becoming greater participants in their healthcare. Patient-centered outcomes research emphasizes decision making between the patient and provider that is collaborative, mutual, and shared. Health literacy is one major factor grounded in informed decision making. Thus, many innovative strategies exist to enhance PCC including methods for increasing health literacy.

Alleviating Barriers to Healthcare Literacy

Considering a patient's health literacy is another crucial aspect to providing PCC. Ratzan and Parker's (2000) definition of **health literacy** is used in the IOM's (2004) consensus report on health literacy as "the degree to which individuals have the capacity to obtain, process, and understand basic health information and services they need to make appropriate health decisions" (p. 31). A patient's basic education and competencies in reading, writing, and mathematics are important components of his or her health literacy as well as skills such as listening and speaking. Those patients and families with limited health literacy skills and knowledge do not have the same resources, ability, or competencies to achieve optimal health services as those who are health literate. Language barriers and poorly understood cultural practices may also adversely impact healthcare communication. Populations vulnerable to low levels of health literacy include ethnic minority groups, recent immigrants, older adults and elderly populations, individuals living with chronic diseases, and populations of people at poverty or even lower socioeconomic class (Center for Health Care Strategies, Inc., 2010).

The issue of health literacy is very complex and requires a multidimensional approach by the interprofessional healthcare team to understand the impact that it has on healthy lifestyles, engagement in health promotion activities, self-efficacy, and optimizing one's potential for well-being. Nurse leaders must recognize that the healthcare system and the educational system, as well as social and cultural factors, all play a role on the impact of health literacy. Healthy People 2020 (U.S. Department of Health and Human Services [HHS], 2011c) has identified improving health literacy as one of its key goals to promoting healthy outcomes and enhancing quality of life. In the past, health literacy was considered a task of educators and viewed from the perspective of the patient's intellectual deficits. Today, health literacy is recognized as a healthcare system's issue.

Health literacy is ensured when nurses and the interprofessional healthcare team reinforce pertinent information with the patient through simple explanations that avoid medical jargon. Patients must understand their role and what it is they need to do to safely follow dietary and healthcare treatments. They must understand why quality of care requires adherence to prescribed medications and the importance of communicating with their provider when encountering difficulties. Healthcare practitioners must encourage patients to ask questions and take an active role in their education to improve care activities. Patients who are well informed and more involved in their care experience better health outcomes (HHS, 2010). Patient initiatives, such as Ask Me 3 (National Patient Safety Foundation, 2011) and Questions Are the Answer (Agency for Healthcare Research and Quality [AHRQ], 2011b) are campaigns designed to promote communication and encourage patients to seek and understand the answers to common questions, that is, What is my main problem? What do I need to do? Why is it important for me to do this? Patient safety can be improved when patients understand their role in their healthcare.

Patient Decision Making

Soliciting the patient's values, needs, and preferences is but one part of assisting them in participatory decision making. Including them in important conversations relative to health status, treatment choice, and evaluation are crucial but how does a nurse actually accomplish this? Fortunately, tools exist that systemically and effectively facilitate this process. One such website is simply called Patient. It offers education about specific conditions and provides pros and cons of treatments typically suggested (patient.info/decision-aids) as a starting point for relevant discussions with their healthcare provider. Additional tools are available through the Mayo Clinic, AHRQ, and HealthITh.gov.

Nurse scholar, Dawn (2015) has examined how to ensure that decision-making aids such as the Patient website encourage interprofessional efforts that help all healthcare providers to hear the needs and wishes of their patients. Her efforts to date have demonstrated lack of interprofessional application of these aids; however, she has facilitated important improvements by bringing important attention to why and how patients make decisions about their healthcare.

EVIDENCE FROM THE LITERATURE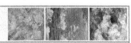

Citation

Stiles, E. (2011). Promoting health literacy in patients with diabetes. *Nursing Standard, 26*(8), 35–40.

Discussion

Patients with low health literacy may struggle with obtaining, understanding, and applying health information. Complex healthcare conditions such as diabetes mellitus are long-term conditions that require good patient understanding to experience positive outcomes. Strategies to help improve low health literacy include a patient-centered approach to improve communication between clinicians and patients with diabetes, providing information to patients in various formats, and improving patient access to services.

Implications for Practice

Nurses play a critical role in assessing and improving health literacy, especially for patients with complex chronic conditions. Culturally appropriate, individualized teaching strategies with tools such as with the use of teach-back methods can reduce the impact of low health literacy, help improve patient-centered care (PCC), and help achieve patient self-management. The "teach-back" method has also been referred to as the "show me" method and is a way for nurses and other members of the interprofessional healthcare team to verify that what was provided as education was received and understood correctly. In the teach-back method, the patient explains to the person giving the education what was taught, thus confirming or validating the information was accurately heard and comprehended.

◼◼◼ LEGISLATION THAT SUPPORTS PATIENT-CENTERED PRACTICES

In March 2010, Congress passed the Patient Protection and Affordable Care Act (ACA). This legislation increases access to health insurance coverage, expands federal health insurance market requirements, and includes measures to improve the delivery and quality of care (www.innovations.cms.gov). The ACA is being implemented in a number of ways through new agency programs, grants, demonstration projects, and regulations. Under the ACA, the Centers for Medicare and Medicaid Innovation has been established to pilot payment and service delivery models driven by the need for quality PCC and fiscal responsibility. The Centers for Medicare and Medicaid Services (CMS, 2012) have established pilot payment and service delivery models driven by the need for quality PCC and fiscal responsibility.

Patient-Centered Medical Home

As healthcare reformers seek to improve outcomes and reduce costs, the patient-centered medical home (PCMH) has become a major strategy in the transformation of primary care and the healthcare system in general (Landon, Gill, Antonelli, & Rich, 2010; Table 7.4). The PCMH concept includes operational characteristics of primary care that are accessible, continuous, comprehensive, family/patient centered, coordinated, compassionate, and culturally sensitive (American College of Physicians [ACP], 2006).

TABLE 7.4 PRINCIPLES OF THE PATIENT-CENTERED MEDICAL HOME

All patients have a personal provider of primary care	Every patient has a provider trained to deliver continuous, comprehensive care from the first patient contact throughout an ongoing patient–provider relationship
The healthcare team is directed by primary care provider	Under the leadership of the personal primary care provider, an interprofessional healthcare team takes responsibility for the ongoing care of patients
The personal provider is responsible for all the patient's healthcare needs	A personal primary care provider takes the lead on providing or coordinating patient care with qualified professionals to meet all of the patient's healthcare needs throughout the stages of life, that is, acute care, chronic care, preventive services, and end-of-life care
The personal provider ensures coordinated/ integrated care	Across the continuum of care, the personal primary care provider implements interventions to ensure that the patient receives culturally appropriate care at the right time and place (hospital, subspecialty care, home health, nursing home) for level of need
The personal provider pursues quality and safety of care	The personal primary care provider, along with other interprofessional healthcare team members, advocates for the patient in the pursuit of optimal patient-centered outcomes guided by use of the following: • Evidence-based medicine and clinical decision-support tools • Continuous QI • Active patient participation in decision making and use of patient feedback to ensure expectations are being met

(continued)

TABLE 7.4 PRINCIPLES OF THE PATIENT-CENTERED MEDICAL HOME (*continued*)

	• Information technology to support optimal patient care, performance measurement, patient education, and improved communication • Accreditation/certification of the personal primary care provider's practice to demonstrate its ability to deliver PCC consistent with the Medical Home model • Patient and family involvement in QI activities
Patients have enhanced access to care	Open efforts are made to increase availability of providers as well as other members of the interprofessional healthcare team through flexible scheduling, extended office hours, and expanded communication options
Proper payment to providers	Payment structure should reflect the added value provided to patients under the care of a patient-centered Medical Home model.

PCC, patient-centered care; QI, quality improvement.

Source: American Academy of Family Physicians (AAFP), American Academy of Pediatrics (AAP), American College of Physicians (ACP), American Osteopathic Association (AOA). (2011). *Joint principles of the patient-centered medical home*. Retrieved from https://medicalhomeinfo.aap.org/Pages/default.aspx

Patient-Centered Primary Care Collaborative

In 2006, the Patient-Centered Primary Care Collaborative (PCPCC) emerged after several large national employers sought the assistance of the American Academy of Family Physicians (AAFP), and other primary care physician groups to address the issue of a failing system of comprehensive primary care. Goals of the PCPCC were to enable improvements in patient–physician relations and develop a more effective and efficient model of care delivery. The PCPCC has taken a significant interest in the development and advocacy of the PCMH model as a means to ensure the delivery of only the highest standards of effective and efficient PCC (PCPCC, 2011).

Health Home Model

The same ACA that supports the Medical Home initiative also provides financial incentives for the development of Health Homes (CMS, 2012). Health Homes are designed to be patient-centered systems of care that enable access to and coordination of care throughout the healthcare continuum, that is, primary, acute, behavioral, and long-term community-based care. The Health Home model expands on the Medical Home model by moving beyond primary care to better meet the needs of patients with multiple chronic conditions. By enhancing coordination and integration of medical and behavioral healthcare, Health Homes provide comprehensive care for patients.

The Health Home model supports the CMS's approach to improving healthcare by improving the patient's care experience, improving the health of populations, and reducing the costs of healthcare (CMS, 2010). The implementation of Health Homes is expected to reduce emergency department use, reduce hospital admissions and readmissions, reduce healthcare costs, and reduce reliance on long-term care facilities, while improving overall patient satisfaction and quality outcomes.

◼◼ DISCHARGE PLANNING AND CARE CONTINUITY

As healthcare reforms and payment structures attempt to balance the efficiency and efficacy of care, acute healthcare systems are facing shorter lengths of stay and rapid patient turnover. These factors can all too often contribute to fragmented patient care, for example, patients discharged while still recovering from an illness or disease exacerbation. The acuity of the patient's condition may still require continued care services and careful monitoring by his or her primary care provider and healthcare team. Patients transitioning between care settings such as hospitals and rehabilitation centers are at risk for potentially avoidable hospitalizations and increased healthcare spending (Naylor, Aiken, Kurtzman, Olds, & Hirschman, 2011). There is a call for improved patient communication handoffs to avoid common mistakes that can occur as the patient transitions from one level of care to another (Ventura, Brown, Archibald, Goroski, & Brock, 2010). Avoiding patient rehospitalization is a key priority for hospitals with higher than expected readmission rates as they will now be facing financial penalties enacted by the ACA (Hansen, Young, Hinami, Leung, & Williams, 2011). Hospitals are implementing various initiatives and comprehensive programs such as Project BOOST (Better Outcomes for Older Adults through Safe Transitions; Society of Hospital Medicine, 2012) and Project RED (Re-Engineered Discharge; Boston University School of Medicine, 2012) to facilitate safe patient discharges that will support patients in their transition from hospital to home and prevent unnecessary readmissions to the hospital (AHRQ, 2011a). These programs also provide toolkits with various interventions and practices that can help healthcare providers be successful, that is, risk assessment tools and how to implement specific discharge strategies. Despite using these tools, discharge planning is complex and must be individualized to each patient.

Continuity of care is aided by the effective transition between levels of care, use of care transition, improved health literacy, and coordination models designed to improve the quality of care by reducing fragmentation of care and enhancing coordination and continuity of care for patients with multiple health and social needs as they receive care across the continuum (Cloonan, Wood, & Riley, 2013). These models often use a number of patient-centered approaches such as patient navigators, advocates, and medication reconciliation.

Patient Navigators

Patient navigators are clinical staff members who are paired with a patient to support, educate, and facilitate the patient's interactions throughout the experience of care within a hospital during the outpatient treatment. The concept of patient navigation has developed into a process of advocacy and engagement in the provision of high-quality PCC (Koh, Nelson, & Cook, 2011). For example, patient navigators are frequently used in oncology where patients typically need to take in a great deal of information about their diagnosis and treatment as well as coordinate care among many providers such as oncologists, their nurses, radiologists, and social workers. A navigator is assigned to each patient upon admission. This relationship is maintained until the patient is discharged. Patient navigation is designed to reduce patient-care barriers and improve patient satisfaction and health outcomes. However, because this initiative is fairly new, more research and evaluation are needed to demonstrate the extent to which this initiative has been effective.

Patient Advocates

As discussed earlier, **patient advocacy** is a hallmark of PCC and healthcare professionals. In addition, integral to the care provided by the interprofessional team, healthcare organizations are making every effort to ensure patients are well-informed and take an active role in their care. As a result, some hospitals have created patient advocate positions. These patient advocate positions provide a means to increase the flow of information to patients and staff, address patient concerns, and provide emotional support to patients and families. Patient advocates serve as a central point of contact for patients, families, physicians, nurses, and other healthcare staff, and assist patients by responding to foreseeable or preventable breaks in service. Patient advocates are an integral part of ensuring that meaningful services are available to all patients. They enhance patient and staff communication and improve patient-care services rendered. For example, a patient advocate can help a patient scheduled for surgery seek all options to anesthesia. They can help the patient formulate the questions he or she need answers to. The advocate can also help ensure the patient's wishes are carried out when the patient cannot speak for himself or herself. The patient can also request the patient advocate accompany him or her to testing and examinations when allowed. The patient advocate can be someone supplied by the hospital and may be a nurse or social worker, however, the position does not require medical or healthcare training. The patient advocate may also be a friend or family member of the patient. The key to this person and/or position is that the person be someone the patient trusts and someone who can effectively communicate for the patient if unable to speak for himself or herself.

EVIDENCE FROM THE LITERATURE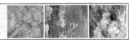

Citation

Buila, S. M. D., & Swanke, J. R. (2010). Patient-centered mental health care: Encouraging caregiver participation. *Care Management Journal, 11*(3), 146–150.

Discussion

Caregivers play a vital role when caring for loved ones suffering from mental illness. Viewing caregivers as partners within a patient-centered approach to care can improve the quality of care provided. Five major themes emerged from caregiver participants in the suicide prevention workshop discussed in this article. The five themes were that (a) caregivers needed to be included in the mental healthcare of their family member, (b) expressed concerns related to diagnosing process, (c) stated a need for improved communication with professionals, (d) articulated a desire for individualized holistic care, and (e) stated a need for service and resource information.

(continued)

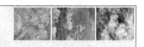

EVIDENCE FROM THE LITERATURE
(*continued*)

Implications for Practice

Nurses and other members of the interprofessional team play an integral part in the treatment of mental illness, particularly in their ability to integrate caregivers into the plan of care. Supporting the perspective of caregivers and recognizing their role as partners in care services will enhance the overall care provided to patients with mental illness.

CRITICAL THINKING 7.3

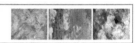

Teresa is a 10-year-old patient diagnosed with juvenile diabetes. She has been hospitalized four times in the past year for complications related to diabetic diet noncompliance. Teresa is an only child who resides with her parents and maternal grandmother of Italian immigrant descent. She and her family have been in America for 8 years, Teresa and her parents have mastered the English language, and Teresa has been a very good student. Her parents both work at the same factory on the assembly line. A number of interprofessional team members have counseled Teresa and her parents on the risks involved with diabetes and dietary noncompliance. Teresa and her parents seem to understand the importance of following her prescribed diabetic diet. As Teresa's nurse, you notice at this hospitalization that Teresa's grandmother spends a great deal of time with her and appears quite agitated by the fact that her granddaughter is "not getting better." She expresses concern to you about Teresa being readmitted to the hospital yet again.

1. Within a patient-centered environment, how would you approach Teresa's grandmother?
2. Considering Teresa and her parents seem to understand the importance of her dietary intervention, how can the interprofessional healthcare team collaborate in gathering potential missing information about Teresa's care to discover the cause for her multiple readmissions?

INFORMATION TECHNOLOGIES TO SUPPORT PCC

With the growing use of technology, nurses are keenly aware that the landscape for healthcare providers has challenged the human connection and patient relationship more than ever before. However, with PCC and collaborative relationships among the interprofessional healthcare team and the patient, personalized and meaningful services can be provided with the patient in control of his or her care. The electronic health record (EHR) creates an opportunity for the interprofessional healthcare team to ensure the patient remains focal to the healthcare delivered as well as facilitate effective collaboration between the team and the patients themselves. As patient-care providers become more adept at electronic data sharing for the provision of continuity of care, many providers offer patients access to their healthcare record online and encourage them to take responsibility for its accuracy. For example, if a patient accesses his or her EHR online and discovers the list of allergies is incomplete, the patient will be expected to update and correct the list. Obviously, inaccurate patient information can lead to negative patient outcomes and healthcare errors.

Personal Health Record

Several initiatives have emerged to help patients build their own personal health record (PHR) such as Microsoft Health Vault (Microsoft, 2012). The Josie King Foundation created a paper and electronic version of a patient journal as a tool to help patients and their families record details of their care along with the questions to ask and important things to remember (Josie King Foundation, 2012). Hospitals can order the journals to provide to patients and their families and/or patients can request a journal for themselves at the Josie King website located at www.josieking. org/carejournals. These initiatives are drivers of patient safety and quality care by empowering patients with specific tools to facilitate active engagement in their own healthcare.

Online Health Information

Patient-driven research (PDR) is an evolving phenomenon that began in the Internet's earliest days. From access to online support groups to access to world-renowned medical centers, patients have access to an incredible amount of online health information they can now use to become an active member of their care team. This access to information gives patients valuable information regarding their conditions, treatment options, best practices, as well as the healthcare organizations known for their clinical excellence of care delivery. Patient-driven online healthcare information allows interested patients to be more informed about their choices and raises their level of expectations for quality care and safety when seeking healthcare services.

Online Patient Communities

Many online communities exist offering opportunity for patients to share experiences and learn about diseases and treatments. The term "e-patient" has been coined to identify this new breed of informed healthcare consumers who are *e*quipped, *e*nabled, *e*mpowered, and *e*ngaged in their health and healthcare decisions. Healthcare has responded to this trend through the development of important resources such as the Society for Participatory Medicine and Sharecare, thus facilitating a new level of partnership between patients and their healthcare teams (Gee et al., 2012).

Participatory medicine is a model of care to support a cooperative approach by all members of the healthcare team, that is, patients, families, and healthcare professionals, across the full continuum of care. Healthcare providers are expected to encourage and value patients and families as responsible drivers of their health and not as passengers. Providers who practice participatory medicine promote clinical transparency through the exchange of information and through support for the e-patient movement (Society for Participatory Medicine, 2011).

Sharecare (www.sharecare.org) was launched in 2010 by the founder of WebMD, Jeff Arnold, as an interactive, social question-and-answer platform for consumers of healthcare as well as healthcare professionals. Sharecare has enlisted the nation's leading health experts, care providers, organizations, and brands to become part of the health and wellness dialogue. Sigma Theta Tau, the International Honor Society of Nursing, is one of the major content contributors for Sharecare. Users of Sharecare have free access to high-quality, relevant answers to their health questions. These answers are provided by experts, along with interactive health and wellness tools that allow patients to take action on what they have learned as an empowered, informed participant of their own care.

PATIENT-CENTERED MEASURES AND MONITORS OF QUALITY HEALTHCARE

Population-focused healthcare is care based on the health status and needs assessment of a target group of individuals who have one or more personal or environmental characteristic in common, such as determined by demographics or geography. Public health core functions of assessment and policy development guide the work of population-focused healthcare. The ultimate goal of these policies is improved patient care that is more effective in treating the underlying causes of disease. By examining trends in the etiology and intervention of larger groups, population-focused healthcare provides information to healthcare providers that allow them to deliver care that is comprehensive, individualized, and ultimately more effective. The U.S. Department of Health and Human Services (HHS) is the lead agency responsible for providing essential human services to Americans, particularly those least able to care for themselves. Together with 12 operating divisions and over 300 programs, the HHS is charged with protecting the health of all Americans (HHS, 2011d).

Strategy for Quality Improvement in Healthcare

The secretary of the HHS has established a National Strategy for Quality Improvement in Health Care to set priorities that guide the nation to increase access to high-quality, patient-centered, affordable healthcare for all Americans (HHS, 2011b). See Table 7.5 for priorities.

TABLE 7.5 DEPARTMENT OF HEALTH AND HUMAN SERVICES NATIONAL STRATEGIES FOR QUALITY IMPROVEMENT IN HEALTHCARE PRIORITIES

PRIORITY	ACTIONS
1. Give safer care	• Exercise relentless effort to reduce risk for injury from care • Aim for ZERO harm to patients • Create healthcare systems that reliably provide high-quality care
2. Deliver patient- and family-centered care	• Give patients and families an active role in their care • Adapt care to individual and family situations, cultures, languages, disabilities, and health literacy levels
3. Promote effective communication and coordination of care	• Develop processes and use technology to provide seamless care, that is, electronic health record, e-prescribing, telemedicine • Eliminate healthcare gaps and duplication of care • Use effective care models to facilitate coordination and communication across the continuum of care

(continued)

TABLE 7.5 DEPARTMENT OF HEALTH AND HUMAN SERVICES NATIONAL STRATEGIES FOR QUALITY IMPROVEMENT IN HEALTHCARE PRIORITIES (*continued*)

PRIORITY	ACTIONS
4. Promote effective prevention and treatment of leading causes of mortality (priority, cardiovascular disease)	• Practice key interventions for cardiovascular disease, that is, ABCS—aspirin, blood pressure control, cholesterol reduction, and smoking cessation
5. Work with communities to use best practices	• Create strong partnerships among local healthcare providers, public health professionals, and individuals • Provide clinical preventive services and increase adoption of evidence-based interventions
6. Provide more affordable quality care	• Ensure the right care is provided at the right time for the right patient • Reduce healthcare-acquired conditions • Reform payment structures, reduce waste • Establish health insurance exchanges to improve cost of insurance for individuals and small businesses

Source: U.S. Department of Health and Human Services (HHS). (2011b). *National strategy for quality improvement in health care.* Washington, DC: Author. Retrieved from http://www.health care.gov/law/resources/reports/nationalqualitystrategy032011.pdf

PATIENT SATISFACTION

Patient satisfaction has been an important aspect of feedback used by care providers for internal quality improvement (QI) efforts. Medicare, Medicaid, and private insurance companies are beginning to place a financial value on patient satisfaction feedback. Tangible, measurable patient outcomes, such as infection rates, are an important indicator of the quality of care patients have received. However, patient satisfaction with the care that has been provided is now recognized as another quality indicator. This knowledge is powerful feedback regarding how respected and valued patients felt as well as how engaged they were relative to their plan of care.

REAL-WORLD INTERVIEW

There are a number of healthcare settings implementing services with the patient in the center of all care being provided. It is not unique to nursing services. One acute care hospital where I serve on the Board focuses on fostering relationships with the patient and family as they provide care to meet the patient's needs. The patient is an active participant in rounds and most staff find it very rewarding to work in a caring environment with the patient central to all services. The hospital was introduced to a relationship-based model for care and found there were many success stories from patients and families as well as the staff who embraced forming caring relationships with their patients. The hospital has developed a comprehensive program that helps

(*continued*)

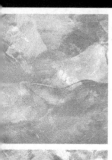

ensure each service within the hospital keeps the patient central to what they do—from housekeepers to surgeons. Besides employee satisfaction, implementing a relationship-based focus on patient-centered care (PCC) has greatly influenced patient satisfaction.

Esther Bankert, Board Member
Faxton/St. Luke's Health Care
Utica, New York

The QSEN competencies for PCC provide a structured guide for developing and assessing a nurse's ability to integrate the patient and/or the patient's designee as the primary source for determining care. These competencies include measures of knowledge, skill, and attitudes. Simply listing these measures does not guarantee the accomplishment of this complex competency. Clearly, the goal to keep the patient's preferences, values, and needs paramount starts with a culture focused on the specific intention of soliciting a patient's voice, honoring it, and ensuring it is respected. Resources exist to assist institutions. An innovative company providing such resources is Planetree whose mission is to provide education to hospitals and other healthcare organizations seeking to create and ensure patient-centered, healing environments (Planetree, 2017). Specifically, they focus on five key areas: cultural transformation, patient activation, staff engagement, leadership development, and performance improvement. Providing education to all levels of an organization, Planetree facilitates a cultural shift that hallmarks the focus on the patient, first and always. A comprehensive program is designed, implemented, and monitored thatdeliberately seeks and listens to the patient's wants and needs. Monitoring the successful implementation of such initiatives is the responsibility of the institution. Many tools are available and used but two surveys are used most often in hospitals, measuring patient success as a measure within the institution as well in comparison to other hospitals: Hospital Consumer Assessment of Healthcare Providers and Systems (HCAHPS) and Press Ganey.

Hospital Consumer Assessment of Healthcare Providers and Systems

In 2005, the National Quality Forum, a national organization of healthcare stakeholders, consumer organizations, public and private purchasers, physicians, nurses, hospitals, accreditation/certification bodies, supporting industries, healthcare researchers, and QI organizations endorsed the HCAHPS (pronounced H-CAPS) survey. The intent of this survey was to provide a standard instrument to be used by hospitals across the nation to measure the patients' satisfaction with their hospital experience. HCAHPS asks a core set of questions to assess patient satisfaction with their care by nurses, doctors, and other members of the interprofessional healthcare team; responsiveness of hospital staff; pain management; communication about medicines; and cleanliness and quietness of hospital environment. These standardized questions permit valid comparisons of patient-care experience at hospitals locally, regionally, and nationally. The HCAHPS survey is focused on three areas:

1. The patients' perception of care that permits objective and meaningful comparisons of hospitals on topics important to patients.

2. Public reporting of results, which provides an incentive for hospitals to improve the quality of care.

3. Public reporting, which also enhances accountability in healthcare by increasing transparency of the quality of the care provided (CMS, 2011a).

Since 2008, HCAHPS patient satisfaction scores have been available to the public on the CMS Hospital Compare website that can be found at www.medicare.gov/HomeHealthCompare/search.aspx.

Press Ganey

Press Ganey is another survey tool used by most hospitals to gauge patient satisfaction (www.pressganey.com). Its survey actually includes the HCAHPS questions to provide a comprehensive assessment of what the patient experienced and felt while hospitalized, collecting both objective and subjective data. While the HCAHPS focuses on measuring "how often a service is provided," Press Ganey aims to capture how well that service was delivered and perceived by the patient (www.pressganey.com/solutions/clinical-quality).

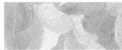

KEY CONCEPTS

- Patient-centered care (PCC) "recognizes the patient or designee as the source of control and full partner in providing compassionate and coordinated care based on respect for patient's preferences, values, and needs" (Quality and Safety Education for Nurses, 2012, p. 1).
- Pettetier and Stickler (2014) identify the absolute need and commitment to PCC by healthcare facilities based on respect for patient self-determination (or right to make decisions for oneself) and autonomy (right to self-govern based on values).
- PCC is based on the unique values held by the patient, which can be based on many aspects of the person including their physical condition, culture, gender identification, generation or age, educational level, socioeconomic status, moral development, religion, and/or spirituality.
- Advocacy refers to any activity that ultimately assists a patient in receiving the "best" care depending on the patient's needs and wishes. Patient empowerment reflects a form of self-directed advocacy that enables and motivates patients to bring about changes and make decisions to manage and improve their health (Bann et al., 2010).
- Empathy involves the ability to understand and share the emotional experience observed in another person. Sympathy by contrast is defined as emotional concern for another (Kunzmann, 2011).
- There are a number of behaviors that facilitate empathetic communication and thus promote PCC. Likewise, there are nonempathetic communication behaviors that hinder communication and thereby impede PCC (Table 7.2).

- Sometimes the verbal and nonverbal components of a patient's communication are incongruent and provide conflicting messages (Table 7.3).
- Expressions of caring can be perceived differently across cultures.
- The use of language interpreters can provide a safe space where patients can freely express their concerns and be understood through the interpreter, calming their fears and apprehensions in an unfamiliar situation and setting (e.g., CTS Language Link, www.ctslanguagelink.com).
- Through the patient-centered model of care, the healthcare industry is called upon to develop innovative strategies to support patients and caregivers in becoming greater participants in their healthcare.
- Populations vulnerable to low levels of health literacy include ethnic minority groups, recent immigrants, older adult and elderly populations, individuals living with chronic diseases, and populations of people at poverty level or an even lower socioeconomic class (Center for Health Care Strategies, Inc., 2010).
- Healthy People 2020 (HHS, 2011c) has identified improving health literacy as one of its key goals to promoting healthy outcomes and enhancing quality of life.
- Patients who are well informed and more involved in their care experience better health outcomes (HHS, 2010).
- Patient initiatives, such as Ask Me 3 (National Patient Safety Foundation, 2011) and Questions Are the Answer (AHRQ, 2011b) are campaigns designed to promote communication and encourage patients to seek and understand the answers to common questions: What is my main problem? What do I need to do? Why is it important for me to do this?
- One website, called Patient, offers education about specific conditions and provides pros and cons of treatments typically suggested (patient.info/decision-aids) as a starting point for relevant discussion with the healthcare provider. Additional tools are available through the Mayo Clinic, AHRQ, and HealthITh.gov.
- In March 2010, Congress passed the Patient Protection and Affordable Care Act (ACA). This legislation increases access to health insurance coverage, expands federal health insurance market requirements, and includes measures to improve the delivery and quality of care (www.innovations.cms.gov).
- The Patient-Centered Medical Home (PCMH), Patient-Centered Primary Care Collaborative (PCPCC), and Health Homes (CMS, 2012) are designed to provide more comprehensive care for patients.
- Hospitals are implementing various initiatives and comprehensive programs such as Project BOOST (Better Outcomes for Older Adults through Safe Transitions; Society of Hospital Medicine, 2012) and Project RED (Re-Engineered Discharge; Boston University School of Medicine, 2012) to facilitate safe patient discharges that will support patients in their transition from hospital to home and prevent unnecessary readmissions to the hospital (AHRQ, 2011a).
- Continuity of care is aided by models that often use a number of patient-centered approaches such as patient navigators, advocates, and medication reconciliation.
- Several initiatives have emerged to help patients, for example, Microsoft Health Vault (Microsoft, 2012), and the Josie King Foundation patient journal (Josie King Foundation, 2012, www.josieking.org/carejournals).
- Participatory medicine is a model of care to support a cooperative approach by all members of the healthcare team, that is, patients, families, and healthcare professionals across the full continuum of care, for example, Sharecare (www.sharecare.org).
- Population-focused healthcare is care based on the health status and needs assessment of a target group of individuals who have one or more personal or environmental characteristics in common, such as determined by demographics or geography.

- The Secretary of HHS has established a National Strategy for Quality Improvement in Health Care to set priorities that guide the nation to increase access to high-quality, patient-centered, affordable health care for all Americans (HHS, 2011b) (Table 7.5).
- Medicare, Medicaid, and private insurance companies are beginning to place a financial value on patient satisfaction feedback.
- An innovative company providing PCC resources is Planetree, with focus on five key areas: cultural transformation, patient activation, staff engagement, leadership development, and performance improvement.
- Hospital Consumer Assessment of Health Care Providers and Systems (HCAHPS) patient satisfaction scores have been available to the public on the CMS Hospital Compare website (www.medicare.gov/HomeHealthCompare/search.aspx) since 2008.
- Press Ganey is another survey tool used by most hospitals to gauge patient satisfaction (www.pressganey.com).

KEY TERMS

E-patient
Empathetic communication
Health literacy
Patient advocacy

Participatory medicine
Patient-centered care
Population-focused healthcare
Self-concept

REVIEW QUESTIONS

1. A nurse will attend a seminar discussing patients with family/significant others at the center for all nursing and interprofessional care services. The nurse knows that which of the following will most likely be the primary topic?

   A. Primary care
   B. Medical Homes
   C. Interprofessional team approach
   D. Patient-centered care (PCC)

2. The nurse wants to use a patient-centered approach to perform patient care. Which of the following best describes the nurse's approach?

   A. Developing friendships with patients as a means of providing better care
   B. Creating an environment of coworkers committed to helping each other
   C. Providing care through the eyes of the patient
   D. Understanding the nurse's role and its relation to other care providers

3. The nurse is preparing to review discharge instructions with a patient. The nurse instructs the patient regarding her medications and wound care for her foot. What indicates to the nurse the level of understanding the patient has regarding discharge instructions?

   A. The patient signs the discharge instruction sheet.
   B. When asked by the nurse, the patient denies any questions or concerns.
   C. The patient asks for new prescriptions for the pharmacy.
   D. The nurse observes the patient changing the dressing on her foot wound.

4. When rounding, the nurse discovers that a patient on isolation has soiled the bed. Upon inquiry, the patient indicated that he did not want to bother the nurse because she was busy. The nurse tells the patient to use the call bell any time. How can the nurse most effectively communicate that she is available to the patient?

A. Remind the patient frequently to use the call bell.
B. Ensure that all the patient's needs have been met before leaving the patient's room, avoid appearing rushed, and let the patient know when the nurse will return.
C. Go in and out of patients' rooms to ensure the patients are aware that the nurse is available.
D. Make sure the call bell is within the patient's reach every time the nurse leaves his room.

5. The nurse is caring for a patient who has multiple chronic conditions and has been hospitalized twice in the last month. The patient has a complex medication regimen, limited family support, and admits to having missed his last two physician appointments because he did not have a ride. What is the benefit of a referral to a health home for this patient?

A. Physicians with lower rehospitalization rates operate Health Homes.
B. Complex cases are managed through skilled nursing facilities until patients are independent again.
C. Home care services are covered for patients regardless of ability to pay.
D. Comprehensive care management enables access to and coordination of care.
E. None of the above

6. A nurse is reviewing discharge instructions with a patient. The patient asks the nurse about a cardiac medication he forgot to mention to the physician because the medication is not listed on the discharge instructions. Which action by the nurse is most appropriate when reconciling discharge medications?

A. Explain to the patient that he should follow up with his primary physician within 7 days to review the medication regimen.
B. Contact the physician to notify him of the discrepancy and receive direction regarding the discharge instructions before discharging the patient.
C. Instruct the patient to take only the medications listed on the discharge instructions.
D. Advise the patient to continue taking the medication until he sees his primary physician.

7. A patient newly diagnosed with breast cancer is asking in-depth questions about her diagnosis and sharing what she has found online that has worked for other patients. The nurse recognizes that this patient represents a growing number of informed healthcare consumers. Which intervention by the nurse demonstrates support for the patient's involvement in her care?

A. Caution the patient about inaccurate information that may be available on the Internet.
B. Instruct the patient to only follow the advice of her medical provider.
C. Advise the patient to begin building a personal health record (PHR).
D. Explain to the patient the importance of regular checkups to identify any changes in condition.
E. All of the above

8. Which of the following actions demonstrates understanding of the role of the nurse in patient satisfaction? Select all that apply.

    A. The nurse discusses the plan of care with the patient and family.
    B. The nurse inquires about the patient's comfort with the room temperature and desire for a meal because dinner has already been served on the unit prior to arrival.
    C. At the change of shift, the nurse makes rounds with the oncoming nurse and introduces the new nurse to the patient.
    D. The nurse obtains permission for the patient's pet to visit after the nurse overhears the patient express that she misses her dog and is afraid she will not see it again.
    E. The nurse tells the patient to fill out the patient survey she will receive after discharge and to make sure to rate her experience as excellent if the nurse met her needs.
    F. A, B, C, D
    G. None of the above

9. A non-English-speaking patient arrives in the ED and is noted to be crying quietly. Which of the following is the most important for the nurse to consider in initially providing care for this patient?

    A. Expressions and interpretations of caring may be perceived differently across cultures.
    B. Therapeutic touch is a universal communication of caring.
    C. Cultural competence includes looking patients in the eye and communicating in their language even if through an interpreter.
    D. When patients have specific cultural beliefs, nurses should consider them as part of the patient's care.

10. The nurse manager in the surgical step-down unit at a large metropolitan hospital would like to evaluate the perceived effectiveness of pain management for prior patients on the unit. The nurse knows that which of the following measures would best assist the nurse manager in understanding past patients' experiences?

    A. Home health compare data
    B. Value-based performance data
    C. Hospital Consumer Assessment of Health Care Providers and Systems (HCAHPS) data
    D. Sentinel events reports

REVIEW ACTIVITIES

Review Activity 7.1

Review the study "The Art of Holding Hand: A Fieldwork Study Outlining the Significance of Physical Touch in Facilities for Short-Term Stay" by Bundgaard, Sorensen, and Nielsen (2011).

Explain how the simple act of holding the patient's hand can instill safety and trust for the patient undergoing an invasive procedure.

What expressions would convey to you the patient is anxious or experiencing discomfort?

How can the nurse or doctor communicate reassurance to the patient while participating in the procedure?

Review Activity 7.2

To practice effective interpersonal skills within a patient-centered environment, one school tested the effects of pairing students during clinical rotations with the assignment of caring for two patients. Refer to Bartges's article, "Pairing Students in Clinical Assignments to Develop Collaboration and Communication Skills" (2012) in *Nurse Educator, 37*(1), 17–22.

Role-play a scenario whereby student pairs collaborate on patient assignments and together review the patient's records. Each student pair will round with the healthcare team and, at the completion of the shift, report out to a second pair of students who will be picking up the same assignment on the next shift.

Reflect upon your experience and describe the collaborative strategies each used to gather pertinent information about your patient.

Describe communication processes you experienced that were barriers and enhancers to effectively collaborating with the interdisciplinary team while caring for your patient.

Discuss one takeaway each student learned from this experience while working with a peer colleague.

Review Activity 7.3

Refer to the mentor–mentee program described by authors Latham, Ringl, and Hogan (2011). Professionalization and retention outcomes of a university: Service mentoring program partnership. *Journal of Professional Nursing, 27*(6), 344–353.

Nurse mentors in the workplace are often sought to support new nurses or nursing students in the practice setting. Formal and informal mentoring programs are developing across academic settings to enhance their partnerships with service.

Discuss the strategies suggested in the study by Latham et al., which formalized the mentor–mentee relationship between the student nurse and staff member.

What are some of the arguments leaders of acute care organizations express in opposition to using staff to mentor student nurses in the workplace?

As a champion to mentoring programs for nursing students and new nurses, what convincing arguments would you present to nurse leaders and the healthcare team in your healthcare centers?

CRITICAL DISCUSSION POINTS

1. Patient-centered care (PCC) recognizes the unique needs, values, and preferences of the patient and coordinates care services within a partnership between the patient and interprofessional team with compassion and respect.
2. Expressions of caring and the interpretation of caring acts are perceived differently across cultures.

3. Empathetic communication embodies respect for another person's feelings, values, and perspective.
4. Collaboration means to work jointly together and share expertise among members of the patient's healthcare team.
5. Physical illness, disease, and injury impact a person's psychosocial self-concept.
6. Promoting health literacy is one strategy of supporting patient-centered healthcare.
7. The Medical Home is a result of the Patient Protection and Affordable Care Act (ACA).
8. Continuity of care can be augmented with effective discharge planning.
9. Nurses and healthcare professionals can facilitate PCC by understanding their role in providing care that supports patient advocacy, continuity, and collaboration with the patient as a member of the interprofessional team across the continuum of care.
10. Nursing plays a significant role in patient satisfaction by ensuring the patient's values and preferences are incorporated into the care that is meaningful to the patient.
11. Quality improvement (QI) in healthcare is a major focus in America that requires an interprofessional approach to support programs and initiatives designed to develop and guide "e-patients" (equipped, enabled, empowered, and engaged) in a journey to a healthier nation.
12. Measurement of patient satisfaction can provide valuable feedback to the interprofessional team regarding the delivery of PCC.
13. During your last clinical experience, what patient-centered care (PCC) initiatives are underway on the nursing unit or within the department of nursing?
14. What PCC resources are available to nurses within the nursing unit or department of nursing where you have your clinical rotation?
15. How has PCC improved for patients and families in your clinical site?
16. What information from the electronic health record (EHR) helps you give PCC to patients in your clinical site?
17. Does the health system use PCC initiatives; how do the nurses feel about PCC initiatives within their work environment?
18. How are nurses involved in decision making affecting PCC at the health system?
19. How are patients included in PCC initiatives in your clinical site? What is the role of the nurse in PCC initiatives?
20. If a nurse has an idea that will improve PCC initiatives, where would he or she take that idea within the organization?

EXPLORING THE WEB

1. Explore the Quality and Safety Education for Nurses (QSEN) website specifically reviewing the Competency of Patient-Centered Care. Find their specific definition for patient-centered care (PCC) at qsen.org/competencies/pre-licensure-ksas/. From there, describe the attributes of PCC. Finally, discuss how administration can support nurses and healthcare providers collaboration to provide PCC in acute and long-term care facilities.
2. Explore the web for professional sites such as Future of Nursing; Robert Wood Johnson Foundation, Institute of Medicine (IOM) at campaignforaction.org/ for two goals of the future of nursing in relation to PCC.
3. Browse the web on any healthcare topic. Access the Internet and complete a basic search on the healthcare topic of your choice. Be sure to include sites such

as WebMD and Sharecare. How can you determine if the information is valid? Evaluate if the information provided is at an appropriate level for healthcare consumers. Provide rationales for your answers.

4. Explore websites offering patient decision-making tools including www.shared-decisions.mayoclinic.org, www.ahrq.gov/professionals/education/curriculum-tools/shareddecisionmaking/index.html, and www.healthit.gov/sites/default/files/nlc_shared_decision_making_fact_sheet.pdf. List pros and cons of each tool offered.

REFERENCES

Agency for Healthcare Research and Quality (AHRQ). (2011a). *Preventing avoidable readmissions.* Retrieved from http://www.ahrq.gov/qual/impptdis.htm

Agency for Healthcare Research and Quality (AHRQ). (2011b). *Questions are the answer.* Retrieved from http://www.ahrq.gov/questions

American Academy of Family Physicians (AAFP), American Academy of Pediatrics (AAP), American College of Physicians (ACP), American Osteopathic Association (AOA). (2011). *Joint principles of the patient-centered medical home.* Retrieved from https://www.aafp.org/dam/AAFP/documents/practice_management/pcmh/initiatives/PCMHJoint2011.pdf

American College of Physicians (ACP). (2006). *The advanced medical home: A patient-centered physician-guided model of health care.* Philadelphia, PA: American College of Physicians.

Asimakopoulou, K., Gilbert, D., Newton, P., & Scambler, S. (2012). Back to basics: Re-examining the role of patient empowerment in diabetes. *Patient Education and Counseling, 86*(3), 281–283.

Bann, C. M., Sirois, F. M., & Walsh, E. G. (2010). Provider support in complementary and alternative medicine: Exploring the role of patient empowerment. *Journal of Alternative and Complementary Medicine, 16*(7), 745–752.

Bartges, M. (2012). Pairing students in clinical assignments to develop collaboration and communication skills. *Nurse Educator, 37*(1), 17–22.

Boston University School of Medicine. (2012). *Project RED (Re-Engineering Discharge).* Retrieved from http://www.bu.edu/fammed/projectred/index.html

Bradshaw, A. (1999). The virtue of nursing: The covenant of care. *Journal of Medical Ethics, 25*(6), 477.

Buila, S. M. D., & Swanke, J. R. (2010). Patient-centered mental health care: Encouraging caregiver participation. *Care Management Journal, 11*(3), 146–150.

Bundgaard, K., Sorensen, E. E., & Nielsen, K. B. (2011). The art of holding hand: A fieldwork study outlining the significance of physical touch in facilities for short-term stay. *International Journal for Human Caring, 15*(3), 34–41.

Burks, D. J., & Kobus, A. M. (2012). The legacy of altruism in health care: The promotion of empathy, prosociality, and humanism. *Medical Education, 46*(3), 317–325.

Center for Health Care Strategies, Inc. (2010). *Health literacy implications of the affordable care act.* Retrieved from http://www.chcs.org/usr_doc/Health_Literacy_Implications_of_the_Affordable_Care_Act.pdf

Centers for Medicare and Medicaid Services (CMS). (2010). *Health homes for enrollees with chronic conditions.* Retrieved from http://www.cms.gov/smdl/downloads/SMD10024.pdf

Centers for Medicare and Medicaid Services (CMS). (2011a). *HCAHPS: Hospital care quality information from the consumer perspective.* Retrieved from https://www.cms.gov/Medicare/Quality-Initiatives-Patient-Assessment-Instruments/HospitalQualityInits/HospitalHCAHPS.html

Centers for Medicare and Medicaid Services (CMS). (2012). *Center for medicare and Medicaid innovation.* Retrieved from http://www.innovations.cms.gov

Cloonan, P., Wood, J., & Riley, J. (2013). Reducing 30-day readmissions: Health literacy strategies. *Journal of Nursing Administration, 43*(7–8), 382–387.

Dawn, S. (2015). Engaging patients using an interprofessional approach to shared decision making. *Canadian Oncology Nursing Journal, 25*(4), 455–469.

Decety, J., & Michalska, K. J. (2010). Neurodevelopmental changes in the circuits underlying empathy and sympathy from childhood to adulthood. *Developmental Science, 13*(6), 886–899.

Gee, P. M., Greenwood, D. A., Kim, K. K., Perez, S. L., Staggers, N., & DeVon, H. A. (2012). Exploration of the e-patient phenomenon in nursing informatics. *Nursing Outlook, 60*(4), e9–e16.

Hansen, L. O., Young, R. S., Hinami, K., Leung, A., & Williams, M. V. (2011). Interventions to reduce 30-day rehospitalization: A systematic review. *Annals of Internal Medicine, 155*(8), 520–528.

Hoyt, S. (2010). Florence Nightingale's contribution to contemporary nursing ethics. *Journal of Holistic Nursing, 28*(4), 331–332.

Institute of Medicine (IOM). (2001). *Crossing the quality chasm: A new health system for the 21st century.* Washington, DC: National Academies Press.

Institute of Medicine (IOM). (2004). *Health literacy: A prescription to end confusion.* Washington, DC: National Academies Press.

Josie King Foundation. (2012). *Josie King Foundation: Creating a culture of patient safety, together.* Retrieved from http://www.josieking.org

Koh, C., Nelson, J., & Cook, P. (2011). Evaluation of a patient navigation program. *Clinical Journal of Oncology Nursing, 15*(1), 41–48.

Kunzmann, R. (2011). Age differences in three facets of empathy: Performance-based evidence. *Psychology of Aging, 26*(11), 66–78.

Landon, B., Gill, J., Antonelli, R., & Rich, E. (2010). Using evidence to inform policy: Developing a policy-relevant research agenda for the patient-centered medical home. *Journal of General Internal Medicine, 25*(6), 581–583.

Latham, C., Ringl, K., & Hogan, M. (2011). Professionalization and retention outcomes of a university: Service mentoring program partnership. *Journal of Professional Nursing, 27*(6), 344–353.

Microsoft. (2012). *Microsoft health vault.* Retrieved from https://international.healthvault.com/us/en

Miles, A., & Mezzich, J. (2011). The care of the patient and the soul of the clinic: Person-centered medicine as an emergent model of clinical practice. *International Journal of Person Centered Medicine, 1*(2), 207–222.

National Patient Safety Foundation. (2011). *Ask me 3.* Retrieved from http://www.npsf.org/askme3

Naylor, M. D., Aiken, L. H., Kurtzman, E. T., Olds, D. M., & Hirschman, K. B. (2011). The care span: The importance of transitional care in achieving health reform. *Health Affairs, 30*(4), 746–754.

Patient-Centered Outcomes Research Institute. (2012). *Patient-centered outcomes research definition: Response to public input.* Retrieved from http://www.pcori.org

Patient-Centered Primary Care Collaborative (PCPCC). (2011). *History of the collaborative.* Retrieved from https://www.pcpcc.org/content/history-0

Pettetier, L. R., & Stichler, J. F. (2014). Patient-centered care and engagement. *The Journal of Nursing Administration, 44*(9), 473–480.

Planetree. (2017). *The formula.* Retrieved from http://www.planetree.org

Press Ganey. (2017). *Clinical quality: Manage improvement across the continuum.* Retrieved from http://www.pressganey.com/solutions/clinical-quality

Quality and Safety Education for Nurses (QSEN). (2012). *Evidence-based practice.* Retrieved from http://www.qsen.org

Ratzan, S., & Parker, R. (2000). Introduction. In C. R. Selden, M. Zorn, S. C. Ratzan, & R. M. Parker (Eds.), *National library of medicine current bibliographies in medicine: Health literacy.* NLM Pub. No. CBM 2000–1. Bethesda, MD: National Institutes of Health, U.S. Department of Health and Human Services.

Society of Hospital Medicine. (2012). *Project BOOST*. Retrieved from http://www.hospitalmedicine.org/AM/Template.cfm?Section=Publications&CONTENTID=27659&TEMPLATE=/CM/HTMLDisplay.cfm

Society for Participatory Medicine. (2011). *Society for participatory medicine*. Retrieved from http://www.participatorymedicine.org

Stiles, E. (2011). Promoting health literacy in patients with diabetes. *Nursing Standard*, *26*(8), 35–40.

Taylor, S. (2011). *Health psychology*. New York, NY: McGraw-Hill.

U.S. Department of Health and Human Services (USDHHS). (2010). Agency for Healthcare Research and Quality. *National health care quality report*. Washington, DC. Retrieved from http://www.ahrq.gov/qual/nhqr10/nhqr10.pdf

U.S. Department of Health and Human Services (USDHHS). (2011b). *National strategy for quality improvement in health care*. Washington, DC: Author. Retrieved from https://www.medicaid.gov/affordable-care-act/index.html

U.S. Department of Health and Human Services (USDHHS). (2011c). Office of Disease Prevention and Health Promotion. *Healthy people 2020*. Washington, DC: Author. Retrieved from http://www.healthypeople.gov/2020/topicsobjectives2020/overview.aspx?topicId=18

U.S. Department of Health and Human Services (USDHHS). (2011d). *U.S. Department of Health and Human Services: About HHS*. Washington, DC: Author. Retrieved from http://www.hhs.gov/about

Ventura, T., Brown, D., Archibald, T., Goroski, A., & Brock, J. (2010). Improving care transitina and reducing hospital readmissions: Establishing the evidence for community-based implementation strategies through the care transitions theme. *The Remington Report*, *18*(1), 24–30.

SUGGESTED READING

Agency for Healthcare Research and Quality (AHRQ). (2011b). *Questions are the answer*. Retrieved from http://www.ahrq.gov/questions

American Medical Association, Ethical Force Program. (2006). *Improving communication-improving care*. Retrieved from http://www.ama-assn.org/ama1/pub/upload/mm/369/ef_imp_comm.pdf

American Nurses Association. (2001). *Code of ethics for nurses with interpretive statements*. Retrieved from https://www.nursingworld.org/practice-policy/nursing-excellence/ethics/code-of-ethics-for-nurses/

Balon, J., & Thomas, S. (2011). Comparison of hospital admission medication lists with primary care physician and outpatient pharmacy lists. *Journal of Nursing Scholarship*, *43*(3), 292–300.

Centers for Medicare and Medicaid Services (CMS). (2011b). *HCAHPS: Patients' perspectives of care survey*. Retrieved from https://www.cms.gov/hospitalqualityinits/30_hospitalhcahps.asp

Chunchu, K., Mauksch, L., Charles, C., Ross, V., & Pauwels, J. (2012). A patient-centered care plan In the HER; Improving collaboration and engagement. *Families, Systems & Health*, *30*(13), 199–209.

Epstein, R., Fiscella, K., Lesser, C., & Stang, K. (2012). Why the nation needs a policy push on patient-centered health care. *Health Affairs*, *29*(8), 1489–1495.

Holmstrom, I., & Roing, M. (2009). The relation between patient-centeredness and patient empowerment: A discussion on concepts. *Patient Education and Counseling*, *79*, 167–172.

Institute of Medicine (IOM). (2004). *Health literacy: A prescription to end confusion*. Washington, DC: National Academy of Sciences.

Jaen, C. R., Ferrer, R., Miller, W., Palmer, R., Wood, R., Davila, M., . . . Stange, K. (2010). Patient outcomes at 26 months in the patient-centered medical home national demonstration project. *Annals of Family Medicine*, *8*(1), S57–S67.

Koh, H., Berwick, D., Clancy, C., Brach, C., Harris, L., & Zerhusen, E. (2012). New federal policy initiatives to boost health literacy can help the nation move beyond the cycle of costly "crisis care." *Health Affairs, 31*(2), 434–443.

Koloroutis, M. (2004). *Relationship-based care: A model for transforming practice.* Minneapolis, MN: Creative Health Care Management.

Levinson, W., Lesser, C., & Epstein, R. (2010). Developing physician communication skills for patient-centered care. *Health Affairs, 29*(7), 1310–1318.

Marks, D. F., Murray, M., Evans, B., & Estacio, E. V. (2011). *Health psychology: Theory, research, and practice.* Los Angeles, CA: Sage.

Miles, A., & Mezzich, J. E. (2011). Person-centered medicine: Identifying the way forward. *The International Journal of Person Centered Medicine, 1*(2), 205–206. doi:10.5759/ijpcm.v1i2.60

Nelson, K. M., Helfrich, C., Sun, H., Hebert, P. L., Liu, C, Dolan, E., . . . Fihn, S. D. (2014). Implementation of the patient-centererd medical home in the verterans health administration: Associations with patient satisfaction, quality of care, staff burnout, and hospital and emergency use. *Journal of the American Medical Association, 174*(8), 1350–1358.

New York State Department of Health. (2011). *Medicaid health homes.* Retrieved from http://www.health.ny.gov/health_care/medicaid/program/medicaid_health_homes

Nosbusch, J., Weiss, M., & Bobay, K. (2010). An integrated review of the literature on challenges confronting the acute care staff nurse in discharge planning. *Journal of Clinical Nursing, 20,* 754–774.

Patient-Centered Outcomes Research Institute. (2012). *Patient-centered outcomes research definition: Response to public input.* Retrieved from http://www.pcori.org

Pettetier, L. R., & Stichler, J. F. (2014). Patient-centered care and engagement. *The Journal of Nursing Administration, 44*(9), 473–480.

Sharecare. (2011). *Sharecare.* Retrieved from http://sharecare.org

U.S. Department of Health and Human Services (USDHHS). (2011a). *Administration implements Affordable care act provision to improve care, lower costs.* Retrieved from https://www.ahrq.gov/workingforquality/reports/2011-annual-report.html

Watson, J. (2012, February 6). *Transforming health care one nurse, one caregiver, one organization, at a time.* World Caring Science Institute. Retrieved from www.watsoncaringscience.org

Webster, D. (2013). Promoting therapeutic communications and patient-centered care using standardized patients. *Journal of Nursing Education, 52*(11), 645–648.

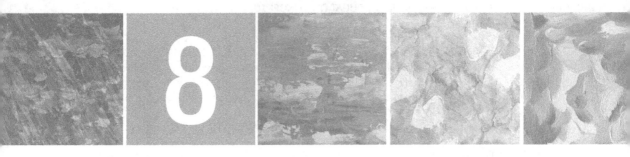

8

INTERPROFESSIONAL TEAMWORK AND COLLABORATION

Gerry Altmiller

It's less of a thing to do ... and more of a way to be. (Unknown Participant, 2007)

Upon completion of this chapter, the reader should be able to

1. Define interprofessional team.
2. Describe how a rapid response team (RRT) contributes to patient safety.
3. Identify the benefit of collaborative interprofessional teams on patient outcomes.
4. Describe resources interprofessional teams can employ to improve quality and safety for patients.
5. Identify the characteristics of effective interprofessional teams.
6. List the three steps of the Team*STEPPS* Delivery System.
7. Describe how informatics supports the interprofessional team's ability to more efficiently and effectively solve problems.
8. Describe how constructive feedback and reflection contribute to positive patient outcomes.
9. Discuss strategies the nurse can implement to include the patient as a partner on the interprofessional team.
10. Discuss strategies and techniques to overcome challenges to teamwork and maximize effective interprofessional communication.

A patient's family approaches the nurse's station and verbalizes concerns regarding their family member's care. They are worried about the patient's lack of energy following surgery to correct a bowel obstruction. They are concerned because the patient is elderly and has not been out of bed for 2 days. He is not eating well and he has diabetes. They ask to speak to the people in charge of the patient's care.

- *What do you know about the members of the interprofessional team caring for the patient?*
- *How will you bring the patient's immediate problems to the appropriate team member's attention?*
- *How will you convey the family's concerns to the interprofessional team?*
- *How can the interprofessional team work together to address this patient's needs?*

With the increasing complexity of patient care, it is clear that no one person can address a single patient's needs. It takes an interprofessional team of people working together, each contributing their individual expertise for the well-being of the patient. Care for the patient extends beyond the hands-on care provided by direct caregivers. To be effective, patient care requires the coordinated services of many people, some not even directly involved with the patient, yet all focused on one thing, a positive outcome and experience for the patient.

This chapter describes what an interprofessional team is and discusses the characteristics that make a team most effective. It describes how at the very center of the interprofessional team is the patient and the patient's family and how their individual preferences influence the decisions that the team makes as they assist the patient in achieving optimal patient outcomes. Within this goal of putting the patient front and center of the interprofessional healthcare team, strategies for how best to include the patient as a partner are presented. This chapter highlights resources that can be utilized as well as strategies that individuals and institutions can implement to create an environment where effective interprofessional communication supports patient safety and improves the overall quality of the care provided to patients, including the use of rapid response teams (RRTs). With the increasing emphasis on quality and safety, techniques to improve communication between interprofessional healthcare team members continues to be of great importance. Tools, techniques, and strategies for communication aimed at facilitating patient safety and quality of care are described, including the use of reflection by the nurse and other members of the interprofessional healthcare team as a means of improving patient outcomes. Likewise, Team*STEPPS* is presented as an effective way to ensure interprofessional healthcare teams are able to communicate with each other to promote situational awareness and patient safety. Strategies to create and develop effective team functioning are identified in this chapter. In addition, this chapter discusses how the World Wide Web has increased the availability of resources to support improved interprofessional communication and the dissemination of information. Informatics has contributed to effective teamwork by making information available at a moment's notice so that team members can exchange ideas to solve problems (Figure 8.1).

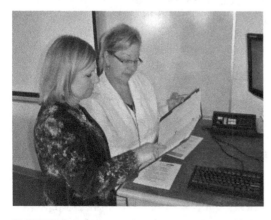

FIGURE 8.1 Interprofessional collaboration on the patient care unit.

Nursing holds a key position on the healthcare team, contributing to the plan of care, delivering nursing services, and providing that vital link between the patient, the patient's family, and the other members of the healthcare team. Skilled communication between the nurse and other members of the interprofessional healthcare team promote the exchange of clear and concise information, which allows the team to react quickly and appropriately to meet patients' needs.

WHAT IS AN INTERPROFESSIONAL TEAM?

A team is a group of individuals who work together for a common goal. In healthcare, the interprofessional team consists of people who have a stake or interest in and contribute to the well-being of the patient. An interprofessional team not only includes those directly involved in the patient's physical care such as the physicians, nurses, and family members, but it also includes those who provide support services such as pharmacists, social workers, dieticians, and those from departments such as housekeeping, radiology, the laboratory, transport services, and physical and occupational therapy. It is important to recognize the valuable contribution that of all these interprofessional team members make to the patient's care.

RAPID RESPONSE TEAMS

Interprofessional teams in the hospital setting may be brought together to focus on identified problems and find solutions. This can happen on a patient care unit or in other areas of the hospital. One common example of an effective team in the hospital is an **RRT**. An RRT is a team that includes specific healthcare professionals with specialized skills, who can mobilize and deliver immediate patient assessment and intervention if needed at the patient's bedside any time of day or night, 7 days a week at the beginning signs of deterioration in the patient's health status. The RRT is separate from a "code" or resuscitation team that is also composed of specialized interprofessional team members who would respond to cardiac and/or respiratory arrest. RRTs were formed based on recommendations by the Institute for Healthcare Improvement (IHI) to improve safety and quality, with the intention of preventing deaths outside of the ICU (IHI, 2012). RRTs may be structured differently within institutions, but most RRTs consist of a physician, critical care nurse, and respiratory therapist, along with other designated interprofessional members, as needed. Expert communication skills are required by RRT members because the patient's safety and well-being depends on the rapid and accurate exchange of pertinent and clear information between team members coming together in a concerted effort to aid the patient. RRTs support an institution's nurses by providing access to immediate assistance for any patient with a deteriorating condition. RRTs may be summoned to a patient's bedside by anyone, including family members. Providing RRT support allows for early intervention at the first sign of deterioration in patients, before they become critically ill or experience a cardiac arrest.

BENEFITS OF COLLABORATIVE INTERPROFESSIONAL TEAMS

At the center of the interprofessional healthcare team is the patient and the patient's family. Patient-centered care ensures that the patient is an integral part of the team and is central in all interactions and decisions. With patient-centered care, the interprofessional team acknowledges patient preferences regarding care and acknowledges individual health values and priorities. Without the patient, there would be no need for the team.

Like patients, nurses have not always been considered members of the interprofessional healthcare team; traditionally they have taken direction from hospital administrators and physicians rather than directly contributing to a collaborative plan of care. Historically, nurses were charged with direct patient care and focused mostly on providing patient hygiene under the direction of the physician. Differences in educational requirements prevented even routine tasks such as obtaining a patient's blood pressure from being delegated to the nurse. Nurses did not have a role in advocating for the patient and physicians did not confer with nurses regarding any aspect of the patient's care. The interprofessional relationship was strictly one of orders being dictated by the physician team member and orders being carried out by the nursing team member.

Gender issues have also contributed to the lack of interprofessional **collaboration** or the ability to effectively work together. In the past, males traditionally assumed the physician role while nurses have primarily been female. Much has changed in recent decades with both males and females assuming roles as physicians and nurses, independent of gender. Females still dominate the nursing profession; however, with the U.S. Department of Labor reporting that in 2011, males made up only 9% of the nursing workforce (U.S. Department of Labor, 2013). In comparison, females were reported to make up 36% of the physician workforce (U.S. Department of Labor).

Economic issues have also contributed to the lack of interprofessional collaboration. Nurses represent the largest segment of the hospital-based employee workforce and have been paid as hourly workers by the hospital. Physicians have been community based and have managed their practice as a business, directly billing their patients and the insurance companies. Some of this is changing as the expanding roles of nurses have created opportunities for hospital-based nurses and for advanced practice nurses in all areas of healthcare. Both of these groups of RNs have increased their education and have contributed to bridging the gap between nurses and physicians. Greater requirements in prelicensure education of nurses have also resulted in a bedside nurse that is able to assess, plan, implement, and evaluate care provided to patients, making the nurse a valuable team member.

Nursing knowledge is based on science combined with the art of caring for the individual needs of patients. Nursing brings a holistic perspective to patient care. The connection of the nurse to the patient and family through close and continued interaction allows nurses to understand and advocate for patient concerns and needs regardless of their practice level. Nurses can build rapport between patients and the team and facilitate collaboration between the interprofessional healthcare disciplines involved in the patient's care. Nurses' knowledge of the patient experience allows them to identify subtle changes in the patient's condition and act quickly to prevent complications of illness. The ability of the nurse to function proactively helps to reduce unnecessary costs to hospitals as well as improve patient satisfaction and outcomes.

Nurses need to recognize the value of this perspective and acknowledge the positive impact they have on patient outcomes. It is important that nurses articulate the value of this positive effect on patient satisfaction as well as the financial benefit that nurses bring to the institutions they serve to enhance their role as contributing team members and to advance the profession of nursing.

TABLE 8.1 THE FUTURE OF NURSING: LEADING CHANGE, ADVANCING HEALTH

FOUR KEY RECOMMENDATIONS

1. Nurses should practice to the full extent of their education.
2. Nurses should achieve higher levels of education through an improved education system that promotes seamless academic progression.
3. Nurses should be full partners with physicians and other healthcare professionals in the redesign of healthcare.
4. Better data collection and information infrastructure are necessary for effective workforce planning and policy making.

Recognizing the value of nursing, the Institute of Medicine (IOM), now known as the National Academy of Medicine, in collaboration with the Robert Wood Johnson Foundation (RWJF), published its report, *The Future of Nursing: Leading Change, Advancing Health* (IOM, 2010). This report identified the barriers that prevent nurses from being able to respond to the rapidly changing healthcare system. It also validated the important role that nurses play in the delivery of seamless, high-quality, affordable healthcare to all. The four key recommendations from the report were focused on the role that nursing should have in providing care (Table 8.1).

Advancing Healthcare Through Improved Education

Although educational differences exist among interprofessional team members, it is important to recognize that each team member brings a perspective to the team that represents specialized knowledge from his or her discipline. For physicians, the educational requirements include a baccalaureate degree with an additional 4 years of medical school, followed by a year of internship in clinical practice, and 2 years of residency. Medical specialization adds additional years of training and fellowship. For nurses, there are varied levels of educational requirements for entry into practice. These include a 3-year diploma school education, a 2-year associate degree education, and a 4-year baccalaureate degree education as well as master's completion programs. Other healthcare disciplines have varied educational degree requirements as well. No matter the educational requirements, each healthcare discipline needs to be able to collaborate with others to provide the highest quality care for the patient. While concepts of interprofessional collaboration are included in the educational process of each healthcare discipline, Hood et al. (2014) notes that purposeful planning and early integration of interprofessional learning would foster an enhanced group dynamic as well as a shared commitment to collaboration with recognition of the value of other disciplines.

To support the appreciation of each healthcare discipline's perspective, expertise, and values, many programs now include an integration of interprofessional education as part of their curriculum. **Interprofessional education** is the opportunity for multiple healthcare disciplines to learn together in the same learning environment simultaneously, gaining a greater understanding for each discipline's role and contributions. A common example of this is medical and nursing students taking an ethics class together or participating in a communication exercise as part of an orientation program.

REAL-WORLD INTERVIEW

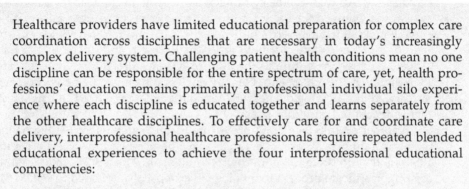

Healthcare providers have limited educational preparation for complex care coordination across disciplines that are necessary in today's increasingly complex delivery system. Challenging patient health conditions mean no one discipline can be responsible for the entire spectrum of care, yet, health professions' education remains primarily a professional individual silo experience where each discipline is educated together and learns separately from the other healthcare disciplines. To effectively care for and coordinate care delivery, interprofessional healthcare professionals require repeated blended educational experiences to achieve the four interprofessional educational competencies:

- Understand the scope of responsibilities of each team member.
- Maintain ethical conduct and quality of care within the team to develop respect and trust.
- Communicate effectively with patients, families, and healthcare team members.
- Utilize teamwork behaviors in executing patient care requirements.

Complex healthcare work environments are driven by little understood human factors including intricacies of communication and behavior. These are important for sharing critical information and coordination among the team. Knowing what each healthcare discipline can contribute during the stress of a healthcare intervention is a critical factor in delivering safe care. A well-developed self-awareness allows team members to function alternately as leader or follower, as appropriate to the situation and individual competence. Healthcare is a team sport involving multiple individuals in the delivery of safe care.

Gwen Sherwood
Professor and Associate Dean for Academic Affairs
University of North Carolina at Chapel Hill School of Nursing
Coinvestigator, Quality and Safety Education for Nurses (www.qsen.org)
Chapel Hill, North Carolina

STRATEGIES FOR MAXIMIZING EFFECTIVE INTERPROFESSIONAL TEAMS

The changing socialization of physicians and nurses as well as other disciplines has allowed for the formation of interprofessional teams that not only care for patients but also tackle some of the toughest problems facing healthcare today. In part, this change has come from changes in traditional gender roles as well as the attainment of baccalaureate and master's degrees by more and more nurses. Working together, physicians and nurses have developed work processes to address quality and safety on all levels of patient care.

Methods such as **root cause analysis** (RCA) are employed to identify problems within the healthcare system. With RCA, teams work together to systematically investigate serious adverse events and identify the root cause and contributing factors that lead to error, patient injury, or a negative outcome so that those factors can be corrected. An RCA can be conducted to identify mechanisms within the healthcare system that allowed for the error or near miss to occur. A **near miss** is an event that could have resulted in an error but was caught in time before it could cause injury. This reporting process allows for both individual growth and development for the nurse as well as correction within the healthcare system's practices to prevent future errors. RCA discovers the root of a problem by not stopping at the first answer it arrives at for its cause, but by delving deeper into why the problem occurred, asking questions until there are no more questions to ask.

Another process used to improve quality and safety is the Six Sigma method. Six Sigma is a quality assurance strategy developed in corporate America in the mid-1980s by the Motorola Corporation (Stanton et al., 2014). Six Sigma, used to improve existing healthcare processes, involves five steps, also referred to as DMAIC: define; measure; analyze; improve; and control. During the define step of Six Sigma, potential team members are identified that are knowledgeable about the healthcare process or service that has been identified as needing improvement. These team members must have a clear understanding of what the expectation and needs are so they know where to aim the improvement. During the measure step of Six Sigma, the problem is investigated and data are gathered to determine how, when, and where the problem is occurring. The analyze step of Six Sigma allows the team to look for trends and patterns of the healthcare problem from the data so they can identify a root cause. During the improve step of Six Sigma, solutions are identified and implemented, and finally, during the control step of Six Sigma, control mechanisms such as retraining or monitoring systems that ensure that the problem does not occur again are put in place.

RESOURCES FOR INTERPROFESSIONAL TEAMWORK AND COLLABORATION

Nowhere is interprofessional teamwork and collaboration more important than in providing required healthcare to patients in need. Although all members of the interprofessional healthcare team possess specific expertise that would benefit the patient, if they were unable to coordinate those skills and connect vital services together, the patient would not have the best possible outcome. Team members must work together to provide coordinated care to achieve the best results.

Patients are at greater risk during transitions between care. **Handoff** is a term used to describe the communication method that the interprofessional team uses to transfer patient care information to one another between shifts or between patient care units or hospitals. In healthcare, poor outcomes occur when there are breakdowns in communication, poor teamwork, or inefficient communication "handoffs" that create situations that can lead to errors. Effective interprofessional teams involved in direct patient care have common goals of high quality and safety, and ensuring that information about the patient is communicated accurately and completely supports those goals during transitions of care.

Interprofessional teams in healthcare may be focused on more long-term projects. These interprofessional teams may be assembled to address a number of concerns which may include anything from quality improvement (QI) processes to planning for the future of the healthcare institution. Although the work of these types of interprofessional teams may seem slower and more deliberate, the principles that guide them are the same as teams that respond to patient emergencies. For example, a long-term goal of a hospital might be to increase the number of baccalaureate-prepared RNs to 80% within 10 years. Collaboration between hospital administration, finance, nursing leadership, and broad representation from nursing staff, all using effective teamwork and communication strategies, would be needed to conduct the same steps of assessment, definition of problem, goal setting, implementation, and evaluation that are part of the nursing process to achieve goals.

CHARACTERISTICS OF EFFECTIVE INTERPROFESSIONAL HEALTHCARE TEAMS

Effective interprofessional teams are able to think reflectively about the situation at hand considering past experiences, contemplate options from all perspectives, and deliberate the options in an atmosphere of mutual respect. In high-functioning, successful interprofessional teams, members can voice concerns and opinions, creating a group dynamic where all members contribute and share in the decision making. Clear, focused communication and respectful negotiation decrease the potential for misunderstandings and promote camaraderie among the team members.

Accountability and Stages of Team Development

Forming, storming, norming, and *performing* are terms used to describe the stages experienced by teams as they progress from formation to functioning as high-performance teams (Tuckman, 1965). The forming stage is generally a short phase when team members are introduced and objectives are established. As the team moves into the storming stage, team roles become clarified and processes as well as structures for the team are established. It is within this process that the details of the approach being used to accomplish the goals or assignment are decided upon. The workload of the task becomes clear during this storming phase and can overwhelm the team members. Conflicts may arise and members build relationships with other team members as they work through conflict resolution. In this storming stage, teams will fail if work processes and team relationships have not been well established.

In the norming stage, team members develop a stronger commitment to the team's goals and assume responsibility for the team's progress. Individuals show leadership in specific areas and team members come to respect each other's roles. As members become socialized as a team, they are able to provide constructive feedback to each other. It is important to note that teams can pass back and forth between the storming and norming stages as new tasks are assigned to the team. The performing stage is realized through achievement of the team's shared vision of the goal. At this point, teamwork feels easier and members can for the most part join and leave the team without affecting the team's performance. The progress achieved from the members' hard work establishes the team as a high-performance team.

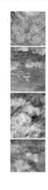

CASE STUDY 8.1

The manager of a critical care unit wants to implement self-scheduling among his large staff. He appoints two staff members from the night shift, two staff members from the day shift, one assistant manager, and one nurse aide to a committee with the goal of developing rules to guide the self-scheduling process. The committee is scheduled to meet weekly until all self-scheduling rules are developed and the self-scheduling process can be put in place. Immediately, tensions run high in the committee as there is disagreement about the number of Fridays that must be worked by each staff member and the number of weekends that must be worked in a 6-week schedule. Through negotiation, agreement is reached on the committee regarding these issues. Just when they believe that they have all issues resolved, there is disagreement among the committee members regarding the number of schedule changes management can make to accommodate unit needs. This is a very heated topic and the negotiation for this continues for 3 weeks. Eventually, it is resolved with agreement by all. It is decided that the scheduling committee will remain intact, assist with the transition for staff, and manage the scheduling process. Committee members will work together to cover the unit needs.

1. *What team stage is identified as the team begins to work to resolve the number of Fridays and weekends that will be required by each staff?*
2. *What team stage is identified when the committee decides to remain intact to assist with the transition and manage the scheduling process?*

Delegation

Willingness to assist colleagues is pivotal to interprofessional teamwork and collaboration. Teamwork requires that members can effectively delegate work to each other. In patient care, it is essential that delegated tasks are within the scope of practice of the individual to whom the task is being delegated. For example, inserting an indwelling urinary catheter could be delegated by a nurse to another nurse. It could not be delegated to a nursing assistant. When delegating, the nurse employs the following steps: assess and plan; communicate what needs to be done; ensure availability to assist and support; and finally, evaluate effectiveness and give feedback (National Council of State Boards of Nursing, 2016).

With all delegation, clear communication of what needs to be done and confirmation of understanding from the individual being delegated to is essential to ensure patient safety. The nurse, who is delegating, needs to provide an opportunity for clarification and questions. If an outcome does not meet expectations, the nurse should lead the discussion with those involved to identify reasons for the unexpected outcome and determine what could be learned from the experience to improve care and to ensure a successful outcome in the future.

Crew Resource Management

Crew resource management (CRM) refers to educating individuals that work in high-stress systems where the human aspect of operations can create an increased potential for error. Originating in the aviation industry for the cockpit crew, CRM develops communication, leadership, and decision-making safety strategies to combat the potential for human error that is inherent in high-stress systems and its devastating effects. The healthcare industry shares an interest in interprofessional teamwork and clear communication with the aviation industry to prevent catastrophic events. Healthcare has applied many CRM strategies to the daily interactions and continuous QI processes of the interprofessional healthcare team. CRM communication, leadership, and decision-making safety strategies focus on cognitive and interpersonal skills to promote situational awareness.

Situational awareness is having the right information at the right time alongside the ability to analyze that information to appropriately and effectively take action. Having this awareness, allows for all team members to be conscientious of the facts in any given situation. The vehicle for this attentiveness is effective communication between interprofessional healthcare team members.

TEAM*STEPPS*

Within healthcare, Team*STEPPS* is a program developed to provide training for effective communication techniques similar to those promoted by CRM. The program is designed to teach interprofessional teams how to communicate with each other to promote situational awareness and patient safety. Specifically Team*STEPPS* is

- A powerful solution to improving patient safety within an organization
- An evidence-based teamwork system to improve communication and teamwork skills among healthcare professionals
- A source for ready-to-use materials and a training curriculum to successfully integrate teamwork principles into all areas of the healthcare system
- Scientifically rooted in more than 20 years of research and lessons from the application of teamwork principles (Agency for Healthcare Research and Quality [AHRQ], n.d., p. 2)

Developed in collaboration with the Department of Defense, the Agency for Healthcare Research and Quality (AHRQ) initiated Team*STEPPS* to augment the effort and abilities of interprofessional teams specially to ensure the highest patient outcomes within healthcare institutions and systems. By focusing on a three-phased process of team development, the program optimizes resources within a team, provides a framework for resolving conflict and enhancing communications, and provides the basis to effectively address potential barriers to effective patient safety and quality care.

AHRQ lists the three phases of Team*STEPPS* as (a) assessment; (b) planning, training, and implementation; and (c) sustainment. Assessment involves pretraining evaluation to determine the willingness and capacity of an organization to change. Within this phase of the process, an interprofessional team is established that is made up of a cross-section of healthcare leaders and professionals within the organization itself. This phase also involves conducting a comprehensive site assessment that identifies areas of weakness and needs relative to teamwork. From this assessment, the second phase of Team*STEPPS* is initiated; a training program is developed to effectively overcome the deficiencies of the team as well as maximize its strengths. Once this education has occurred, the third and final phase can be initiated. The long-range goal of the third phase is to maintain and continually improve teamwork efforts throughout the organization. Through coaching, feedback, and reinforcement of strategies taught,

TABLE 8.2 SITUATION, BACKGROUND, ASSESSMENT, AND RECOMMENDATION

SBAR	MEANING	EXAMPLE
S	Situation: Describe what is happening with the patient	Doctor, I am calling about Mrs. Smith, your patient admitted yesterday to room 304 with respiratory distress.
B	Background: Explain the background of the patient's circumstances	She was comfortable during the evening after being placed on 2 L oxygen by nasal cannula and receiving 20 mg of furosemide (Lasix) intravenously, but is now complaining of shortness of breath.
A	Assessment: Identify what data you have regarding the situation	Her respiratory rate is 28. Pulse is 110/min and her oximetry measures 91%. She has crackles in the lower third of her lung fields bilaterally. She is laboring to breathe.
R	Recommendation: Identify what you think needs to be done to correct the situation	I think she may need her furosemide (Lasix) dose increased.

SBAR, situation, background, assessment, and recommendation.

teamwork and communication skills can be continually reinforced and built upon as opportunities for improvement in clinical and administrative situations throughout the organization.

Situation, Background, Assessment, and Recommendation

A framework for communication that has been implemented in many healthcare settings is SBAR, an acronym for the words *situation, background, assessment, and recommendation* (AHRQ, n.d.). It was developed by the military and is now applied to healthcare as a means to relay significant information regarding a patient's condition or to be used as patients' care is communicated and handed off from one caregiver to another (Table 8.2).

ADDITIONAL TECHNIQUES FOR EFFECTIVE COMMUNICATION WITHIN INTERPROFESSIONAL TEAMS

Clear and open communication among team members allows ideas to be shared and counteracts the potential for human errors of judgment. Techniques such as cross-monitoring require that team members listen carefully to the details being communicated and provide correction for the team if needed. **Cross-monitoring** is the process of monitoring the actions of other team members for the purpose of sharing the workload and reducing or avoiding errors (AHRQ, n.d.). An example of this technique can occur during grand rounds where interventions are discussed by a group of physicians, nurses, pharmacists, and other healthcare providers. Decisions verbally agreed upon can sometimes be missed as orders are articulated for the patient. A nurse asking for clarification of an order he or she recalls differently is an example of cross-monitoring.

Other communication techniques can be used to bring attention to patient situations. A callout is used to communicate important information to the entire team simultaneously (AHRQ, n.d.). In a callout, the team member would callout to others for assistance. For example, during a resuscitation effort, also known as a code, a nurse monitoring the patient's blood pressure might assertively state the changing status to the medical resident. Typically, the callout is then followed by a check back, which verifies receipt of the information and provides feedback and appropriate response. In this example, the resident might acknowledge the callout by asking for medication to be given to stabilize the patient's blood pressure. Check back requires the receiver verbally acknowledge the message to provide opportunity for correction if needed.

The two-challenge rule states that if an individual does not believe that his or her first attempt to bring attention to a concerning patient situation has been successful, the individual is obligated to make a second attempt to make the problem known to others on the team (AHRQ, n.d.). The two-challenge rule is designed for when team member's input is ignored purposely. It is the obligation of the person to bring it forward again to make sure it is not ignored. An example of the two-challenge rule is when a nurse tells a physician about a concern she has for the patient, like a low urine output, and the physician does not address it for one reason or another. The nurse is obligated to bring it forward again.

Another tool that can be used to advocate for a patient is CUS, which is an acronym for the words *concerned, uncomfortable*, and *safety* (AHRQ, n.d.). Frequently, nurses are expected to advocate for their patients but they may not know how to do so. CUS is a tool that assists the nurse in taking an assertive stance to do what the nurse believes is needed for the patient. For example, in the case of a larger than recommended dose of medication being ordered for a patient, the nurse may approach the ordering provider and state, "I'm concerned with the dose that has been ordered. I am uncomfortable giving such a large dose to this patient because of her renal condition. I don't think it is safe."

STRATEGIES FOR EFFECTIVE COMMUNICATION WITHIN INTERPROFESSIONAL TEAMS

Time-outs are mandated in the operating room (OR) and procedure suites by The Joint Commission to help ensure patient safety (The Joint Commission, n.d.). Time-outs can also be initiated during any procedure at the bedside. The time-out is an opportunity for everyone in the room to stop and ensure that the correct patient is having the correct procedure done to the correct site. The time-out requires that everyone stop his or her clinical work and devote his or her attention to the patient. Another safety strategy the team can employ is the use of safety huddles. Safety huddles allow those caring for the patient to review pertinent information and the plan of care. It is similar to a team huddle used in sports and ensures everyone is aware and working toward the same goals for the patient. An example of when a huddle would facilitate effective, coordinated care is when medications need to be altered due to change in a patient's status. Responding to an adverse reaction of a patient to a specific medication for instance would best be handled with a focused, coordinated approach by as many of the interprofessional team members as possible.

All of the aforementioned communication strategies are developed by the AHRQ which provides reference videos for clinicians, administrators, and educators demonstrating Team*STEPPS* tools, strategies, and techniques at its website, www.ahrq.gov/professionals/education/curriculum-tools/teamstepps/instructor/videos/index.html (Table 8.3).

TABLE 8.3 AVAILABLE TOPICS FOR REFERENCE AND EDUCATION ON AHRQ TEAM*STEPPS* WEBSITE

SBAR	Provides a standardized framework for communication, that is, situation, *background*, *assessment*, and *recommendation*.
Cross-monitoring	Involves listening to other team members to identify correct and incorrect information. This allows the team to self-correct healthcare errors before they occur.
Callout	Asks for help from other team members.
Two-challenge rule	Obligates team members to make a second attempt to have a concern heard when their first attempt to bring attention to a concern is not acknowledged.
CUS	Advocacy strategy using the words concerned, *u*ncomfortable, *s*afety.
Check back/read back	Verbally calling out and repeating back information to confirm it is understood correctly.
Handoff	Transferring responsibility for a patient's care from one unit to another or from one individual to another.

CUS, concerned, uncomfortable, and safety; SBAR, situation, background, assessment, and recommendation.

CRITICAL THINKING 8.1

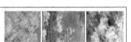

The nurse calls the physician to report that a patient has suddenly developed hives while receiving an IV dose of antibiotic. The hives are covering most of his back. The physician tells the nurse that he does not think that the antibiotic is the cause and that she should just continue to monitor the patient. The nurse is concerned that the hives may be the beginning of a serious allergic reaction.

1. What safety strategy would be most effective for the nurse to use to advocate for the patient in this situation?

Another way that team members can work to prevent errors is by reporting them to other members of the healthcare team. Timely reporting of errors and near misses, also known as close calls where an error could have occurred but was stopped before it caused harm, provides an opportunity for the team to learn from them. In most cases, errors and near misses are not the result of a single person's actions. They are often the result of a failure within a healthcare system. By reporting all errors or near misses, the need for an RCA can be evaluated more completely and effectively and actions can be taken to ensure the same situation does not put patients at risk in the future.

USE OF INFORMATICS FOR EFFECTIVE PROBLEM SOLVING

Minimizing the potential for errors is the goal of everyone on the healthcare team. Participating in behaviors that guard against error and protect patients is a fundamental part of daily healthcare practice. There are many available web resources funded by government agencies and national healthcare organizations that are designed to improve teamwork and collaboration, prevent error, promote patient safety, and

TABLE 8.4 WEB RESOURCES FOR TEAMWORK AND COLLABORATION, ERROR PREVENTION, PATIENT SAFETY, AND QI

RESOURCE	WEBSITE ADDRESS
Team*STEPPS*	www.ahrq.gov/professionals/education/curriculum-tools/ teamstepps/instructor/videos/index.html
Patient Safety Network	psnet.ahrq.gov
The National Database of Nursing Quality Indicators	nursingandndnqi.weebly.com/ndnqi-indicators.html
ISMP	www.ismp.org
The Future of Nursing Report	www.nationalacademies.org/hmd/Reports/2010/The-Future-of-Nursing-Leading-Change-Advancing-Health.aspx
QSEN	www.qsen.org
The Joint Commission	www.jointcommission.org

ISMP, Institute for Safe Medication Practices; QSEN, Quality and Safety Education for Nurses.

improve the quality of the care that patients receive. Nurses, as well as other team members, can access these resources to learn about strategies that address quality and safety as a way to improve their practice and keep patients safe from errors (Table 8.4).

Communication and Interprofessional Teamwork in QI

All members of the interprofessional healthcare team have an obligation to improve patient care processes and outcomes by focusing on communication and QI. **Debriefing** is the process of reviewing performance effectiveness following challenging patient care situations. Utilizing strategies such as debriefing allows the interprofessional team to evaluate the effectiveness of their communication and teamwork and to identify areas where improvement is possible. It is during debriefing that constructive feedback is given and received. All team members should feel comfortable to participate in this process. Individuals may differ in how they provide feedback to peers, but feedback, whether positive or negative, should always be an unbiased reflection of what occurred, opening the door to a discussion of evidence-based practice (Clynes & Raftery, 2008). Constructive feedback should carefully detail events as they occurred and avoid opinion.

Constructive feedback recounts events, offering options for improvement. Constructive feedback is most effective when focused on a task, a process used, or on self-regulation, because that focus contributes to learning; feedback focused on the individual is less effective because it does not increase learning (Hattie & Timperley, 2007). For instance, feedback such as "It was wise to gather your supplies before you went into the patient's room" focuses on the task. Feedback such as "Your explanation to the patient before you began allowed the patient to trust you" focuses on the healthcare process. Feedback such as "It is good that you realized you broke sterile technique and changed your gloves" focuses on self-monitoring. All of these support knowledge development. Feedback such as "You did a good job" focuses on the individual and is least effective because it does not add to one's understanding of what aspects of his or her practice were effective and "a good job." Although it is difficult to give and receive unflattering feedback, team members must understand that feedback is essential for growth. Feedback is the mechanism that allows one to make continual adjustments in practice. Receiving feedback is often the catalyst for change and should be viewed as an opportunity for growth. Sometimes when receiving feedback that is perceived as negative, it challenges the team member to consider the validity of the comments made, particularly considering whether the same feedback has been provided previously by other sources. If after consideration, feedback is perceived as inaccurate, the team member can ask for examples of poor performance and focus on improvement, asking the person providing feedback how he or she feels improvement can be achieved.

Auditing Patient Care and Outcomes

Teams can work together to conduct audits and other organizational studies that measure quality, safety, and patient outcomes which can have a significant impact on the process of QI. Collecting and analyzing data regarding patient care practices and patient outcomes allows the team to document differences between the actual system's performance and the goals of the organization. By documenting differences, changes can be made to narrow the gap between the two and improve team performance for quality of care and patient safety.

REFLECTION AND FEEDBACK

Communication and interprofessional teamwork skills are a huge part of the protection from injury and complications that nurses provide for patients. These skills help not only when interacting with patients and healthcare team members to solve problems but also when nurses reflect on patient care events and discuss ways to improve outcomes. Providing feedback to team members allows the team to identify strengths and weaknesses, make changes to the healthcare system, and adjust practice for individual growth and development.

Self-evaluation of one's communication and decision making is a crucial element of professional growth and strengthens one's ability to contribute to the team's decisions by employing strong clinical judgment. As discussed

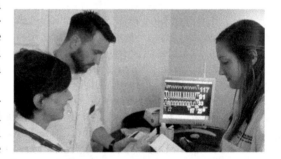

FIGURE 8.2 Monthly staff meeting.

earlier in the chapter, reflection supports confidence in decision making and provides an opportunity for the individual to consider his or her interactions with others and determine what actions enhanced a positive outcome and what actions worked against it. Reflecting on clinical situations and their outcomes allows team members to make positive changes to improve practice (Figure 8.2).

Tanner Model of Thinking Like a Nurse

Tanner's model of Thinking Like a Nurse (2006) demonstrates how clinical judgment is developed through reflection, enhancing critical thinking skills. These skills are essential to develop as one gains expertise in protecting patients through situational awareness and mindfulness. **Mindfulness** in this context implies staying focused with the ability to see the significance of early and weak signals as well as to take strong and decisive action to prevent harm (Weick & Sutcliff, 2001). Tanner's model stems from review of approximately 200 studies focused on the nurses' development of clinical judgment. From her review, she concluded that

- Clinical judgments are more influenced by what nurses bring to the situation than the objective data about the situation at hand.
- Sound clinical judgment rests to some degree on knowing the patient and his or her typical pattern of responses, as well as an engagement with the patient and his or her concerns.
- Clinical judgments are influenced by the context in which the situation occurs and the culture of the nursing care unit.

EVIDENCE FROM THE LITERATURE

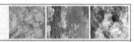

Citation

McBride, A. B. (2010). Toward a roadmap for interdisciplinary academic career success. *Research and Theory for Nursing Practice: An International Journal, 24*(1), 74–86.

Discussion

The complexity of today's health problems requires more than the knowledge of one provider. This necessitates an interprofessional collaborative approach. Identified by the Institute of Medicine (IOM) as a core competency of all health-care professionals, interprofessional collaboration has different meanings to different people. Examples of interprofessional collaboration include understaffed hospital personnel working together during the night shift to ensure patient safety or nurses and physicians discussing a patient plan to decrease complications or multiple disciplines working in partnership for education and research endeavors to decrease mortality and morbidity within their institution.

One of the barriers to achieving interprofessional collaboration has been the socialization of the separate healthcare disciplines, which has been focused on how they differ from one another. Up until recently, each healthcare discipline was taught without interacting with the other healthcare disciplines; each establishing its own distinct body of knowledge.

Implications for Nursing

Nursing has built a large body of knowledge based on scientific research. Nursing's strengths include its holistic orientation to the patient and its ability to facilitate the bridging of disciplines and boundaries, thus supporting interprofessional collaboration. The reward of interprofessional collaboration is an expanded perspective where multiple healthcare disciplines work together to develop new models of care, new methods of care delivery, and breakthroughs in disease management, and health promotion. Through interprofessional collaboration, knowledge obtained from research can be translated into practice for the benefit of human health. The nursing profession is in a key position to support collaboration between all healthcare professionals from all disciplines as they move forward to meet the core competencies identified by the IOM.

- Nurses use a variety of reasoning patterns alone or in combination.
- Reflection on practice is often triggered by a breakdown in clinical judgment and is critical for the development of clinical knowledge and improvement in clinical reasoning (Tanner, 2006, p. 204).

STRATEGIES TO INCLUDE THE PATIENT AS PARTNER

Communication between the healthcare team, the patient, and the patient's family during times of stress and illness can be challenging but it is essential to safety and a key factor in patient satisfaction. Patients and families look to the nurse to provide a personal connection with the team. In addition, many patients and families look to the nurse as a source of information. The nurse should use language that is understandable to the patient and provide patient-centered information that allows the patient to assume a role of partnership rather than dependency. The nurse plays a pivotal role in including the patient, providing explanations, and providing access for the patient to communicate with other members of the interprofessional team. To promote the patient's partnership with the interprofessional healthcare team, the nurse can create connections for the patient to other members of the team, such as providing information regarding when the physician usually makes rounds. The nurse can encourage the patient and family to write down their questions for the physician and put the questions in the chart so that the physician may address them.

Developing Enhanced Communication Skills

The nurse must possess strong communication skills to contribute to effective team functioning. Communication is the interactive process of exchanging information. Effective communication is clear, precise, and concise, with no ambiguities. Safety is enhanced when the communication sender uses the proper terminology and provides an opportunity for clarification. Ideally, in response, the receiver of the communication acknowledges the message as heard and understood.

Many barriers can interfere with communication, such as knowledge gaps, education levels, culture, language barriers, or stress. It is important for nurses to develop strategies to identify and overcome these barriers. Nonverbal cues, such as the patient's facial expression, eye contact, and body posturing, may signal a message from the patient, but when safety is a priority such as it is in healthcare, interpreting nonverbal cues only is not an acceptable technique for communicating. Any perception one develops from nonverbal communication must be verified verbally to maintain a safe environment.

Effective communication is essential to maintaining a safe and protected environment for patients. Ineffective communication continues to be identified as the root cause for many sentinel events reported to The Joint Commission (2016), which explains why improving communication is a safety priority for the next decade. Students and nurses who are new to practice may find team interaction intimidating for several reasons, including that they do not clearly understand the culture of healthcare communication, they have known knowledge gaps, and they have not yet gained enough experience in the healthcare setting from which they can draw. Recognizing what information needs to be communicated to which individuals on the team and in what time frame is essential to developing effective communication skills. Regularly scheduled meetings of key team members help to ensure effective communications. Quality and safety in patient care are strongly influenced by the ability of the healthcare team to communicate clearly without uncertainty, in a timely manner, and to contribute to the healthcare team's productive, efficient approach to patient care.

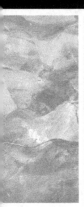

REAL-WORLD INTERVIEW

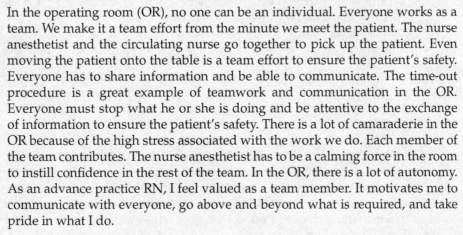

In the operating room (OR), no one can be an individual. Everyone works as a team. We make it a team effort from the minute we meet the patient. The nurse anesthetist and the circulating nurse go together to pick up the patient. Even moving the patient onto the table is a team effort to ensure the patient's safety. Everyone has to share information and be able to communicate. The time-out procedure is a great example of teamwork and communication in the OR. Everyone must stop what he or she is doing and be attentive to the exchange of information to ensure the patient's safety. There is a lot of camaraderie in the OR because of the high stress associated with the work we do. Each member of the team contributes. The nurse anesthetist has to be a calming force in the room to instill confidence in the rest of the team. In the OR, there is a lot of autonomy. As an advance practice RN, I feel valued as a team member. It motivates me to communicate with everyone, go above and beyond what is required, and take pride in what I do.

Daniel Boucot
Rancocas Anesthesia Associates
Kennedy Health System
Sewell, New Jersey

Strategies for Communication in Difficult Situations

Challenging patient care situations such as patient resuscitations, difficult patient procedures, rapid response efforts, or end-of-life events require extreme attention and clarity. Unnecessary conversation should cease during these situations and all communication should focus on the situation at hand without distractions. To ensure patient safety at these times, communication senders and receivers should continually verify their communication using read backs or check backs. For example, during a difficult labor and delivery, the physician might assertively request many urgent medications and interventions. In this chaotic and unnerving scenario, it is essential that the nurse and other healthcare professional verify what orders and instructions are being relayed by repeating them to those giving the orders. In addition, documentation must be clear and accurate during these times so as to provide a written account of events. It is during these types of challenging patient care situations that communication with patients and families can sometimes be overlooked. This can be avoided by including the patient in decision making whenever possible and appointing someone on the team to provide updates to the family. Family presence at patient resuscitations is becoming more commonplace. Institutions that support this practice designate a member of the team, frequently a nurse, to support the family and explain the interventions and actions of the healthcare team's efforts. Supporting the family during such a high-stress, high-stakes event requires skillful communication that is clear, accurate, and compassionate.

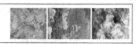

CRITICAL THINKING 8.2

During a patient resuscitation, the nurse pulling supplies from the code cart discovers that supplies are missing. When the code has ended, the nurse reviews the documentation form to determine who stocked the cart last.

1. What would be the best approach for the nurse to initiate a discussion with coworkers about the incorrectly stocked cart?
2. What aspects should the nurse focus on during the discussion?
3. How can the nurse create a learning experience for coworkers in this instance?

Managing Conflict

It is vital to patient safety that the lines of communication remain open among all those involved in the patient's care. When there is disruption in the smooth flow of communication among team members, it is important to address it promptly before it becomes a more prolonged barrier to communication. Destructive events such as physicians who will not respond to pages, nurses who are resistant to carrying out legitimate orders, or pharmacists who do not move quickly to fill STAT or urgent orders prescriptions, create difficult communications among healthcare providers that can negatively impact patient care (Table 8.5). It is important to address misunderstandings and conflicts promptly so that they do not become long-standing barriers to communication. Team members must be vigilant in fulfilling their ethical duty to work together for the patient's well-being.

Negative or difficult communication in the work environment can come from patients, families, physicians, other nurses, or any person involved in the operations of the institution. Physicians who yell, do not answer calls, and display disrespect and condescension toward colleagues make it uncomfortable to practice. Miscommunications between the interprofessional team can put patients at risk. Stressed patients, families, and/or staff can act out frustrations and aggression. It is important that all members of the interprofessional team respect the expertise of each individual, giving each the power to speak up and provide input in decision making with the team. Those in leadership roles should work to equalize the power structure so that all feel safe to contribute (Rittenmyer, Huffman, Hopp, & Block, 2013).

Horizontal Violence

One of the most troubling conflicts for nurses is nurse-to-nurse aggression, also known as lateral violence or horizontal violence (Rittenmeyer et al., 2013). Horizontal violence is uncivil behavior toward colleagues that may manifest as making faces or raising eyebrows in response to comments, making snide remarks, withholding information that interferes with a colleague's ability to perform professionally, refusing to help, or appearing not available to give help. Scapegoating (blaming one person for all negative things that have happened), criticizing, breaking confidences, fighting among nurses, and excluding peers from dialogue and activities are all forms of horizontal violence and result in injury to the dignity of another (Griffin, 2004). Nurses can experience

TABLE 8.5 MANAGING DIFFICULT COMMUNICATIONS

HEALTHCARE PROVIDER	COMMUNICATION ISSUE	THE NURSE'S BEST COMMUNICATION APPROACH
Physician	Not answering page	Call physician's office or overhead page to solve immediate problem; later discuss with physician that the patient's needs are the primary concern and give the reason for the page.
Physician	Speaking in an angry condescending manner	Maintain calm and keep focus on the patient; state your primary concern is to solve the patient's immediate need. Identify the patient's need clearly and succinctly.
Pharmacist	Not filling STAT orders quickly	Maintain calm and explain patient's immediate need.
Unlicensed assistive personal	Not following through with delegated duties	Explore reasons for why duties were not completed. If needed, make adjustment to workload. Develop plan for future communication regarding delegated duties.
Nurse	Rolls eyes and sighs during report; indicates irritation with you	Respond in civil tone, stating that you sense there is something the nurse wants to say and that you learn when people are direct. Ask nurse to please be direct with his or her concerns.
Nurse	Does not provide assistance when needed	Explore reasons for lack of assistance; be quick to volunteer to help others so they will be just as quick to return the favor when you need help.
Nurse	Resistant to carrying out legitimate orders	Explore concerns related to orders; develop plan. Offer assistance to peers when able.

STAT.

physical consequences (loss of sleep, weight loss, irritable bowel syndrome) and/or psychological consequences (depression, anxiety, and loss of confidence) as a result of lateral violence (Becher & Visovsky, 2012). In addition, lateral violence can interfere with continuity of care and be detrimental to patients and to the institutions that provide care.

When encountering lateral violence, nurses should respond to it in a manner that focuses on consensus building rather than respond emotionally with anger. If a communication becomes angry or difficult, the nurse can refocus the interaction on the patient's safety and well-being. Refocusing on the patient's needs will take the focus off of the power struggle that occurs when people are angry. In addition to protecting one's self, nurses have an obligation to report behaviors that compromise patient safety or the well-being of coworkers to their supervisor or someone else in authority to adequately address the problem. Conflicts and negative behaviors place patients at risk because they serve as a distraction preventing nurse from functioning at their best. In addition, conflicts can keep nurses from communicating concerns to physicians, from asking questions when they are unsure, and from asking for help when critical situations arise.

Besides horizontal violence between and among nurses themselves, nurses can experience hostile work conditions from physicians, patients, or their families. The nurse can utilize refocusing or de-escalation strategies with physicians, patients, and families as well. Again, an effective tool to de-escalate difficult or angry communication is to bring the focus of the conversation back to the patient. Refocusing the discussion back on the patient's needs takes the focus off any perceived power struggle and helps everyone to refocus on the priorities at hand. Nurses can enlist the support of more senior colleagues when conflicts arise with team members. Other useful neutralizing techniques include listening attentively to others and demonstrating concern. Nurses can reduce negative situations by identifying people that are receptive to their questions and are willing to serve as resources. It is important for nurses to set the example by ending conversations where coworkers are being discussed in a negative manner.

New-to-practice nurses are more vulnerable to horizontal violence and hostile work conditions in the healthcare environment due to their lack of experience. Addressing these conditions as soon as possible frequently puts an end to it. However, it is important not to be confrontational in one's approach. An effective tactic against horizontal violence is to develop **de-escalation** strategies for these encounters, which can decrease the intensity, and stress of the situation. When confronted with nonverbal innuendos such as eyebrow raising, rolling of eyes, and long sighs by peers, one can be direct and say, "I sense that there is something that you want to say to me. I learn best when people are direct. It's okay if you are direct with me" (Griffin, 2004). This type of response directly addresses the horizontal violence in a civil manner without aggression. It indicates to the violator that his or her body language is perceived as negative and that it is preferable for the recipient to discuss the reason for it rather than ignore it. It should be said in earnest and not with anger to de-escalate the situation and open the lines of communication. When de-escalation strategies are not successful, Griffin and Clark (2014) suggest using the CUS acronym stating "I'm concerned with the way you are speaking to me, I'm uncomfortable with where this conversation is going, and I don't think it is safe for us to continue." Using this strategy allows the exchange to end in a civil manner before it escalates further.

Those in leadership positions have a crucial role in creating a workplace environment where horizontal violence and hostile communications are not tolerated. Promoting a team structure where power is shared among all members improves decision making and workload distribution (Rittenmeyer et al., 2013). Leaders need to set the standard for realistic expectations regarding workload so that their staff can meet those expectations and have a sense of accomplishment and satisfaction with their work and their work environment rather than feeling discouraged. Nursing leaders within the organization have an obligation to their direct care nurses to establish policies that discourage horizontal violence and help staff feel comfortable in confronting such behavior without fear of retaliation (Rittenmeyer et al).

CRITICAL THINKING 8.3

A new-to-practice nurse who is on orientation is assigned a complex patient to care for with his preceptor. During a stressful exchange, the preceptor states, "You're way too slow! You are never going to make it here if you don't pick up the pace."

1. What strategies for difficult communications would be most appropriate to use in this instance?
2. When should the new-to-practice nurse address this with the preceptor?
3. What would be the new-to-practice nurse's best communication approach with the preceptor?

Communicating With Preceptors

Preceptors are experienced nurses who provide orientation and support to new-to-practice nurses as they learn the roles and responsibilities of a new job. Preceptors have increased responsibilities of caring for patients while providing instruction to new nurses. They are frequently chosen for this important role because of their expertise in caring for patients and because they exemplify professional behaviors. New-to-practice nurses rely heavily on their preceptors to guide them in learning how to communicate with other team members and become a productive member of the healthcare team. Communicating with team members requires that nurses maintain a professional presence and act with confidence. During the orientation period, communication can be intimidating for the new nurse. It is difficult to feel like a valued member of the team when one is not sure about what to anticipate next. It can be a stressful time for both the preceptor and the orientee, particularly during challenging patient care situations. To diffuse any stressful communication, an honest and open exchange between the preceptor and the orientee at a quiet moment later will provide an opportunity to clarify concerns and reach an understanding about expectations. The new nurse can open the discussion by identifying his or her desire to learn and understand the situation. New nurses need to maintain realistic expectations regarding their knowledge base and expertise and seek feedback that will help them develop skill and effective clinical judgment. Accepting that he or she has knowledge gaps will allow the new nurse to ask questions without injury to self-esteem. Collaboration skills improve as the nurse develops a better understanding of the work expectation and unit routine.

CRITICAL THINKING 8.4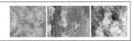

The nurse is caring for a patient with an extensive burn injury. The patient has a decreased white blood cell count and is scheduled for skin grafting at the end of the week. The patient is receiving a regular diet but has a poor appetite and has not been able to eat enough to meet his required calorie intake.

1. How can the nurse involve the patient and the family to address the patient's nutrition?
2. Which members of the interprofessional team would have the expertise to address the patient's nutritional status?
3. How can the interprofessional team work together to meet the patient's nutritional needs?

Cognitive Rehearsal

It is most important to continually promote an environment of respect and collaboration. Nurses must challenge themselves to use respectful negotiation when disagreements occur between members of the healthcare team and to remain civil in the face of incivility as part of their professional development. Cognitive rehearsal is one strategy that the nurse can use when confronted with incivility from a coworker or another person. Cognitive rehearsal is a prepared response that one practices ahead of time that would address a negative comment or situation in a civil manner. It allows one to not react emotionally but to pause and respond with a rehearsed, intellectually driven, civil response. For instance, if a coworker harshly criticizes the speed with which you

REAL-WORLD INTERVIEW

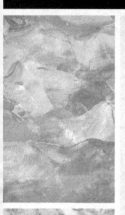

Being a new nurse had its challenges. I had worked as an extern and then as a technician, but when I transitioned to an RN, I realized how much I was responsible for and had to learn quickly how to deal with the stress. The hardest part was knowing the right thing to do for the patient and who I could comfortably go to for questions. Even though I felt I had a good education, it took a good year to feel comfortable with my practice and confident with my knowledge and skills. I was hired at the same time as another nurse and we supported each other during orientation. My hospital also had a nurse residency program and it helped me to know that my peers on other units were having the same feelings and difficulties that I was having. In the program, we talked about communication and about working with complex patient and family situations. We supported each other a lot through my first year of nursing practice.

Katie Bicknell
Children's Hospital of Pennsylvania
Philadelphia, Pennsylvania

complete a task, rather than react emotionally and become hurt and angry, you might respond by saying, "This is different from how I learned. Can you help me to understand how you complete it so quickly?"

As mentioned earlier, reflection and the ability to gain insight into one's actions can facilitate powerful, effective change. Specifically, reflecting on your ability to communicate with colleagues and other members of the interprofessional team provides an opportunity to consider behaviors that build consensus among colleagues and behaviors that create barriers to communication and interfere with safe patient care. During reflection, one should ask oneself, "What went well?" "What could have gone better?" "What could I have done to improve this situation?"

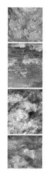

CASE STUDY 8.2

You and a senior colleague are assigned to the same patient room. You are caring for the patient in Bed B and she is caring for the patient in Bed A. You notice that the patient in Bed A is sleeping. On the bedside table, there is a filled medication syringe and an empty vial labeled heparin, 10,000 units/mL. You carry the medication syringe and heparin out to the nurse's station and state to your colleague, "These were on the bedside table." She takes them from you and states, "Yes, I have to remember to give the heparin to him when he wakes up" and returns them to the patient's bedside table.

1. *What standard is your colleague violating?*
2. *Recognizing that your colleague did not react to your implied concern for the patient's safety and the standard of practice, what communication strategy would you implement to maintain this patient's safety?*
3. *How can you address practice concerns like this from an organization's point of view to prevent this type of practice?*

Hospital and Nursing Leadership

Hospital and nursing leadership have a significant influence on how teams function. Leaders can set the tone for communication, role model effective conflict management, and create and foster an environment that facilitates safety and quality care. Nurse managers, preceptors, and other leaders within the healthcare organization can support new-to-practice nurses by providing effective feedback. Nurses can approach leaders to facilitate needed change when a chain of command authority is needed. Most leaders continually assess their environment as well as the people that report to them to determine if adequate support is provided for their subordinates to do their jobs. However, leaders can miss subtle signs of trouble or inefficiency. In that case, nurses must take it upon themselves to approach the leader to ask for help. Effective communication and team building help ensure the message for requesting help or clarification will be heard.

The responsibility of the nurse manager to serve as a role model for team building and collaboration cannot be understated. The nurse manager will be the leader that direct care nurses will have the greatest amount of interaction with, making it essential that he or she demonstrate active listening and partnership in solving problems. Engagement is supported by feedback that builds rather than tears down so skills in delivering and receiving constructive feedback can be demonstrated by the nurse manager so that others can emulate them. Behaviors that demonstrate respect and collegiality will build and sustain a civil work environment and set the expectation for the interprofessional team.

Interprofessional teamwork and collaboration is essential to ensure quality healthcare for patients and maintain safety. Nurses are valued members of the interprofessional healthcare team. Nurses' contribution to the patient's care include knowledgeable assessments, reflective thinking, effective planning, thoughtful interventions based on evidenced-based practice, and careful evaluation of care. Nurses' communication skills play a pivotal role in team building. Nurses who communicate concerns and address problems enhance their ability to prevent errors, achieve positive patient outcomes and patient satisfaction, and improve the system in which they work.

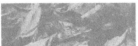

KEY CONCEPTS

1. An interprofessional healthcare team consists of people who have a stake or interest in and contribute to the well-being of the patient, for example, physicians, nurses, family members, those who provide support services, such as pharmacists, social workers, dieticians, and those from departments such as housekeeping, radiology, the laboratory, transport services, and physical and occupational therapy.

2. A rapid response team (RRT) is a team that includes specific healthcare professionals with specialized skills, who can mobilize and deliver immediate patient assessment and intervention if needed at the patient's bedside any time of day or night, 7 days a week at the beginning signs of deterioration in the patient's health status.

3. Recognizing the value of nursing, the Institute of Medicine (IOM), now known as the National Academy of Medicine, in collaboration with the Robert Wood Johnson

Foundation (RWJF), published its report, *The Future of Nursing: Leading Change, Advancing Health* (IOM, 2010). The four key recommendations from the report were focused on the role that nursing should have in providing care (Table 8.1).

4. To effectively care for and coordinate care delivery, interprofessional healthcare professionals require repeated blended educational experiences to achieve four interprofessional educational competencies, that is, understand the scope of responsibilities of each team member, maintain ethical conduct and quality of care within the team to develop respect and trust, communicate effectively with patients, families, and healthcare team members, and utilize teamwork behaviors in executing patient care requirements.

5. Root cause analysis (RCA) discovers the root of a problem by not stopping at the first answer it arrives at for its cause, but by delving deeper into why the problem occurred, asking questions until there are no more questions to ask.

6. Six Sigma, used to improve existing healthcare processes, involves five steps, also referred to as DMAIC.

7. In healthcare, poor outcomes occur when there are breakdowns in communication, poor teamwork, or inefficient communication "handoffs" that create situations that can lead to errors.

8. *Forming, storming, norming,* and *performing* are terms used to describe the stages experienced by teams as they progress from formation to functioning as high-performance teams (Tuckman, 1965).

9. When delegating, the nurse employs the following steps: assess and plan; communicate what needs to be done; ensure availability to assist and support; and finally, evaluate effectiveness.

10. Originating in the aviation industry for the cockpit crew, crew resource management (CRM) develops communication, leadership, and decision-making safety strategies to combat the potential for human error that is inherent in high-stress systems and its devastating effects.

11. Situational awareness is having the right information at the right time alongside the ability to analyze that information to appropriately and effectively take action. The vehicle for this attentiveness is effective communication between interprofessional healthcare team members.

12. TeamSTEPPS is a program designed to teach interprofessional teams how to communicate with each other to promote situational awareness and patient safety (AHRQ, n.d., p. 2).

13. Situation, background, assessment, and recommendation (SBAR; AHRQ, n.d.) was developed by the military and is now applied to healthcare as a means to relay significant information regarding a patient's condition or to be used as patients' care is communicated and handed off from one caregiver to another (Table 8.2).

14. Time-outs are an opportunity for everyone in the room to stop and ensure that the correct patient is having the correct procedure done to the correct site.

15. Safety huddles allow those caring for the patient to review pertinent information and the plan of

16. Cross-monitoring, callout, two-challenge rule, concerned, uncomfortable, and safety (CUS), check back/read back, and handoff are developed by the AHRQ which provides reference videos for clinicians, administrators, and educators demonstrating TeamSTEPPS tools, strategies, and techniques at its website, www.ahrq.gov/professionals/education/curriculum-tools/teamstepps/instructor/videos/index.html (Table 8.3).

17. Timely reporting of errors and near misses, also known as close calls where an error could have occurred but was stopped before it caused harm, provides an

opportunity for the team to learn from them. In most cases, errors and near misses are often the result of a failure within a healthcare system.

18. There are many available web resources funded by government agencies and national healthcare organizations that are designed to improve teamwork and collaboration, prevent error, promote patient safety, and improve the quality of the care that patients receive (Table 8.4).

19. Debriefing is the process of reviewing performance effectiveness following challenging patient care situations.

20. Feedback, whether positive or negative, should always be an unbiased reflection of what occurred, opening the door to a discussion of evidence-based practice (Clynes & Raftery, 2008). Constructive feedback should carefully detail events as they occurred and avoid opinion.

21. Teams can work together to conduct audits and other organizational studies that measure quality, safety, and patient outcomes which can have a significant impact on the process of quality improvement (QI).

22. Providing feedback to team members allows the team to identify strengths and weaknesses, make changes to the healthcare system, and adjust practice for individual growth and development.

23. Self-evaluation of one's communication and decision making is a crucial element of professional growth and strengthens one's ability to contribute to the team's decisions by employing strong clinical judgment.

24. Tanner's model of Thinking Like a Nurse (2006) demonstrates how clinical judgment is developed through reflection, enhancing critical thinking skills.

25. Mindfulness implies staying focused with the ability to see the significance of early and weak signals as well as to take strong and decisive action to prevent harm (Weick & Sutcliff, 2001).

26. Communication between the healthcare team, the patient, and the patient's family during times of stress and illness can be challenging but it is essential to safety and a key factor in patient satisfaction.

27. Many barriers can interfere with communication, such as knowledge gaps, education levels, culture, language barriers, or stress. It is important for nurses to develop strategies to identify and overcome these barriers.

28. Effective communication is essential to maintaining a safe and protected environment for patients. Ineffective communication continues to be identified as the root cause for many sentinel events reported to The Joint Commission (2016).

29. Destructive events such as physicians who will not respond to pages, nurses who are resistant to carrying out legitimate orders, or pharmacists who do not move quickly to fill STAT prescriptions, create difficult communications among healthcare providers that can negatively impact patient care (Table 8.5).

30. One of the most troubling conflicts for nurses is nurse-to-nurse aggression, also known as lateral violence or horizontal violence (Rittenmeyer et al., 2013).

31. New-to-practice nurses are more vulnerable to horizontal violence and hostile work conditions in the healthcare environment due to their lack of experience.

32. Preceptors are experienced nurses who provide orientation and support to new-to-practice nurses as they learn the roles and responsibilities of a new job.

33. Reflection and the ability to gain insight into one's one actions can facilitate powerful, effective change.

34. Hospital and nursing leadership have a significant influence on how teams function.

KEY TERMS

Collaboration
Cross monitoring
Debriefing
De-escalation strategies
Hand-off
Interprofessional education

Mindfulness
Near miss
Rapid Response Teams
Root cause analysis
Situational awareness

REVIEW QUESTIONS

1. A nurse receives a telephone order from a physician for specific x-ray tests. The nurse established the identity of the patient involved and the name of the ordering physician. Which of the following should she do next?

   A. Write the order on the order sheet in the chart.
   B. Repeat what the physician says and then write it down on the order sheet.
   C. Ask the physician to directly place the order with the radiology department.
   D. Write the order on the order sheet and then perform a read back to the physician to verify the order is accurate.

2. The nurse is informed that an RRT will be initiated at the hospital to better meet the needs of patients. Which of the following best describes the way in which the nurse should utilize the RRT?

   A. Provide support for medical-surgical nurses and decrease the number of patient arrests requiring ICU admission.
   B. Rapidly move patients through the hospital system at time of transfer.
   C. Notify the attending physician of the client's deteriorating status.
   D. Provide immediate assistance to patients in the ICU.

3. The nurse is transferring a patient from the ICU to the step-down patient care unit. When the ICU nurse calls report to the receiving unit, what is the best way for the nurse to provide the handoff information?

   A. Situation, Background, Assessment, Requirements
   B. Situation, Background, Assessment, Recommendations
   C. Systems, Background, Activities, Recommendations
   D. Systems, Background, Activities, Requirements

4. The nurse pages a physician due to the patient's change in status. When the physician calls the unit, the physician yells at the nurse for interrupting dinner. Which of the following would be the nurse's best approach?

   A. Tell the physician that she is going to report him to the nursing supervisor.
   B. Tell the physician that she is doing her job and does not deserve to be yelled at.
   C. Refocus the communication on the patient and the reason for the call.
   D. Apologize for interrupting the dinner and page his partner.

5. The nurse attends an interprofessional meeting to discuss the care of a patient who is a paraplegic after an automobile accident. Which of the following best describes the purpose of assembling an interprofessional team?

   A. To provide multiple perspectives to contribute to the patient's care and well-being
   B. To divide the work appropriately among disciplines
   C. To ensure that the physician controls the patient outcome
   D. To provide support in difficult patient care situations

6. Following a serious medication error that resulted in patient injury, a nurse is assigned to a team assembled to investigate the cause. The nurse knows which of the following represents the best method for doing so?

   A. Root cause analysis
   B. Debriefing
   C. Six Sigma
   D. Crew resource management

7. The nurse on the oncology unit cares for a patient who frequently comments that she would like better pain control through the night. The nurse tells the patient that a note will be placed on the front of the patient's chart alerting the physician in case the nurse misses the physician during her rounds. Which of the following represents a better process to ensure the patient's needs are met?

   A. Nursing rounds
   B. Team huddle
   C. Debriefing
   D. Root cause analysis

8. A patient's family is angry about their family member's deteriorating condition and tells the nurse that they are not satisfied with the patient's care. Which of the following would be the most appropriate action by the nurse?

   A. Notify the hospital administration
   B. Explain to the family that the patient's condition is complex and that the patient is receiving appropriate care
   C. Convey understanding and notify members of the healthcare team so that a family meeting with the team can be provided
   D. Ask the family members why they feel that way

9. Which of the following processes would best assist the nurse to increase expertise, adjust practice, and improve self-regulation?

   A. Conduct a RCA
   B. Elicit constructive feedback from others
   C. Participate in debriefing
   D. Use the CUS technique

10. Skilled communication is essential to patient safety for which of the following reasons?

    A. Patients need to be convinced to receive specific treatments.
    B. Nurses need to explain procedures to patients.
    C. Miscommunication is responsible for many harmful events in the hospital.
    D. Poor quality is associated with poor communication.

REVIEW ACTIVITIES

1. A patient calls the nurse into the room and complains of shortness of breath. The patient was admitted yesterday for pulmonary edema and has been successfully treated with nasal oxygen at 4 L, and furosemide (Lasix) 40 mg IV every 12 hours. The nurse determines that the patient's respiratory rate is 30, the pulse oximetry reading is 91%, and auscultation of the lungs reveals crackles halfway up the back. Using SBAR technique, provide report to the physician regarding the previously mentioned patient.
2. The nurse believes the dose of a medication ordered for a patient is too high and may be dangerous for the patient to receive. What communication strategy would the nurse implement to verbalize this? How would it be implemented?
3. The nurse receives a critical lab result via telephone from the laboratory. What safety strategy should the nurse implement to ensure safety regarding the lab value?

CRITICAL DISCUSSION POINTS

1. During your last clinical experience, what interprofessional teamwork and collaboration initiatives were underway on the nursing unit or within the department of nursing?
2. What interprofessional teamwork and collaboration resources are available to nurses within the nursing unit or department of nursing where you have your clinical rotation?
3. How has interprofessional teamwork and collaboration improved for patients and families in your clinical site?
4. How do the nurses feel about the culture of interprofessional teamwork and collaboration within their work environment?
5. How are nurses involved in interprofessional teamwork and collaboration in the health system?
6. How are patients, nurses, and the interprofessional team included in daily interprofessional rounds in your clinical site?
7. If a nurse has an idea that will improve the interprofessional teamwork and collaboration regarding patient care delivery, where would he or she take that idea within the organization?
8. Interprofessional teams include physicians and nurses that provide direct patient care but also include the patient, family members, and many others who provide support services such as pharmacists, dieticians, social workers, and physical and occupational therapists.
9. All members of the interprofessional team should be valued for their contribution of a specific expertise to the plan of care for the patient.
10. Interprofessional education as well as quality and safety standards can improve the collegial interactions of members of the team.
11. Attention to quality and safety improvement have resulted in national organizations promoting the implementation of processes such as RCA, Six Sigma, and RRTs to raise the standard of care.
12. The human factors associated with providing healthcare contribute to the potential for errors but effective teams incorporate safety strategies to communicate, monitor each other's work, and prevent injury to patients.
13. Good communication skills for exchanging information and delegating are an essential element of successful teamwork and collaboration.

14. Giving and receiving feedback provides an opportunity for individuals and teams to identify areas for improvement and alter their practice.

15. Healthcare team members have an ethical duty to work together for the patient's well-being.

16. Difficult or strained communications place patients at risk because team members are afraid to ask questions or confirm practice standards.

17. Nurses can promote teamwork and prevent communication barriers by using strategies to de-escalate tense situations, by framing their communications in safety language, by using cognitive rehearsal, and by reflecting on events to consider opportunities for building consensus.

QSEN WEBSITE EXERCISES

1. Introduction to the QSEN Competencies. Review presentation available at: qsen .org/quality-and-safety-education-for-nurses-an-introduction-to-the-competencies-and-the-knowledge-skills-and-attitudes/

Discussion: This PowerPoint presentation is a brief overview for individuals that are unfamiliar with the IOM/QSEN competencies and wish to introduce ideas that promote development of the knowledge, skills, and attitudes that support the competencies. It includes direct links to helpful resources such as the First Touch website, to Infection Control Bundles at The Joint Commission website, and to the Team*STEPPS* video collection at the Agency for Healthcare Research and Quality website.

2. Giving and Receiving Constructive Feedback. Review this 18-minute narrated presentation to learn how to give and to receive constructive feedback to improve practice and build teamwork: qsen.org/giving-and-receiving-constructive-feedback/

Discussion: This is a narrated presentation focused on helping students to understand the importance of learning to give and to receive constructive feedback. Key points include understanding constructive feedback's role in quality improvement and patient safety, and learning to view constructive feedback as an opportunity for improvement. Students may listen to it online, at home, or in the classroom with a faculty member. The presentation can be loaded into Electronic Course Frameworks and assigned. If assigned as an out of class activity, faculty can have students blog or post in discussions about what they gained from the presentation.

EXPLORING THE WEB

1. Go to qsen.org and find the Teamwork and Collaboration Competency. Review the knowledge, skill, and attitude a graduate nurse should exhibit. Then go to the Publication tab and review the various articles, toolkits, and other resources. Do you find something that could help you with a current group of people/ classmates/colleagues you are working with?

2. Access the web resources in Table 8.4.

3. Review the websites listed in Table 8.4. What do you identify as the consistent theme or focus of all of these websites?
4. What strategies do you see on these websites that would enhance teamwork?

REFERENCES

Agency for Healthcare Research and Quality (AHRQ). (n.d.). *TeamSTEPPS™ fundamentals course: Module 1. Introduction: Instructor's slides.* Retrieved from https://www.ahrq.gov/teamstepps/instructor/fundamentals/module1/igintro.html

Becher, J., & Visovsky, C. (2012). Horizontal violence in nursing. *Medsurg Nursing, 21*(4), 210–213.

Clynes, M. P., & Raftery, S. E. C. (2008). Feedback: An essential element of student learning in clinical practice. *Nurse Education in Practice, 8*, 405–411.

Griffin, M. (2004). Teaching cognitive rehearsal as a shield for lateral violence: An intervention for newly licensed nurses. *The Journal of Continuing Education in Nursing, 3*(6), 257–263.

Griffin, M., & Clark, C. (2014). Revisiting cognitive rehearsal as an intervention against incivility and lateral violence in nursing: 10 years later. *Journal of Continuing Education in Nursing, 45*(12), 535–542.

Hattie, J., & Timperley, H. (2007). The power of feedback. *Review of Educational Research, 77*(1), 81–112.

Hood, K., Cant, R, Baulch, J., Gilbee, A., Leech, M., Anderson, A., & Davies, K. (2014). Prior experience of interprofessional learning enhances undergraduate nursing and healthcare students' professional identity and attitudes to teamwork. *Nurse Education in Practice, 14*, 117–122.

Institute for Health Care Improvement (IHI). (2012). *Deploy rapid response teams.* Retrieved from http://www.ihi.org/explore/RapidResponseTeams/Pages/default.aspx

Institute of Medicine (IOM). (2010). *The future of nursing: Leading change advancing health.* Retrieved from http://nationalacademies.org/HMD/Reports/2010/The-Future-of-Nursing-Leading-Change-Advancing-Health.aspx

The Joint Commission. (n.d.). *The universal protocol for preventing wrong site, wrong procedure, and wrong person surgery: Guidance for health care professionals.* Retrieved from http://www.jointcommission.org/assets/1/18/UP_Poster.pdf The Joint Commission. (2016). Sentinal events statistics released for 2015. *Joint Commission Perspectives, 36*(4).

McBride, A. B. (2010). Toward a roadmap for interdisciplinary academic career success. *Research and Theory for Nursing Practice: An International Journal, 24*(1), 74–86.

National Council of State Boards of Nursing. (2016). *National Guidelines for Nursing Delegation.* Retrieved from https://www.ncsbn.org/NCSBN_Delegation_Guidelines.pdf

Petri, L. (2010). Concept analysis of interdisciplinary collaboration. *Nursing Forum, 45*(2), 73–81.

Rittenmeyer, L., Huffman, D., Hopp, L. & Block, M. (2013). A comprehensive systematic review on the experience of lateral/horizontal violence in the profession of nursing. The JBI Database of Systematic Reviews and Implementation Reports. 11. 362. doi:10.11124/jbisrir-2013-1017.

Stanton, P., Gough, R., Ballardie, R., Bartram, T., Bamber, G., & Sohal, A. (2014). Implementing lean management/six sigma in hospitals: Beyond empowerment and work intensification? *The International Journal of Human Resource Management, 25*(21), 2926–2940.

Tanner, C. A. (2006). Thinking like a nurse: A research based model of clinical judgment in nursing. *Journal of Nursing Education, 4*(6), 204–211.

Tuckman, B. (1965). Developmental sequence in small groups. *Psychological Bulletin, 63*(6), 384–99. doi:10.1037/h0022100

Unknown participant. (2007, June). *Quality and safety education for nurses collaboration.* Chicago, IL.

U. S. Department of labor. (2013). *Occupations by gender shares of employment.* Retrieved from https://www.dol.gov/wb/stats/occ_gender_share_em_1020_txt.htm

Weick, K. E., & Sutcliffe, K. M. (2001). *Managing the unexpected.* San Francisco, CA: Jossey-Bass.

SUGGESTED READINGS

Agency for Healthcare Research and Quality (AHRQ). (2011). *Preventing avoidable readmissions*. Retrieved from http://www.ahrq.gov/qual/impptdis.htm

Altmiller, G. (2012). The role of constructive feedback in patient safety and continuous quality improvement. *Nursing Clinics of North America, 47*(3), 365–374. doi:10.1016/j.cnur.2012.05.002

American Nurses Association (ANA). (2015). *Code of ethics for nurses with interpretive statements*. Retrieved from http://nursingworld.org/MainMenuCategories/EthicsStandards/CodeofEthicsforNurses/Code-of-ethics.pdf

Barr, H. (2002). Interprofessional education, today, yesterday and tomorrow. Retrieved from https://www.unmc.edu/bhecn/_documents/ipe-today-yesterday-tmmw-barr.pdf

Carter, P. (2010). Six sigma. *American Association of Occupational Health Nurses Journal, 58*(12), 508–510.

Cronenwett, L., Sherwood, G., Barnsteiner, J., Disch, J., Johnson, J., Mitchell, P., . . . Warren, J. (2007). Quality and safety education for nurses. *Nursing Outlook, 55*(3), 112–131. doi:10.1016/j.outlook.2007.02.006

Douglas, M. (2016). Bridging gaps in rapid response systems. *Nursing Management, 47*(12), 26–31. doi:10.1097/01.NUMA.0000508260.11605.47

Halbesleben, J. R. B., Wakefield, D. S., & Wakefield, B. J. (2008). Work-arounds in the health care setting: Literature review and research agenda. *Health Care Manager Review, 33*(1), 2–12. doi:10.1097/01.HMR.0000304495.95522.ca

Institute of Medicine (IOM). (2003). *Health professions education: A bridge to quality*. Washington, DC: National Academies Press.

Leach, L. S., & Mayo, A. M. (2013). Rapid response teams: Qualitative analysis of their effectiveness. *American Journal of Critical Care, 22*(3), 109–210. doi:10.4037/ajcc2013990

Lim, F., & Pajarillo, E. J. Y. (2016). Standardized handoff report form in clinical nursing education: An educational tool for patient safety and quality of care. *Nurse Education Today, 37*(3), 3–7. doi:10.1016/j.nedt.2015.10.026

Smith, P. L., & McSweeney, J. (2017). Organizational perspectives on rapid response team structure, function, and costs. *Dimensions of Critical Care Nursing, 36*(1), 3–13. doi:10.1097/DCC.0000000000000222

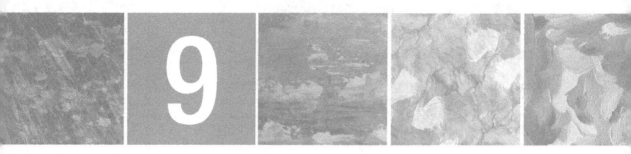

9

INFORMATICS

Beth A. Vottero

The biggest waste in the healthcare system is not unnecessary treatment or duplicated test results; it is that we collect data and never use it again.

—Chris Lehmann, Vanderbilt University Professor of Pediatrics and Biomedical Informatics

Upon completion of this chapter, the reader should be able to

1. Define nursing informatics.
2. Explore the data, information, knowledge, and wisdom framework that guide nursing informatics.
3. Differentiate between an electronic medical record (EMR) and an electronic health record (EHR).
4. Discuss evolving national initiatives that encourage use of EHRs.
5. Explore the utility of patient portals in providing healthcare.
6. Explain the role telehealth plays in the care of the homebound or rurally located patients.
7. Describe how to evaluate the quality of health-related content on websites and applications.
8. Explain technology initiatives that support the delivery of safe patient care such as clinical decision support systems and clinical alerts.
9. Differentiate among the concepts of privacy, confidentiality, and security.
10. Discuss the future of health informatics.

I n November 2007, actor Dennis Quaid and his wife Kimberly walked into Cedars-Sinai Medical Center to visit their newborn twins: Thomas Boone and Zoe Grace. To the Quaids' horror, they were immediately greeted by a nurse who informed them that the twins had been given an overdose of heparin (10,000 U/mL rather than 1,000 U/mL) not only once, but twice during the hospitalization. Once the error was noticed, the children were treated with protamine sulfate and they apparently suffered no long-term effects of the incident. The Quaids subsequently sued the drug company for using drug labels on the high- and the low-concentration heparin vials that were very similar and could cause confusion. Although they did not sue the hospital, they did ask that the hospital review its policies and procedures (Rosen, 2008).

- *What other healthcare professionals had an influence on this medication error?*
- *What are some low-technology and high-technology interventions that could have prevented this medication error?*
- *What types of policies and procedures may have not been followed that allowed such an error to have occurred.*

A relatively new specialty in healthcare is the growing field of informatics. This growth is due in part to the expanding capacity of technology leading to breakthroughs in communication and analytics. Healthcare has embraced the known abilities and the potential of technology in supporting high-quality, safe patient care nationwide. The full impact of technology on healthcare delivery will never be known due to the continuing evolutionary nature of the field. Health informatics is the collective term applied to various interprofessional health workers who focus on collecting, storing, retrieving, transmitting, and analyzing health data to support high-quality patient care. While still a new specialty, nursing informatics has grown to become a critical asset within health informatics.

This chapter defines nursing informatics and the data, information, knowledge, and wisdom model that guides nursing informatics as a specialty as well as presents the sciences contributing to nursing informatics: computer science, cognitive science, and nursing science. The impact of existing and emerging national initiatives is discussed relative to nursing practice such as changes to Meaningful Use, Medicare Access and CHIP Reauthorization Act (MACRA), and publicly reportable data. From that vantage point, the role of technologies in hospitals and other healthcare systems is explored. In addition to inpatient examples of nursing informatics, the role telehealth plays in outpatient care is discussed. Health information technologies designed to support the delivery of high-quality patient care are explored. Federal laws that protect identifiable information are detailed, providing differentiation among the concepts of privacy, confidentiality, and security. Finally, the future of informatics is discussed.

◼◼◼◼ NURSING INFORMATICS DEFINED

While informatics is simply the science of collecting, managing, and retrieving information, **nursing informatics** is "the specialty that integrates nursing science with multiple information and analytical sciences to identify, define, manage, and communicate data, information, knowledge, and wisdom in nursing practice" (American Nurses Association [ANA], 2015). Information and analytical sciences that make up nursing informatics include, but are not limited to, computer science, cognitive science, the science of terminologies and taxonomies (including naming and coding conventions), information management, library science, heuristics, archival science, and mathematics (ANA, 2015). Management of health records dominates the discussion of health informatics; however, computer technology offers a variety of ways to record and retrieve information to support the evidence-based needs and actions of the interprofessional team including:

- Patient-decision support tools
- Laboratory and x-ray results reporting and reviewing systems
- Quality improvement (QI) data collection/data summary systems
- Disease surveillance systems
- Electronic bed boards that monitor bed availability
- Simulation laboratories

Quality and Safety Education for Nurses (QSEN) describes informatics as the use of "information and technology to communicate, manage knowledge, mitigate error, and support decision making" (Cronenwett et al., 2007). Newly licensed nurses are expected to possess informatics knowledge, skills, and attitudes that reflect the ability of the nurse to competently provide high-quality, safe patient-centered care in a technology-rich nursing care environment (Cronenwett et al., 2007).

CRITICAL THINKING 9.1

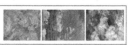

A common misconception about nursing informatics is that the specialty involves computer programming, computer system design, and networking. If someone said that nursing informatics requires the nurse to know how to program a computer, how would you respond?

METASTRUCTURE OF NURSING INFORMATICS

Nursing informatics draws from a variety of sciences such as information science, computer science, cognitive science, library science, and information management as well as human factors engineering. The guiding structure for nursing informatics, also known as the metastructure, was built upon the way nurses interact and use clinical information systems. In the ANA description, "data, information, knowledge, and wisdom" form the metastructure, which increases in complexity as work increases in interactions and interrelationships (2016). Both the sciences and the metastructure form the framework for understanding nursing informatics. Figure 9.1 illustrates the data, information, knowledge, and wisdom metastructure.

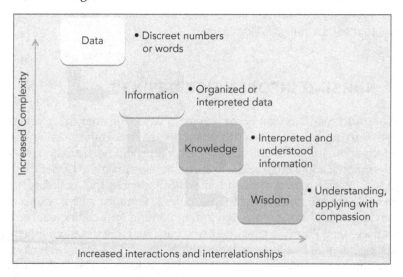

FIGURE 9.1 Data, information, knowledge, wisdom metastructure.

The ANA Scope and Standards for Nursing Informatics Practice describe what constitutes each component of the metastructure (Table 9.1).

TABLE 9.1 DATA TO WISDOM METASTRUCTURE COMPONENTS

METASTRUCTURE ELEMENT	DESCRIPTION	EXAMPLE
Data	Discrete points collected and described objectively without interpretation from a variety of sources and includes numbers or words	Data collected for one point in time during an assessment include the following: Heart rate: 76 Blood pressure: 118/64 Respiratory rate: 18 Mental state: alert and oriented Eye and hair color: brown eyes, blonde hair
Information	Data that have been organized, structured, and interpreted	Heart rate assessment findings collected over the entire hospitalization that are trended using a graph to show highs and lows in the data
Knowledge	Synthesized information so that relationships are identified and formalized	Heart rate and blood pressure findings for the morning assessment prior to a beta-blocker dose then looking at the same assessment findings 4 hours after the medication dose to see if it had an affect on heart rate and blood pressure findings. Includes reviewing the same information from previous mornings to see the effect
Wisdom	The appropriate use of knowledge to manage and solve individual patient problems with consideration for how and when to apply knowledge to complex patient problems	Heart rate is 62 and blood pressure is 104/58 at 9 a.m. The trends over the past 2 days for both vitals show that medications do lower both the heart rate and blood pressure within 1 hr of taking the dose. The beta-blocker dose is due at 10 a.m. The patient is scheduled for a treadmill stress test at 11:00 a.m. The patient's 10 a.m. medications are metoprolol 50 mg (Lopressor) and furosemide 40 mg (Lasix). The nurse is concerned that the medications may lower the blood pressure too much and that the medications may also affect the treadmill stress test results. The nurse calls the physician to discuss concerns and ask if the medications should be held until after the test.

Source: Adapted from American Nurses Association. (2015). *Nursing informatics: Scope and standards of practice* (2nd ed.). Silver Spring, MD: Nursebooks.org.

CASE STUDY 9.1

Denise is a new nurse on a medical-surgical unit. She is just beginning to become comfortable providing nursing care to her assigned patients. She starts her day by receiving a shift report on each of her patients. The shift report is delivered at the bedside allowing Denise to introduce herself and start a plan of care for the day with input from the patient. After report, she looks up the patient's laboratory results in the computer, noting both normal and abnormal findings. Denise then completes a thorough nursing assessment on each patient and documents her findings in the electronic documentation record. Today Denise is providing nursing care for a 63-year-old man admitted 2 days ago with heart failure and diabetes. Today the vital signs are blood pressure 90/54, heart rate 82, and respirations of 20. She knows the patient is due for a dose of Lopressor 50 mg PO and Lasix 80 mg PO.

1. *What questions or concerns do you have based on these data?*
2. *What additional data do you need to create information based on the Data to Wisdom Metastructure?*

Denise reviewed the electronic medical record (EMR) and noted the following abnormal findings.

	Yesterday 6 a.m.	Yesterday 11 a.m.	Yesterday 4 p.m.	Yesterday 10 p.m.	Today 6 a.m.	Today 10 a.m.	Today 4 p.m.
Glucose	148	104	298	423	116	312	469
B-Type naturetic peptide (BTNP)	620				280		
Potassium (K+)	3.2				4.2		

Denise looked at the patient's medications including the following information:

• *Lasix 80 mg PO BID (orally twice a day) at home. Lasix 80 mg IVP BID (intravenous pyelogram twice a day) given yesterday as a one-time dose*
• *Levamir 72 u SQ BID (subcutaneous twice a day) at home. The same dose is resumed while the patient is in the hospital*
• *Lopressor 50 mg BID (twice a day) at home. The same dose is resumed while the patient is in the hospital*

(continued)

CASE STUDY 9.1 *(continued)*

Vital signs charted on the patient and medications given over the past 2 days included:

	Yesterday 6 a.m.	Yesterday 12 p.m.	Yesterday 6 p.m.	Today 12 a.m.	Today 6 a.m.	Today 12 p.m.	Today 6 p.m.
Blood pressure	88/52 Lopressor 50 mg Levamir 72 u Lasix 80 mg IVP	112/80	96/58 Lopressor 50 mg Levamir 72 u Lasix 80 mg PO	102/62	102/84 Lopressor 50 mg Levamir 72 u Lasix 80 mg PO	124/78	90/54
Heart rate	88	72	74	72	90	96	78
Respirations	20	18	18	16	16	18	

Denise takes the following actions based on the information provided. She calls the physician to relate the blood glucose reading and asks for a sliding scale insulin dose in addition to the normal Levamir dose. Denise requests that the nursing assistant records strict intake and output levels and documents findings in the EMR every shift. Denise gives the patient the regularly scheduled medications of Lasix, Levamir, and Lopressor.

Answer the following questions based on the given data.

1. *What is the difference between having data from one assessment and having trended data over several days during the hospitalization? Why is it important to have access to trended data?*
2. *Why did Denise give the patient his scheduled dose of Lopressor and Lasix if the blood pressure was 98/60? What might be her rationale?*
3. *How does technology help change data to information? Information to knowledge? Knowledge to wisdom?*
4. *How did Denise demonstrate knowledge and wisdom in providing care for her patient?*

▬▬ ▬ EMR AND EHR

The Health Care Information Management and Systems Society (HIMSS) discriminates between an EMR and an EHR. An **electronic medical record** is a legal record of what happened to a patient during one care encounter at a healthcare organization (HIMSS, 2006). For example, an EMR includes data from one hospital stay, one physician visit, or one instance of accessing healthcare. The EMR is confined to one point in time or one range of dates. In contrast, an **electronic health record** is a longitudinal electronic record of patient health information generated by one or more encounters in any care delivery setting (Centers for Medicare and Medicaid

Services [CMS], 2012). Included in this record are patient demographics, provider progress notes, health problems, medication lists, vital signs, the patient's past medical history, past or current immunizations, laboratory data, and radiology reports. In order for an EHR to exist, there must be an EMR in place that captures data from the healthcare encounter. The EHR has the ability to generate a complete record of a clinical patient encounter, as well as supporting other care-related activities including evidence-based decision support, quality management, and outcomes reporting.

EHRs will form the basis of the National Health Information Network (NHIN), which is a plan that will enable the exchange of patient information electronically from one healthcare provider to another healthcare provider. NHIN will allow the healthcare provider to access previous information such as the patient's disease history, the list of medications, the known allergies, and the prior test results. The electronic exchange of patient information will eliminate delays that occur when paper records must be copied and sent to another provider. The NHIN will also help exchange patient information between healthcare providers and public health authorities. For example, submission of reports to government vaccination registries and the reporting of communicable diseases will be done from the EHR. The reports will be done at the same time care is provided (in real time) so agencies charged with protecting the health of the public will be able to act quickly. If a particular lot of a vaccine is recalled, health authorities will know which patients to contact. If a virulent strain of influenza occurs, health authorities can issue public health warnings and close some public places to prevent further spread of the disease. The electronic information exchange within NHIN must protect patient privacy and the content of the data. Healthcare providers have a legal and ethical duty to maintain the confidentiality of patient information. For patient safety, data cannot be altered in any way. For example, information regarding a medication must maintain the same name, dose, frequency, and route of administration as it is being transmitted to another provider. No one should be able to capture data en route and change them.

The Department of Health and Human Services (HHS) predicts that the NHIN will enhance the quality of care by reducing healthcare errors (especially those related to medications), eliminating the need for duplicate testing, thus subjecting the patient to less risk and reducing delays that occur from lack of information. If the efficiency and effectiveness of care is improved, the costs of providing care should be reduced.

At the time of the 1991 IOM report (see Real-World Interview 9.1), the banking industry already used highly sophisticated electronic information systems with the ability to exchange information among banks with relative ease. Other industries such as the airlines industry also had initiated advanced electronic information systems that included the ability to make reservations and do flight scheduling. The airlines had access to information about all the passengers on each plane, the names of the staff members, and other important details about each flight. The 1991 IOM report urged healthcare organizations to look at the technology used by other industries and make investments in electronic information systems that would address some of the problems associated with paper records and to move to electronic patient records. With electronic patient records, information could be more easily exchanged in real time (i.e., as it is happening) among healthcare providers, with legible records, and documentation done at the point of care. Care could be streamlined with more efficient methods of data collection, and computer programs could be written to improve safety issues such as medication interactions.

REAL-WORLD INTERVIEW

Recently, we created new workflows and job descriptions based on community and population health needs. The core team is comprised of a physician, a nurse manager, two nurse navigators, an actuary, and a clinical informatics analyst. The goals are based on best available evidence and determined by large studies such as healthy people 2020. The physician helps to determine the measures that could be moved in a significant manner to measure care. The actuary determines goals set at intervals throughout the change process. The manager determines the expected scope and expansion rate to provider offices. The nurse navigators work with the providers and the patients to achieve the goals. As a clinical informatics analyst, I build, maintain, and update the software program to accommodate and measure results in a meaningful way. We are a small close-knit group who acknowledge the contributions each member. Sometimes there can be a different "pitch" regarding the upcoming changes. Some providers will only listen to another physician without regard to the best practice presented by another colleague. Some providers are particularly competitive, so I will individually address documentation changes that have the biggest effect in the shortest amount of time.

Elaine Brown, RN
Clinical Informatics Analyst
LaPorte Regional Health

NATIONAL INITIATIVES SUPPORT FOR EHRS

Although work in the informatics discipline started many decades ago, a landmark 1991 report by the Institute of Medicine (IOM) brought national attention to the topic of informatics. The report titled *The Computer-Based Patient Record: An Essential Technology for Health Care* stated it was time for the healthcare industry to catch up with other industries with regard to its use of information technology (Dick & Steen 1991; IOM, 1997). In 1991, almost all healthcare records were on paper. If a patient visited three different physician offices, there would be a paper healthcare record in each office. Similarly, if the patient were hospitalized, there would be yet another paper healthcare record at the hospital. The result was as follows:

- No one healthcare provider had a coordinated and complete view of the patient's health status; therefore, optimum care was more difficult to ensure.
- No one healthcare provider knew exactly what tests had been performed on the patient; thus, there was duplicate testing that wasted healthcare dollars, created an inconvenience for patients, and, in some cases, subjected patients to unnecessary risks.
- Paper healthcare records were mostly handwritten and frequently illegible; thus, important information about patients was not readable and mistakes in care resulted. In particular, physician orders for medications were sometimes incorrectly interpreted and/or sent to the pharmacy resulting in the wrong medications being given and/or incorrect doses being administered.
- Human intervention was required to predict when adverse drug reactions might occur due to contraindications and/or certain drug combinations. As the number of available medications grew, it became more difficult for humans to remember all the important aspects of each medication.

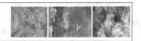

CRITICAL THINKING 9.2

A 65-year-old man comes to the ED via ambulance after being in a car accident. He is currently unresponsive and has no family members present. He does have a wallet and identification and his car had out of state plates. Without a medical record of past history, medications, test results, or previous medical diagnoses, it is difficult to know how to treat the patient. At this hospital they do have links to a national EHR database. By entering his name and birthdate, the healthcare provider can see that the patient has a history of an ischemic stroke and is on Coumadin. The patient also has diabetes and a history of heart failure. The healthcare provider can review the patient's current medications, previous test results, past history, and assessment findings.

1. How does having access to a patient's previous medical records improve patient care?
2. Why do you think the EHR is not currently in place in the United States?
3. Create a concept map with the patient at the center that shows how an EHR can impact the delivery of safe, high-quality patient care.

- Paper healthcare records were sometimes lost, resulting in no information being available about the patient. In the case of a healthcare emergency, the treatment team sometimes had to treat the patient symptomatically or just on the basis of findings at that time and without knowledge of the patient's past history, what medications the patient was on, or what chronic diseases the patient had.
- Patients who had not been seen before by a healthcare provider had no healthcare history on file with that provider. It was a manual process to try to obtain copies of records from other providers. There was a delay in receiving these records so there were also some delays in care.
- Documentation of the care given was a time-consuming process for all members of the healthcare team. Time spent documenting care left less time to actually care for the patient.

Progress on implementing electronic patient records has been slow, in part because of concerns for patient privacy and the perceived lack of funding for information technology. In 2001, the IOM published a series of landmark reports called the *Quality Chasm* series in which it identified ways the healthcare system could change to reduce the number of errors. The 2001 report titled *Crossing the Quality Chasm: A New Health System for the 21st Century* devoted an entire chapter to information technology (Committee on Quality of Health Care in America, 2001). Among the recommended changes for healthcare technology were the following:

- **Computerized provider order entry** (CPOE)-automated reminder systems to improve compliance with clinical practice guidelines
- Computer-assisted diagnosis
- Computer-assisted patient management
- Computer-assisted patient education
- Computerized clinical decision support systems (CDSSs; National Research Council, 2001, p. 164)

To effectively address this list of recommended changes, the computer system is used as a tool to alert the healthcare provider to problems with the patient; to remind the provider about clinical practice guidelines, allergies, or potential adverse effects of drug combinations; to help the provider arrive at an accurate diagnosis and an effective treatment plan; and to present educational information to patients either by an onsite computer or via the Internet.

Committee on Patient Safety and Health Information Technology

A 2011 IOM report titled *Health Information Technology and Patient Safety: Building Safer Systems for Better Care* identified a series of characteristics that computer software developers should consider to make electronic information systems easier for the healthcare professional to use.

The suggestions made included the following characteristics:

- The data within the system are accurate, timely, reliable, and native.
- The system is easy to navigate and use as well as one with which users want to interact.
- The system, as well as data displays, are simple and intuitive to the user.
- The evidence at the point of care is available to aid clinical decision making.
- The system works only to enhance workflow, automate mundane tasks, and streamline work rather than increase physical or cognitive workload.
- The time required for upgrades is minimal and limited.
- The data are easily imported and exchanged between systems (Committee on Patient Safety and Health Information Technology, 2011, p. 62).

Native, Accurate, Reliable, and Timely Data

The Committee's work clearly focused on increasing the efficiency and efficacy of computer and electronic information systems to aid and augment the work of the clinician and healthcare professional. The Committee wanted to ensure the highest standards for protecting patient information. For example, in the first bullet in the preceding list, "native data" is that information entered directly into the electronic computer system. Native data might include information about vital signs entered by the nursing staff; whereas imported data would include data coming from another electronic information system such as the electronic laboratory result information system. In most healthcare organizations, laboratory tests are done on a completely different electronic system specific to the laboratory within the healthcare organization, or a laboratory outside the organization does them. For the data to be considered "accurate and reliable," the data could not have been changed in any way. Within this requirement, assurance is needed that no one is able to hack into the computer system and/or alter the data.

The Committee also recognized the importance of "timely" data. Data are timely if available as soon as they are created. For example, laboratory test results are needed immediately for patients in critical-care units such as intensive care. Once a blood chemistry test such as the serum level of potassium is completed, the information must be relayed to the healthcare provider immediately, especially if it is abnormal. For example, if the potassium level in a patient is low, IV administration of potassium would probably be necessary (low potassium levels may cause the patient's heart to beat irregularly). Quality care depends on having the results as soon as possible so interventions can be taken as the patient's condition warrants. A laboratory result sent 2 weeks after the blood chemistry was drawn will be of little use in caring for the intensive care patient.

Easy to Use

An electronic record system must be easy to learn and easy to use so healthcare providers will want to use it as part of patient-care activities. Healthcare providers will not want to work with electronic systems that are difficult to learn and that do not make sense to them. The way information is entered and used in the electronic system should match the way the provider works. For example, a provider might have a standard set of questions to ask a patient with diabetes. The electronic record system should have the same set of questions in the same order so the provider can easily add the patient's answers as they are given. In some cases, a checklist of probable answers can be listed in the electronic patient record so all the provider has to do is check off the applicable answer. Ideally, providers should be able to customize the electronic record system to match the way they do their work.

Intuitive Displays

The Committee suggested that the computer system incorporates "simple and intuitive" data displays referring to what is usually on a computer screen or a smartphone. Intuitive data displays are those that present the information in the form the user needs it. For example, a nurse might want to see the blood pressure readings displayed in a table, whereas a physician might prefer that same information be displayed on a graph. If either the physician or the nurse wants to change the display format, it should be easy to toggle or change between the table and the graph. The master electronic information system will need to know what device the user has, so that the information will be properly displayed on their device. Some information such as graphs can easily be read on a personal computer (PC) screen but may not be easily adapted to small displays such as on a smartphone.

Navigation

Another characteristic the Committee suggested was that EHRs be easy to "navigate." Navigation refers to the way the computer user moves from one part of the electronic patient record to the next part. For example, if a nurse wants to look first at patient assessment data and then look at the care plan data, it should be easy to make that move in the patient's electronic record. This is usually done through a navigation bar that may be on the side of the screen or across the top of the screen.

Evidence at the Point of Care

Availability of "evidence at the point of care" was yet another characteristic suggested by the Committee. Evidence at the point of care refers to the availability of scientific evidence at the bedside or in the exam room to aid the provider. The availability of this evidence to aid with decision making is crucial to providing quality care. For example, the provider may be confronted with an unusual clinical situation and may want to consult the existing professional literature on that topic. The provider should be able to access the literature or "evidence" from the same computer or workstation they are using to enter data into the patient's EHR. In another instance, a wound care nurse who is treating a stage IV decubitus ulcer may want to see the latest articles available in full text from the National Library of Medicine. The nurse should be able to access those articles at the patient's bedside without having to go to the organization's library. This process is known as knowledge utilization, a method of bringing evidence to the bedside. Informatics is uniquely positioned to provide this knowledge utilization feature.

Another means of providing evidence at the point of care is to base assessment findings and interventions on the best available evidence. Ideally, when the nurse selects an intervention, an option for viewing the evidence that supports the intervention is displayed. The convenience of having the best available evidence supporting patient care interventions at the bedside, where care is provided, is the optimal scenario. Although we are not quite optimizing technology to support evidence-based nursing care at the bedside, there is a push toward making this a reality. This is one way that electronic documentation can facilitate the use of evidence at the point of care.

Enhance Workflow

Electronic information systems transform data into information that is meaningful for the user. A simple example of the electronic transformation of data into information is the list of deposits and withdrawals made to a bank account. The transactions of deposits and withdrawals are the data. When those transactions result in an addition and/or subtraction of the money in the account, the data are processed electronically and information results. The information is the balance in the bank account. The balance information guides the owner of the bank account in managing finances. Likewise, in healthcare when information is combined with experience and understanding, it becomes knowledge that can be used to make informed decisions (LaTour & Maki, 2010). Knowledge becomes wisdom when it is "applied in a practical way or translated into actions" (Kenney & Androwich, 2012, p. 63) and state that a nurse is applying knowledge in a practical way when a patient care plan is developed (p. 124).

Limit Inefficiencies

Electronic information systems should introduce efficiencies in the way work is done so no new physical demands will be placed on the nurse. For example, a nurse should not have to travel to a separate computer or be required to be in a library to access scientific literature. Likewise, it is important not to make the nurse's work anymore mentally demanding than it already is. Rather than creating a delay in patient care, new electronic technologies should enhance patient care efficiently for all involved. Information in healthcare is expanding exponentially and although healthcare providers are highly educated, no one provider can be expected to know everything. Point-of-care technology, for example, provides reliable information to fill the knowledge gap of providers at the time they need it most—while they are interacting with the patient.

All electronic information systems will need some downtime for routine hardware and software updates and/or maintenance. The computer will not be available during those times. However, this downtime should be for a short duration of time and the nursing and healthcare staff need to know when this downtime will occur. Planned downtime is usually in the middle of the night when the least number of users will be affected. As healthcare is delivered round the clock, any necessary downtime should be for a relatively short duration. Healthcare facilities try to prevent excessive downtime by having backup generators for power failures and by running parallel computer systems so if one computer system goes down, another computer system immediately kicks into action. Disaster planning requires that provisions be made for unusual situations such as hurricanes, power outages, and other large-scale problems. Accreditation standards also require healthcare facilities to determine how they will provide essential services under extreme conditions.

"Provisions" and "essential services" must include protecting data within electronic health systems from unauthorized access or getting lost due to systems failure.

Exchange of Information

Since patients are often treated across many different healthcare organizations, it should be quick and easy to obtain information from another organization. The coordination of the access and exchange of patient information occurs through the establishment of **health information exchanges** (HIEs), where a patient's vital health data are shared electronically on both regional and national levels (HealthIT.gov, 2014). HIEs usually operate on a regional level such as by cities or counties since most health information is shared among local healthcare providers. HIEs are not-for-profit organizations formed by a variety of vested healthcare professionals from healthcare organizations, institutions, and practices. At the regional level, these HIEs are referred to as regional health information organizations (RHIOs). When health information is shared over a longer distance, it is shared among HIEs. Thus, information about a patient in Syracuse, New York, can be shared with providers in Los Angeles, California. The RHIOs or network of HIEs forms the basis of the NHIN discussed earlier in this chapter. Patients have a choice to sign an authorization to have their information shared or can opt out of the HIE if they do not want their information shared (Bass, 2011).

▰▱▱ HEALTH INFORMATICS LEGISLATION

The reports of the IOM inform Congress about important legislation needed to bring about change in health informatics. As a result, several important laws have been passed to advance the health informatics agenda. These laws include the following:

- Health Insurance Portability and Accountability Act (HIPAA, 1996), which contains important provisions for privacy and security of health information (Pub. L. 104–191, Aug. 21, 1996, 110 Stat. 1936).
- Health Information Technology for Economic and Clinical Health Act (HITECH Act; Pub. Law 111–5, div. A, title XIII, div. B, title IV, February 17, 2009, 123 Stat. 226, 467 [42 U.S.C. 300jj et seq.; 17901 et seq.]), which was part of the American Recovery and Reinvestment Act of 2009 (ARRA; Pub. L. 111–5). The HITECH Act provided billions of dollars of federal money in the form of grants to advance widespread use of health information technology.
- The Patient Protection and Affordable Care Act (PPACA) of 2010 (Public Law 111–148), often called the Affordable Care Act (ACA). The ACA provides ongoing funding for health information technology (www.congress.gov/111/plaws/publ148/PLAW-111publ148.pdf).

Health Insurance Portability and Accountability Act

The **Health Insurance Portability and Accountability Act (HIPAA)** of 1996 is a federal law requiring healthcare providers to use several privacy protections for patients and their records (HHS, 2013). HIPAA protects an individual's identifiable health information that is in oral, written, and/or electronic form. HIPAA also requires that each healthcare facility have a designated privacy officer. There are two aspects to HIPAA, information privacy and security of private health information.

Information Privacy

Information privacy is the patient's right to limit the amount of personal healthcare information accessible to and known by others (HIPAA, 1996). Within this right of patients, providers are mandated to maintain confidentiality. Confidentiality is the duty the provider has to hold patient information private. Although the patient's right to information privacy is not stated in the U.S. Constitution, various court cases such as *Griswold v. Connecticut* (1965) interpret sections of the Bill of Rights (the first 10 amendments to the Constitution) as giving the patient this right. In particular, the fourth amendment to the Constitution, which protects against unreasonable search and seizure of papers and effects, is thought to provide information privacy. Attention to privacy is extremely important because if patients think their privacy will not be protected, they will be reluctant to share information needed to provide quality care. An excellent online resource for staff training on privacy is available from the National Institutes of Health (NIH). Courses relevant for the new or novice nurse include NIH Information Security Awareness Course and NIH Privacy Awareness Course. Users can take the course on the website (irtsectraining.nih.gov/publicUser.aspx) and receive a certificate of completion.

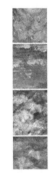

CASE STUDY 9.2

A patient complains to the nurse about the amount of personal data collected in the admissions office. The patient states that too much data are collected and he is concerned about the protection of his privacy.

1. *What should the nurse explain to the patient about the amount of personal data collected?*
2. *What should the nurse explain to the patient about how his data are protected?*

Security

HIPAA requires that healthcare organizations have specific measures in place to safeguard patient's health information. First, there must be access controls in place such as passwords and PIN numbers to limit unauthorized access to sensitive patient information. Second, health organizations must encrypt patient health information, meaning information cannot be read or understood unless the person is authorized and has a decryption key. Most times, the decryption key is linked to the person's password or PIN number. **Security** is the set of protections placed on a computer system to prohibit unauthorized access and to prevent any loss or distortion of the data (HIPAA, 1996). HIPAA also requires that security measures be in place in an organization and that there is a designated security officer. The NIH training website (irtsectraining.nih.gov/publicUser0.aspx) also offers a course to the public on the topic of computer security.

The Health Information Technology for Economic and Clinical Health Act

The **HITECH Act** is a federal law that provides money to healthcare providers, institutions, and organizations to encourage the use of EHRs (HHS, 2017). However, the federal government also wanted to make sure its money was wisely spent. It will only give providers enhanced payments if they use certified EHRs. In addition, the provider must show the EHR is being used in a meaningful way.

To assist providers in determining if their use of the EHR met the federal expectation, the CMS of the HHS developed criteria showing meaningful use.

As new healthcare legislation is enacted, both HITECH and Meaningful Use are being integrated into the newer laws. This does not mean that the objectives of each act are no longer relevant—they are still required of healthcare organizations and providers and have been integrated within other regulations. The Medicare Access and CHIP Reauthorization Act (MACRA) of 2015 includes requirements from the EHR Merit-Based Incentive Payment System, or MIPS, began in January of 2017 and includes requirements for reimbursement and payment based on the following:

- Quality of care
- Resource use
- Clinical practice improvement activities
- Meaningful use of certified EHR technology

Both MACRA and MIPS replace certain initiatives set by the EHR Incentive Program (Meaningful Use) and HITECH so that organizations working toward meeting the requirements can continue moving forward without an interruption in requirements.

Meaningful Use

The CMS (2011) initiated a program called the EHR Incentive Program, also known as Meaningful Use. **Meaningful Use** was an initiative designed to encourage the use of EHRs by using data collected in the clinical setting such as hospitals, clinics, or physician offices, to improve patient-care outcomes (HealthIT.gov, 2015). It was an incentive program from CMS that provided reimbursements based on the ability to meet three stages of the initiative. Stage 1 ran from 2011 to 2012 and involved data capture and sharing. Stage 2 started in 2014 and involved advanced clinical processes based on data. Stage 3 started in 2016 and included improved patient outcomes. Demonstrating achievement of requirements for each stage resulted in substantial reimbursements from the CMS. Select specific criteria for each stage are shown in Table 9.2.

The Meaningful Use initiative was beneficial in forcing healthcare providers and organizations to adopt and integrate EMRs in the care provision setting. Each stage of Meaningful Use is categorized under five major domains:

- Improve quality, safety, and efficiency.
- Engage patients and families.

TABLE 9.2 MEANINGFUL USE STAGE CRITERIA

STAGE 1	STAGE 2	STAGE 3
• Electronically capture health data • Use data to track clinical conditions • Report quality measures and publicly reportable health measures • Use data to engage patients and families in their care	• Rigorous health information exchanges • Increased requirement for e-prescribing and lab reporting • Share patient-care summaries across care settings • Increased patient-controlled data	• Improved quality, safety, and efficiencies based on electronic information • Develop decision supports for high-priority conditions • Patient access to self-management tools • Access to comprehensive patient data through health information exchanges • Improve population health

Source: https://www.healthit.gov/providers-professionals/how-attain-meaningful-use.

- Improve care coordination.
- Improve public and population health.
- Ensure privacy and security for personal health information.

Although the EHR Incentive Program has ended, the initiatives from the program are still required for reimbursement from CMS. Major outcomes from the initiative include using electronically captured health data to improve quality of care processes and patient outcomes, clinical decision supports, e-prescribing, and improved patient engagement in healthcare decisions through patient portals.

Data Capture to Improve Quality

Data are continuously captured during patient-care encounters through patient assessments and documentation of interventions. Using these data to improve healthcare processes is a key part of Meaningful Use. Consider all the data captured during one patient care encounter. Data could include height, weight, age, heart rate, blood pressure, respiratory rate, lung sounds, level of consciousness, oxygenation, orientation, level of activity, ability to ambulate, color of urine, frequency of bowel movements, and so on. This vast amount of data is inputted into a computer documentation system and placed by the program into logical categories. The data in the categories can be extracted into trends within a category (heart rate data over time) or compared against other data using reports. A report can combine data from different categories to determine relationships or cause and effects.

For example, a patient is admitted to a hospital and is on bed rest. Nursing care based on the evidence includes skin care and turning the patient every 2 hours to prevent hospital-acquired pressure ulcers. The nurse would document that the patient is on bed rest, turning the patient every 2 hours, and that skin care is provided. By documenting each of these items the electronic system is able to run reports on the data. This is also a measure of quality nursing care; therefore, a report could be generated to include the number of patients on bed rest who are turned every 2 hours. An example of findings might show that of the 70 patients on bed rest, 55 patients had documentation in their record of being turned every 2 hours. To calculate a percentage, 55 divided by 70 is 0.786, or 79%. The unit can say that patients on bed rest are turned every 2 hours 79% of the time. If theigoal is to have 100% of patients on bed rest turned every 2 hours then the data show that a problem exists. This same measure can occur every month to give a trended report of compliance.

Clinical Decision Support Systems

A **clinical decision support system** (CDSS) is an integrated database of clinical and scientific information to aid healthcare professionals in providing care (Agency for Healthcare Research and Quality [AHRQ], 2016). The CDSS is designed to look at a set of data and then lead the user through a decision-making process. For example, asking the user a set of questions that narrow possible choices to one choice that is the most effective. A CDSS might be used to arrive at a correct diagnosis or it might be used to determine the most effective treatment plan for the patient. Clinical decision supports can take the form of alerts, alarms, hard stops (the nurse is unable to continue charting until a specific item is addressed), clinical guidelines, order sets, and clinically relevant evidence to support decisions. For example, a doctor might be treating a patient who is a recovering drug addict with postoperative pain. By using the CDSS on the hospital's health information system, the provider is able to enter assessment data and confounding factors such as opiate addiction to decide the best alternative medication to prescribe.

For example, a hospital collects data on patient falls per month. Upon admission and once a day afterward, every patient receives a fall risk assessment. When using the fall risk assessment tool the results are categorized into low, medium, or high risk for falls. The hospital has a set group of interventions for patients who score at either the medium- or high-risk categories. To meet stage 1 of meaningful use, the hospital would integrate the interventions with the fall risk assessment. When the nurse completes a patient fall risk assessment in the electronic documentation system and the finding is high risk, specific interventions based on the best available evidence automatically appear. The nurse must select the interventions in place for the patient before moving forward with the electronic charting. This form of clinical decision support not only reminds the nurse of evidence-based interventions needed for the patient, but also requires implementing the evidence-based interventions before continuing with charting.

CRITICAL THINKING 9.3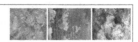

View the video at youtu.be/zoxpuzH4B_0 (or go to YouTube and search for the video titled "Clinical Decision Support for Evidence-Based Care"). Watch the short 11-minute video that demonstrates the use of a CDSS for the "Safe and Sound" program.

1. How was a CDSS used in the video?
2. How did the CDSS demonstrate integrating evidence-based practice to guide decision making?

---

e-Prescribing

An objective of Meaningful Use included e-Prescribing by clinicians in both the hospital and clinical setting. Whenever the letter "e" precedes a word it means "electronic." The goals of e-Prescribing were to reduce redundancies, prevent errors in transcription, increase efficiencies in medication acquisition, and share medications across all care settings. To achieve this goal, a nation-wide computerized sharing of medication data among all pharmacies, healthcare organizations, and clinics was established. This allowed the sharing of medication across all healthcare settings. Once data sharing was in place, all healthcare providers in all settings had to use e-Prescribing in order to capture all medications.

For example, a patient provides a home medication list upon admission to the hospital. During the course of the hospitalization some medications are discontinued, new medications are added, and doses changed. Upon discharge, the medication list may look completely different than when the patient was admitted. The hospital physician uses e-Prescribing to order all medications from the patient's pharmacy to be used at home. The new medication list is sent electronically to the pharmacy so that the new medications can be prepared. Additionally, the new medication list is also electronically stored and sent to all the patient's physicians. After discharge the patient will see his or her primary and specialty physicians. During each physician visit, the new medication list is available for review or revision based on the patient's health needs. The seamless sharing of medications helps facilitate consistent and patient-centered care during every healthcare encounter.

Patient Portals

One objective of Meaningful Use was to create **patient portals** that allow patients timely access to health data and education (CMS, 2016). Electronic documentation vendors along with healthcare organizations create access controls to allow healthcare organizations to decide what and how much information to allow patients to access electronically. Although the objective did not specify what information should be available, the objective did require that patients use the information to make informed health decisions.

For example, a patient sees an orthopedic physician about knee pain. The physician orders a MRI diagnostic test. During the appointment, the nurse asks the patient to sign up for the patient portal, explaining that the patient can access health information through the portal. The patient signs up for the portal and establishes a login and password. The patient has the MRI the next week and is scheduled to see the physician in 2 weeks. A day after the MRI the patient receives an email from the patient portal system that a new test is available to view. The patient accesses the patient portal and is able to review the MRI report. When the patient attends the appointment with the physician the patient is able to discuss MRI findings and ask questions based on the report.

Standards for Interoperability

Interoperability is an agreed-upon standard of communication among hardware and software companies that allows for the effective exchange of patient information among various health information systems (HIMSS, 2017). HITECH and Meaningful Use both rely on systems to be interoperable in order for the regulations to work. For example, different hospitals use different EMR vendors; however, with interoperability standards in place, these various EMRs are able to exchange patient information seamlessly and accurately. The telephone system is an excellent example of interoperability. Regardless of the type of phone used or the service vendor selected, anyone is able to communicate via phone. That is because all the phone makers and all the service providers adhere to a common set of standards. The same level of interoperability is needed for the computer exchange of health information.

Many computer standards are currently available to facilitate communication between different health information systems and even more standards are under development. Policies, procedures, and development of standards for health information systems arecoordinated by the American National Standards Institute (ANSI; ansi.org) and its Healthcare Information Technology Standards Panel (HITSP; www. hitsp.org). Standards development groups include representatives from government, the healthcare industry, and health informatics system vendors.

The NHIN is a federal certification program in place to make sure vendors develop EHR products that meet interoperability and formatting standards. The ANSI sets the standards; however, the federal government provides the certification that the health information system meets meaningful use provisions.

For an EHR product to be certified, the vendor must submit the product for a technical evaluation by an expert panel from a certifying organization recognized by the federal government. Medicare and Medicaid are currently offering enhanced payments to healthcare providers who adopt certified EHRs. These financial incentives are being used to speed EHR adoption so the vision of an NHIN can become a reality.

The NHIN would be a structure that would allow for secure sharing of confidential healthcare information among healthcare providers across the country.

TELEHEALTH

The Health Resources and Services Administration (HRSA) of the HHS defines **telehealth** as the use of electronic information and communications technologies to support and facilitate clinical- and population-based healthcare, patient health education, and health administration from long distances (2015). Technologies include videoconferencing, the Internet, imaging sharing, streaming media, and wireless communications (www.hrsa.gov/ruralhealth/telehealth/).

Telehealth uses some type of computer or communication device at both the sending end and the receiving end of the communication. Cameras and microphones may also be used to send pictures and sound. Technology allows a patient's home to serve as an extension of the healthcare facility in that it removes time and distance barriers in the provision of healthcare services (Dewsburys, 2012). The typical telehealth scenario has nurses interacting with patients over telephone systems. The patients are usually in their homes and they may have home monitoring equipment connected to their phone lines. This monitoring equipment is used to gather data on the patient such as blood pressure, pulse oximetry, blood glucose, and weight. Originally, only telephones with landlines were used but now it is possible to use mobile devices such as cellular phones, satellite phones, phones connected over television cable systems, and the Internet (Dewsburys, 2012).

Some telehealth devices prompt the patient at a certain time of the day to obtain specified data for transmittal to the healthcare provider. For example, the patient may attach a blood pressure cuff to his or her arm, press a button, and then wait while the cuff inflates. The monitoring device records the blood pressure and transmits it over phone lines to the nurse who usually works for a home care agency. A pulse oximeter is attached to the patient's finger and, again, the data are transmitted to the nurse. For patients with conditions such as congestive heart failure, it is important to check the patient's weight to determine if he or she is retaining fluid. Thus, a scale may also be attached to the monitoring device. Patient data may be transmitted through cables attached to the home monitoring station or the data may be transmitted wirelessly to the station.

On the receiving end, a nurse uses a telehealth computer workstation to monitor the data coming in from the patient. The telehealth computer software will provide alerts if any information falls outside the parameters set for that patient. The nurse will usually phone the patient after the data arrive to discuss how the patient is feeling and to see if there are any problems that need to be addressed. If the nurse is unable to reach the patient, the nurse may contact family members and/or call 911 to check on the patient. The home health agency may also send a nurse to the patient's home.

One of the many benefits of telehealth use is among patients with chronic diseases. For example, identification of small changes that may signify a problem before it becomes life-threatening is critical. Telehealth can draw prompt attention to the patient's healthcare status to decrease the risk of exacerbation of the disease. Telehealth can improve patient outcomes and can be delivered at a lower cost than home healthcare. Along with reducing the burden on patients to travel to receive healthcare, Anguita (2012) notes other benefits of telehealth. These include increased patient independence, increased collaboration with other community organizations, and increased opportunities for nurses to provide education to patients and families.

EVIDENCE FROM THE LITERATURE

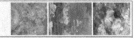

Citation

Totten, A. M., Womack, D. M., Eden, K. B., McDonagh, M. S., Griffin, J. C., Grusing, S., & Hersh, W. R. (2016, June). *Telehealth: Mapping the evidence for patient outcomes from systematic reviews* (Technical Briefs, No. 26). Rockville, MD: Agency for Healthcare Research and Quality. Retrieved from https://www.ncbi.nlm.nih.gov/books/NBK379320/

Discussion

The purpose of this report was to create an overview of the body of evidence about telehealth for use by decision makers and to assess the impact of telehealth on clinical outcomes. Fifty-eight systematic reviews met the authors' inclusion and exclusion criteria. The authors created an evidence map based on findings from the included studies using weighted estimates of effect. The authors found that sufficient high-quality evidence exists to support the effectiveness of telehealth for specific uses with some types of patients, including:

- Remote patient monitoring for patients with chronic conditions
- Communication and counseling for patients with chronic conditions
- Psychotherapy as part of behavioral health

The most consistent benefit was found when telehealth was used for communication and counseling with patients and the remote monitoring of chronic conditions such as cardiovascular and respiratory diseases, with improvements in outcomes such as mortality, quality of life, and reductions in hospital admissions.

Implications for Practice

The use of telehealth for patient populations with a high risk for readmission such as heart failure or chronic obstructive pulmonary disease can help reduce hospitalizations and improve quality of life. For chronic conditions, both remote monitoring and communications with health providers were found to have a positive effect on outcomes.

CASE STUDY 9.3

A newly hired nurse is assigned to work at the telehealth workstation. The nurse is monitoring the data coming in from home-based patients, checking to see if there are any situations that require nurse intervention, and taking action as appropriate. One patient with type 2 diabetes reports fasting blood glucose of 52. Another patient who has congestive heart failure and normally reports in on a daily basis does not transmit any data.

(continued)

> **CASE STUDY 9.3** *(continued)*
>
> **1.** *What is the best course of action for the nurse to take regarding the patient with diabetes?*
> **2.** *How should the nurse proceed regarding the lack of information obtained from the patient with heart failure?*

HEALTH-RELATED WEBSITES

A growing number of consumers use the Internet as a handy way to access health-related information. Some health-related Internet sites provide high-quality information to help consumers understand health problems, make informed health decisions, and provide insights about healthcare expectations. Although the information is convenient and generally accessible, most health-related information on the Internet is not monitored for quality. The average consumer generally may not have the knowledge to judge the quality of the source or the health information found on the Internet. This raises concerns about the type of information available to guide consumer health decisions.

An expectation of nurses is that they have the knowledge to guide patients toward accessing the best and highest quality health-related websites available on the Internet. There are several types of website evaluation tools available with varying levels of reliability and validity. One widely recognized website evaluation tool specific to health-related sites was developed by the Health on the Net Foundation (HON). HON is a nonprofit, nongovernmental, and international foundation that developed a set of criteria to judge the quality of health information available on the Internet. There are a set of eight principles for evaluating a health website. The HON Foundation uses the eight principles to certify if the principles are met. If the website does meet the standards they are considered HON certified and can display the HON logo on their website. To note, the user can click on the symbol and see how the website meets the criteria. The principles include the following:

1. Authority: The qualifications of the authors or contributors are clearly stated.
2. Complementarity: A statement is included on the website that states the information is not meant to replace the advice of a healthcare provider.
3. Privacy: Confidentiality of personal information.
4. Information: Information is marked with date of last modification and external references.
5. Justification: Claims made on the website have supporting justification.
6. Contact: Website contact information is clearly stated.
7. Disclosure: All funding sources are clearly described.
8. Advertising: Website clearly discloses advertising sources and funding as well as differentiates between advertising and website content (www.hon.ch/HONcode/Patients/Visitor/visitor.html#accreditation).

Healthcare applications have also gained popularity with mHealth (mobile health information). Criteria for appraising the quality of health-related applications are varied in the literature with almost all agreeing upon certain characteristics. Using a structured and standardized approach to appraising mobile health applications is critical to ensuring patients are guided to appropriate information. The following is a list of characteristics typically used to appraise health-related mobile applications.

1. Confidentiality and security of health information
2. Graphics and layout appeal, ease of use
3. Engagement, entertainment, and customization of information
4. Functional design
5. Quality of information presented, attribution to experts
6. Subjective quality (BinDihm, Hawkey & Trevena, 2014; Stoyanov et al., 2015)

Nurses should be familiar with the need to appraise health-related websites and mobile applications. Understanding this need and possessing skills in appraisal help the nurse guide patients in selecting appropriate electronic medical information.

TECHNOLOGIES AND INFORMATION SYSTEMS IN HOSPITALS

A hospital has many information systems that feed into the EHR and that support healthcare safety and quality. Among the information systems of most interest to nursing staff are admission/discharge/transfer (ADT) and patient registration systems; messaging/communication technology; CPOE; bar-code medication administration (BCMA); and radio frequency identification (RFID).

CRITICAL THINKING 9.4

Watch the short 4-minute video at youtu.be/DAQ2CnjL7tQ. You can also access the video by going to YouTube and searching for "Beacon Community Program: Improving Health Through Health Technology." When watching the video, take note of how technology improves the quality and safe delivery of patient care.

1. What technological advances have improved communication in the healthcare setting?
2. Why is it important to understand technology advances in the patient care setting?

The ADT and patient registration systems are used to collect demographic data about patients being admitted to the hospital or being registered as outpatients. ADT systems are used for inpatients; patient registration systems are used for outpatients. Demographic data contain facts that identify a patient as a unique individual. They include name, address, phone numbers, date of birth, sex, race, ethnicity, religion, and insurance information. In addition, ADT and patient registration systems collect dates and times healthcare services were provided. If a patient is transferred from one inpatient unit to another, the ADT system will track the change. Data accuracy in these systems is extremely important to make sure appropriate care is given to the correct patient.

Communication Technologies

In almost every hospital patient care setting you will find that nurses carry assigned phones on their person. The phones are linked to the hospital phone system to facilitate communication between the nurse and others, such as the unit secretary, the patient, other hospital departments, and other care providers. The intent of the phone is to facilitate direct communication with the nurse and to eliminate delays in communication and miscommunication about the patient-care team. Of concern is that the phones can cause an additional distraction or interruption to the nurse, which may result in delay of care or errors (Koong et al., 2015).

Technology that facilitates communication includes more than phones; another major type of communication technology is the EMR. Most EMR systems have an area for notes from the interprofessional team about care of a patient. This form of communication enhances patient care by sharing information among the healthcare workers who need it at the point of care. For example, a nurse can access dietary education, physical therapy, and respiratory therapy notes on a patient. Having this information available at the point of care helps the nurse identify any gaps in care or additional education needed.

Computerized Physician Order Entry

A **computerized physician (provider) order entry** (CPOE) is considered any system that allows the physician to directly transmit an order electronically to a recipient (AHRQ PSNet, 2017). The CPOE is a software component of an EMR that allows the clinician to enter patient-care orders directly into the computer system, thus eliminating any illegibility problems that can potentially occur with handwritten orders. Patient orders can be entered from any location so there is no longer a need for verbal orders or telephone orders. In addition, the CPOE issues alerts about various aspects of the patient's condition. For example, the CPOE might alert the clinician to a low heart rate currently being experienced by a patient. The CPOE also checks orders against the hospital formulary to determine if a medication is stocked by the hospital pharmacy and then checks known allergies, medication–medication interactions, and appropriate dosages of medication. Delays in care are avoided because orders for lab tests are immediately transmitted to the lab, medication orders are immediately transmitted to the pharmacy, and blood transfusion orders are immediately transmitted to the blood bank.

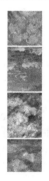

CASE STUDY 9.4

The nursing staff at your hospital is upset because computerized provider order entry (CPOE) was implemented 3 months ago. However, only about half of the healthcare providers are using the new system. The rest of the healthcare providers continue to handwrite orders as well as only give verbal and/or telephone orders. This creates confusion for the nursing staff because they have to remember which providers are using the new system. For providers not using the new CPOE system, the nurses must read the handwritten orders and make sure they are properly executed. In addition, the nurses feel that they have a greater liability when they receive verbal or telephone orders and the physician has not yet signed them.

1. *What should the nurses do in this situation?*
2. *What could have prevented this problem?*

Bar-Code Medication Administration

Bar-code medication administration (BCMA) links the electronic medication administration record (eMAR) with medication-specific identification in the form of bar codes to help with compliance of the five "rights" of medication administration: right patient, right dose, right route, right time, and right medication (healthit.ahrq.gov/ ahrq-funded-projects/emerging-lessons/bar-coded-medication-administration). BCMA is a system that receives orders from the CPOE system, which prints bar-coded labels that contain the patient's identification number (usually the patient's healthcare record number). BCMAs may also print the specifics of the medication order (i.e., name of the medication and dose). The patient identification bar-code label is then attached to the medication sent from the pharmacy to the nursing unit. Before the nurse administers the medication, the bar code on the patient's wrist bracelet is scanned and the bar code on the medication packet is scanned. The computer system will check to make sure that the packet contains the right medication for the patient and that the medication is being given according to the clinician's order; that is, the right time and frequency, right dose, and the right route of administration (Sharma, 2018). Poon et al. (2010) studied an academic medical center and found BCMA systems reduced the number of potential adverse drug events by more than half.

Radio Frequency Identification

Radio frequency identification (RFID) is a technology that uses radio waves to transfer data from an electronic tag to an object for the purpose of identifying and tracking the object (Ajami & Rajabzadeh, 2013). The use of RFID tags in healthcare involves a small computer chip worn on the patient's body like a bracelet or necklace. The RFID device transmits radio waves that can be picked up by sensors located throughout a healthcare facility. A common application of RFID is with Alzheimer's patients in a nursing home setting. RFID technology used in the patients' wrist bracelets can be used to sound an alarm when patients try to leave the unit or when an external door is opened. The computer chip used in an RFID can also store much more information than a bar code so an RFID provides the ability to have even more detail about the patient in a medication administration system. This additional information comes at a higher cost than associated with bar-code technology.

RFID chips are used in surgical sponges to determine if any sponges are left in the patient at the end of the surgical procedure. This RFID technology ensures the patient will not have to return to surgery to remove a missed sponge (Lazzaro et al., 2017). It also protects the healthcare facility from liability and unnecessary costs. The CMS (2008) determined it would no longer pay for higher costs of hospitalization associated with events such as objects left in an operative wound. Surgical sponge RFID chips help healthcare facilities meet the goal of zero sponges left postsurgery.

Technology in Direct Patient Care

Electrophysiological monitoring technology collects vital signs and other related data such as heart rhythms about the patient and immediately sends them to the EHR to give the clinician faster access to the data. The EHR can also issue clinical alerts to the clinician. The alerts might be present when the clinician signs on to the EHR or the

EHR might send an electronic page, an email message, or a phone call to the clinician. The EHR systems eliminate the transcription errors that occur when vital signs data are handwritten and then later documented in the record.

Smart Healthcare Devices

The miniaturization of computer chips allows their use in a number of healthcare devices. These devices are called smart devices because they are able to monitor certain parameters about a patient and transmit that information to the healthcare provider. In some cases, the smart devices are programmed to take corrective action when problems occur. An implantable cardioverter defibrillator (ICD) is one example. If the patient experiences ventricular tachycardia or ventricular fibrillation, the smart device will immediately evaluate the situation and deliver an electric impulse to the heart. If the heart rhythm does not convert to an acceptable level, the smart device will deliver another, stronger impulse (National Heart, Lung, and Blood Institute, 2012). These smart devices save lives because they can identify and/or treat abnormal conditions much faster than the healthcare provider can.

Other common devices with smart technology include infusion pumps and implantable insulin pumps. Smart pumps are IV pumps in the clinical setting that are programmed with a library database of IV medications (Harrison, 2016). Each medication has hard limits (i.e., the clinician cannot program the pump to deliver more than a specified range) and soft limits (an alert is given when a range of medication dose is reached but the pump will continue to deliver the medication). When used correctly, smart pumps have shown to reduce medication errors (Stephenson, 2016).

In each case, a computer processor is an essential component of the smart device. The use of smart devices will continue to expand with the advent of nanotechnology. According to the National Nanotechnology Initiative (2012), a nanometer is one billionth the size of a meter. It describes nanotechnology as the science involved with understanding, manipulating, and manufacturing materials of this small size. This will make it possible to have extremely small computer processors for smart devices.

TO ALERT OR NOT TO ALERT

Although automatic EHR alerts within hospitals can be very helpful, care should be taken in the electronic system design and implementation to make sure the physicians and the nursing staff are not receiving too many alerts. Otherwise, a problem known as alarm fatigue can occur. Alarm fatigue happens when the nurse becomes desensitized to the alarm because of the high volume of alarms that occur in the clinical setting that results in staff ignoring the alerts (Turmell, Coke, Catinella, Hosford, & Majeski, 2017). Staff may try to turn the alerts off and can become increasingly annoyed with the system. The actual users of the electronic system should determine which alerts will be the most beneficial to them. For example, in a cardiac ICU the interprofessional team may determine cardiac parameters they want alarms for such as heart rates decreasing or increasing by 10%. The presence or absence of an alert does not relieve the nurse or the providers of the duty to provide quality care. Alerts are only tools. The responsibility to deliver quality care remains with the healthcare professional rather than the device.

EVIDENCE FROM THE LITERATURE

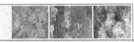

Citation

Rouleau, G., Gagnon, M., Côté, J., Payne-Gagnon, J., Hudson, E., & Dubois, C. (2017). Impact of information and communication technologies on nursing care: Results of an overview of systematic reviews. *Journal of Medical Internet Research*, *19*(4), e122. Retrieved from http://www.jmir.org/2017/4/e122/

Discussion

An overview of systematic reviews was conducted to understand how nursing care is influenced by information and communication technologies (ICTs). Twenty-two qualitative, mixed methods, and quantitative reviews met inclusion criteria and were reviewed. Findings from all reviews were synthesized into nursing care indicators that were influenced by ICT and included the following: time management; time spent on patient care; documentation time; information quality and access; quality of documentation; knowledge updating and utilization; nurse autonomy; intra- and interprofessional collaboration; nurses' competencies and skills; nurse-patient relationship; assessment, care planning, and evaluation; teaching of patients and families; communication and care coordination; perspectives of the quality of care provided; nurses' and patients' satisfaction or dissatisfaction with ICTs; patient comfort and quality of life related to care; empowerment; and functional status.

Implications for Practice

The 19 nursing indicators identified as influenced by ICTs should be kept in mind when considering implementing new technologies that affect nurses.

CRITICAL THINKING 9.5

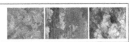

The nurse is reviewing orders and completing the medication reconciliation in the EHR on a patient just admitted to the medical–surgical floor. Medication reconciliation is a process for double checking medications, where the nurse verifies that the details of the medications written on the provider's orders match those recorded in the medication administration record used by the nurse. During the reconciliation process, several system alerts go off.

1. Does the use of electronic health records (EHRs) guarantee error-free patient care?
2. What types of nursing behavior regarding the use of EHRs might contribute to jeopardizing patient safety?
3. What are the dangers of excessive system alerts in computer charting systems? How can the nurse guard against the potential effect?

FUTURE OF INFORMATICS

Nursing curricula at both the undergraduate and graduate level are changing to include more knowledge of informatics. This is due in large part to the work of the Technology Informatics Guiding Educational Reform (**TIGER**), which is a national plan to enable practicing nurses and nursing students to fully engage in the unfolding digital electronic era in healthcare. The purpose of the initiative is to identify information/knowledge management best practices and effective technology capabilities for nurses. TIGER's goal is to create and disseminate action plans that can be duplicated within nursing and other multidisciplinary healthcare training and workplace settings and is focused on using informatics tools, principles, theories, and practices to enable nurses to make healthcare safer, more effective, efficient, patient-centered, timely, and equitable (TIGER, 2012, para. 1).

Today's nurse must be prepared to embrace rapidly changing technology. Technology in all forms, including informatics, is the future of healthcare that, when used properly, can effectively help to ensure patient safety and quality of care by nurses.

CRITICAL THINKING 9.6

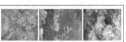

It has been a very busy shift and the nurse is a bit overwhelmed with five assigned patients. It is 6 hours into the shift and the nurse has only charted initial assessments. She must remain in a room to monitor an IV medication but believes she can also begin charting, even if just for the patient whose room she is in. The challenge is the patient's family is also in the room.

1. What team members would have important input on this team?
2. What principles should the nurse consider in completing bedside charting in the presence of the patient's family?

KEY CONCEPTS

1. EMRs are used to document one instance of care, whereas EHRs follow a person from birth to death.
2. EMRs and EHRs are replacing paper records as a result of a federal initiative.
3. When properly implemented, EHRs improve the quality of care and reduce healthcare costs.
4. EHR is the preferred term that will be replacing the term EMR as a national health record is implemented.
5. Several different information systems in a hospital feed data to the EHR.
6. Telehealth keeps patients in their homes, improves patient outcomes, reduces the number of hospital days used, and reduces healthcare costs.
7. Nurses should participate in the development of computer system alerts to make sure they are useful and not an annoyance. Nurses retain responsibility for the care they provide, regardless of the presence or the absence of an alert.

8. The HIPAA and its rules on privacy and security apply to EMRs and EHRs. Nurses have a duty to protect patient privacy.
9. Nursing curricula must change to incorporate the study of new technologies.
10. Lifelong learning is essential for practicing nurses to keep up with technology.

KEY TERMS

Bar-code medication administration
Clinical decision support system
Computerized provider order entry
Electronic health record
HIPAA

HITECH
Medical identity theft
Radio frequency identification
Telehealth
TIGER

QSEN ACTIVITIES

1. A self-paced module that illustrates the professional responsibilities inherent in informatics: qsen.org/heath-informatics-and-technology-professional-responsibilities/
2. Electronic health record case studies: qsen.org/effectively-using-ehrs-with-interdisciplinary-teams-improving-health-quality-of-care/

REVIEW QUESTIONS

1. The nurse is caring for a patient and preparing to administer scheduled medications. Which of the following represents a benefit of using informatics technology with regard to medication administration?
   A. Automated medication systems alleviate the need for cross-checking allergies.
   B. Using automated medication systems prevents medication errors.
   C. Automated medication systems provide decision-making aids that alert the nurse to potential problems.
   D. Automated medication administration systems prevent the nurse from administering the wrong medication.

2. The nurse uses the electronic medical record (EMR) to review key components of the patient's health. What most directly impacts the nurse's ability to effectively utilize the EMR?

   A. The functional design of the EMR system as described by the manufacturer.
   B. The national guidelines for every nurse using an EMR system.
   C. The state and federal initiatives mandating the use of EMR systems.
   D. Local policies, training, and institutional guidelines on the EMR.

3. The facility is using a newly implemented electronic medical record (EMR) for patient care. The nurses have expressed some frustrations with the high volume of system alerts that are generated throughout the day. Which of the following demonstrates the most appropriate response to excessive alerts by the nurse?

   A. Turn alerts off so they do not slow down the data processing capability.
   B. Report excessive alerts to the software designer.

C. Collaborate with the nurse informaticist in the institution to make necessary adjustments.

D. Just ignore the alerts and they will eventually go away.

4. The nurse wants to decrease the rate of medication errors for patients and advocates for use of a computerized provider order entry (CPOE) system. Which of the following best indicates the benefit of CPOE systems?

A. Eliminates the need for the nurse to decipher illegible handwriting.

B. Assists the nurse in receiving verbal orders from the providers.

C. Eliminates the need for the nurse to chart.

D. Takes the guesswork out of knowing when to call the provider.

5. A patient presents to the ambulatory surgery clinic for scheduled rhinoplasty. During the admission interview, the patient notes a history of an allergic reaction to an antibiotic medication 3 years prior. The patient states that she does not know the name of the drug. Which of the following actions is best for the nurse to take?

A. Call the surgeon and share that the patient's allergy history remains incomplete.

B. Ask the patient to describe what the pills looked like.

C. Consult the patient's EHR.

D. Chart that the patient has an allergy to antibiotics.

6. A nurse on the cardiac unit overhears the licensed practical nurse explain to a coworker how to check the status of patients in the labor and delivery unit even though the computer system should not provide this access. Where does the responsibility for system security reside to guard against this type of access?

A. With the nurse who will maintain patient privacy and avoid Health Insurance Portability and Accountability Act (HIPAA) violations.

B. With the nurse informaticist who will make certain the electronic medical record (EMR) maintains confidentiality.

C. With the federal government who will make sure no laws are violated.

D. With the designated security officer who will make sure the entire system is secure.

7. One feature of some electronic medical records (EMRs) is decision-making pop ups. For example, the nurse will be alerted to the patient's medication allergies when administering medications. Which of the following best describes the potential work place benefit for the nurse?

A. It is time saving and eliminates the need to ask the patient about allergies.

B. It is safer and provides a double check opportunity for the nurse to remember to ask the patient.

C. It helps with communication and eliminates cross checking with Pharmacy.

D. It is cost-effective and reduces the time the nurse spends in transcribing medications.

8. The nurse is preparing a patient for discharge. Which of the following represents the nurse's most effective application of the information technology at the bedside?

A. Accessing the best available evidence in preparation to answer the patient's questions upon discharge.

B. Using the computer to print a list of websites that may be of interest to the patient.

C. Posting the patient's questions to a social media website and compiling the response for the patient.

D. Referring the patient to his or her healthcare provider so the provider can answer the patient's questions.

9. The nurse is monitoring the telehealth computer and notices that the patient's pulse oximetry reading drops below 90%, which is the predetermined action criterion for this patient. Which of the following depicts the most appropriate next step the nurse should take?

A. Call the patient's family and alert them to administer oxygen immediately.

B. Call 911 to send emergency responders to the home.

C. Call the patient and assess how the patient is feeling and what is currently happening.

D. Call the primary care provider to obtain treatment orders.

10. Nurses need to increase awareness of the implementation of technology and informatics in patient care. Which of the following best represents a collaborative effort to ensure best practices in nursing informatics?

A. HIPAA

B. TIGER

C. VISTA

D. EHR

REVIEW ACTIVITIES

1. Search the web for position descriptions for a Nurse Informaticist. Consider the education requirements, position description, and required experience. Compare your findings with other classmates. What similarities did you find? What differences?

2. Form groups of three to five students. Create a brochure that helps explain the patient portal to a patient or family member. Consider the literacy level, understanding, knowledge, and prior experience of your patient population. Present your brochure to the class.

3. Go to Health on the Net (www.healthonnet.org/HONcode/Conduct.html). Review the HON code of conduct for health-related websites. Select a website or a health-related application and examine the content based on the HON principles. Select a website or application that does not currently have HON certification (can typically be seen at the bottom of the webpage by the HON Code symbol found on the website). What suggestions can you give to improve the website or application? Does the HON code work for applications as well as it works for websites? How would you evaluate the quality of health-related information on an application?

CRITICAL DISCUSSION POINTS

1. Consider a recent clinical experience. Describe how the data, information, knowledge, and wisdom framework were used in practice (e.g., technology supported

gathering and communicating data, transformed data to information, helped the nurse take the information and use knowledge in patient care, and how technology did or could help the nurse use wisdom when providing care).

2. Discuss the use of the EHR and the EMR when providing patient care. Explain how each might facilitate the delivery of safe patient care.

3. Patient portals are becoming mainstream for communicating with patients in the community setting. What are the benefits and drawbacks of using patient portals for nurses? For patients? For providers (e.g., physicians)?

4. Access the Why Not the Best website at www.whynotthebest.org. Compare two different hospitals on the key indicators provided. What do the data tell you about the outcomes from care provided in the selected area? Does the website provide a clear picture of patient-care outcomes? If yes, why? If no, what is missing?

▪▪▪ EXPLORING THE WEB

1. Visit the HealthIT Buzz Blog at www.healthit.gov/buzz-blog. This blog is run by the Office of the National Coordinator (ONC) of Health Information Technology. It contains blogs on the latest topics in health informatics. Follow the links to read three blogs. Be prepared to participate in a class discussion on these topics.

2. Visit the ONC's YouTube channel on www.youtube.com/user/HHSONC. Watch five videos about patients and their experiences with health information technology. Most videos are only 2 to 3 minutes long.

3. Prepare a list of five benefits that patients might experience as a result of the implementation of this health information technology. Draft a one-page, double-sided, trifold brochure that could be given to patients to educate them on the topic. Title the brochure "Health IT and You." Insert photos or graphics as you think appropriate.

▪▪▪ REFERENCES

Agency for Healthcare Research and Quality (AHRQ). (2016). *Clinical decision support*. Rockville, MD: Agency for Healthcare Research and Quality. Retrieved from http://www.ahrq.gov/professionals/prevention-chronic-care/decision/clinical/index.html

Agency for Healthcare Research and Quality, Patient Safety Network (AHRQ PSNet). (2017). *Computerized provider order entry*. Retrieved from https://psnet.ahrq.gov/primers/primer/6/computerized-provider-order-entry

Ajami, S., & Rajabzadeh, A. (2013). Radio frequency identification (RFID) technology and patient safety. *Journal of Research in Medical Sciences, 18*(9), 809–813.

American Nurses Association (ANA). (2015). *Nursing informatics: Scope and standards of practice* (2nd ed.). Silver Spring, MD: Author.

American Recovery and Reinvestment Act of 2009 (ARRA) (Pub. L. 111–5).

Anguita, M. (2012). Opportunities for nurse-led telehealth and telecare. *Nurse Prescribing, 10*(1), 6–8. doi:10.12968/npre.2012.10.1.6

Bass, D. (2011). Opting for opt out: How one HIE manages patient consent. *Journal of AHIMA, 8*(5), 34–36.

BinDihm, N. F., Hawkey, A., & Trevena, L. (2014). A systematic review of quality assessment methods for smartphone health apps. *Telemedicine and eHealth, 21*(2), 97–104. doi:10.1089/tmj.2014.0088

Centers for Medicare and Medicaid Services (CMS). (2008). *Medicare and Medicaid move aggressively to encourage greater patient safety in hospitals and reduce never events*. Retrieved from https://www.cms.gov/Newsroom/MediaReleaseDatabase/Press-releases/2008-Press-releases-items/2008-07-313.html

Centers for Medicare and Medicaid Services (CMS). (2011). *Eligible professional meaningful use table of contents core and menu set objectives.* Retrieved from https://www.cms.gov/EHRIncentivePrograms/Downloads/EP-MU-TOC.pdf

Centers for Medicare and Medicaid Services (CMS). (2012). *Electronic health records.* Retrieved from https://www.cms.gov/medicare/e-health/ehealthrecords/index.html

Centers for Medicare and Medicaid Services (CMS). (2016). *EHR incentive programs 2015 through 2017.* Retrieved from https://www.cms.gov/Regulations-and-Guidance/Legislation/EHRIncentivePrograms/Downloads/2016_PatientElectronicAccess.pdf

Committee on Quality of Health Care in America. (2001). *Crossing the quality chasm: A new health system for the 21st century.* Washington, DC: National Academy Press. Retrieved from http://books.nap.edu/openbook.php?record_id=10027&page=R1

Cronenwett, L., Sherwood, G., Barnsteiner J., Disch, J., Johnson, J., Mitchell, P., ... Warren, J. (2007). Quality and safety education for nurses. *Nursing Outlook, 55*(3), 122–131. doi:10.1016/j.outlook.2007.02.006

Dewsburys, G. (2012). Telehealth: The hospital in your home. *British Journal of Healthcare Assistants, 6*(7), 338–340. doi:10.12968/bjha.2012.6.7.338

Dick, R. S., & Steen, E. B. (Eds.). (1991). *The computer-based patient record.* Washington, DC: National Academies Press.

Griswold v. Connecticut, 381 U.S. 479. (1965).

Harrison, L. T. (2016). Nursing informatics: Safely managing smart pumps in the clinical setting. *Nurse Manager, 47*(6), 20–22. doi:10.1097/NAQ.0b013e31820fbdc0

Health & Human Services (HHS). (2017). *HITECH act enforcement interim final rule.* Retrieved from https://www.hhs.gov/hipaa/for-professionals/special-topics/HITECH-act-enforcement-interim-final-rule/index.html

Health Information Technology for Economic and Clinical Health Act (HITECH Act) (Pub. L. 111 5, div. A, title XIII, div. B, title IV, February 17, 2009, 123 Stat. 226, 467 [42 U.S.C. 300jj et seq.; 17901 et seq.]).

Health Insurance Portability and Accountability Act (HIPAA). (1996). (Pub. L. 104–191).

Health Resources Services Administration (HRSA). (2015). *Telehealth programs.* Retrieved from https://www.hrsa.gov/rural-health/telehealth/index.html

Healthcare Information Management and Systems Society (HIMSS). (2006). *Electronic medical records vs. electronic health records: Yes there is a difference.* Retrieved from http://www.himss.org/electronic-medical-records-vs-electronic-health-records-yes-there-difference-himss-analytics

Healthcare Information Management and Systems Society (HIMSS). (2017). *HIMSS dictionary of healthcare information technology terms, acronyms and organizations* (4th ed., p. 75). Boca Raton, FL: CRC Press.

HealthIT.gov. (2014). *Health information exchange (HIE).* Retrieved from https://www.healthit.gov/providers-professionals/health-information-exchange/what-hie

HealthIT.gov. (2015). *Meaningful use definition & objectives.* Retrieved from https://www.healthit.gov/providers-professionals/meaningful-use-definition-objectives

Institute of Medicine (IOM). (1997). *The computer based patient record: An essential technology for health care.* Retrieved from https://www.nap.edu/read/5306/chapter/1

Kenney, J. A., & Androwich, I. (2012). Nursing informatics roles, competencies, and skills. In D. McGonigle & K. G. Mastrian (Eds.), *Nursing informatics and the foundation of knowledge* (2nd ed., pp. 121–145). Burlington, MA: Jones & Bartlett Learning.

Koong, A. Y. L., Koot, D., Eng, S. K., Purani, A., Yusoff, A., Goh, C. C., ... Tan, N. C. (2015). When the phone rings: Factors influencing its impact on the experience of patients and healthcare workers during primary care consultation: a qualitative study. *BMC Family Practice, 15*(6), 1–8. doi:10.1186/s12875-015-0330-x

LaTour, K. M., & Maki, S. M. (Eds.). (2010). *Health information management concepts, principles and practice* (3rd ed.). Chicago, IL: American Health Information Management Association.

Lazzaro, A., Corona, A., Iezzi, L., Quaresima, S., Armisi, L., Piccolo, I., ... Di Lorenzo, N. (2017). Radiofrequency-based identification medical device: An evaluable solution for surgical sponge retrieval? *Surgical Innovation, 24*(3), 268–275. doi:10.1177/1553350617690608

National Heart, Lung, and Blood Institute. (2012). *What is an implantable cardioverter defibrillator?* Retrieved from http://www.nhlbi.nih.gov/health/health-topics/topics/icd

National Nanotechnology Initiative. (2012). *What it is and how it works*. Retrieved from http://www.nano.gov/nanotech-101/what

National Research Council. (2001). *Appendix A: Report of the technical panel on the state of quality to the quality of health care in America committee. Crossing the quality chasm: A new health system for the 21st century*. Washington, DC: The National Academies Press. Retrieved from http://www.nap.edu/openbook.php?record_id=10027&page=225

Patient Protection and Affordable Care Act (PPACA) of 2010 (Public Law 111–148).

Poon, E. G., Keohane, C. A., Yoon, C. S., Ditmore, M., Bane, A., Levtzion-Korach, O., … Gandhi, T. K. (2010). Effect of bar-code technology on the safety of medication administration. *The New England Journal of Medicine, 362*(18), 1698–1707. doi:10.1056/NEJMsa0907115

Rosen, I. (2008, March 16, 2008; updated August 22, 2008). *60 minutes*. New York, NY: CBS News.

Sharma, L. (2018). Evidence Summary. Medication Administration Errors: "Rights" of Administration. The Joanna Briggs Institute EBP Database, JBI10648.

Stephenson, N. (2016). Evidence summary. Medication safety: Smart infusion pumps. *The Joanna Briggs Institute EBP Database*, JBI15505.

Stoyanov, S. R., Hides, L., Kavanagh, D. J., Zelenko, O., Tjondronegoro, D., & Mani, M. (2015). Mobile app rating scale: A new tool for assessing the quality of health mobile apps. *JMIR mHealth and uHealth, 3*(1), e27. doi:10.2196/mhealth.3422

Technology Informatics Guiding Educational Reform (TIGER). (2012). Retrieved from http://www.himss.org/getinvolved/technology-informatics-guiding-education-reform-tiger-initiative

Totten, A. M., Womack, D. M., Eden, K. B., McDonagh, M. S., Griffin, J. C., Grusing, S., & Hersh, W. R. (2016, June). *Telehealth: Mapping the evidence for patient outcomes from systematic reviews* (Technical Briefs, No. 26) [Internet]. Rockville, MD: Agency for Healthcare Research and Quality. Retrieved from https://www.ncbi.nlm.nih.gov/books/NBK379320/

Turmell, J., Coke, L., Catinella, R., Hosford, T., & Majeski, A. (2017). Alarm fatigue: Use of an evidence-based alarm management strategy. *Journal of Nursing Care Quality, 32*(1), 47–54. doi:10.1097/NCQ.0000000000000223

SUGGESTED READING

Akridge, J. (2010). Carts roll with the flow of healthcare challenges. *Healthcare Purchasing News, 34*(8), 52–62. Retrieved from https://www.highbeam.com/doc/1G1-234312957.html

Bedouch, P., Allenet, B., Grass, A., Labarère, J., Brudieu, E., Bosson, J., & Calop, J. (2009). Drug-related problems in medical wards with a computerized physician order entry system. *Journal of Clinical Pharmacy & Therapeutics, 34*(2), 187–195. doi:10.1111/j.1365–2710.2008.00990.x

Chaffee, B., & Zimmerman, C. (2010). Developing and implementing clinical decision support for use in a computerized prescriber-order-entry system. *American Journal of Health-System Pharmacy, 67*(5), 391–400. doi:10.2146/ajhp090153

Flood, L., Gasiewicz, N., & Delpier, T. (2010). Integrating information literacy across a BSN curriculum. *Journal of Nursing Education, 49*(2), 101–104. doi:10.3928/01484834–20091023-01

Green, S., & Thomas, J. (2008). Interdisciplinary collaboration and the electronic medical record. *Pediatric Nursing, 34*(3), 225.

Headlines from the NLN. (2008). Informatics in the nursing curriculum: A national survey of nursing informatics requirements in nursing curricula. *Nursing Education Perspectives, 29*(5), 312–317.

Health & Human Services (HHS). (2013). *Summary of the HIPAA security rule*. Retrieved from https://www.hhs.gov/hipaa/for-professionals/security/laws-regulations/index.html

HealthIT.gov. (n.d.). *EHR incentives and certifications*. Retrieved from http://www.healthit.gov/providers-professionals/meaningful-use-definition-objectives

HealthIT.gov. (2013). *Policy, regulation and strategy: Clinical decision support*. Retrieved from https://www.healthit.gov/policy-researchers-implementers/clinical-decision-support-cds

McIntire, S., & Clark, T. (2009). Essential steps in super user education for ambulatory clinic nurses. *Urologic Nursing, 29*(5), 337–343.

Murphy, J. (2011). Nursing informatics: Engaging patients and families in eHealth. *Nursing Economics, 29*(6), 339–341.

Patient Protection and Affordable Care Act (PPACA) of 2010 (Public Law 111–148). Retrieved from https://www.gpo.gov/fdsys/pkg/PLAW-111publ148/pdf/PLAW-111publ148.pdf

Russo, M. (2008). eMAR and mobile computing: Why nursing homes need to get wired now. *Nursing Homes: Long Term Care Management, 57*(1), 32. Retrieved from https://www.iadvanceseniorcare.com/article/emar-and-mobile-computing-why-nursing-homes-need-get-wired-now

Schleyer, R., & Beaudry, S. (2009). Data to wisdom: Informatics in telephone triage nursing practice. *AAACN Viewpoint, 31*(5), 1. Retrieved from https://www.aaacn.org/sites/default/files/members/viewpoint/sepoct09.pdf

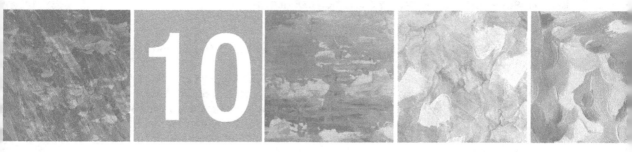

10

BASIC LITERATURE SEARCH STRATEGIES

Kimberly J. Whalen

For clinicians to get the answers they need to provide the best care to their patients, they must choose appropriate databases; design an appropriate search strategy using keyword, title, and subject headings; use limits; and successfully navigate in the databases they are searching. In addition, clinicians must consider the cost of *not* searching for the best evidence. Commitment to finding valid, reliable evidence is the foundation for developing the skills that foster a sound search strategy which, in turn, helps to reduce frustration and save time.

—(Melnyk and Fineout-Overholt, 2015)

Upon completion of this chapter, the reader should be able to

1. Describe the importance of developing basic literature search strategies when looking for the best available evidence.

2. Explain how research topics and questions are used to search the literature.

3. Explain how the patient/population, intervention, comparison, outcome, time (PICOT) model for structuring evidence-based practice clinical questions is used to search the literature.

4. Identify high-quality electronic databases and online resources for basic literature searches.

5. Identify high-quality patient-care information tools including point-of-care databases and practice guideline sources for basic literature searches.

6. Utilize keywords and subject headings in electronic databases and online resources.

7. Utilize Boolean Operators and other search techniques in electronic databases and online resources.

8. Develop broad literature search strategies.

9. Access high-quality evidence resources for lifelong learning.

Y ou are spending time on a surgical inpatient unit as one of your clinical rotation assignments. You observe that peripheral IV catheters are left in patients for 3 days prior to being changed. In a previous clinical rotation at a different organization, you recall that the policy for changing peripheral IV catheters was to change them every 4 days. You ask your preceptor about this as part of your efforts to better understand which organization has the safer practice. The preceptor appreciates your question and reports wondering the same thing. The preceptor comments that patients often dread having their IVs restarted on the third day when most of them are going home the next day. You and your preceptor decide to speak with your nurse manager about looking into the recommended practice for the timing for peripheral IV catheter changes. You review the literature and find that many studies report no increase in infection rates, infiltration risk, and so on, if an IV is changed every 96 hours instead of every 72 hours. You and your preceptor summarize key points from the literature, determine the expected cost savings from fewer IV replacements, and highlight the potential impact on patient satisfaction. You present your findings to the nursing practice committee. As a result, nursing practice is modified to reflect the best evidence for a safe experience for patients requiring peripheral IV catheters.

1. *What opportunities are there in nursing to ask questions about current practice?*
2. *What opportunities are there in nursing to facilitate dissemination of information?*
3. *What other nursing actions should you take when adopting practice changes like this?*

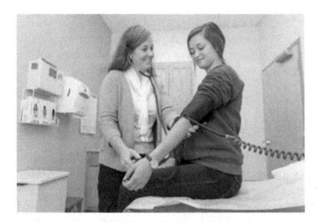

FIGURE 10.1 A nurse at work in a student health center.

Basic literature search strategies are used to search the literature for research and evidence that will improve patient care and fill knowledge gaps. High-quality literature searches are needed to ensure that the most up-to-date research and best available evidence are being used to shape patient care. Nurses and healthcare delivery institutions use research to shape practice and ensure that the care delivered is at the forefront in terms of safety and quality. "As evidence-based practice becomes more integrated into routine care, systematically searching of the literature is essential to making informed clinical decisions. To uncover all the evidence and get the most unbiased sense of what is known about a particular phenomenon or caregiving practice, a clear method of searching that is systematic is needed" (McGrath, Brown, & Samra, 2012). This highlights the need for nurses to have skills in basic literature search strategies.

This chapter discusses the importance of basic literature search strategies as they relate to nursing. How to form research questions and use a structured patient/population, intervention, comparison, outcome, time (PICOT) model for searching the literature is described. High-quality electronic databases, point-of-care databases, and practice guideline sources are explored. Search strategies including the use of keywords, subject headings, Boolean Operators, and other search techniques are described. Techniques and support for broad literature search strategies are identified. Finally, the chapter identifies literature search resources for lifelong learning.

BASIC LITERATURE SEARCH STRATEGIES

Healthcare practitioners use basic literature search strategies to answer a clinical question or explore a research question (Boss & Williams, 2014). Librarians and other experienced literature searchers approach the literature search process differently than novice or inexperienced searchers. Experienced searchers think about the

---

CRITICAL THINKING 10.1

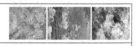

Using an internet search engine, search for a professional nursing organization that represents the clinical practice area you are interested in, for example, Emergency Nurses Association. Visit the professional organization's webpage to see what kind of literature they create, share, or publish.

1. What are some topics currently being discussed by the professional organization?
2. If the organization publishes a professional journal, what is the journal title?
3. How can research and information published by organizations like the one selected be useful to your practice?

---

topic of interest and plan their systematic search before beginning the literature search (Stillwell, Fineout-Overholt, Melnyk, & Williamson, 2010b). Nurses who follow a similar approach to the literature search process can decrease the time a literature search takes and increase the relevancy of search results.

DEVELOPING RESEARCH TOPICS AND QUESTIONS

According to Melnyk and Fineout-Overholt, the first step of the evidence-based practice (EBP) process is to cultivate and maintain a spirit of inquiry within the nursing profession. Nurses should be encouraged to demonstrate a spirit of inquiry by questioning what is known and not known about a topic of interest, clinical care, and unit-based or institutional practice. Nurses should start by reviewing the policies and practices related to patient-centered care within their organization. Gathering additional information through literature searches can help a nurse better understand the topic or research question. A preliminary research topic can be as simple as pain management in children. Research topics are used at the start of a literature search process. Once the searcher begins to understand an area of interest more, a research question is often developed. A preliminary research question developed from the pain management in children topic can be as simple as, "What are nonpharmacologic ways to manage postoperative pain in children?" Once the topic or question to be researched is identified, an experienced literature searcher would conduct a simple and broad preliminary literature search for published information using the most relevant words or phrases. This simple and preliminary literature search provides the searcher with a better understanding of the topic or question and provides a sense of the information available. After a review of the results, the literature searcher would refine the topic or question further, adjust the keywords or phrases used, rerun the search, review the results again, and repeat the process as often as necessary until the results are

EVIDENCE FROM THE LITERATURE

Citation

Baker-Rush, M. (2016). Reducing stress in infants: Kangaroo care. *International Journal of Childbirth Education*, *31*(4), 14–17.

Discussion

Evidence-based practice (EBP) involves either testing a new idea against existing practice or extending a proven EBP into real-world use. Research studies are one type of evidence used to inform EBP. The study of the care of preterm infants is a good example of how ongoing research and published studies can shape and inform patient-centered care.

Beginning in the 1970s, nurses in neonatal intensive care units (NICUs) began experimenting with what is sometimes called *kangaroo care*. Kangaroo care is a technique practiced on newborn, usually preterm, infants wherein the infant is held skin-to-skin with an adult. The NICU nurses explored whether there would be a positive difference in fragile preterm infants' conditions if there were skin-to-skin contact between parents and preterm infants.

Initial studies demonstrated improved social development (Kramer, Chamorro, Green, & Kundston, 1975), food intake, and weight gain (Rausch, 1981; White & Labarba, 1976) in neonates, all of which lead to decreased lengths of stay, resulting in significant cost savings for both families and institutions (Field et al., 1986). By 2002, research studies indicated that positive cognitive, perceptual, and motor development in the infant were attributed to kangaroo care (Feldman, Eidelman, Sirota, & Weller, 2002). Trials continue today to test variations of physiologic and developmental milestones (Scher et al., 2009) and have even extended the use of kangaroo care to help manage pain (Cong, Ludington-Hoe, & Walsh, 2011; Johnston et al., 2008). Forty years of developing, testing, and extending the evidence of the beneficial effects of kangaroo care is an example of EBP within NICU settings.

Implications for Practice

Investigating new and improved ways to care for different patient populations is what continues to elevate patient-centered care. As evidenced from the earlier example, this can start with a simple question and lead to years of research, knowledge generation, best practice dissemination, and evidence utilization in clinical practice. The culture of inquiry is important to the profession of nursing as it encourages bedside practitioners to consistently question the efficacy of their current practice. This inquiry leads to improvements in care and improvements in patient outcomes.

relevant. An experienced literature searcher would repeat this process with as many sources of information as appropriate for the topic, the question, and the needs of the research.

USING THE PICOT MODEL TO STRUCTURE QUESTIONS

A slightly more sophisticated way to inquire about a topic is to develop a clinical question using the PICOT (pronounced *peak-'at*) model. Use of the **PICOT** model is an effective way to systematically identify and retrieve nursing and healthcare published studies (Table 10.1); the "P" represents the patient or population of interest, "I" represents the intervention of interest, "C" represents the comparison of interest, "O" represents the desired outcome of interest, and "T" represents the amount of time the outcome will be observed. The PICOT model ensures that a literature search question remains organized and all aspects are addressed within the search strategy. An example of a PICOT question is, "Does treatment of patients with type 2 diabetes with weight loss surgery result in maintained weight loss of 20 pounds or more compared to traditional patient management with pharmaceuticals, diet, and exercise over a 2-year period of time?" The "T" representing time can be difficult to search with so it is often left out of the question and subsequently the search. When that occurs, the question model is called PICO (pronounced *peak-o*). Even without the "T" represented, the model helps to provide the structure to transition a question into a systematic literature search.

Generating Synonyms

While thinking about a topic or question of interest, or while developing a PICOT question, it can be helpful to think of related and relevant synonyms. A synonym for weight loss surgery could be gastric bypass surgery. A synonym for body weight could be body mass index (BMI). Creating a list of synonyms and related terms will help to locate information that uses any of the related terms within the literature. While this may broaden the search results it will also capture relevant literature that might have otherwise been missed. Keeping track of synonyms that work well and do not work well throughout the search process will help the searcher identify the proper term or terms to use.

TABLE 10.1 PICOT MODEL

(P) Patient/Population of interest	Answers the question, "who?"	Example: Patients with type 2 diabetes
(I) Intervention of interest	Answers the question, "what?"	Example: Weight loss surgery
(C) Comparison	Used to describe the intervention of interest	Example: Compared to management with pharmaceuticals, diet and exercise
(O) Outcome	Used to describe desired outcome	Example: Maintain weight loss of 20 pounds or more
(T) Time	Used to describe the amount of time the outcome will be observed	Example: Over 2 years

Sources: Developed with information from Stillwell, S. B., Fineout-Overholt, E., Melnyk, B. M., & Williamson, K. M. (2010a). Evidence-based practice, step by step: Asking the clinical question: A key step in evidence-based practice. *American Journal of Nursing, 110*(3), 58–61; Thomson, J. S., Currier, A., & Gillaspy, M. (2014). Basic literature search strategies. In P. Kelly, B. A. Vottero, & C. A. Christie-McAuliffe (Eds.), *Introduction to quality and safety education for nurses* (pp. 309–338). New York, NY: Springer Publishing.

Deciding Where to Search

After a topic's research question using PICOT or PICO has been drafted, the next step is to consider where the best sources of information are. Nursing information can be found within textbooks, book chapters, scholarly journals, trade publications, professional association reports, white papers, online publications, and so on. Textbooks, and many other sources, tend to take a long time to be published so the information is not always the most recent. Trade publications and many other sources tend not to be peer reviewed so the information contained has not always been evaluated by experts prior to publication. Since the nursing profession favors scholarly, peer-reviewed journal articles and professionally published information, this chapter focuses on selecting high-quality electronic databases and online tools.

There are a few electronic databases with professionally published literature that are free, but most require a subscription and fee. Due to cost, access to electronic databases is usually provided by large organizations such as universities, hospitals, and libraries, or through a resource website, such as a university library web page. An institutional login is often required. The cost of an electronic database varies greatly by institution. Cost is based on factors such as number of students (for a university) or beds (for a hospital) and the nature of the institution (community college, nursing school, medical school, etc.). Personal subscriptions to these types of electronic databases are not usually practical or even possible. Literature searchers may not have access to all electronic databases but access to even a few can make a significant difference to a literature search and clinical practice.

ELECTRONIC DATABASES FOR SEARCHING THE LITERATURE

There are two main types of electronic databases: bibliographic databases or indexes as they are often called and full-text databases. **Bibliographic databases** provide a basic record, or citation, for an article and often provide an abstract or brief summary of the article; they do not necessarily contain the complete text of the article itself. **MEDLINE** is the U.S. National Library of Medicine's (NLM's) bibliographic database, indexing thousands of journals in the fields of medicine, nursing, dentistry, veterinary medicine, healthcare systems, and the preclinical sciences. The Cumulative Index to Nursing and Allied Health Literature **(CINAHL)**, is another bibliographic database that indexes thousands of journals in the fields of nursing, biomedicine, alternative/complementary medicine, consumer health, and numerous allied health fields. CINAHL's name contains the word "index," which is a clue that not everything within the database is available in full text. Whether you will be able to access the full text of an item found in a bibliographic database depends on the institutional subscription. Bibliographic databases like MEDLINE and CINAHL are very important for EBP because they allow the user to search a wide range of relevant literature without limiting the results only to articles the user can access in full text.

Full-text databases provide the complete text of an article as well as the article citation. When using a full-text database, search results will still be presented in a list with basic information about each article, but unlike a bibliographic database, the user should be able to access the complete text of search results. Though MEDLINE and CINAHL are considered bibliographic databases, they are available via subscription to institutions with varying levels of full-text access. MEDLINE with Full Text and CINAHL Plus with Full Text are two of the levels of full-text access available for purchase by institutions.

The best type of database to use depends on the needs of the user. Involvement in a large-scale research study would require searching multiple bibliographic databases and full-text databases because it would be necessary to see all research relevant on the topic to create a good study design, to ensure that the idea in question has not already been studied, and to ensure that there are no major safety concerns. A student in need of one or two recent scholarly peer-reviewed articles about a topic might only need access to one or two full-text databases.

Depending on your institution, the bibliographic databases and full-text databases might be connected so citations and abstracts in a bibliographic database could be linked to the full text of an article available in another full-text database. Taking time to explore the databases and resources available through your library will ensure you are using the resources effectively. Taking time to email or meet with your librarian will ensure you are accessing all of the information available.

Access to Databases

Databases can be confusing. They can be bibliographic or full text. Most contain a combination of citations, abstracts, and full-text content. Some databases also provide free Internet access to content. The same database, CINAHL, CINAHL Plus, CINAHL Plus with Full Text, and so on, can be purchased with a differing amount of full-text content and can also be purchased from different companies including EBSCO and ProQuest. These differing levels of access and different providers can make accessing databases and accessing literature confusing.

MEDLINE is one of the most confusing databases of all. MEDLINE requires paid subscription access through companies including OVID and EBSCO. The MEDLINE search screen, search capabilities, and access to the full-text content of the more than 25 million citations varies by subscription. MEDLINE, MEDLINE Complete, and MEDLINE with Full Text can each be purchased. Most of the same citations contained within MEDLINE can also be accessed through PubMed (www.ncbi.nlm.nih.gov/pubmed). **PubMed** provides free Internet access to MEDLINE citations and abstracts, access to citations from journal articles not indexed within the MEDLINE database, citations from journals before the MEDLINE database began indexing the journal, articles from journals that submit their full text directly to PubMed Central, and citations for National Center for Biotechnology Information (NCBI) books. Though PubMed provides limited access to full-text articles, it is an excellent resource for those who do not have subscription access to electronic databases through their college, university, hospital, or organization.

Select Electronic Databases and Search Engines

Table 10.2 provides basic information about select electronic databases and search engines for literature searching. This is not intended to be an exhaustive list; rather, it is a snapshot of some of the resources available.

TABLE 10.2 SELECT ELECTRONIC DATABASES AND SEARCH ENGINES

ELECTRONIC DATABASES

CINAHL (www.ebscohost.com/nursing/products/cinahl-databases) is a bibliographic database that indexes the contents of nursing and allied health publications, including journals, dissertations, and other materials. While MEDLINE indexes content from a wide variety of medical, nursing, and scientific fields, CINAHL is more nursing-focused, making it essential for nursing literature searches.

The Cochrane Library (www.cochrane.org) is a collection of six databases including Cochrane Systematic Reviews, a full-text database of systematic reviews on a wide variety of clinical topics designed to help practitioners make healthcare decisions. Thousands of clinicians, researchers, providers, and consumers across the world have been adding to the library of evidence-based reviews since 1993.

JBI EBP Database (joannabriggs.org/) is similar to the Cochrane Library. The JBI EBP database provides systematic reviews, Best Practice Information Sheets, Evidence Summaries, and Evidence-Based Recommended Practices. The original focus of JBI was nursing; this emphasis remains but in recent years JBI has expanded to include evidence-based tools for medical and allied health researchers, clinicians, academics, quality managers, and consumers. The Institute began in 1996.

Embase (www.elsevier.com/online-tools/embase) is a bibliographic database indexing peer-reviewed literature in the biomedical and pharmaceutical sciences. Embase contains more than 1,800 journal titles not indexed by MEDLINE, Google, or Google Scholar.

MEDLINE (www.ovid.com/site/catalog/databases/901.jsp) is the U.S. NLM database of journal articles related to biomedicine. The NLM is a component of the National Institutes of Health. Literature from the life sciences and biomedicine dates back to 1809. PubMed is the NLM's free publicly available version of MEDLINE.

NCBI (www.ncbi.nlm.nih.gov/), a resource of biomedical literature from MEDLINE, life science journals, and online books.

PsycINFO (www.apa.org/pubs/databases/psycinfo/index.aspx) is a bibliographic database of peer-reviewed literature in the fields of mental health and the behavioral sciences from the American Psychological Association. Historical records and summaries date as far back as the 1600s with one of the highest DOI matching rates in the publishing industry. Journal coverage, which spans from the 1800s to the present, includes international material selected from periodicals in dozens of languages. References for books, book chapters, and dissertations are included along with journal article citations and full text.

PubMed (www.ncbi.nlm.nih.gov/pubmed/) is the the NLM's free publicly available version of MEDLINE. PubMed provides access to more than 25 million citations found within MEDLINE and in some cases links to the full text available for free from publishers or funding organizations.

SEARCH ENGINES

Google (www.google.com) is a general search engine. One should never feel bad about using it to find basic and preliminary knowledge about a topic or research question; search engines can provide quick access to general information. It is very important to avoid situations where a search engine is the only tool used during a literature search.

Google Scholar (scholar.google.com) is a separate Google search engine focused on retrieving scholarly literature. It is very important to avoid situations where a search engine is the only tool used during a literature search.

CINAHL, Cumulative Index to Nursing and Allied Health Literature; EBP, evidence-based practice; JBI, Joanna Briggs Institute; NCBI, National Center for Biotechnology Information; NLM, National Library of Medicine.

PATIENT-CARE INFORMATION TOOLS FOR SEARCHING THE LITERATURE

Most patient-care information tools are accessed online. Some are accessed at the bedside to provide immediate information for patient diagnosis, treatment, and procedure. Patient-care tools can be divided into two types, point-of-care databases (Table 10.3) and practice guidelines (Table 10.4). Both are similar in that they are designed to provide objective, evidence-based information to assist healthcare practitioners in clinical decision making. Like electronic databases, most point-of-care databases are only available by subscription. **Point-of-care databases** contain evidence summaries, literature reviews, and enhanced content such as pictures, videos, and patient education materials. Content from many point-of-care databases is accessible on handheld devices including smartphones and tablets. Point-of-care databases are designed to provide quick and accurate access to patient-centered care information. They include current summaries, reviews, pictures, videos, and so on, and are intended to be used at the bedside or during clinical decision making. Content is updated daily to ensure that practitioners are connected to the most recent evidence. Though access to point-of-care databases is beneficial, not all of them use the same processes to search, select, and appraise, nor do they describe their information in the same way, so literature searchers should be aware of the database's processes before use. Access to point-of-care databases is often funded by hospitals, medical centers, or physician practices, and some can be purchased as an individual subscription by a practitioner. Point-of-care databases are rarely available within college, university, or public libraries.

TABLE 10.3 SELECT POINT-OF-CARE DATABASES

Lippincott's Nursing Advisor (lippincottsolutions.com/solutions/advisor) is a point-of-care tool developed specifically for nursing; it includes drug information, patient education handouts, evidence-based care guidelines, and care plans.

Clinical Key for Nursing (www.clinicalkey.com/nursing/) is a point of care tool that connects nurses to clinically relevant information from books, journals, and practice guidelines.

DynaMed (www.dynamed.com/home/) is an evidence-based, point-of-care reference database for nurses, nurse practitioners, physicians, residents, and other healthcare professionals.

Essential Evidence Plus (www.essentialevidenceplus.com) is a point-of-care database that utilizes a unique evaluation criteria called POEMs—Patient-Oriented Evidence that Matters—to determine if the content is worthy of addition to the database.

UpToDate (www.uptodate.com) is designed primarily for healthcare practitioners; it is a point-of-care tool containing frequently updated information on hundreds of conditions and treatments and patient education materials.

TABLE 10.4 SELECT PRACTICE GUIDELINE TOOLS

U.S. National Library of Medicine, National Institutes of Health, PubMed	www.ncbi.nlm.nih.gov/pubmed
Guidelines International Network	www.g-i-n.net
Registered Nurses' Association of Ontario	www.rnao.ca/bpg

Select Practice Guidelines

Practice guidelines are summaries of information developed by practitioners, professional organizations, expert groups, and others who synthesize information about a clinical topic, procedure, or scenario and make recommendations for clinical practice. The full text of guidelines can often be found on professional organizations' websites or published within scholarly peer-reviewed journal articles.

Once the literature searcher selects the appropriate database or information sources to be searched, the next step in the process is to identify the keywords, phrases, or subject headings to be used in the search.

CRITICAL THINKING 10.2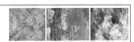

Go to nccih.nih.gov/health/providers/clinicalpractice.htm. Find a clinical practice guideline for a healthcare condition that you are interested in.

1. What is the title of the clinical practice guideline?
2. What patient-care recommendations mentioned in the clinical practice guideline have you seen within a clinical experience or in current practice?
3. Is the organization you selected an authoritative source within the profession?

LITERATURE SEARCHING WITH KEYWORDS AND SUBJECT HEADINGS

A literature search can be done with keywords and with subject headings. A **keyword** is a search term that uses your own personal natural language to search the literature. A **subject heading** is a search term or phrase that represents a concept used consistently in data organization and retrieval. Subject headings are part of a larger system of controlled vocabulary, one that is structured as a hierarchy with broad terms and narrow subtopic terms.

Keyword Searching

Keyword searching allows the searcher to enter any keywords or groups of keywords into an electronic database. The electronic database matches the words exactly as entered; it does not evaluate the usefulness or relevancy of the words to the focus of the literature search (Sherwill-Navarro, 2010). Through practice and patience, a literature searcher will become better at evaluating the relevancy of search results and determining if the keyword or keywords being used are appropriate.

Different electronic databases use different search screens and processes. In PubMed, for example, you would accomplish a keyword search by entering each of your keywords in the PubMed search bar. After each search, click on *Advanced*. Then, on the *Results* screen, scroll down to *History* and click *Add* to combine search results together. A keyword search done on June 1, 2017, within PubMed for *type 2 diabetes* retrieved 141,121 articles; then, a keyword search for *diet* retrieved 444,659 articles. When the searcher clicked on *Advanced* on the *Results* screen, scrolled down to *History*, and clicked on *Add* to combine the two search topics of *type 2 diabetes and diet* together, the combined search identified 19,061 articles.

Most electronic databases and online resources use similar techniques for phrase searching. **Phrase searching**, where a specific phrase is enclosed within quotes in the literature search box, for example, "gastric bypass surgery," is used to ensure that more than one word is found within the search results. For example, to find the exact phrase, *gastric bypass surgery*, the literature phrase searcher would enter "gastric bypass surgery" within the search box. To find the exact phrase *pressure ulcer*, the phrase searcher would enter "pressure ulcer" within the search box. The search from the previous paragraph was rerun on June 1, 2017, within PubMed using phrase searching. A phrase search for "type 2 diabetes" retrieved 93,392 articles; then a keyword search for *diet* retrieved 444,659 articles. When the phrase searcher clicked on *Advanced* on the *Results* screen, scrolled down to *History* and clicked on *Add* to combine the two search topics together, the combined search identified 13,469 articles. Almost 6,000 articles fewer were retrieved because phrase searching located the exact *type 2 diabetes* phrase. Phrase searching can help find fewer but more relevant search results.

Subject Headings/MeSH Subject Headings

Electronic literature databases usually employ a subject heading system. These systems attach an index term to information using a single, controlled vocabulary subject heading, regardless of the keywords or phrases used within the information written by the author. The NLM introduced subject headings back in the 1950s. **Medical subject headings (MeSH)**, is the current controlled vocabulary thesaurus of biomedical terms used to describe the subjects of each piece of literature in MEDLINE. MeSH contains approximately 28,000 subject heading descriptors and is updated regularly to reflect changes in medical terminology. MeSH subject headings are arranged hierarchically (Table 10.5) by subject categories with more specific subject headings arranged beneath broader subject headings. The MeSH hierarchy in its entirety is available at meshb.nlm.nih.gov/search.

Anyone who has used hashtags within social media tools including Twitter or Instagram has used subject headings. Hashtags categorize content within social media just like subject headings categorize content within electronic databases and Internet resources. When tagging a tweet with a photo taken while on a vacation, a user might tag it #vacation. The same hashtag, #vacation, is likely to have been used by others

TABLE 10.5 MESH SUBJECT HEADING STRUCTURE

Education
Education, Nonprofessional
  Health Education
    Consumer Health Information
    Health Education, Dental
    Health Fairs

to tag their tweets or photographs related to vacations. There may be other similar hashtags, such as #roadtrip or #springbreak, which further categorize the same tweet or photo. When you search for vacation tweets or photographs, a search for the #vacation hashtag will retrieve other items tagged with the same hashtag. Like hashtags, using subject headings makes searching more efficient and precise because it groups similar information together (Sherwill-Navarro, 2010). Because of the efficiency and precision in which subject headings search for similar information, it is important to learn how to search the literature using them.

MeSH headings are commonly used within nursing and medical databases. Many electronic databases make this hierarchy of subject headings clearly visible while searching, although the location of the hierarchy will vary from database to database. The MeSH hierarchy of headings is visible within MEDLINE, the Cochrane Library, and many other electronic databases and Internet resources. Other databases use a slightly different set of subject headings. CINAHL's subject heading structure, called CINAHL Headings, is a system of controlled vocabulary similar to MeSH. PsycINFO's information is indexed by a thesaurus developed by the American Psychological Association. It too is similar to MeSH.

Because of the controlled vocabulary and structure, a literature searcher wishing to find articles on *weight loss surgery* in an electronic database using a controlled subject heading vocabulary will not need to search with the keywords, *weight loss surgery, weight loss surgeries, gastric bypass,* and so on. Instead, the literature searcher can identify and search using the relevant subject heading in that database. In PubMed, the MeSH subject heading for *weight loss surgery* would be *bariatric surgery*. Specific categories within *bariatric surgery* include *gastric bypass, gastroplasty,* and *lipectomy*. Subheadings within *bariatric surgery* include *complications, economics, epidemiology, mortality, nursing, pharmacology,* and *therapy*. If the *complications* subheading is selected, literature that does not discuss complications will be eliminated from the search results. Subject heading searches identify relevant and focused literature while keyword searches tend to be broader and include less-relevant results (Anders & Evans, 2010).

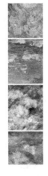

CASE STUDY 10.1

A nurse, a nutritionist, and a physical therapist have been caring for an overweight young adult patient with type 2 diabetes. They all are aware that type 2 diabetes is a widespread disease and traditional treatments often fail to provide adequate control. The patient has heard discussions on television about weight loss surgery providing better outcomes than traditional management with pharmaceuticals, diet, and exercise. The interprofessional team decides to conduct a literature search to find information related to the intervention options.

1. *How will exploring the evidence be useful to the patient? To the interprofessional team?*
2. *What keywords or MeSH terms could be used in the literature search?*
3. *How will literature results be shared with the patient?*

UTILIZING BOOLEAN OPERATORS AND OTHER SEARCH TECHNIQUES

Almost all electronic databases make use of Boolean logic to define relationships between relevant terms in literature searches. **Boolean Operators** are terms such as AND, OR, or NOT that are used to expand or limit literature search results. A literature search in an electronic database, using the words, *Weight Loss Surgery* AND *Type 2 Diabetes* makes use of the Boolean Operator AND. The specific attributes of the AND and OR Boolean Operators are frequently confused. The AND Boolean Operator means that all terms linked by the AND operator must be present in the literature to be included in the search results. When a search uses the AND operator, as in Figure 10.2, only the small amount of literature containing the words *Type 2 Diabetes* AND the words *Weight Loss Surgery* will be returned in the search results. When a search uses the OR operator, as in Figure 10.3, all literature containing either the words *Type 2 Diabetes* OR the words *Weight Loss Surgery* will be returned in the search results. The use of the OR Operator can, at times, return a large amount of results. The NOT Boolean Operator will eliminate all literature containing the term that follows the NOT operator from the literature search results, for example, *Type 2 Diabetes* OR *Weight Loss Surgery* NOT *Type 1 Diabetes*. Literature containing the words Type 2 Diabetes or Weight Loss Surgery will be returned, but literature containing the words Type 1 Diabetes will not be returned in the search results. Literature searchers should be cautious when using the NOT operator because it eliminates literature that contains terms regardless of their context. Inappropriate use of the NOT operator can eliminate relevant and useful literature. Table 10.6 contains examples of how Boolean Operators and search techniques can be applied within the CINAHL database.

Literature Search Limits

When using electronic databases, be sure to look for literature search limits. **Literature search limits** will edit search results to only include those search results that meet your limiting criteria, for example, articles published in the last 5 years. Literature searchers should include search limits later in the search process, not within the broad initial search (Sherwill-Navarro, 2010). Every database has slightly different search limits, but common search limits include the following:

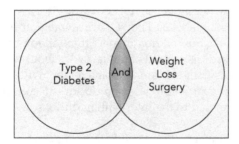

FIGURE 10.2 Using the *AND* Boolean Operator. Search results will include only literature that includes both phrases.

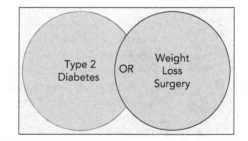

FIGURE 10.3 Using the *OR* Boolean Operator. Search results will include all literature that includes either phrase.

TABLE 10.6 BOOLEAN OPERATORS AND SEARCH TECHNIQUES

KEYWORDS/PHRASES	SEARCH RESULTS	END RESULT
weight loss AND type 2 diabetes	1,630	
"weight loss" AND "type 2 diabetes"	1,119	Quotes around phrases ensure the words in the phrase are found next to each other as an exact phrase.
"weight loss" OR "lose weight" AND "type 2 diabetes"	1,132	The *OR* Boolean Operator searches for both phrases within results.
"weight loss" OR "lose weight" AND "type 2 diabetes" NOT surgery	964	The *NOT* Boolean Operator excludes all results that include the word(s) after it.

- Limit results to English language publications. Note that larger electronic databases often index and provide full-text results in many languages.
- Limit results to scholarly peer-reviewed sources. Note that larger electronic databases often include scholarly and nonscholarly sources including newspaper articles and trade publications.
- Limit results by the date of publication, for example, current year, past 5 years, and so on.
- Limit results to the type of publication, for example, randomized controlled trials, literature reviews, meta-analyses, practice guidelines, and so on.

Even the most basic of literature search limits can lower the number of literature search results considerably. It is often best to start with basic literature search limits, for example, limit to English language and limit by publication date. Literature searchers should add more specific literature search limits as needed within subsequent searches.

REAL-WORLD INTERVIEW

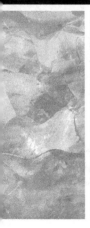

The more chances nurses have to practice their literature searching skills, the better they will get at it. A well-planned and executed literature search can be both sensitive and specific—sensitive enough to identify what is important and specific enough so results are targeted and not overwhelming. I wish all nurses were aware of how the Boolean Operators *AND* and *OR* work. Boolean Operators translate to most databases and Google so a basic understanding is useful. Identifying and using synonyms within a literature search is also important. Databases are not that smart and only search for exactly the keywords and phrases searched, so a good list of synonyms can often lead to finding the best evidence.

(continued)

REAL-WORLD INTERVIEW (*continued*)

New nurses might also not be aware of how librarians can collaborate with nurses, physicians, and clinical teams to improve patient-centered care. At our library, we have established a program called Evidence in Action Rounds. A librarian joins the interprofessional team to talk about a patient of interest. The next day, the librarian presents the evidence found and briefly demonstrates the literature search process. The patient-care team then utilizes the evidence in practice. Though this program only focuses on one patient at a time, the evidence found can impact patient care for many.

Stephanie J. Schulte, MLIS
Associate Professor and Head
Research and Education Services
Health Sciences Library
The Ohio State University
Columbus, Ohio

Other Literature Search Techniques

Other literature search techniques (Table 10.7) can improve the quality of literature search strategies and results. Literature searchers should be cautioned, however, that **truncation** and **wildcard symbols** can vary based on the database or tool. Inappropriately placed search techniques can result in poor results, so use the techniques wisely.

CRITICAL THINKING 10.3

You are a nurse on a rehab unit. You and a physical therapist from your interprofessional team notice that others, including physicians, other nurses, and other physical therapists, are not washing their hands as often as they should. You and your colleague think this is leading to an increase in infection rates and would like to determine the best ways to improve hand washing practices on your unit.

1. How can this research topic be modified into a question using the PICOT model?
2. What databases or online resources would you search for information?
3. What keywords or exact phrases would you use in a preliminary search of the literature?

Citation Chasing

Once a literature searcher finds a relevant piece of literature, it is wise to look through its references for other relevant literature that might otherwise have been overlooked. Look at the other article titles, journal titles, book chapter titles, books, and so on listed in the literature's references. Use the citation information provided within the references to locate the full text of the references of interest. This

TABLE 10.7 OTHER LITERATURE SEARCH TECHNIQUES

TECHNIQUE	SYMBOL EXAMPLE	END RESULT
Phrase searching	" "	Term for a literature search for exact phrases by putting quotation marks (" ") around a phrase, e.g., *pressure ulcer"*
Truncation	*	Term for a literature search for variations of the same word at one time, e.g., nurs* finds nurse, nurses and nursing
Wildcards	?	Term for a literature search for alternative spellings of the same word, e.g., behavio?r finds behavior or behaviour

process, called **citation chasing**, uses a citation or reference from one literature source to find the citation and then the full text for other relevant literature sources. Citation chasing helps ensure that valuable information is not missed during a literature search.

Hand Searching

Literature can be missed even after a sophisticated database search and citation chasing, which is why hand searching is a common practice for experienced searchers. **Hand searching** is the process of electronically or physically browsing a relevant journal cover-to-cover to locate literature. Most journal publishers have a website for each journal that describes the scope of the journal, its publication timeline, author submission criteria, subscription costs, and so on. These websites often provide an archive of journal issues and contents. Common headings to look for on a journal website would be *Archive* or *Previous Issues*. Then, click on or page through to the table of contents. Skim article titles, abstracts, and any full-text literature that appears relevant. Researchers conducting systematic reviews and other in-depth analyses regularly conduct a hand search of key journals for a period of years as part of their evidence-gathering process.

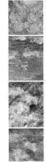

CASE STUDY 10.2

You are a nurse in a pediatrician's office with many newborn patients. Some new patients' parents are concerned about vaccinations causing harm to their children and are refusing to have their children vaccinated. The physician you work with has asked you to help find authoritative and current professional information about vaccinations so she can develop a vaccination policy for the office.

1. *What are two to three authoritative and professional information sources you would search for information?*
2. *What are one to two types of information sources you would not include in your search?*
3. *How will you share the results with your physician? And with the parents of the patients?*

DEVELOPING BROAD LITERATURE SEARCHES

When searching electronic databases for literature, especially when using databases that employ a controlled vocabulary such as subject headings, it is best to start your search broadly. An initial search that is broad helps to identify what literature is available on the topic before a search using every keyword, subject heading, and limiter is applied. A broad literature search helps gain an initial sense of how much published literature exists on the topic before the searcher begins to narrow results (Bartels, 2013). If you were working with a research question that, for example, had four keywords, it is often best to initially search for the one or two more core keywords to see how many relevant search results are returned. For example, if you are interested in finding evidence to indicate whether or not weight loss surgery is a more effective treatment option for type 2 diabetes compared to traditional treatments specifically with normal-weight or nonobese patients, it would be best to initially search an electronic database for the phrases "weight loss surgery" AND "type 2 diabetes." If a large enough data set is returned, add the additional phrase of "ideal body weight" OR "normal body weight." If the literature is abundant, add the additional phrase of "traditional treatment." If the initial phrases return a small set of literature, adding more phrases, and thus limiting your search further, will not be helpful. Table 10.8 illustrates a narrow PubMed search with limited results.

When searching with subject headings, it is beneficial to conduct an initial search with a broad subject heading, since more specific subtopics will automatically be included in the literature search. For example, in the MEDLINE electronic database, a literature search using the subject heading *bariatric surgery* will automatically include the subject heading *gastric bypass*, a specific type of bariatric surgery. It is also beneficial to search for information about each individual subject heading separately before combining search results. Adding more subject headings, keywords, phrases, and limiters to subsequent searches will refine and focus the results.

Checking for Usefulness and Relevancy

Once literature search results have been returned, they should be evaluated for usefulness and relevancy. A preliminary review of the article titles and abstracts will enhance the literature searcher's understanding of the topic. During the literature review, the searcher should consider whether the results are what the searcher needs to find. Are the results relevant to the patient population or clinical scenario or intervention of interest? Are results too broad? Too narrow? Are there enough results? Not enough? There is no exact number, or number range, of search results that tell the literature searcher when a search is accurate and appropriate. If a research topic or question is a popular topic that is researched and written about often, there will be much literature to find. If a research topic or question has not been researched or written about much, or if research was conducted many years ago, there might not be much literature to find. Through practice and patience, a literature searcher will become more knowledgeable about the research topic or question and therefore better at crafting an accurate literature search to identify relevant search results. If search results do not appear relevant, several strategies can help improve the search results:

- Check the subject headings used in the literature search. Are they too broad for what you are seeking? Too specific? Not relevant enough? It may be necessary to

TABLE 10.8 SEARCHING PUBMED WITH A NARROW SEARCH

QUESTION: IS AN INSULIN PUMP A GOOD CHOICE FOR A PATIENT WITH TYPE 2 DIABETES WHO IS HAVING PROBLEMS KEEPING BLOOD GLUCOSE UNDER CONTROL?

1. Start by brainstorming possible search terms for this topic, e.g.,
   - Insulin pump
   - Uncontrolled blood glucose
   - Type 2 diabetes
2. Identify electronic databases available for your literature search. Databases frequently chosen for nursing-related literature searching include the following:
   - CINAHL
   - MEDLINE
   - PubMed
3. Access the database and begin a preliminary search
   e.g., PubMed (www.ncbi.nlm.nih.gov/pubmed).
   Within PubMed, click the Advanced search link at the top of the database under the search box. Type your first keyword phrase, identified earlier in Step 1; e.g., type *"insulin pump."*
   Note that when a literature search for the phrase *"insulin pump"* was done on June 1, 2017, in PubMed, 1,730 items were found.
4. Type another phrase from Step 1 into the search box; e.g., type *"uncontrolled blood glucose."*
   Note that when a literature search for the phrase *"uncontrolled blood glucose"* was done on June 1, 2017, in PubMed, 44 items were found.
   Now within the History section, *Add to search builder* both searches and click *Search*. Note that when the search was combined on June 1, 2017, in PubMed, two items were found.
5. Limit your literature search further, as needed, by choosing filters from the left column of the PubMed search results page, e.g., choose the following:
   - *Free full text* within the *Text availability* section
   - *5 years* within *Publication dates* section
   Note that when these search limits were applied to the aforementioned literature search, one item was returned. This is a very small number of results so the literature searcher should go back to Step 3 and adjust the search terms used. The phrase *"uncontrolled blood glucose"* might not be the best way to describe the patient scenario. The searcher might need to go back to Step 1 and brainstorm new keywords or phrases. What other keywords should be tried? Perhaps *"blood glucose"* and *control*? Or *"glucose levels"* and *control*? What other keywords might work?
   Note that it often takes multiple adjustments to create an effective search. Do not give up along the way!

CINAHL, Cumulative Index to Nursing and Allied Health Literature.

Source: Developed with information from Thomson, J. S., Currier, A., & Gillaspy, M. (2014). Basic literature search strategies. In P. Kelly, B. A. Vottero, & C. A. Christie-McAuliffe (Eds.), *Introduction to quality and safety education for nurses* (pp. 309–338). New York, NY: Springer Publishing.

select additional subject headings or subheadings. For example, *glucose metabolism disorders* and *diabetes mellitus, lipoatrophic* are both subject headings that are related to *diabetes mellitus, type 2. Glucose metabolism disorders* is a broader MeSH subject heading than *diabetes mellitus, type 2. Diabetes mellitus, lipoatrophic* is a more specific MeSH subject heading than *diabetes mellitus, type 2. Drug therapy, diet therapy*, and *genetics* are all subheadings that can be used with the subject heading *diabetes mellitus, type 2.*

- If a few individual search results are relevant, but the overall set of search results do not seem relevant, examine the entire database entry for the relevant individual search results including subject headings and abstract, if available. Most databases that make use of subject headings show which subject headings were used to index the article within the database entry. Clicking the title of the article in the search results usually brings up the complete database entry with article details. Seeing how one highly relevant article is indexed can provide clues for improving a literature search. This technique is called pearl growing. **Pearl growing** examines the complete record of one highly relevant article to see which subject headings have been attached to it, thus identifying relevant subject headings to be used in subsequent literature searches.

- Remember that while searching with subject headings is preferable, some topics need to be searched with keywords, phrases, and synonyms. To find literature about family involvement in palliative care, a literature searcher will soon determine that there is no MeSH heading for family involvement, so searching for phrases including "family involvement" OR "family participation" OR "family-centered" OR "family presence" could be the best way to identify relevant articles.

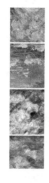

CASE STUDY 10.3

While conducting a basic literature search for information about whether cinnamon has an effect on glycemic levels in adults, you find that you do not have much recent information in your search results. So far, you have only searched one electronic database, CINAHL, using the keyword *cinnamon* and the exact phrase *"glycemic levels."* You have also been limiting search results to information published within the last year.

1. *What might be wrong with the initial search strategy?*
2. *How could you broaden the search using additional synonyms and Boolean Operators?*

Once the literature searcher is confident in the search results, accessing the full text is the next step. If the full text is not available within the institution's subscription, the searcher should see if full text is freely available within PubMed, Google Scholar, or elsewhere on the Internet. Due to funding from U.S. federal agencies and other grant makers, some published research literature must be made freely available to the public. If the full text is not accessible, the literature searcher should find out whether his or her institution participates in a shared resources system, most often called interlibrary loan. **Interlibrary loan** is a system through which institutions can share full-text literature with other institutions.

Library and Librarian Support

The most valuable resource for searching the literature for peer-reviewed and professional information is your institution's library and, specifically, the librarians (Eresuma & Lake, 2016). Check to see if your institution has an on-site or an online library. Speak to your librarian about your library's journals and electronic databases. Librarians within hospitals and healthcare centers often conduct literature searches for nurses, doctors, social workers, patients, patient family members, and other clinicians. If your institution does not have a library or reference librarian on-site, you may have

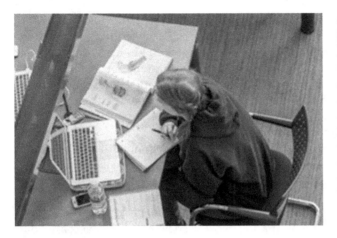

access to one from another location. Some organizations gain access to library services through a university or healthcare system affiliated with a school of nursing. Public libraries are also a viable option for stand-alone healthcare institutions that lack library resources. Healthcare questions are common at public libraries, so, many public librarians are well versed in healthcare electronic databases and how to conduct a literature search.

Figure 10.4. A nursing student studying.

Administrative and Computer Support

Administrative and computer support for literature searches is a resource that is increasingly necessary for working nursing professionals. Administrative support can take the form of making computers and library resources available or providing time away from patient care to access and examine the literature. Administrative support can provide funding for paid time away from the unit, mentorship, statistician support, or money to conduct original research studies. Often, scholarships through charitable boards or endowments are offered to those who aim to investigate and improve patient-centered care. Some of these scholarships and supports are offered for broad research interests, such as best practices, while others are offered to support certain patient populations, that is, patients with cancer, neonates, and so on. An important recommendation for novice nursing researchers is to seek a mentor who has the ability to coach a researcher through the research process and assist in securing funds, resources, or other necessary support. Mentors can also help navigate discussions about literature search results and change in practice recommendations with nurse managers and members of the interprofessional team.

Many healthcare organizations have a specific department or committee responsible for the advancement of nursing practice through research and EBP. Contact this department or committee to find out how it supports the access and use of literature for patient-centered care. Searching the literature requires access to a computer with Internet connectivity and access to electronic databases. Some electronic databases discussed in this chapter are free (e.g., PubMed at www.ncbi.nlm.nih.gov/pubmed) but most are only available through an institution with a subscription. Find out whether there are funds at your healthcare organization or elsewhere to support nurses interested in literature search efforts.

■■ RESOURCES FOR LIFELONG LEARNING

Learning how to search for literature within electronic databases and online tools can be difficult (Table 10.8). Online tutorials, videos, and webinars developed by the companies that sell electronic databases can help to improve search skills and strategies. PubMed's *PubMed for Nurses* tutorial can be completed in 30 minutes (www.

nlm.nih.gov/bsd/disted/nurses/cover.html). EBSCO Information Services has a YouTube channel of database videos and search guides (www.youtube.com/user/ebscopublishing). All of these tools and tutorials can keep nurses up to date on basic literature search skills, databases, and patient-care information tools.

Another way to keep up to date is through database features that save literature searches and provide email alerts of new information that meet the search criteria. PubMed has a free self-registration feature called My NCBI. My NCBI allows a literature searcher to save complex search strategies with limits and will automatically run the searches at a later time. The service sends an email with new results to the literature searcher on a predetermined schedule. Literature searches are saved on the NLM servers, not on a specific computer, so they can be accessed anywhere with Internet access. CINAHL and PsycINFO via the EBSCO platform, MEDLINE via the OVID platform, and most databases on the ProQuest platform also allows literature searchers to create an account and save searches that can be accessed and rerun on demand.

Another way to keep up to date is through email alert services offered through professional organizations or information providers. Examples include the following:

- The American Nurses Association (ANA) offers ANA SmartBrief, a regular news update service that is free to nonmembers. Sign up at www.smartbrief.com/ana.
- Medscape offers medical news, journal articles, and expert perspective news updates for free. Register at www.medscape.com/nurses.

Taking advantage of free training resources, features that save a search within electronic databases, and e-mail alert services can make it easy to stay current on topics of interest with a minimum of time and effort (Sherwill-Navarro, 2010).

KEY CONCEPTS

1. Developing a good research question is necessary to ensure a clear, purposeful research direction.
2. Basic literature search strategies are used to search electronic literature databases for healthcare literature using keywords and subject headings.
3. While searching with subject headings is preferable, some literature search topics are better searched with keywords in one's own natural language.
4. Using Boolean Operators, synonyms, and search techniques such as truncation and phrase searching can help identify important content in electronic literature databases.
5. Once literature has been retrieved from relevant electronic databases, it must be evaluated to determine how useful and relevant it is to the situation to which it will be applied.
6. The PICOT model for searching the literature helps organize a search and ensure that all aspects of the research question are addressed.
7. There are several high-quality electronic databases for searching scholarly peer-reviewed professional journals and professionally published information sources.

8. If available, patient-care information tools, for example, point-of-care databases and practice guidelines, should be searched within basic literature searches.
9. It is often better to first approach a literature search broadly and then narrow the search after the initial literature search results are returned.
10. Lifelong learning can be facilitated with the use of resources on the Internet.

KEY TERMS

Bibliographic databases
Boolean Operators
CINAHL
Citation chasing
Full-text databases
Hand searching
Interlibrary loan
Keyword
MeSH
MEDLINE

Pearl growing
Phrase searching
PICOT and PICO
Practice guidelines
PubMed
Search limits
Subject heading
Truncation
Wildcards

REVIEW QUESTIONS

1. Which of these literature search strategies includes a Boolean Operator? Select all that apply.

   A. Safety NOT security
   B. Ginger OR cinnamon
   C. Communicat*
   D. Stroke AND heart attack
   E. "Glucose levels"

2. From past clinical experiences, a nurse has noticed that postoperative patients who ambulate early require less pain medication. The nurse would like to initiate an ambulation protocol on the unit. What should the nurse's first action be?

   A. Meet with physicians to have them add early ambulation to the postoperative order set.
   B. Encourage colleagues to integrate early ambulation into their patients' postoperative care.
   C. Perform a literature search to see if there is evidence to validate the efficacy of early ambulation of postoperative patients to control pain.
   D. Suggest a pilot study that compares current practice to early ambulation.

3. After working with a few adult patients recently diagnosed with high cholesterol, the nurse notices that patients who grow herbs are more likely to manage their cholesterol without medication than patients who do not grow their own herbs. The nurse wonders if encouraging herb gardening is an intervention recommended in the literature. Which statements are accurate? Select all that apply.

   A. It is only necessary to search for literature with one Internet search engine, since most search engines cover everything available on the Internet.

B. Not all published research can be found with an Internet search engine.

C. In order to find the greatest amount of literature, it is necessary to consult more than one bibliographic database, full-text database, or patient-care information tool including the Joanna Briggs Institute, the Cochrane Library, MEDLINE with Full Text, Cumulative Index to Nursing and Allied Health Literature (CINAHL) Plus with Full Text, PubMed, UptoDate, and National Guideline Clearinghouse (NGC).

D. It is only necessary to search for literature within one bibliographic database like PubMed, MEDLINE, or CINAHL, since most bibliographic databases include research relevant to every topic.

E. Nurses should not question what is known or not known about an intervention.

4. A novice nurse researcher seeks to better understand the potential implications of a different wound dressing technique on postsurgical healing. A research mentor is assisting the nurse in developing a patient/population, intervention, comparison, outcome, time (PICOT) question. Which question best demonstrates the PICOT model?

A. For postprocedural patients, does dressing the flap with a moist bandage, rather than a dry bandage, decrease healing time?

B. For patients who have undergone a flap procedure following a single mastectomy, does dressing the flap with a moist bandage, rather than a dry bandage, decrease healing time over a 7-day period?

C. Does dressing a surgical site with a moist bandage, rather than a dry bandage, decrease healing time?

D. For patients who have undergone a flap procedure following a single mastectomy, does dressing the flap with a moist bandage decrease healing time?

5. The Chief Nursing Officer at your hospital has asked you to participate on a research team that will investigate the most effective models for assigning patients to the nursing staff for care. A member of the team suggests performing a literature search to see if any previous research has been done on models that base patient assignments on patient location instead of patient acuity. Why is this literature search important?

A. Searching the literature could help provide methods for the research study design, help avoid duplicating previous research, and identify patient assignment models to study further.

B. A literature search can help protect against legal liability in the event of a patient-care accident, even if no further action is taken.

C. A literature search can eliminate the need to conduct original research since patient-care models will be described within the research results.

D. A literature search would not be important in this scenario.

6. The interprofessional team on a general medical–surgical floor is interested in improving the outcomes of patients who have a tracheostomy. The first step would be which of the following?

A. Review your hospital's current policy and practice for how best to care for patients with a tracheostomy.

B. Review available literature for best practices.

C. Solicit the thoughts and opinions of experts around you.

D. Implement a best practice highlighted in a medical–surgical nursing journal.

7. Before conducting a literature search in Medline, PubMed, or CINAHL, it is important to remember which of the following?

   A. In most cases, the best search results will be returned if you search using multiple keywords, exact phrases, subject headings, and limiters all together in your initial search.
   B. In most cases, it is preferable to search using the electronic database's system of controlled vocabulary subject headings.
   C. In most cases, the best search results will be returned if you search an electronic database with one keyword.
   D. In most cases, the best search results will be returned if you search an electronic database with one specific phrase.

8. You are searching for evidence in an electronic database and notice that it makes use of a system of controlled vocabulary. Because of this, it is usually best to do which of the following?

   A. Combine all search terms on the same search command line, as one normally would with an Internet search engine.
   B. Disregard the system of controlled vocabulary and search using your natural language of keywords.
   C. When the database allows it, break your search question down into separate subject headings and search for each subject heading separately before combining search results.
   D. Maximize results by searching using many subject headings in the initial search.

9. Members of a nursing unit are planning to search the literature but their research question is very broad and involves many concepts. Searches of this type are best approached in which of the following ways? Select all that apply.

   A. To maximize results, search for all concepts together within the initial search.
   B. Initially search for one or two core concepts and add more specific concepts, keywords, subject headings, and limiters in subsequent searches.
   C. Search only for the initial keywords identified by the nursing team. No other keywords, synonyms, subject headings, or limiters will be needed for the literature search.
   D. Work with the nursing team to create a PICO or PICOT question based on the research question. The structured model will help organize the literature search question and make sure that all the important concepts are addressed within the search strategy.
   E. Simplify the research question. Simple initial questions and simple initial searches can help the team begin to understand the research available in the area of interest. A more specific question can be developed later.

10. You are working with a principal investigator on a large-scale study to improve how frequently used nursing supplies and equipment are ordered and stored throughout your organization. You have been asked to conduct a literature search to look for scholarly peer-reviewed journal articles discussing best practices. What source of information will best serve your needs?

    A. Bibliographic databases
    B. Bibliographic and full-text databases

C. Full-text databases

D. The Internet

E. A collection of relevant print journals

REVIEW ACTIVITIES

1. Some literature searches work better with subject headings than with keywords and exact phrases. For example, try to find evidence to support the use of aspirin with patients who have had a heart attack. Try searching this topic using PubMed (www.PubMed.gov). Type *"myocardial infarction" AND aspirin* into the search bar at the top of your computer screen. See how many results you get. Assess the usefulness and relevancy of those results. Then click the medical subject headings (MeSH) link found in the drop-down box under PubMed, just left of the main search box. Instead of typing both terms together with the Boolean Operator *AND* in between, type one term at a time, search for it, select the best match from the MeSH results on the left side of the screen, click the link *Add to search builder* on the screen, and repeat the process until you are ready to click the *Search PubMed* button to run the search. Assess the usefulness and relevancy of the results returned from the MeSH search. What did you find? Which of the searches yielded more relevant and useful results?

2. You are working with the nurse manager. She is looking for research on the ideal patient-to-staff ratio for night shift charge nurses who practice in a neonatal intensive care unit (NICU). In this situation, it is probably best to start by looking for research evidence with the phrases *"patient-to-staff ratio" AND "intensive care."* Once you see the number, quality, and relevancy of the search results returned, adjust the search using additional synonyms, keywords, exact phrases, and truncation symbols including *"staff ratio*," staffing, "charge nurs*," "night shift*," "neonatal intensive care,"* or *NICU*. Try the search in Cumulative Index to Nursing and Allied Health Literature (CINAHL) and/or PubMed. How many results were you able to find in each database? Adjust the search as appropriate. Which keywords, phrases, MeSH, or CINAHL subject headings used identified the most relevant evidence?

CRITICAL DISCUSSION POINTS

1. How does the culture of the clinical environment affect a nurse's spirit of inquiry? How does it affect a nurse's ability to question current nursing practice?

2. What resources are needed for direct care nurses to regularly be able to engage in basic literature search activities?

3. Consider all the different kinds of information sources available including books, magazines, newspapers, websites, videos, and so on. Why do you think the nursing profession focuses so much attention on information published within scholarly peer-reviewed professional journals and electronic databases?

4. During your last clinical experience, did you see any nurses or members of the interprofessional team using information to guide their patient-centered care? What databases or tools did the information come from?

5. How are point-of-care databases different from bibliographic and full-text databases?

6. How are practice guideline sources different from bibliographic and full-text databases?
7. After you complete your nursing degree, how do you plan to keep up to date on patient-centered care practices?

QSEN ACTIVITY

1. Explore the Professional Organizations information listed on the QSEN site, qsen.org/faculty-resources/organizations. Name one organization listed that you would consider an authoritative source for nursing information. Do any of the organizations publish professional journals, point-of-care databases, or practice guidelines?
2. The Quality and Safety Education for Nurses (QSEN) competency for evidence-based practice (EBP) is defined as "Integrate best current evidence with clinical expertise and patient/family preferences and values for delivery of optimal health-care." Go to the QSEN competencies page at qsen.org/competencies/pre-licensure-ksas/ and find the knowledge, skills, and attitudes targets for the EBP competency. What is one knowledge target that relates to this chapter? One skills target that relates to this chapter? One attitudes target that relates to this chapter?

EXPLORING THE WEB

1. Review the *Picking a PICO* guide for nursing from Southern Illinois University Edwardsville library (libguides.siue.edu/c.php?g=333872&p=2244149). Use the templates to practice creating PICO and patient/population, intervention, comparison, outcome, time (PICOT) questions of interest.
2. Compare the various Cumulative Index to Nursing and Allied Health Literature (CINAHL) database subscriptions including CINAHL Complete, CINAHL Plus, and CINAHL with Full Text available from EBSCO Information Services (health.ebsco.com/products/the-cinahl-database). Which of the subscriptions, if any, are available at your institution?
3. Review the medical subject headings (MeSH) database tutorial from PubMed (www.nlm.nih.gov/bsd/disted/pubmedtutorial/020_490.html). Practice identifying and using MeSH within a search in PubMed.

REFERENCES

Anders, M. E., & Evans, D. P. (2010). Comparison of PubMed and Google scholar literature searches. *Respiratory Care, 55*(5), 578–583.

Baker-Rush, M. (2016). Reducing stress in infants: Kangaroo care. *International Journal of Child-birth Education, 31*(4), 14–17.

Bartels, E. M. (2013). How to perform a systematic search. *Best Practice & Research Clinical Rheumatology, 27*(2), 295–306. doi:10.1016/j.berh.2013.02.001

Boss, C. M., & Williams, B. (2014). Conducting a literature search and review. In Hedges C. & Williams B. (Eds.), *Anatomy of research for nurses* (pp. 97–109). Indianapolis, IN: Sigma Theta Tau International.

Cong, X., Ludington-Hoe, S. M., & Walsh, S. (2011). Randomized crossover trial of kangaroo care to reduce biobehavioral pain responses in preterm infants: A pilot study. *Biological Research for Nursing, 13*(2), 204–216. doi:10.1177/1099800410385839

Eresuma, E., & Lake, E. (2016). How do I find the evidence? Find your librarian—STAT! *Orthopaedic Nursing, 35*(6), 421–423. doi:10.1097/NOR.0000000000000299

Feldman, R., Eidelman, A. I., Sirota, L., & Weller, A. (2002). Comparison of skin-to-skin (kangaroo) and traditional care: Parenting outcomes and preterm infant development. *Pediatrics, 110*(1 pt. 1), 16–26. doi:10.1542/peds.110.1.16

Field, T. M., Schanberg, S. M., Scafidi, C. R., Bauer, C. R., Vega-Lahr, N., Garcia, R., … Kuhn, C. M. (1986). Tactile/kinesthetic stimulation effects on preterm neonates. *Pediatrics, 77*(5), 654–658.

Johnston, C. C., Filion, F., Campbell-Yeo, M., Goulet, C., Bell, L., McNaughton, K., … Walker, C. (2008). Kangaroo mother care diminishes pain from heel lance in very preterm neonates: A crossover trial. *BMC Pediatrics, 8*(13). Retrieved from https://bmcpediatr.biomedcentral.com/articles/10.1186/1471-2431-8-13

Kramer, M., Chamorro, I., Green, D., & Kundston, F. (1975). Extra tactile stimulation of the premature infant. *Nursing Research, 24*(5), 324–334.

McGrath, J. M., Brown, R. E., & Samra, H. A. (2012). Before you search the literature: How to prepare and get the most out of citation databases. *Newborn & Infant Nursing Reviews, 12*(3), 162–170. doi:10.1053/j.nainr.2012.06.003

Melnyk, B., & Fineout-Overholt, E. (2015). *Evidence-based practice in nursing & healthcare* (3rd ed.). Philadelphia, PA: Lippincott Williams and Wilkins.

Rausch, P. B. (1981). Effects of tactile and kinesthetic stimulation on premature infants. *JOGN Nursing, Journal of Obstetric, Gynecologic, and Neonatal Nursing, 10*(1), 34–37.

Scher, M. S., Ludington-Hoe, S., Kaffashi, F., Johnson, M. W., Holditch-Davis, D., & Loparo, K. A. (2009). Neurophysiologic assessment of brain maturation after an 8-week trial of skin-to-skin contact on preterm infants. *Clinical Neurophysiology, 120*(10), 1812–1818. doi:10.1016/j.clinph.2009.08.004

Sherwill-Navarro, P. (2010). Information and life-long learning. In Polifko K. A. (Ed.), *The practice environment of nursing* (pp. 329–356). Clifton Park, NY: Delmar Cengage Learning.

Stillwell, S. B., Fineout-Overholt, E., Melnyk, B. M., & Williamson, K. M. (2010a). Evidence-based practice, step by step: Asking the clinical question: A key step in evidence-based practice. *American Journal of Nursing, 110*(3), 58–61. doi:10.1097/01.NAJ.0000368959.11129.79

Stillwell, S. B., Fineout-Overholt, E., Melnyk, B. M., & Williamson, K. M. (2010b). Evidence-based practice, step by step: Searching for the evidence. *American Journal of Nursing, 110*(5), 41–47. doi:10.1097/01.NAJ.0000372071.24134.7e

Thomson, J. S., Currier, A., & Gillaspy, M. (2014). Basic literature search strategies. In Kelly, P. Vottero, B. A. & Christie-McAuliffe C. A. (Eds.), *Introduction to quality and safety education for nurses* (pp. 309–338). New York, NY: Springer Publishing.

White, J. L., & Labarba, R. C. (1976). The effect of tactile and kinesthetic stimulation on neonatal development in the premature infant. *Developmental Psychobiology, 9*(6), 569–577.

SUGGESTED READINGS

Baumann, N. (2016). How to use the medical subject headings (MeSH). *International Journal of Clinical Practice, 70*(2), 171–174. doi:10.1111/ijcp.12767

Brusco, J. M. (2010). Effectively conducting an advanced literature search. *AORN Journal, 92*(3), 264–271. doi:10.1016/j.aorn.2010.06.008

Coughlan, M., Cronin, P., & Ryan, F. (2013). Selecting a review topic and searching the literature. *Doing a literature review in nursing, health and social care* (pp. 48–61). Thousand Oaks, CA: SAGE.

Facchiano, L., & Snyder, C. H. (2012). Evidence-based practice for the busy nurse practitioner: Part two: Searching for the best evidence to clinical inquiries. *Journal of the American Academy of Nurse Practitioners, 24*(11), 640–648. doi:10.1111/j.1745-7599.2012.00749.x

Fineout-Overholt, E., Melnyk, B. M., Stillwell, S. B., & Williamson, K. M. (2010a). Evidence-based practice, step by step: Critical appraisal of the evidence: Part I. *American Journal of Nursing, 110*(7), 47–52. doi:10.1097/01.NAJ.0000383935.22721.9c

Fineout-Overholt, E., Melnyk, B. M., Stillwell, S. B., & Williamson, K. M. (2010b). Evidence-based practice, step by step: Critical appraisal of the evidence: Part II. Digging deeper—Examining the "keeper" studies. *American Journal of Nursing*, *110*(9), 41–48. doi:10.1097/01.NAJ.0000388264.49427.f9

Fineout-Overholt, E., Melnyk, B. M., Stillwell, S. B., & Williamson, K. M. (2010c). Evidence-based practice, step by step: Critical appraisal of the evidence: Part III. *American Journal of Nursing*, *110*(11), 43–51. doi:10.1097/01.NAJ.0000390523.99066.b5

Finfgeld-Connett, D., & Johnson, E. D. (2013). Literature search strategies for conducting knowledge-building and theory-generating qualitative systematic reviews. *Journal of Advanced Nursing*, *69*(1), 194–204. doi:10.1111/j.1365-2648.2012.06037

Joseph, T., Saipradeep, V. G., Raghavan, G. S., Srinivasan, R., Rao, A., Kotte, S., & Sivadasan, N. (2012). TPX: Biomedical literature search made easy. *Bioinformation*, *8*(12), 578–580. doi:10.6026/97320630008578

Melnyk, B., Fineout-Overholt, E., Stillwell, S., & Williamson, K. (2010). Evidence-based practice: Step by step. The seven steps of evidence-based practice: Following this progressive, sequential approach will lead to improved health care and patient outcomes. *American Journal of Nursing*, *110*(1), 51–53. doi:10.1097/01.NAJ.0000366056.06605.d2

Nourbakhsh, E., Nugent, R., Wang, H., Cevik, C., & Nugent, K. (2012). Medical literature searches: A comparison of PubMed and Google scholar. *Health Information and Libraries Journal*, *29*(3), 214–222. doi:10.1111/j.1471-1842.2012.00992.x

Riesenberg, L. A., & Justice, E. M. (2014). Conducting a successful systematic review of the literature, part 1. *Nursing*, *44*(4), 13–17. doi:10.1097/01.NURSE.0000444728.68018.ac

Smith, M. L., & Shurtz, S. (2012). Search and ye shall find: Practical literature review techniques for health educators. *Health Promotion Practice*, *13*(5), 666–669. doi:10.1177/1524839911432930

Young, S., & Duffull, S. B. (2011). A learning-based approach for performing an in-depth literature search using MEDLINE. *Journal of Clinical Pharmacy and Therapeutics*, *36*(4), 504–512. doi:10.1111/j.1365-2710.2010.01204.x

Younger, P. (2010). Using Google scholar to conduct a literature search. *Nursing Standard*, *24*(45), 40–46, 48. doi:10.7748/ns2010.07.24.45.40.c7906

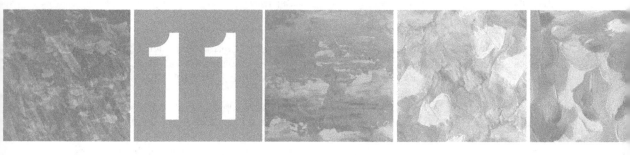

11

EVIDENCE-BASED PRACTICE

Beth A. Vottero

As more knowledge is generated through research, and as the ability to transmit information via such media as the Internet or direct broadcast increases, all professionals in all fields will come under increasing pressure to show that they are abreast of current knowledge, and that they exhibit this through delivering services that are in line with the most recent and rigorous evidence.

Alan Pearson, 2014

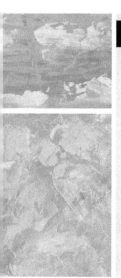

At the completion of this chapter, the reader should be able to

1. Define evidence-based practice (EBP).
2. Explain what is meant by "best available evidence."
3. Describe the significance of a hierarchy of types of evidence that inform an EBP project.
4. Appraise the quality of evidence using appropriate appraisal tools.
5. Explore how clinical expertise is determined.
6. Explain the significance of including patient preferences for EBP.
7. Describe the models and frameworks for EBP.
8. Examine the nurse's role in EBP.
9. Discuss tools for implementing evidence into practice.

At the quarterly nursing practice committee meeting, the nursing research facilitator asks what issues you as a clinician have been concerned about. You think of the recent increase in urinary tract infections (UTI) that you have observed on the surgical unit. You know that as per the Centers for Medicare and Medicaid Services (CMS), there will be no reimbursement for any hospital-acquired UTIs. You wonder if the current standard of practice on the surgical unit regarding care of patients with indwelling catheters is based on best practices. You wonder what the evidence is to support these practices. Is it best practice? How would you find out? What would you do if there were a difference between your organization's practice and the evidence?

In 2011, the Institute of Medicine (IOM) set a target: *"By the year 2020, 90 percent of clinical decisions will be supported by accurate, timely, and up-to-date clinical information, and will reflect the best available evidence"* (IOM, 2011). This prompted all healthcare professionals and healthcare institutions to set a goal to use the best available evidence throughout the healthcare delivery process. This is a lofty goal that requires healthcare workers to develop skills for EBP and knowledge about the steps in the process. These steps include the following:

- *Identifying a clinical problem*
- *Asking a searchable question based on a clinical problem*
- *Searching the literature for the best available evidence*
- *Appraising the quality of the evidence*
- *Determining the level of the evidence based on a hierarchy*
- *Synthesizing the best available evidence into guidance for clinical practice*
- *Implementing the best available evidence into healthcare practice*
- *Evaluating the outcomes from the change*
- *Sustaining the change*

This chapter defines and explores the processes involved in EBP as it relates to bedside nursing practice. This chapter uses a pragmatic approach to explore models that guide EBP and models for implementing evidence into practice for nursing. The role of nurses in EBP projects is detailed. The chapter also explores tools for appraising the quality of the evidence and hierarchies that identify the level of evidence types. Finally, logical descriptions of models that guide implementing evidence into practice are described.

▮▮▮ DEFINING EVIDENCE-BASED PRACTICE

Over the past three decades, the science of nursing has evolved into a research-based practice. While nursing has always been based on research, the introduction of evidence-based practice (EBP) has revolutionized the science aspect of nursing. The first definition of **EBP** was "... integrating individual clinical expertise with the best available external clinical evidence from systematic research" (Sackett, Rosenberg, Muir-Gray, Haynes, & Richardson, 1996, p. 971). The Quality and Safety Education for Nurses (QSEN) initiative has a mission defined as: "The QSEN Institute is a collaborative of healthcare professionals focused on education, practice, and scholarship to improve the quality and safety of healthcare systems" (www.qsen.org/about-qsen/). The QSEN initiative adapted the definition to include best available evidence and patient engagement, defining EBP as "... the delivery of optimal healthcare through the integration of best current evidence, clinical expertise and patient/family values" (QSEN, 2012).

At first glance, EBP does not appear to be complicated. It is when the definition is deconstructed and examined that the complexity becomes apparent. One begins to see how each part contributes to the bigger picture. Best available evidence, clinical expertise, and patient preferences all affect the way evidence is used to make clinical decisions about patient care (Figure 11.1). The busy bedside nurse cannot possibly research the evidence on every clinical problem, nor can the nurse always access the best available evidence. This creates a gap between the evidence and practice. In response to the

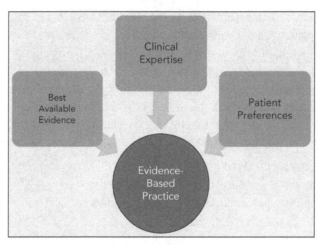

FIGURE 11.1 Evidence-based practice model.

growing need for evidence, the emphasis of EBP is to bring updated and synthesized best available evidence to the busy direct care nurse.

A common mistake regarding EBP is the belief that EBP relies solely on evidence and ignores patient preferences and values (Dicenso, Guyatt, & Ciliska, 2005). This is not true. In addition to the best available evidence, it is important to recognize that clinical expertise and patient preferences are equally important in the provision of evidence-based, optimal care. Each component of the EBP model should be explored and integrated into practice by nurses and other healthcare providers. The following explores each part of the model separately to illustrate why each part is interdependent on each other.

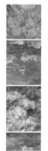

CASE STUDY 11.1

As a nurse on the medical–surgical fl oor, you are caring for an Amish patient with end-stage renal disease (ESRD). The patient's attending physician has been talking about the need to start hemodialysis. The patient is asking you many questions related to this treatment recommendation. After listening to your explanations, which you give based on evidence from the research literature, the patient states that he would prefer to go home, and if he dies, then it is God's will.

1. *Is it appropriate to tell the patient that he needs to do what the physician ordered because dialysis can extend life expectancy?*
2. *Why or why not?*
3. *What would be the most appropriate action to take?*

BEST AVAILABLE EVIDENCE

In efforts to improve patient safety and outcomes, the IOM promotes the goal that 90% of all health decisions be evidence-based by the year 2020 (Olsen, Aisner, & McGinnis, 2007). Melnyk, Fineout-Overholt, Stillwell, and Williamson (2009) suggest that healthcare settings that promote curiosity regarding clinical decision making are optimally situated to discover and incorporate EBP, thereby improving patient outcomes. While all healthcare professionals are challenged by the IOM goal, nurses are uniquely situated to influence evidence-based clinical decisions at the bedside.

The largest component of EBP requires the best available evidence to inform appropriate patient care clinical decisions. Change can occur at the bedside, affecting a care process on a unit, informing policy changes for a healthcare organization, or, on a grander scale, changing state or federal level health policy. The term "**best available evidence**" implies that someone must conduct a thorough search of the literature and then judge the quality of the evidence to determine if it truly is the "best available." "Best" means that there is a need to judge the quality and rank the evidence. "Available" means that an exhaustive search for evidence has occurred. This means that nurses do not use whatever evidence is handy. Rather, the nurse must ensure that the evidence is of the highest quality available. This leads to the question, how do we know what counts as evidence and how do we know it is of high quality?

When searching for the best evidence that is available, the nurse needs to review the quality of evidence. Since the purpose of implementing evidence-based care is to improve patient safety and achieve high-quality outcomes, a nurse or other healthcare provider needs to be certain that enough rigor exists in the research evidence to provide confidence that the evidence is indeed factual and accurate. Rigor refers to the quality of the evidence and infers a high degree of thoroughness and merit or strength. It would be detrimental to patient safety and high-quality outcomes to base changes in patient care on poor quality, erroneous research.

It is important to take a **pluralistic approach** that considers all the literature when searching for evidence (Pearson, Wiechula, Court, & Lockwood, 2007). A pluralistic approach is based on a philosophical view that there is more than one way to look at something. A pluralistic approach is inclusive of all types of evidence, from the highest level of evidence—that is, systematic reviews (SR) using meta-analysis of high-quality randomized controlled trials (RCT)—to the lowest form of nonresearch evidence called expert opinion.

Hierarchies of evidence (also known as **levels of evidence**) provide a visual representation of evidence from the least reliable (at the bottom) to the most reliable (at the top; Ingham-Broomfield, 2016). Hierarchies provide a way to understand the strength and reliability of the evidence based on the type of study or evidence (McNair & Lewis, 2012). An important distinction between strength and reliability of evidence and the quality of evidence must be made. Hierarchies, or levels of evidence, can only tell you the strength of the type of evidence for transfer of the findings to other contexts. It does not tell you anything about the quality of the evidence. The quality of the evidence is determined through appraisal, discussed later in the chapter. There are conflicting representations of what type of evidence is found at what level. For the most part, there is a general consensus on levels of evidence. Table 11.1 displays a synthesis of different hierarchies.

Table 11.1 illustrates how the first level includes the strongest type of evidence. Each level decreases in strength and reliability of evidence. While the higher levels (levels I–IV) describe forms of research evidence, there are other types of evidence that can be used when there is lack of research articles on a topic. For example, a new idea is tried in practice where a nurse wears a yellow vest to reduce interruptions and signify "do not disturb" while removing medications from an electronic medication dispensing system. While this seems appropriate and does not cause harm, what is not known is if wearing the vest actually decreases interruptions during the medication removal

TABLE 11.1 SYNTHESIS OF TYPES AND LEVELS OF EVIDENCE RANKED STRONGEST TO WEAKEST

LEVEL OF EVIDENCE	TYPE OF EVIDENCE
I (strongest) Experimental designs	SRs of RCTs using meta-analyses
	Comprehensive SR of RCTs and other types of studies
	Clinical practice guidelines based on SRs and RCTs
II Quasi-experimental designs	SR of quasi-experimental designs
	Controlled trial without randomization
III Observational and analytical designs	Qualitative SRs of cohort or case studies
	Cohort study
	Case-control study
IV Observational or descriptive studies	Qualitative SRs of descriptive studies using meta-aggregation
	Single descriptive or qualitative study
V (weakest) Text and expert opinion	Expert opinion, reports from committees, grey literature, literature reviews

RCT, randomized control trials; SR, systematic review.

Sources: Compiled with information from Melnyk, B., Fineout-Overholt, E., Stillwell, S., & Williamson, K. (2009). Igniting a spirit of inquiry: An essential foundation for evidence-based practice. *American Journal of Nursing, 109*(11), 49–52; Hopp, L., & Rittenmeyer, L. (2012). *Introduction to evidence-based practice: A practical guide for nursing.* Philadelphia, PA: F.A. Davis; Ackley, B., Ladwig, G., Swan, B.A., & Tucker, S. (2008). *Evidence-based Nursing Care Guidelines.* New York, NY: Elsevier; The Joanna Briggs Institute. (2014). *The JBI approach.* Retrieved from http://joannabriggs.org/jbi-approach.html#tabbed-nav=Levels-of-Evidence

activity. A thorough search of the literature on this topic may only produce one article, written by a nurse, about the experience and perception of reduced interruptions while wearing a yellow vest. This type of evidence is considered expert opinion. While it is one of the lower quality forms of evidence, an argument can be made that it still constitutes evidence and can inform practice in the absence of research evidence.

One piece of evidence may not be enough to change practice. Preappraised evidence includes SRs and clinical practice guidelines. These types of evidence theoretically should include an appraisal of all evidence up to the date the literature was written. For SRs, there should be a section on inclusion and exclusion criteria that detail the data range for the literature search. Clinical practice guidelines will also include a date range for the literature search. This is important so that the user understands how far the date range is for the search and the studies included. For example, an SR on clinical decision support systems in electronic documentation may have a date range of 2000 to 2017. This is appropriate since clinical decision support systems are a relatively new innovation and were not used prior to 2000. If a qualitative SR on patient isolation had a date range of 2000 to 2017, one might suspect that some evidence is missing since isolation has been a healthcare practice since the inception of nursing. A date range of 1970 to 2000 would be appropriate as this range captures the beginning of published evidence.

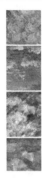

CASE STUDY 11.2

As a nurse in the operating room, you are asked to change the method used to position patients during surgical procedures. You have been educated and trained in the new procedure that is being implemented as an evidence-based change. After several days of using the new positioning technique, you have noticed several patients with increased areas of skin erythema on key pressure points.

1. *Since this change is evidence based, will you just keep utilizing the new method despite concerns?*
2. *Why or why not?*
3. *What would be the most appropriate action to take?*

Evidence Appraisal

Once the best available evidence from the literature is located, the nurse should appraise the quality of the evidence and the generalizability of the information to the practice setting. In other words, is the available evidence strong enough, or rigorous enough, to support a change in patient care practice? Is the evidence strong enough to inform clinical decisions? Also, can the evidence be applied in the nurse's clinical setting? Is the nurse's individual institution willing to adopt change based on its unique situation, availability of resources, and culture of change? These questions drive the appraisal of evidence.

Tools to Appraise Evidence From the Literature

Critical appraisal of evidence is one of the most important steps in EBP. Critically appraising the evidence to determine if it is valid, reliable, and appropriate helps to focus only on high-quality evidence and eliminate evidence that is either not applicable or of low quality. Appraising research can be intimidating, particularly to the new-to-practice nurse. However, tools exist to aid the interprofessional team in judging the quality of the evidence. It is important to understand that every piece of evidence should go through a rigorous appraisal process to judge the quality of the evidence. This action is taken to ensure that only the best available evidence is used to inform clinical decision making and that any proposed changes based on the evidence are defensible. The following are tools to assist both novice and expert nurses and the interprofessional team to appraise different types of evidence.

The Appraisal of Guidelines for Research and Evaluation II Instrument

The Appraisal of Guidelines for Research and Evaluation (AGREE) II Instrument provides a framework to evaluate clinical practice guidelines (The AGREE II Next Steps Consortium, 2009). The AGREE II is both valid and reliable and comprises 23 items organized into six quality domains as follows:

- Scope and purpose
- Stakeholder involvement

- Rigor of development
- Clarity of presentation
- Applicability
- Editorial independence (The AGREE II Next Steps Consortium, 2009)

Each of the 23 items in the quality domains target various aspects of practice guideline quality. The AGREE II also includes two final overall assessment items that require appraisers to make overall judgments of the practice guideline as well as consider how they would rate the 23 items. The AGREE II tool is easy to use for the purposes of the nurse evaluating clinical guidelines for the best available evidence. The tool is free of charge and can be accessed ternet at www.agreetrust.org. A tutorial is included with the tool.

CRITICAL THINKING 11.1

You work on a medical–surgical unit delivering care to patients. You want to be sure your care delivery is based on evidence and is state of the art.

1. How will you, as a new nurse, begin to promote EBP?
2. What contributions can you make to EBP?
3. How can nurses help to overcome potential resistance to EBP?

The Critical Appraisal Skills Program

The Critical Appraisal Skills Program (CASP, 2010) is another available free resource that provides the nurse with tools to judge the quality of various types of research evidence. In contrast to the AGREE II tool for appraising clinical practice guidelines, CASP has different appraisal tools for different types of evidence (see Table 11.3). CASP provides checklists specific to types of research including RCTs, SRs, cohort studies, case-control studies, and qualitative research studies (see Table 11.2). The CASP tools can be located at www.casp-uk.net/. The website also provides tutorials for new users.

TABLE 11.2 RESEARCH TERMINOLOGY

TERM	DEFINITION
Case-control study	A study comparing cases of two study participants in order to identify causes of what makes them different. For example, a case control study might compare two nursing home patients, one with recurrent urinary tract infections (UTI) and one who never had a UTI in order to identify elements that might predict the condition in others (e.g., incontinence, immobility)
Clinical practice guidelines (or practice guidelines)	Statements with recommendations to assist healthcare professionals regarding most appropriate treatment for specific clinical situations. Evidence-based clinical practice guidelines provide the strongest level of evidence to guide practice, and are based on systematic reviews (SRs) of randomized clinical trials or the best available evidence on a specific clinical circumstance or situation

(continued)

TABLE 11.2 RESEARCH TERMINOLOGY (*continued*)

TERM	DEFINITION
Cohort study	A prospective study of two groups conducted over time in order to collect and analyze data in comparison to one another. For example, a cohort study might examine a group of inner city elementary children from birth through age 18 compared to a similar group in a rural setting
Integrative review	An analysis of the literature on a specific topic or concept leading to implications for practice
Meta-analysis	A comprehensive and systematic approach using statistical methods to pool the results of independent studies on a topic that leads to inferences or conclusions about that topic
Mixed methods	A study that uses both quantitative and qualitative study designs
Nonexperimental research	A study in which the researcher collects and analyzes data based on what is observed about a phenomenon without using a comparison
Outcomes research	A study conducted to measure the effectiveness of an intervention. For example, hospitals frequently conduct outcomes research to document the effectiveness of their services by measuring the end results of patient care (e.g., infection rates, rates of readmission)
Prospective study	A nonexperimental study that begins with an examination of assumed causes (e.g., high-fat diet), which then goes forward in time to the presumed effect (e.g., obesity)
Qualitative research	A study that examines a phenomenon with words and descriptions rather than statistics or numbers in order to determine underlying elements and patterns within relationships
Quantitative research	A study that examines a phenomenon with numeric data and statistics rather than words or descriptions in order to determine the magnitude and reliability of relationships between variables or concepts
Randomized controlled trial (RCT)	A study that uses a true experimental design (research that provides an intervention or treatment to research participants who have been randomly chosen to be either in the experimental group receiving a treatment or in the control group where they receive no intervention or treatment)
Systematic review (SR) of the literature	A study that uses an exhaustive and transparent systematic approach to searching all the literature on a topic and then critically examines and synthesizes all the evidence on that specific topic
Text and expert opinion	Opinions from experts or committees; literature reviews, nonresearch articles and editorials are some types of expert opinions

Source: Compiled with information from Hopp, L., & Rittenmeyer, L. (2012). *Introduction to evidence-based practice: A practical guide for nursing*. Philadelphia, PA: F.A. Davis; Melnyk, B., Fineout-Overholt, E., Stillwell, S., & Williamson, K. (2009). Igniting a spirit of inquiry: An essential foundation for evidence-based practice. *American Journal of Nursing, 109*(11), 49–52; Dicenso, A., Guyatt, G., & Ciliska, D. (2005). *Evidence-based nursing: A guide to clinical practice*. St. Louis, MO: Elsevier Mosby.

CRITICAL THINKING 11.2

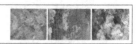

You are a new graduate nurse working on a medical–surgical unit delivering care to patients. You notice that the IV team nurse makes rounds daily and changes all IV catheters that were placed 3 days ago. When you ask her why this is done, she states, "This has been the policy since I started 3 years ago."

1. What action would be appropriate for the new nurse at this time?
2. How will the new nurse accomplish this?
3. Who might be a good resource for the new nurse?

TABLE 11.3 EXAMPLE OF USING A CRITICAL APPRAISAL SKILLS PROGRAM (CASP) TOOL TO APPRAISE AN ARTICLE

EVALUATION OF A SYSTEMATIC REVIEW (SR) UTILIZING THE CASP TOOL

Locate the following article to be reviewed: Baatiema, L., Otim, M.E., Mnatzagnian, G., de-Graft, A., Coombs, J., & Somerset, S. (2017). Health professionals' views on the barriers and enablers to evidence-based practice for acute stroke care: A systematic review. *Implementation Science, 12*(74), 1–15. Retrieved from https://implementationscience. biomedcentral.com/articles/10.1186/s13012-017-0599-3

Be sure to read the article completely and make sure you understand the purpose of the study. Focus on purpose, methodology, and results. Be sure to determine what type of study this article is discussing (e.g., RCT, SR, cohort study, qualitative study). Do this BEFORE you start the evaluation of the study.

Access the appropriate evaluation tool from the CASP website, located at www.casp-uk.net/. On the CASP homepage there are links for various checklists based on the type of study to be evaluated. In this example, the study to be evaluated is an SR. Click on the appropriate link to access the SR evaluation tool. The evaluation tool consists of 10 questions divided into three sections that address whether the results are valid (Section A), what the results are (Section B), and if the results will help with the population of interest to the reviewer (Section C).

Section A

Question 1: Does the review address a clearly focused question?

Yes. This study aims to identify health professionals' views on the barriers and enablers to their use of four evidence-based recommendations for acute stroke care interventions. The authors clearly explain the four evidence-based recommendations for acute stroke care interventions. Additionally, the authors explain that a delay exists in adopting evidence-based interventions in the clinical setting.

Question 2: Did the authors look for the appropriate sort of papers?

Yes. The authors were fully transparent in their search strategy. The authors reported that they conducted a systematic review of databases including MEDLINE, CINAHL, Embase, PsycINFO, Cochrane Library, and AMED. The authors used the PRISMA SR approach. The date range was explained as encompassing the times when evidence-based practice (EBP) occurred. The appropriate key terms were used to locate applicable articles.

(continued)

TABLE 11.3 EXAMPLE OF USING A CRITICAL APPRAISAL SKILLS PROGRAM (CASP) TOOL TO APPRAISE AN ARTICLE (*continued*)

Section B

Question 3: Do you think the important, relevant studies were included?

Yes. The authors used two reviewers to examine abstracts of 8,446 articles with 8,344 articles discarded as not meeting the inclusion and exclusion criteria. For the remaining 102 articles, a three-step approach was used. First, two authors conducted a review of the full text for relevance to the topic. Second, the two authors exchanged articles for review agreement. Third, the rest of the authors reviewed the articles. Agreement on the articles was achieved and 10 studies were identified as meeting all criteria for inclusion. This study considered both qualitative and quantitative study designs.

Question 4: Did the review's authors do enough to assess the quality of the included studies?

Yes. The authors assessed the quality of the articles using a standardized tool. The authors adequately discussed the strengths and weaknesses of each study based on their appraisals of the studies. Seven quantitative and three qualitative studies were included. Weaknesses of some of the studies were reported and the authors did a nice job of explaining and discussing the weaknesses. For the quantitative studies, only one fully described sampling techniques to minimize selection bias, three reported high response rates, and four reported low response rates. All seven were cross-sectional study designs. For the qualitative studies, none of the included studies reported on a philosophical paradigm to situate the study and only two addressed reflexivity (potential reporting bias).

EVALUATION OF AN SYSTEMATIC REVIEW (SR) UTILIZING THE CASP TOOL

Question 5: If the results of the review were combined, was it reasonable to do so?

Yes. The authors explained the use of distribution percentages and weighted frequency for each finding showing the significance of each barrier and enabler for stroke care.

Question 6: What are the overall results of the review?

Six major findings came from a synthesis of the evidence (in order of frequency):

1. *Capacity for organizational change.* Institutional resources, time for professional development in EBP, limited capacity, and workload demands were cited as barriers.
2. *Individual health professionals.* Barriers found with health professionals included lack of awareness, lack of skills or belief in their ability to apply the intervention, and lack of motivation to implement an evidence-based therapy.
3. *Resources and incentives.* Some of the common barriers/enablers reported in both qualitative and quantitative studies were limited physical space to establish stroke units, lack of CT scans, lack of financial resources, limited time, limited stroke beds, and limited staff capacity.
4. *Guideline factors.* Nine of 10 eligible studies reported barriers related to the characteristics or the nature of evidence related to the stroke intervention or guidelines. Despite the evidence, participants expressed doubts in the effectiveness of the guidelines.
5. *Patient factors.* Six studies highlighted factors of late arrival to seek care, patients' or relatives' lack of awareness of early stroke symptoms, or patients' decision for other acute care interventions outside the standardized recommendation.
6. *Professional interactions.* The uptake of evidence is influenced by interactions among health professionals in five studies. Barriers included inadequate communication especially among clinical staff, lack of clinical leadership or support from senior clinicians.

The authors did achieve saturation of themes that arose from the data.

Section C

Question 8: Can the results be applied to the local population you are interested in?

Yes with caveats. All studies were conducted in high-income countries, making the generalizability of the findings questionable. In areas with low resource availability, including

TABLE 11.3 EXAMPLE OF USING A CRITICAL APPRAISAL SKILLS PROGRAM (CASP) TOOL TO APPRAISE AN ARTICLE (*continued*)

rural populations in high-income countries, it may be difficult to apply the results. If using the findings, it is strongly recommended to look at available resources such as personnel, experience, leadership, time, advanced practice nurses, and engagement. Additional material resources identified included the need for additional CT scans, space, and dedicated stroke care staff.

Question 9: Were all important outcomes considered?

Yes. The authors discussed achieving saturation of data, meaning that as they extracted data from the studies, no further new themes were identified. The authors identified barriers from which enablers, or the opposite, could be assumed.

Question 10: Are the benefits worth the harms and costs?

Absolutely. None of the studies included demonstrated any harm to patients. The findings show some benefit and no harm. The findings showed support for additional resources necessary to implement the specific evidence-based guideline for acute stroke care.

Additionally, the study underscored the need for increased attention to patient-level barriers to stroke care. There is an essential need to increase understanding of early recognition of stroke symptoms, what to do when stroke symptoms are present, and why there is a need for emergency care; this can be done through outreach campaigns, education, and engagement.

Overall the SR was comprehensive and well organized. Limitations to the review primarily stem from limitations in the available research. Potential harms to patients from incorporating any of the suggestions appear to be minimal. For these reasons, these findings are appropriate to consider when implementing an evidence-based acute stroke program.

Clinical Expertise

In 1984, Benner published a landmark book in which she disseminated the idea that nurses constantly evolve in their practice along a continuum from novice to expert. This evolution occurs with the acquisition of advanced skills, experience, and understanding of patients, families, and their unique needs as well as with additional education (Benner, 1984). Benner further stated that regardless of how much education a nurse possessed, the nurse could never become an expert without actual clinical experience. In practical terms, what this implies is that based on knowledge and experience, each nurse brings unique perceptions and strengths to the healthcare setting.

There is an expectation in society that nurses will bring theoretical and practical clinical knowledge and expertise to their practice as a credentialed nursing expert. As a professional, there is an assumption that every RN will provide safe and competent care to every patient. **Clinical expertise** develops as the nurse tests and refines both theoretical and practical knowledge in actual clinical situations (Benner, 1984). Hopp and Rittenmeyer (2012) state that clinical expertise is more than the education, skills and experience of a nurse. Clinical expertise must be explicit, or clearly visible to others, so that it can be subjected to analysis and critique. Nurses demonstrate clinical expertise when they assess their patient and the patient's family, consider the setting of the provision of care, make clinical decisions that place the patient's values at the center of care, and coordinate patient care based on available resources. Analysis and critique of clinical expertise most commonly occurs through performance evaluations, competency assessment, certification from a professional organization, or peer evaluations based on standardized nursing performance criteria.

For example, a physically debilitated patient requires assistance transferring from the chair to the bed. The nursing staff used a gait belt to assist with this procedure.

Two nurses, with differing experience and background, can approach the care of this patient differently while at the same time they both ensure the safety and well-being of the patient. A novice nurse, with limited practical experience and knowledge related to the patient, decides to ask the physical therapist to assist her by showing her the proper techniques needed for the safe transfer of the patient to the bed. A more experienced nurse, familiar with proper body mechanics, gait belt transfers, and the patient's physical ability, chooses to assist the patient with the gait belt by herself. Both nurses achieved the same goal of safely transferring the patient to the bed; however, they approached the issue differently based on personal experience and knowledge. This example demonstrates how the individual nurses' varying clinical expertise can impact how care is delivered to this patient. To ensure optimal patient outcomes and patient safety, all nurses need to constantly be aware of their strengths and limitations as they plan and implement care.

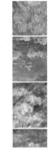

CASE STUDY 11.3

Your head nurse has asked you to investigate what the best EBPs are related to the prevention of pressure sores. The unit protocol for pressure sore prevention was last updated 5 years ago. You implement a search of the literature but are unable to locate any articles relevant to your topic of interest.

1. *What factor has most likely hampered your ability to locate relevant information?*
2. *What is your next step?*
3. *Who can assist you with this?*

Patient Preferences

Patient preferences refer to the involvement of the patient and family with a consideration of their values and beliefs in clinical shared decisions (Hopp & Rittenmeyer, 2012). Some patients like to leave healthcare decisions up to their provider whereas others like full disclosure about their health issues. When patients are included in their healthcare decisions there is an improvement in cognitive (e.g., ability to retain education, memory recall) and behavioral (e.g., the ability to adhere to a prescribed regimen) outcomes (Shay & Lafata, 2015). Evaluating the patient's preferences for inclusion in decisions should be part of providing care to each and every patient. (Chapter 7 explores tools and guides that help assess the patient's preferences to help patients make healthcare decisions.) While considering the patient's preferences seems easy, sometimes patient preferences go against the nurse's own belief system. For example, the patient may continue to smoke after receiving a diagnosis of lung cancer, choose alternative treatments over conventional therapy, refuse life-saving blood transfusions, or decide not to treat a condition altogether. Remaining nonjudgmental and keenly aware and accepting of a patient's wishes are important elements of evidence-based nursing practice.

Shared decision making is an approach that involves both clinicians and patients in considering the best available evidence to make healthcare decisions. Patients are empowered, engaged, and supported to make autonomous decisions about healthcare (Truglio-Londrigan, Slyer, Singleton, & Worral, 2014). A variety of models exist to guide shared decision making. One particular model describes the responsibilities required of the healthcare provider and essential skills needed for shared decision making, as follows:

- Involve the patients either implicitly or explicitly in the decision-making process.
- Explore ideas, fears, and expectations of the problem and possible treatments.
- Describe treatment options with consideration for equilibrium and balance.
- Identify the patient's preferred format for education and provide tailor-made information.
- Check the patient's understanding of information and reactions.
- Include the patient to the extent he or she desires to be involved in the decision-making process.
- Discuss the options and either make or defer the healthcare decision. (Elwyn et al., 2012)

EVIDENCE FROM THE LITERATURE

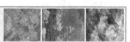

Citation

Truglio-Londrigan, M., Slyer, J. T., Singleton, J. K., & Worral, P. S. (2014). A qualitative systematic review of internal and external influences on shared decision-making in all healthcare settings. *JBI Database of Systematic Reviews & Implementation Reports, 12*(5), 121–194.

Discussion

Knowledge of the influences on shared decision making is important to the healthcare provider when working with patients to make the best decision. A high-quality qualitative SR was conducted on the topic with the objective of finding the best available evidence on meaningfulness of internal and external influences on shared decision making. The findings illustrate factors that influence shared decision making:

- Patient-centered care: care that is developed based on the patient specific knowledge gathered from the patient assessment and based on trust and respect.
- Bridging the knowledge gap: accomplished through assessment inclusive of barriers that inform what information providers must share and how they will share the information. Providers share options, risks, benefits, and potential outcomes to engage patients in shared decision making.
- Dimensions of decision making: shared decision making involves a negotiating process that considers the role that the patient wishes to assume in the experience. The decision-making process may change depending on the variables of the experience, inclusive of the patient, provider, and context.

(continued)

EVIDENCE FROM THE LITERATURE (*continued*)

Implications

The findings of this SR can be used to understand the holistic nature of shared decision making. Healthcare providers need to understand the patient and develop a relationship based on trust and respect. When helping patients make a decision, healthcare providers should determine the best approach to shared decision making for the individual patient, sharing the options, risks, benefits, and potential outcomes in such a way that the patient can fully understand them. Understanding the patient's level of desire to participate in shared decision making is critical to achieving shared decision making. The healthcare provider must also be conscious that the decision-making process can change over time depending on the variables of the experience such as setting, diagnosis, resources, and patient assessment findings.

MODELS AND FRAMEWORKS FOR EBP

Models and frameworks for implementing EBP into healthcare help nurses to understand the complexity of EBP and guide implementation of EBP transfer to practice. Understanding the differences between a model and framework helps nurses to understand how they can help implement EBP into nursing practice. "A model is narrower in scope and more precise than a framework. The concepts within a model should be well-defined and relationships defined. They are representations of the real thing" (Rycroft-Malone & Bucknall, 2010). Each EBP model and framework varies in the approach to implementing evidence and is diverse in its complexity and inclusiveness as well as depth and breadth of approach to EBP. Table 11.4 is a broad overview of EBP models and frameworks and includes a brief description of each.

Some of the process models and frameworks explain the steps of evidence implementation as a process with clear steps and expectations for outcomes making them easier to understand for the novice nurse. Other process models and frameworks address evidence implementation as a complex process that requires consideration of the interplay between multiple variables. Regardless of the type of model, each model and framework helps to guide EBP projects to implement evidence into practice.

There are three general purposes of models and frameworks. First, descriptive models and frameworks attempt to explain the characteristics and properties of a phenomenon. These can be used when you want to understand the cultural factors in a setting that affect how an evidence-based change is accepted by the nursing staff. Second, explanatory models and frameworks explore the cause and effect relationship among the concepts. These can be used when you want to understand how training nurses to use a new evidence-based intervention affects the use of the evidence-based intervention in everyday nursing practice. Third, predictive models and frameworks forecast the behavior of phenomena and their relationships and generate hypotheses. These can be used when planning an evidence-based change to nursing practice to identify if the change has the desired effect on patient outcomes (Rycroft-Malone & Bucknall, 2010).

TABLE 11.4 EBP MODELS

NAME	TYPE	DESCRIPTION
ACE Star Model of Knowledge Transformation (2004)	Process model	Illustrates how evidence moves through cycles, including combining with other knowledge and integrating into practice. www.nursing.uthscsa.edu/onrs/starmodel/star-model.asp
ARCC (1999)	Process model	Guides system-wide implementation and sustainability of evidence-based interventions by removing barriers and supporting facilitators, using mentors and champions (Melnyk, Fineout-Overholt, Stillwell, & Williamson, 2009).
AHRQ Model of Knowledge Transfer	Process model	Synthesizes concepts from different professional models. Knowledge transfer is subject to sequencing of steps and timing of activities and that EBP implementation is impacted by people, processes, and systems (Titler, 2008).
Dissemination and use of research evidence for policy and practice (2002)	Process framework	Describes and depicts the process of informed decision making based on evidence for both health policy and health decisions. Based on the Roger's Diffusion of Innovation Model along with premises of other sciences to facilitate evidence-informed decisions (Rycroft-Malone & Bucknall, 2010).
JBI Model of Evidence-Based Healthcare as a Framework for Implementing Evidence (2005)	Process model	Identifies four components of global evidence-based health: evidence generation, evidence synthesis, evidence/knowledge transfer, and evidence utilization (www.joannabriggs.org/jbi-approach.html).
KTA Framework (2006)	Process model	Assumes knowledge producers and users within a social system or systems are responsive and adaptive in unpredictable ways. The KTA process is iterative, with changes made based on outcomes, using an action cycle to adapt to changes in the process. A planned action model (www.cihr-irsc.gc.ca/e/40618.html).
Ottowa Model of Research Use (1998)	Planned change model	Explores the interplay between research development and use that reflect complexities of knowledge translation. Maintains patients as a central focus. External factors and healthcare environments influence the translation of knowledge into practice (www.nccmt.ca/resources/search/65).
PARiHS	Determinant framework	Implementing research into practice requires consideration of factors such as context, facilitation, and evidence. Each factor is explored on a matrix from high to low in terms of influence on successful implementation (www.nccmt.ca/resources/search/85).

(continued)

TABLE 11.4 EBP MODELS (*continued*)

NAME	TYPE	DESCRIPTION
Rogers' Diffusion of Innovation Framework (1971)	Classic theory	Implementing change in practice requires certain conditions that increase or decrease likelihood of success. Focuses on the individuals impacted by the change and their acceptance or resistance level to the change (www.ou.edu/deptcomm/dodjcc/groups/99A2/theories.htm).
Stetler Model	Process model	Explains a step-by-step process in five stages for implementing evidence into practice: preparation, validation, decision making, application, and evaluation www.nccmt.ca/resources/search/83).
Titler's Iowa Model of Evidence-Based Practice to Promote Quality Care (2001)	Process model	Guides healthcare practitioners in using evidence to improve health outcomes. The model integrates evidence into practice, from identifying triggers or indicators that a need exists through implementing evidence into practice (Rycroft-Malone & Bucknall, 2010).

ACE, Academic Center for Evidence-Based Practice; AHRQ, Agency for Healthcare Research and Quality; ARCC, Advancing Research and Clinical Practice Through Close Collaboration; EBP, evidence-based practice; JBI, Joanna Briggs Institute; KTA, Knowledge to Action; PARiHS, Promoting Action on Research Implementation in Health Services.

Useful Models and Frameworks for Evidence Implementation

Of the models and frameworks presented, there are four that are most frequently used in healthcare: Iowa Model, Roger's Diffusion of Innovation, Joanna Briggs Institute (JBI) Model, and Promoting Action on Research and Implementation in Health Services (PARiHS). Each of these will be explored for applicability to healthcare and nursing practice.

JBI Model

The JBI model focuses on healthcare decisions that consider the feasibility, appropriateness, meaningfulness, and effectiveness of healthcare practices (www.joannabriggs.com). The model holds true to the definition of EBP presented at the beginning of the chapter by describing the EBP process as a combination of the best available evidence, the context of care, the individual patient, and the practitioner's clinical judgment. The model shows EBP as a cyclical process consisting of the following:

- Evidence generation: consideration of international evidence to inform questions about feasibility, appropriateness, meaningfulness, and effectiveness (research, expertise, and discourse).
- Evidence synthesis: a systematized approach to SRs that considers the pluralistic forms of evidence (SR, evidence summary, guidelines).
- Evidence transfer: dissemination of evidence from SRs in formats that are usable to clinicians (active dissemination, systems integration, education).
- Evidence implementation: moving evidence into practice and sustaining the change (context analysis, facilitation of change, evaluation of process and outcome; Jordan, Lockwood, Aromataris, & Munn, 2016).

JBI provides training and assistance for each component of the model knowing that it requires highly skilled and trained healthcare professionals to accomplish all components. Because the basic premise of the model is that implementing evidence-based healthcare depends on the best available evidence, a comprehensive SR training workshop is part of the JBI's resources and is offered worldwide to eligible participants. This is part of the evidence synthesis aspect of the model. Each SR completed by a JBI trainee must meet a structured, standard set of guidelines based on transparency and authenticity of the recommendations produced.

JBI does have a fee-based library through Lippincott. This library includes peer-reviewed, high-quality SRs that are completed by health professionals and librarians who have attended training in SR methodology. Additionally, the library houses best practice information sheets and evidence summaries, which provides recommendations that are condensed from SRs and include the level and quality of evidence used to support ready-to-use practice recommendations.

PARiHS Model

The PARiHS Model focuses on how to move evidence into practice. **Evidence implementation** involves the evolving and imperfect science of moving evidence into practice (Pearson, 2010). The model attempts to make sense of the complexities involved with evidence implementation. There are three components that affect the success of evidence implementation: evidence, context, and facilitation.

- Evidence consists of research, clinical experience, patient experience, and local data.
- Context consists of the culture, leadership, and evaluation (feedback).
- Facilitation consists of those who help move the evidence into practice with consideration of purpose, role, skills, and attributes (National Collaborating Centre for Methods and Tools, 2011).

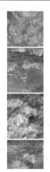

CASE STUDY 11.4

Two patients with identical healthcare histories are diagnosed with Stage IV lung cancer. The nurse is present when the physician explains to each patient the optimal treatment to maximize life expectancies and that mortality for this condition is very high. The nurse uses assessment findings from each patient, considers interactions with the patients, and thinks about the individual characteristics of each patient such as family support, employment, housing, lifestyle, and their values and beliefs about life. She speaks with each patient to discuss options for care. After learning all of the facts related to the disease, treatment, and prognosis, each patient chooses a different treatment course. The first patient states that he has led a good life, is very spiritual, and wishes to die peacefully at home with his family at his side. The second patient states that he has life goals that are unachieved and that he is also very spiritual and his family's support will assist him as he does whatever is necessary to beat the cancer.

1. *Based on the Current Literature 11.1, how did the nurse employ shared decision-making during the interactions with each patient?*
2. *Should shared decision-making include family members? Why or why not?*
3. *How might each patient's decision change the nurse's plan of care?*

Each component is ranked based on criteria on a matrix from high to low. Theoretically, when the evidence, context, and facilitation are all ranked as "high," then evidence implementation and sustaining the implementation should be successful and the more likely the evidence implementation project will be successful.

Rogers' Diffusion of Innovation Framework

Rogers' (2003) Diffusion of Innovation framework is based on the premise that innovations and changes are social phenomena. Rogers stated that if a third of any given group adopts a new practice change based on new evidence, then the rest of the group will follow based on their comfort with the innovation and considering the practice changes the norm. Rogers' Diffusion of Innovation framework entails five steps detailed in Table 11.5.

Nurses can use Rogers' Diffusion of Innovation framework to guide full implementation and adoption of a new EBP process. It is important to identify the types of adopters who are affected by the change as this will affect the success of the change. Types of adopters are explained in Table 11.6.

TABLE 11.5 ROGERS' DIFFUSION OF INNOVATION FRAMEWORK

STEPS	EXPLANATION	APPLICATION
Knowledge	The change/innovation is described to the decision-making unit (individual, team, or organization) who develops a beginning understanding of the suggested change.	CDC guidelines indicate that urinary tract infections in hospitalized patients are decreased when urinary catheters are inserted only when absolutely necessary and left in for no longer than 48 hours.
Persuasion	The change agent(s) work to develop favorable attitudes toward the innovation/change.	An interprofessional performance improvement team provides in-service education to all staff members at initiation of trial of a new evidence-based clinical practice for urinary catheters for 6 months on the surgical unit. The performance team meets with staff every 2 weeks to answer questions and provide support.
Decision	A decision is made to adopt or reject the innovation/change.	Results indicate that over this 6-month period, the number of new catheter-associated urinary tract infections on this surgical unit decreased by 50%.
Implementation/trial	The innovation is put in place. Reinvention or alterations may occur.	The new urinary catheter clinical practice is implemented on all hospital units.
Confirmation	The individual or decision-making unit seeks reinforcement that the decision made was correct, or a decision that was previously made may be reversed.	Over the next 6 months the rate of catheter-associated urinary tract infectionsdecreases by 35%. The new protocol has become the accepted standard of practice.

TABLE 11.6 TYPES OF ADOPTERS

TYPE OF ADOPTER	EXPLANATION
Innovators	Willing to take risks and take the chance that the change will fail; demonstrate a high risk tolerance
Early adopters	Elect to adopt based on an analysis of risk; typically have a high social status and can influence other's opinions of a change
Early majority	Wait to engage in the change until outcomes from the change are known; rarely opinion leaders
Late majority	Demonstrate skepticism about the change and will adopt only after the change is accepted by almost everyone else
Laggards	Focused on tradition and the last to adopt any innovation; difficult to get this group to accept change

Source: Adapted from Rogers, E. M. (2003). *Diffusion of innovation* (5th ed.). New York, NY: Free Press.

Nurses can first work with staff members who are known **innovators** and early adopters of change. Innovators accept change and are willing to try new things. Once the innovators are on board, they then appeal to the early majority. The importance of identifying and engaging the early majority is that they will quickly adopt the change and have an influence on the opinion of others about the change. Positive opinions about any change are critical to influencing others to accept the change and integrate it into practice. This has a significant effect on the success of any change.

The late majority will eventually accept the change as the innovation becomes the norm in practice and any problems are worked out. The final group is the laggards, who either are the last to accept the change or will leave the setting to avoid making the change. While not all will embrace the change in the beginning, some of the later adopters may turn out to be the greatest proponents of the new practice. Therefore, in conducting a pilot, it is smart to approach a unit with known innovators to start the project. Staff on the practice committee may be able to identify these known innovators.

Titler's Iowa Model of Evidence-Based Practice

Using Titler's model as a guide, nurses look for knowledge- and problem-focused triggers from the external professional environment and the internal healthcare organization. **Knowledge-focused triggers** are triggers that stem from the research literature, a

---

CRITICAL THINKING 11.3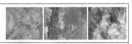

As a nurse with 6 months experience on a pediatric inpatient unit, you have developed an interest in how pain control is addressed for pediatric patients. You feel that improvements could be made to provide improved comfort and decreased anxiety for patients and their parents.

1. How will you explore this issue?
2. Who will need to be involved in a discussion related to the issue?
3. Who could help facilitate the discussion?

TABLE 11.7 TITLER'S IOWA MODEL OF EVIDENCE-BASED PRACTICE

Step 1. Narrow the focus into a researchable question using the PICO format.
Step 2. Search the literature for what is known about this issue.
Step 3. Critically appraise the evidence.
Step 4. Conduct a pilot project.
Step 5. Evaluate the practice decision and outcomes of the pilot project; determine if the change is to be implemented throughout the entire organization.

PICO, patient/population, intervention, comparison, outcome.

new philosophy of care, new national standards, or from professional guidelines (Titler et al., 2001). **Problem-focused triggers** are triggers that stem from internal identification of a clinical problem or local data (Titler et al., 2001). For example, performance improvement and quality data as well as internal and external benchmarking can trigger identification of clinical performance problems. New procedures and treatments driven by technology, as well as by outside regulators, can also trigger the identification of clinical issues. Often these clinical issues are identified at the point of care delivery on patient care units. They are then brought to the unit practice committee and then to the organization-wide practice and quality care committees to be addressed. Once a quality trigger is identified, there are five steps nurses can use to implement Titler's Iowa Model of Evidence-Based Practice to Promote Quality Care (Table 11.7).

Bassett Healthcare, a Magnet® designated facility in Cooperstown, New York, uses Titler's Iowa Model of Evidence-Based Practice to identify and implement EBPs (Figure 11.2).

Bassett Healthcare's Council for the Advancement of Research and Evidence-Based Practice is the main vehicle through which nursing standards of practice are developed and updated. Bassett's Council for the Advancement of Research and Evidence-Based Practice is an interprofessional council, which includes representatives from nursing, the library, the Institutional Review Board, and a representative of the Performance Improvement Department as standing members. The Performance Improvement Department representative acts as a liaison to other institutional interprofessional teams focused on creating and updating standards of practice based on new evidence. Through this EBP implementation process, the interprofessional practice team determines whether the practice change is appropriate to implement throughout the entire organization, and/or where modifications need to be made in practice prior to implementation throughout the organization.

IMPLEMENTING EVIDENCE-BASED CHANGES

There is no doubt that every nurse will be influenced by evidence-based changes during his or her career regardless of setting or type of nursing. Even if you are not part of a team or committee charged with creating the change, you will be affected by the changes in how you provide care. From small changes such as using chlorhexidine instead of betadine preoperatively, to larger and more impactful changes, such as a new process and forms for admitting patients, changes to healthcare processes happen continuously. As a novice nurse, your role in evidence implementation will be small. You may be asked to participate in a small pilot study to investigate the impact of a change or you may be asked for your insights about care provision as someone who provides direct patient care. Regardless, embrace the opportunity to participate in evidence-based changes.

There are two primary sciences that deal with moving evidence into routine clinical practice. **Implementation science** is a science that investigates the

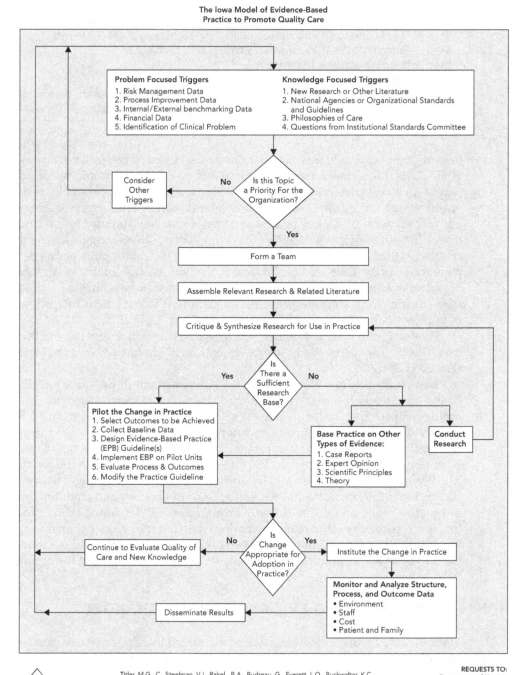

The Iowa Model of Evidence-Based
Practice to Promote Quality Care

FIGURE 11.2 Titler's Iowa model of evidence-based practice.

Used/reprinted with permission from the University of Iowa Hospitals and Clinics. Copyright 2015.

adoption and integration of evidence-based findings, including identification of barriers and facilitators, to successfully integrate the evidence into routine healthcare
(www.implementationscience.biomedcentral.com/about). Implementation science is
also an open source website funded by the Canadian government that provides full-
text access to high-quality SRs concerning best practices for evidence implementation

and sustainability of change. **Translation science** examines variables affecting adoption of evidence-based changes by individuals or organizations designed to improve healthcare decision making (Titler, 2008). While both of these sciences are taught at the graduate level, knowledge of their existence and basic premise is important for every nurse, including the novice nurse. Implementing and sustaining change is predicated on the ability of nurses to maintain vigilance in adhering to any new changes in patient care. Some of the complex variables found in healthcare that both implementation

REAL-WORLD INTERVIEW

With the Centers for Medicare and Medicaid Services' core measure for the evidence-based treatment of severe sepsis and septic shock (SEP-1), many hospitals set up practices to meet the requirements. We chose to address the problem as one committee from a five-hospital system. The purpose of this committee was purely to identify and alleviate gaps between evidence-based practice (EBP) and current practice.

A vital part of EBP implementation is to bring ALL key stakeholders to the table. For implementation of the sepsis EBP project, a group was formed including a chief nursing officer from one of the five hospitals as an executive sponsor, key physicians from internal medicine, intensivists, infection disease and prevention, ED, as well as pharmacy and laboratory leadership, nursing directors from the five emergency and critical care departments, quality directors, social work and case management, spiritual support, and a front-line staff nurse from medical–surgical, critical care and emergency. Several meetings were spent discussing who else needed to have a voice in this practice change to ensure all key stakeholders were included.

The many key and vocal parties often made it difficult to come to important decisions about the practice changes. Several meetings were spent debating the validity of the evidence itself. This is where inclusion of a clinical nurse specialist (CNS) trained in the skill of appraising evidence was key. As a CNS, I had to be both strong and confident in this skill, as this group (especially our physician colleagues) were quite confident in their debate of the evidence. After appraisal of the guideline along with appraisal of key studies used to develop the guideline, the group came to the decision that the guideline was indeed the best evidence.

When implementing EBP improvements to quality care, a few things are important to remember:

1. Prior to any discussion about the practice change itself it is VITALLY IMPORTANT to ensure that all key stakeholders are involved from the very beginning of the project. They must understand why they were invited to the table and the important role they play in the practice change.
2. Having strong evidence and someone who can appraise the evidence and fight for its utilization is the key. The CNS is highly trained in this skill.
3. Sustainable EBP changes do not happen quickly. The implementation of EBP changes often takes over a year from inception to sustained practice change.
4. Knowing the reality that it is never really "done" because evidence based improvements to quality care are always evolving as a result of new evidence.

Julia Sbragia MSN, APRN, ACCNS-AG
Las Vegas, Nevada

science and translational science focus on are characteristics of the setting or context for change: experience, knowledge, and competence of healthcare providers involved with the change; stakeholders with a vested interest in the change and stakeholder engagement strategies; and embedding evidence into routine practice.

Sacred Cows

While it may seem that doing the right thing the right way for the right patient at all times should be second nature, many times making a change from "doing it the way it has always been done" to "basing nursing care on evidence" can be difficult. Known as "sacred cows," there are some healthcare workers who hold on to old practices believing they are the best approach to patient care and resist making change. As a new nurse, you will be faced with these types of individuals. Maintaining a focus on questioning current practice and keeping current with changes to nursing care in your practice setting is important. Vocalizing evidence-based changes and guiding others to question their nursing practice can help to shift the culture from "sacred cows" to nursing care based on current best available evidence.

Evidence-Based Implementation Tools

Many strategies and tools to assist with transferring and embedding evidence into everyday nursing practice exist. High-quality SRs have been conducted on the strategies and tools to scientifically evaluate their effectiveness. You may have already used some of the tools during your clinical experiences without realizing it. Table 11.8 explores some common tools used for evidence implementation.

TABLE 11.8 EVIDENCE IMPLEMENTATION TOOLS

TOOL/ STRATEGY	DESCRIPTION	EXAMPLE
Academic detailing	Using a trained person to deliver focused education to healthcare providers in the practice setting with the intent to change the provider's practice (McElwaine et al., 2016)	Planning frequent, short, 10-minute educational inservices on a new admission form for nurses during each shift.
Audit and feedback	Providing data from clinical practice audits to healthcare providers with dissemination of data occuring in real time (Tuti et al., 2017)	Charting nursing interventions based on evidence and patient responses in the electronic record for patients with ventilator-associated pneumonia occurs for each patient assessment. The data are automatically gathered and trended against previously entered data. The nurse can see graphs that illustrate adherence to evidence-based interventions in real time.

(continued)

TABLE 11.8 EVIDENCE IMPLEMENTATION TOOLS (*continued*)

TOOL/ STRATEGY	DESCRIPTION	EXAMPLE
Bundles	A straightforward set of EBP directives, generally three to five, that when collectively and reliably performed are proven to improve patient outcomes (www.ihi.org/Topics/Bundles/Pages/default.aspx)	An evidence-based care bundle exists for preventing CLABSI. The following actions comprise the bundle: • Hand hygiene • Maximal barrier precautions • Chlorhexidine skin antisepsis • Optimal catheter site selection • Daily assessment of need for the central line (Institute for Healthcare Improvement, 2012) When the actions are taken together, there is statistical evidence that CLABSI rates drop.
Clinical pathways	A structured, multidisciplinary plan that includes evidence-based actions using criterion-based interventions and supports standardizing care (Kinsman et al., 2010)	Clinical pathways are started when a patient with a specific diagnosis is admitted. A patient with heart failure could be placed on a clinical pathway that explains evidence-based interventions such as lab tests, medications, patient education, diagnostic tests as well as milestones to be achieved each day until discharge.
Decision support	Computerized alerts, cues, or reminders to help guide the healthcare provider to deliver care based on the best available evidence (Sahota et al., 2011)	When charting, the nurse is reminded to enter the patient's blood sugar based on the times ordered. If the blood sugar reading is too high or too low, the nurse cannot continue charting until an intervention is done. The charting provides a drop-down list of evidence-based intervention options.
Order sets	A group or "set" of evidence-based orders that are applied to specific patient diagnoses designed to reduce variation and standardize practice (White, Dudley-Brown, & Terhaar, 2016)	An order set is automatically generated for patients with total hip and total knee replacement postsurgery. The order sets include TED hose, sequential compression device, and low molecular weight heparin (dose dependent on weight).
Practice guidelines	Defined as "statements that include recommendations, intended to optimize patient care, that are informed by a systematic review of evidence and an assessment of the benefits and harms of alternative care options" (IOM, 2011, p. 15)	To address the problem of reducing 30-day readmission rates for patients with heart failure, a quality improvement team could use practice guidelines from a high-quality source such as the American Heart Association. Practice guidelines can arise from national initiatives, specialized areas (e.g., Emergency Nurses Association develops guidelines specific for ED nurses), or created by a hospital to address a problem.

TABLE 11.8 EVIDENCE IMPLEMENTATION TOOLS *(continued)*

TOOL/ STRATEGY	DESCRIPTION	EXAMPLE
Protocols	A prescribed set of steps and rules followed for specific patient populations or diagnoses. Conveys more detail than a practice guideline. Helpful to the novice nurse learning to manage complex patients (White, Dudley-Brown, & Terhaar, 2016)	A protocol can be used to communicate expectations for managing complex patient care such as sedation in the ICU, weaning from a ventilator, or recovering a patient in postoperative anesthesia.
Toolkits (practice resources)	A compilation of resources, information, or tools designed to guide users to follow evidence-based recommendations or interventions (AHRQ, 2017)	A "crash cart" or "code cart" found on different units of a hospital is standardized, with the same information, resources, medications, and other tools needed to provide advanced cardiac life support. All carts are set up the same way regardless of where they are located in a hospital. This supports safe patient care in a high-risk situation.

CLABSI, central line-associated bloodstream infections; EBP, evidence-based practice.

CRITICAL THINKING 11.4

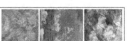

Interview a nurse practicing in the clinical setting and ask what evidence-based nursing practice changes have occurred recently that impact how nurses provide patient care. Ask the nurse if any of the tools and strategies described in Table 11.8 were used to facilitate implementing the evidence-based nursing practice change. Is the nurse familiar with any of the tools and strategies detailed in Table 11.8? Discuss your findings with a classmate.

The Nurse's Role in Evidence Implementation

All nurses can facilitate the implementation of EBP changes. A nurse's willingness to accept a new change is impacted by the nurse's previous experience with change, the nurse's educational preparation, and the length of time and experience the nurse has on the unit where the EBP change will occur. Innovators embracing change stemming from evidence will find it important to educate nurses regarding the science behind any change and encourage them to let go of their old ideas related to delivering patient care, even if a practice is one that has always been done this way. It is also important to include all interprofessional stakeholders in planning the innovation and value their perspectives.

The direct care nurse is in the perfect position to identify the existence of problems with patient care. During a normal workday, a nurse will care for a team of patients and coordinate care with an assortment of interprofessional healthcare providers. These interactions can highlight problems that are perfect for EBP changes. Communicating patient care problems or issues to a person in a position of influence is critical to initiate change. Such positions of influence can include the unit director or manager, the quality representative on the unit or the unit practice council. Becoming familiar with appropriate venues for conveying patient care problems is critical as a new nurse.

CRITICAL THINKING 11.5

As a nurse with six months experience on a pediatric inpatient unit, you have developed an interest in how pain control is addressed for pediatric patients. You feel that improvements could be made to provide improved comfort and decreased anxiety for pediatric patients and their parents. How will you explore this issue? Who will need to be involved in a discussion related to the issue? Who could help facilitate the discussion?

Nurses can promote a positive attitude regarding innovation and embrace the opportunity to assist in the implementation of EBPs, serving as mentors to others and encouraging inquisitiveness regarding best practices. Enlightened users of EBP can provide encouragement to others as they incorporate innovative change.

Practicing in the information age, clinicians are privileged to have the results of scientific evidence at their fingertips through a variety of devices. When considering a change in practice, the issues that arise include the following:

- Giving up old ways of doing and practicing (sacred cows)
- Identifying the best available evidence
- Determining the best available evidence to use for the patient population in a specific practice setting
- Implementing new practice changes in an efficient, organized manner

The EBP frameworks referred to in this chapter are effective guides for professional nurses who choose to take on the challenge of creating an EBP culture with their interprofessional colleagues, promoting safety and quality that leads to excellence in patient care. Knowledge of basic EBP principles is essential for the new nurse. While new nurses are not expected to lead EBP projects, they should be able to engage at a beginner level by identifying patient care problems, collaborate with others to identify the best available evidence, and support implementation of evidence in patient care.

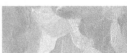

KEY CONCEPTS

1. Evidence-based practice (EBP) promotes the delivery of optimal healthcare through the integration of best available evidence, clinical expertise, and patient preferences.
2. EBP requires a combination of three elements: the best available evidence, the nurse's clinical expertise, and consideration for the patient's preferences.

3. A structured approach to EBP includes: identifying a clinical problem, asking a question based on the problem, searching the literature for the best available evidence, appraising the quality of the evidence, determining the level of evidence based on a hierarchy, synthesizing the evidence into guidance for practice, implementing the change, and sustaining the change over time.

4. Collaborating with reference librarians increases the likelihood of finding the best available evidence on a topic.

5. Examining the type of evidence using a hierarchy of evidence or level of evidence is critical to knowing the strength and reliability of the evidence used to inform a practice change.

6. A standardized appraisal tool, such as Appraisal of Guidelines for Research and Evaluation (AGREE) II and Critical Appraisal Skills Program (CASP) tools, provides a valuable, easy-to-use guide for the nurse to judge the quality of the evidence.

7. EBP models exist to guide changes to nursing practice.

8. Knowledge transfer refers to processes that bridge synthesizing the best available evidence and implementing the evidence into daily nursing practice.

9. Implementation science is an emerging field of study that uses research to identify strategies that are shown to increase the likelihood of successfully making and sustaining a change in clinical practice.

KEY TERMS

Best available evidence
Clinical expertise
Evidence-based practice (EBP)
Evidence implementation
Hierarchies of evidence
Implementation science

Knowledge-focused triggers
Patient preferences
Pluralistic approach
Problem-focused triggers
Shared decision making
Translation science

REVIEW QUESTIONS

1. You are a member of a clinical practice interprofessional team that is looking at the best available evidence to reduce hospital-acquired pressure ulcers on the medical–surgical unit. Which of the following actions by the team demonstrate using the best available evidence?

    A. Conducting a thorough search of the literature using Google to find evidence.
    B. Searching all nursing databases for evidence on the care of hospital-acquired pressure ulcers.
    C. Conducting a thorough search of the literature using CINAHL and MEDLINE.
    D. Using an article based on guidelines from the medical–surgical nursing professional organization.

2. The nurse is giving a presentation to coworkers regarding the patient benefits of adopting policies based on evidenced—based practice (EBP). Which of the following benefits of EBP should be included in the presentation? Select all that apply.

    A. Improved quality of care
    B. Improved cost savings

   C. Decreased patient satisfaction
   D. Decreased lengths of stay
   E. Improved patient outcomes
   F. Decreased cost savings

3. The nurse cares for a patient who has been diagnosed with recurring lung cancer. The oncology unit has a nurse-led support group for improving quality of life for cancer patients. The patient declines participation stating that he is a private person and he is not interested in participating in a group. Which of the following is the best response by the nurse?

   A. "The grieving process will bring you through many phases. Many patients experience denial initially. If you change your mind at a later date, let me know."
   B. "This program is based on research that found that support groups help cancer patients cope with their disease. I suggest that you consider coming to the next meeting anyway."
   C. "I will bring over another patient who says the program has been life-changing so you can make an informed decision."
   D. "What types of support have you found helpful in dealing with trying situations in the past?"

4. The nurse is gathering evidence on interventions to reduce the risk for falls for patients who are at high risk for falls. The nurse finds a variety of types of evidence. All evidence types are appraised using the appropriate tool and found to be high quality. Which of the following are inappropriate types of evidence to use considering all listed types of evidence are found?

   A. Systematic literature review
   B. Report from a national committee on fall prevention
   C. Clinical practice guidelines
   D. Editorial
   E. Systematic review using meta-analysis
   F. Meta-analyses of randomized, controlled trials
   G. Case studies
   H. Qualitative study

5. The nurse is gathering the best available evidence on interventions to reduce hospital-acquired pressure ulcers. Which of the following would be considered the highest level of evidence?

   A. Clinical practice guideline
   B. Randomized control trial
   C. Phenomenological study
   D. Meta-analysis systematic review

6. The nurse is involved in a task force to design patient care plans using evidence. Which of the following statements is true regarding evidence-based practice (EBP)?

   A. All patients should receive the same care based on evidence.
   B. Lower level evidence (levels IV or V) should not be used to impact patient care decisions.
   C. Patient values are a key component of EBP.

   D. All systematic reviews (SR) are considered the highest level of evidence.

   E. Given the ease of access to scientific data, EBP can be quickly incorporated into care plan design.

   F. Evidence from a textbook publisher is considered high quality.

   G. Clinical practice guidelines should not be used to develop care plans.

   H. If an SR is found during the search, the person can stop the literature search.

7. The nurse wants to implement evidence-based practice (EBP) in the care of patients on the unit. Identify the correct order to implement EBP.

   A. Measure outcomes from the change

   B. Appraise the evidence

   C. Ask a searchable question

   D. Incorporate the change into practice

   E. Sustain the change

   F. Create a change based on the evidence

   G. Identify a clinical problem

   H. Locate the best available evidence

   I. Determine level of evidence

8. A nurse is leading an interprofessional team working on strategies to improve patient satisfaction in the ED. A social worker is part of the team and asks the nurse, "Why do we have to appraise all the research articles we found. Isn't it good enough to use the findings from the articles since they are all research?" What would be the most appropriate way for the nurse to respond?

   A. "We need to know which of the articles have the best evidence."

   B. "By appraising the evidence, we will find out the level of each article."

   C. "The appraisal will direct us on what evidence supports each intervention."

   D. "Appraisal helps us determine the quality of the evidence."

9. The ED nurse reads an article that states that patient morbidity and mortality are increased when patients are given plasma volume expanders in the initial treatment of hypovolemic shock. The nurse is concerned about patient outcomes in the ED as plasma volume expanders are often prescribed. What is the best action by the nurse?

   A. Narrow the issue to develop a searchable PICO question and then conduct a search of the literature. Contact a local university to use their library database resources.

   B. Contact the chief of emergency medicine and nurse manager to request creating an interprofessional team to investigate the clinical problem.

   C. Discuss the article with the unit practice council. Request that the issue be taken to the next nursing quality committee.

   D. Post the article in the breakroom. Make copies of the article and place it in conspicuous areas to disseminate the information.

10. A team of nurses in the ICU worked on an evidence-based practice project to eliminate the use of restraints for all patients. When implementing the change, the team shared the evidence that supported eliminating restraint use for patients by posting information in break rooms. The team conducted 10-minute educational inservices for all staff on all shifts in the ICU. Restraints were eliminated as an option for charting in the documentation system and were no longer available or stocked on the unit. Finally, restraint use was eliminated from all clinical pathways, policies, and order sets as an option and replaced with other de-escalation techniques. Based on the information, which evidence implementation tools were used by the ICU nurse team to eliminate the use of restraints?

A. Audit and feedback
B. Protocols
C. Clinical pathways, policies, and order sets
D. Decision support
E. Bundles
F. Academic detailing

REVIEW ACTIVITIES

1. Use information presented in this chapter about the evidence-based practice (EBP) process and required skills to create an interview guide. Use the guide you created to interview a nurse about his or her experiences with EBP projects. You can ask a nurse you know or one you have contact with during your clinical experiences. Examine your findings against the knowledge and skills required for nurses to participate in EBP.
2. Go to the website WhyNotTheBest (www.whynotthebest.org/contents). Review the list of case studies and select one of your choice. Look at the information presented, paying particular attention to how evidence was used to make the change and how nurses were involved as part of the team. Based on what you have learned in the chapter, would you make any changes to the project? What suggestions would you give?
3. Form groups of five to 10 students, depending on the number and availability of library databases. Conduct a search of the literature to identify barriers and facilitators to EBP by new nurses in a hospital setting. Inclusion and exclusion criteria can be set by the students but all articles must be peer reviewed. Each student should search a different database and all evidence should be appraised using the appropriate tool. As a group, combine all findings from the best available evidence into categories of barriers and facilitators. From each list, the group can come up with strategies to overcome barriers and to enhance facilitators. Share your group's findings with the class. Retain your findings to help you assimilate into nursing practice after graduation.

CRITICAL DISCUSSION POINTS

1. The definition of evidence-based practice (EBP) includes three distinct areas: best available evidence, the nurse's clinical judgment, and patient preferences. How would you prioritize the three areas for a successful EBP project? Which area has the greatest impact? Which area is most likely to be forgotten during EBP projects? How will you make sure that all three areas are considered for an EBP project?
2. When you look through the literature for information on a topic for an assignment, are you locating the best available evidence? Why or why not? What might you do to ensure that you are capturing the best available evidence on a topic?
3. Think about your last clinical experience. How did you demonstrate consideration for your patient's preferences? What changes can you make in the future to include the patient's preferences when providing care?

4. Locate one peer-reviewed article on a nursing topic of your choice. Select the appropriate appraisal tool (Critical Appraisal Skills Program [CASP] or Appraisal of Guidelines for Research and Evaluation [AGREE] II) to examine the quality of the evidence. What judgments can you make about the quality of the evidence? Would you use the evidence to inform a change in your clinical practice?

5. What is the importance of using a hierarchy of evidence to determine the types of evidence for an EBP project? Locate one hierarchy online by searching for "nursing evidence hierarchies" or "levels of evidence" using www.google.com and explain why the hierarchy appeals to you.

6. Why is it important to use a model or framework to guide an EBP project or change in practice? Select one model or framework and discuss the benefits and challenges of using the model or framework to guide an EBP change to practice and evidence implementation.

7. Compare and contrast the terms "evidence implementation" and "knowledge transfer." What are the similarities? What are the differences?

QSEN ACTIVITIES

1. Go to the QSEN website (www.qsen.org) and search for the teaching strategy, Using Evidence to Address Clinical Problems (www.qsen.org/USING-EVIDENCE-TO-ADDRESS-CLINICAL-PROBLEMS/). Follow the directions on the teaching strategy page to help students identify how to use evidence during clinical rotations.

2. Locate "Nurse as the leader of the team huddle. An unfolding oncology case study" on the QSEN website (www.qsen.org/nurse-as-the-leader-of-the-team-huddle-an-unfolding-oncology-case-study/). Focus on the identification of evidence-based interventions for the patient in the case study as well as the patient's preferences. PowerPoint and YouTube videos accompany the unfolding case study.

3. As a nurse on the medical–surgical inpatient floor, you have noticed several patients have experienced phlebitis at the site of insertion of IV catheters. You start to wonder if there are EBP changes that could be made to decrease the incidence of phlebitis. Locate two articles and use the appropriate CASP or AGREE II tool to appraise the quality of the evidence. Explain why you selected the two articles including the level of evidence from the evidence hierarchy. How would you use the evidence to create guidance for interventions to reduce the incidence of phlebitis?

4. Access a nursing policy from your clinical laboratory experience. Review the evidence that supports the policy. Conduct a literature search on the topic of the policy. Is the evidence currently used to support the policy the best available evidence? Is there better evidence available? What changes would you propose to the policy based on your findings?

EXPLORING THE WEB

1. The Cochrane Collection (www.cochrane.org) produces systematic reviews (SR) and other types of evidence reports. Holdings can be searched by topic or key word.

2. The Joanna Briggs Institute (www.joannabriggs.org) produces peer-reviewed high-quality SRs, evidence summaries, and best practice series that tend to be nursing focused. Holdings can be searched by topic or key word.

3. Access a few of the EBP models and frameworks outlined in Table 11.4. Review the characteristics of each type. Consider how each model and framework might fit into clinical practice settings.
4. Go to the Indiana Center for Evidence Based Nursing Practice (ICEBNP) at www. ebnp.org/evidence. Review the tools available to assist nurses with EBP.
5. Go to the open access website Implementation Science (implementationscience. biomedcentral.com). This is a grant-funded website from Canada that houses high-quality SRs, evidence summaries, research, and reports from around the world. Search the site using the tool labels listed in Table 11.8 as key words. Locate and read the evidence that supports the tools.
6. Go to the following website to further develop your knowledge of evidence-based healthcare: EBM Education Center of Excellence, North Carolina: www.library. ncahec.net.

REFERENCES

Ackley, B., Ladwig, G., Swan, B. A., & Tucker, S. (2008). *Evidence-based nursing care guidelines*. New York, NY: Elsevier.

Agency for Healthcare Research and Quality (AHRQ) (2017). Toolkit for Using the AHRQ Quality Indicators. Rockville, MD. Retrieved from http://www.ahrq.gov/professionals/ systems/hospital/qitoolkit/index.html

The AGREE II Next Steps Consortium. (2009). *Appraisal of guidelines for research and evaluation II instrument*. The AGREE Research Trust. Retrieved from http://www.agreetrust.org

Benner, P. (1984). *From novice to expert: Excellence and power in clinical nursing practice*. Menlo Park, CA: Addison-Wesley.

Critical Appraisal Skills Program (CASP). (2010). Retrieved from http://www.casp-uk.net/

Dicenso, A., Guyatt, G., & Ciliska, D. (2005). *Evidence-based nursing: A guide to clinical practice*. St. Louis, MO: Elsevier Mosby.

Elwyn, G., Frosch, D., Thomson, R., Joseph-Williams, N., Lloyd, A., Kinnersley, P., … Barry, M. (2012). Shared decision making: A model for clinical practice. *Journal of General Internal Medicine*, 27(10), 1361–1367. doi:10.1007/s11606-012-2077-6

Hopp, L., & Rittenmeyer, L. (2012). *Introduction to evidence-based practice: A practical guide for nursing*. Philadelphia, PA: F.A. Davis.

Ingham-Broomfield, B. (2016). A nurses' guide to the hierarchy of research designs and evidence. *Australian Journal of Advanced Nursing*, 33(3), 38–43. Retrieved from https://www. researchgate.net/publication/301605361_A_nurses%27_guide_to_the_hierarchy_of_ research_designs_and_evidence

Institute for Healthcare Improvement. (2012). How-to Guide: Prevent Central Line-Associated Bloodstream Infections. Cambridge, MA. Retrieved from http://www.ihi. org/resources/Pages/Tools/HowtoGuidePreventCentralLineAssociatedBlood streamInfection.aspx

Institute of Medicine (IOM). (2011). *Clinical practice guidelines we can trust*. Washington, DC: The National Academies Press. Retrieved from http://www.nationalacademies.org/hmd/ Reports/2011/Clinical-Practice-Guidelines-We-Can-Trust.aspx

The Joanna Briggs Institute. (2014). *The JBI approach*. Retrieved from http://joannabriggs.org/ jbi-approach.html#tabbed-nav=Levels-of-Evidence

Jordan, Z., Lockwood, C., Aromataris, E., & Munn, Z. (2016). The updated JBI model for evidence-based healthcare. *The Joanna Briggs Institute*. Retrieved from http://joannabriggs. org/jbi-approach.html

Kinsman, L., Rotter, T., James, E., Snow, P., & Willis, J. (2010). What is a clinical pathway? Development of a definition to inform the debate. *BMC Medicine, 8*, 31. doi:10.1186/1741-7015-8-31

McElwaine, K. M., Freund, M., Campbell, E. M., Bartlem, K. M., Wye, P. M., & Wiggers, J. H. (2016). Systematic review of interventions to increase the delivery of preventative care by primary care nurses and allied health clinicians. *Implementation Science, 11,* 50. Retrieved from https://implementationscience.biomedcentral.com/articles/10.1186/s13012-016-0409-3

McNair, P., & Lewis, G. (2012). Levels of evidence in medicine. *International Journal of Sports Physical Therapy, 7*(5), 474–481.

Melnyk, B., Fineout-Overholt, E., Stillwell, S., & Williamson, K. (2009). Igniting a spirit of inquiry: An essential foundation for evidence-based practice. *American Journal of Nursing, 109*(11), 49–52. doi:10.1097/01.NAJ.0000363354.53883.58

National Collaborating Centre for Methods and Tools. (2011). *PARiHS framework for implementing research into practice.* Hamilton, ON: McMaster University. (Updated 30 March, 2011). Retrieved from http://www.nccmt.ca/resources/search/85

Olsen, L., Aisner, D., & McGinnis, J. M. (Eds.). (2007). *The learning health care system: Workshop summary (IOM roundtable on evidence-based medicine).* Washington, DC: The National Academies Press.

Pearson, A. (2010). The Joanna Briggs Institute model of evidence-based health care as a framework for implementing evidence. In J. Rycroft-Malone & T. Bucknall (Eds.), *Models and frameworks for implementing evidence-based practice: Linking evidence to action* (chap. 9). Sigma Theta Tau International. Malden, MA: Wiley-Blackwell.

Pearson, A., Wiechula, W., Court, A., & Lockwood, C. (2007). A re-constitution of what constitutes "evidence" in the health care professions. *Nursing Science Quarterly, 20*(1), 85–88 doi:10.1177/0894318406296306

Quality and Safety Education for Nurses (QSEN). (2012). *Evidence-based practice.* Retrieved from http://qsen.org/competencies/pre-licensure-ksas/

Rogers, E. M. (2003). *Diffusion of innovation* (5th ed.). New York, NY: Free Press.

Rycroft-Malone, J., & Bucknall, T. (2010). *Models and frameworks for implementing evidence-based practice: Linking evidence to action.* Sigma Theta Tau International. Malden, MA: Wiley-Blackwell.

Sackett, D. L., Rosenberg, W. M., Gray, J. A., Haynes, R. B., & Richardson, W. S. (1996). Evidence based medicine: What it is and what it isn't. *British Medical Journal, 312*(7023), 71–72.

Sahota, N., Lloyd, R., Ramakrishna, A., Mackay, J. A., Prorok, J. C., Weise-Kelly, L., ... Brian Haynes, R. (2011). Computerized clinical decision support systems for acute care management: A decision-maker-researcher partnership systematic review of effects on process of care and patient outcomes. *Implementation Science* (6)91. doi:10.1186/1748-5908-6-91

Shay, L. A., & Lafata, J. E. (2015). Where is the evidence? A systematic review of shared decision making and patient outcomes. *Medical Decision Making: An International Journal of the Society for Medical Decision Making, 35*(1), 114–131. doi:10.1177/0272989X14551638.

Titler, M. G. (2008). The evidence for evidence-based practice implementation. In R. G. Hughes (Ed.), *Patient safety and quality: An evidence-based handbook for nurses.* Rockville, MD: Agency for Healthcare Research and Quality (US). Retrieved from https://www.ncbi.nlm.nih.gov/books/NBK2659/

Titler, M. G., Kleiber, C., Steelman, V. J., Rakel, B. A. Budreau, G., Everett, L.Q., ... Goode, C. (2001). The IOWA model of evidence-based practice to promote quality care. *Critical Care Nursing Clinics of North America, 13*(4), 497–509. doi:10.1188/14.CJON.157-159

Truglio-Londrigan, M., Slyer, J. T., Singleton, J. K., & Worral, P. S. (2014). A qualitative systematic review of internal and external influences on shared decision-making in all health care settings. *JBI Database of Systematic Reviews & Implementation Reports, 12*(5), 121–194. doi:10.11124/jbisrir-2012-432

Tuti, T., Nzinga, J., Njoroge, M., Brown, B., Peek, N., English, M., Paton, C., & van der Veer, S. N. (2017). A systematic review of electronic audit and feedback: Intervention effectiveness and use of behavior change theory. *Implementation Science, 12*(61). doi:10.1186/s13012-017-0590-z

White, K. M., Dudley-Brown, S., & Terhaar, M. F. (2016). *Translation of evidence into nursing and health care* (2nd ed.). New York, NY: Springer Publishing.

SUGGESTED READINGS

Carter, M. J. (2010). Evidence-based medicine: An overview of key concepts. *Ostomy Wound Management, 56*(4), 68–85.

Ferguson, L. M., & Day, R. A. (2007). Challenges for new nurses in evidence-based practice. *Journal of Nursing Management, 15*(1), 107–113. doi:10.1111/j.1365-2934.2006.00638.x

Fineout-Overholt, E. (2008). Synthesizing evidence: How far can your confidence meter take you? *AACN Advanced Critical Care, 19*(3), 335–339. doi:10.1097/01.AACN.0000330385.64637.5d

Gerrish, K., McDonnell, A., Nolan, M., Guillaum, Y., Kirshbaum, M., & Tod, A. (2011). The role of advanced practice nurses in knowledge brokering as a means of promoting evidence-based practice among clinical nurses. *Journal of Advanced Nursing, 67*(9), 2004–2014. doi:10.1111/j.1365-2648.2011.05642.x

National Council of State Boards of Nursing (NCSBN). (2017). *Evidence-based nursing education*. Retrieved from https://www.ncsbn.org/668.htm

Rauen, C., Vollman, K., Arbour, R., & Chulary, M. (2008). Challenging nursing's sacred cows. *American Nurse Today, 3*(4), 23–26.

Van Achterberg, T., Schoonhoven., & Grol, R. (2008). Nursing implementation science: How evidence-based nursing requires evidence-based implementation. *Journal of Nursing Scholarship, 40*(4), 302–310. doi:10.1111/j.1547-5069.2008.00243.x

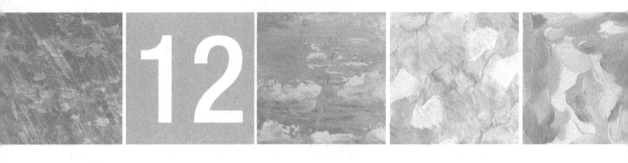

12

PATIENT SAFETY

Christine Rovinski-Wagner and Peter D. Mills

Fundamentally, nursing is doing things for patients that, if well, they could do themselves. Nurses are a human connection between the complex health care system and the patient. From bed baths to managing intra-aortic balloon pumps, nurses meet patient care requirements through empathy and applied science, matching interventions with assessed needs. This blend of empathy, healthcare system expertise, and scientific application puts nurses in a unique position to recognize risk and prevent patient harm (Douglas Howard, personal communication, 2017).

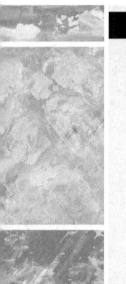

Upon completion of this chapter, the reader should be able to

1. Define safety.
2. Discuss the quality measures of structure, process, and the monitoring of outcomes related to a safe healthcare system.
3. Describe the components necessary for the nurse and interprofessional team to create a culture of safety in a healthcare environment, that is, leadership, measurement, risk identification and reduction, and teamwork.
4. Describe how utilization management (UM) supports a culture of safety.
5. Discuss the overuse, underuse, and misuse of healthcare services.
6. Describe the difference between a person approach and a system approach to patient care safety.
7. Discuss strategies that reduce variation in healthcare delivery and standardize the provision of safe patient care.
8. Identify characteristics of organizations that sustain and spread healthcare safety.
9. Discuss current safety initiatives in healthcare.
10. Discuss safety initiatives for healthcare staff.

M r. Williams is an 82-year-old man with resolving pneumonia. He lives alone and has residual right-sided weakness from an old cerebral vascular accident. During the 2 days that Mr. Williams has been under your care, you have observed him borrowing salt from his roommate's tray, forgetting to use his walker, and insisting on reusing another patient's cloth handkerchiefs because he states that using cloth is better for the environment. The physical therapy and social work consults have not been completed.

1. *What actions could you take to engage Mr. Williams in appropriate self-care management?*
2. *What actions could you take as a nurse to support Mr. Williams's safety?*
3. *What actions could you take within your healthcare system to support Mr. Williams's safety?*

In this chapter, we define and discuss safety and describe four components necessary for the nurse and interprofessional team to create a culture of safety in a healthcare environment: leadership, measurement, risk identification and reduction, and teamwork. We discuss quality structures, processes, and the monitoring of outcomes related to a safe healthcare system. The role of utilization management (UM) in supporting patient safety and the overuse, underuse, and misuse of healthcare services is discussed. The difference between a person approach and a system approach to the process of eliminating harm to patients and improving patient safety is reviewed. We introduce strategies that reduce variation in healthcare delivery and standardize the provision of safe patient care. Characteristics of organizations that sustain and spread healthcare safety are identified. We discuss current safety initiatives in healthcare, such as reduction of workforce bullying, healthcare rankings, safe staffing, medication safety, nurses with **impairing conditions**, hand hygiene, safe patient handling and mobility (SPHM), suicide prevention, environmental safety, safe patient handoffs, and **rapid response teams** (RRTs). Finally, we discuss safety for healthcare staff.

STRUCTURES, PROCESSES, AND OUTCOMES IN A SAFE HEALTHCARE SYSTEM

Safety is the process of minimizing risk of harm to patients and providers through both system effectiveness and individual performance (QSEN Institute, 2017). Safety does not occur naturally or without effort. Nurses utilize their leadership and management skills to work with the interprofessional team to set up or structure healthcare systems to provide safe outcomes for patients. Nurses also use safe activities or processes to achieve safe, high-quality outcomes. Nurses use all these structure and process resources to create, nurture, and sustain safe outcomes. In a safe healthcare system, nurses and the interprofessional team identify and fix quality problems before a patient and/or staff is harmed. When a nurse accepts a patient care assignment, the nurse will develop and/or use a healthcare system's elements of safe, high-quality structures and processes to ensure safe, high-quality patient outcomes (Table 12.1).

When a nurse comes on duty to the emergency department (ED) and is assigned four empty patient rooms, the nurse checks the healthcare system's safety structures, that is, supplies, suction equipment, and patient monitors in the four rooms. The nurse verifies that safe healthcare processes are in place and checks her assignment and responsibilities with the physician, other nurses, and nursing assistive personnel. Then the nurse is ready for the arrival of a patient needing emergency healthcare, having ensured that the structures and processes are in place to ensure the outcomes of patient safety and quality patient care. "Maintaining safety reflects a level of compassion and vigilance for patient welfare that is as important as any other aspect of competent health care" (Stone, Hughes, & Dailey, 2008).

TABLE 12.1 NURSING IN A SAFE, HIGH-QUALITY HEALTHCARE ENVIRONMENT

QUALITY MEASURE	EXAMPLE
Structure—The setting where healthcare occurs. Includes physical facility structures, ventilation systems, hospital equipment, human resources, staffing, etc.	• The patient environment, staffing, and access to the interprofessional team and supervisor are set up and structured to ensure patient safety and quality care before beginning patient care. • Quality patient standards are put in place by the nurse and interprofessional team to ensure delivery of quality patient care with a high degree of reliability. • A just, fair-minded spirit that realizes that errors are often system problems, not just individual problems, is in place so that when errors in patient care occur, review of the entire system that led to the error occurs, not just review of the performance of the individual involved. • Patient care assignment sheets are in place to communicate elements of patient care to the interprofessional team.
Process—All actions in healthcare delivery. Includes the process of diagnosis and treatment, the technical way care is delivered, and the interpersonal way care is delivered.	• The nurse utilizes hospital policies that reflect the Five Rights of Delegation (National Council of State Boards of Nursing, 2015). The Five Rights of Delegation specify leadership and supervisor involvement, chain of command, and the actions to take when delegating care. They also specify follow-up and remediation when indicated. • The nurse and interprofessional team follow evidence-based policy and procedure, patient care standards, guidelines, bundles, and so on, when giving patient care. • The nurse and interprofessional team set priorities when delivering patient care processes to ensure patient safety.
Outcomes—The effects of healthcare on patients and staff. Includes changes in patient and staff knowledge, behavior, health status, cost, and patient satisfaction.	• The nurse and interprofessional team monitor the following outcomes on an ongoing basis: patient clinical outcomes, patient satisfaction, patient safety, staff safety, staff satisfaction, staff adherence to policy and procedure and evidence-based standards, and key healthcare structures and processes.

Financial Consequences

Safety has major financial consequences for patients, providers, insurers, family, and/ or caregivers. One study suggested that the potentially preventable complications of urinary tract infection (UTI) and pneumonia resulted in a five-patient increase in the average daily census in a hospital as well as a two to three times longer lengths of stay for these patients, the extra lengths of stay costing up to $3,000,000 for a 9-month period (Lagoe, Johnson, & Murphy, 2011). The length of hospital stay is also associated with an increase in risk of harm to patients including hospital-acquired infections and death. The way to improve safety is to learn about the causes of error and to use this knowledge to design safe systems of care to reduce the incidence and harm from errors.

A CULTURE OF SAFETY

Safety flourishes best when it is part of an organization's culture of safety. The term, **culture** broadly relates to the norms, values, beliefs, and assumptions shared by members of an organization or a distinctive subculture within an organization (Schein & Schein, 2016). The term **culture of safety** refers to the extent to which individuals and groups will:

- Commit to personal responsibility for safety
- Act to preserve, enhance, and communicate safety concerns
- Strive to actively learn, adapt, and modify both individual and organizational behavior based on lessons learned from mistakes
- Strive to be honored in association with these values (von Thaden & Gibbons, 2008)

There are four important components of a culture of safety in healthcare: leadership, measurement, risk identification and reduction, and teamwork (Table 12.2). A healthcare organization that wants to strengthen its culture of safety may also incorporate the components of high reliability organizations (HROs): preoccupation with failure, reluctance to simplify, sensitivity to operations, commitment to resilience, and deference to expertise. HROs are organizations that achieve a culture of safety in dangerous environments, for example, aviation, and nuclear energy. HROs are discussed more in Chapter 4.

Nurses who role-model behaviors that support a culture of safety recognize and honor when others do the same are demonstrating nursing leadership, regardless of their positions. A culture of safety in a healthcare organization allows for the greatest reduction in accidental harm to patients. A culture of safety allows for healthcare delivery that is replicable, or can be reproduced in another healthcare organization, and reliable regardless of the day of the week, area of patient care, patient transfers, or patient background. In other words, a healthcare organization with a culture of safety can be relied upon to deliver the right care to the right patient at the right time in the right setting.

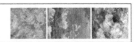

CRITICAL THINKING 12.1

A hospital identified a steady increase in the occurrence of hospital-acquired catheter-associated urinary tract infections (CAUTIs) during a 3-month period. Review of the medical records revealed the average length of inpatient stay for these patients was over 5 days, two nurses did most of the urinary catheter insertions, and more than half of the patients were postoperative hip replacement. Further review of all medical records for postoperative hip replacement patients from the same 3-month period revealed that about a third of these patients experienced a urinary tract infection (UTI). The hospital and nursing leadership decide that an improvement team should be formed to address reduction of CAUTI incidence.

1. Who should be included on the CAUTI length of stay team and why?
2. How should the association between the two nurses and the increase in UTIs be addressed?

TABLE 12.2 BEHAVIORS SEEN IN A CULTURE OF SAFETY IN HEALTHCARE

CULTURE OF SAFETY IN HEALTHCARE	BEHAVIORS
Leadership	• Responding with a system approach to safety disruptions, for example, when a nurse exhibits reckless behavior by not wearing gloves during dressing changes on an infected methicillin-resistant Staphylococcus aureus wound, leadership would consider the availability of gloves, staffing ratios, etc., as well as the need for nursing reeducation and competency testing. • Encouraging nurses and all staff to assume leadership and report any unsafe conditions that could lead to patient falls. • Being sensitive to reports of any deviations from standard safety protocols even if this slows down work, for example, encouraging incident reports about safety near misses. New misses are unplanned occurrences that did not result in injury, illness or damage, but had the potential to do so.
Measurement	• Designing the healthcare system to encourage development of evidence-based practices and measuring the outcomes of evidence-based practices as they are developed and implemented. • Ensuring that removing steps from a healthcare process will not cause more or other adverse events and tracking the number of adverse events after the steps are removed.
Risk identification and reduction	• Identifying risks and reducing the possibility that an adverse event can happen, for example, adding safe patient handling instructions to a care plan for a patient with right-sided weakness. • Designing healthcare systems to avoid errors before they cause harm or result in an adverse event, for example, by using a checklist to guide nurses in the timely use of preoperative antibacterial cloths.
Teamwork	• Watching each other's back and working together to ensure patient safety. • Engaging patients in health promotion/disease prevention through interprofessional and patient-centered strategies. • Empowering the people with the greatest expertise in a specific area to help resolve a potential safety concern rather than always deferring to the person with the highest rank, for example, on a safety quality improvement team, including staff who actually use the healthcare processes being examined.

Leadership

Nursing leadership in a culture of safety acknowledges the high-risk nature of the organization's activities and empowers all nurses and employees to report safety hazards. Nursing leaders create and sustain a blame-free environment. Employees feel confident that there will be no negative consequences in communicating safety problems to supervisors. Nurse leaders support the idea that every nurse is a leader and manager responsible for safe, high-quality care. If a patient's safety is threatened, nurses speak up and work with the interprofessional team and administration to manage the environment for patient safety. Nurses are personally involved in seeking and understanding gaps in patient safety, making safety a priority, and committing organizational resources needed to close any performance gaps in providing

TABLE 12.3 LEADERSHIP ACTIVITIES THAT SUPPORT A CULTURE OF SAFETY

LEADERSHIP GROUP	ACTIVITIES SUPPORTING A CULTURE OF SAFETY
Hospital boards	Include safety as a standing item on board agenda. Establish an organizational baseline measure of safety culture performance. Include representatives with clinical expertise on the board.
Hospital administration and nurse leaders and managers	Integrate patient safety into every activity in the organization. Create an annual patient safety award to recognize outstanding teamwork in making patient care safer. Listen to the bedside nurse to identify obstacles that are encountered in daily work and continue to enhance patient safety and staff competencies. Implement policies that ensure that nurses are safe and have adequate resources at work. Provide clinical nursing supervision. Include nurses in decisions that affect their work environments.
Peer review committees	Focus on clinical practice measured against professional standards. Review and evaluate patient records for quality and appropriateness of services ordered or performed by their professional peers. Identify practice patterns that indicate a need for more knowledge.
Staff nurse leaders	Motivate and encourage staff nurse leaders to deliver safe, high-quality patient care through timely and meaningful feedback. Maintain competency in evidence-based practice. Utilize opportunities for professional development.

safe, high-quality care consistently. In a culture of safety, successful hospital boards and nursing leaders use specific measures of safe performance to monitor quality improvement (QI). They hold all nurses accountable for high levels of quality and safety, they learn from best practices in the healthcare field, and they implement new knowledge within their organizations. Healthcare and nursing leaders in cultures of safety are sensitive to the daily operations of their organizations and they encourage nursing leadership and collaboration across the organization's hierarchies, reporting structures, and interprofessional roles (Table 12.3).

NURSE LEADER AND MANAGER

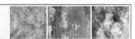

Capt. Mary Lee Mills, (Ret.), USPHS, MSN, MPH, RN, CNM, overcame racial, gender, class, and societal barriers to dramatically improve public health and nursing. Her portrait is featured with 33 distinguished African Americans at the Smithsonian Institution in Washington, DC. Read more about her at www.nursingworld.org/halloffame.

Measurement

The second component of a culture of safety is measurement. Measurement provides information and feedback to leadership and clinicians about a culture of safety and its clinical outcomes. Nurses promote a culture of safety by posting outcome graphs and safety dashboards (Figure 12.1) on their units. When the nurses look at this dashboard, they can see the trend-line dashes that show a decrease in falls from the first quarter of 2015 to the first quarter of 2017. This trend tells the staff that the activities undertaken to reduce the number of falls has been effective but that further work is needed to continue to reduce fall events. A data display or dashboard is designed to help facilities identify and target areas for QI and promote safe practices.

Clinical outcomes associated with patient safety such as patient falls and risk-adjusted mortality and morbidity are measured, tracked, and analyzed in a culture of safety. In-hospital mortality in healthy patients who were not expected to die based on the condition of the patient upon admission is reviewed. Measurement and analysis of how and what clinicians feel about their work environment are also reviewed and can predict whether nurse and patient safe outcomes will be positive or negative. A positive culture of safety is associated with fewer adverse events.

Measurement in a culture of safety will often include use of the Institute for Healthcare Improvement (IHI) Global Trigger Tool for Measuring Adverse Events, available at www.ihi.org/resources/Pages/IHIWhitePapers/IHIGlobalTriggerTool WhitePaper.aspx (Griffin & Resar, 2009).

The IHI Global Trigger Tool methodology includes a retrospective review of a random sample of patient records using "triggers" (or clues) to identify possible adverse events. The IHI Global Trigger Tool includes a specific list of triggers and their definitions; detailed information on using the methodology; and step-by-step instructions for establishing a review team and using the tool to accurately identify adverse events (harm) and measure the rate of adverse events over time.

Triggers can identify the need to examine a patient care record more carefully to determine if there were any problems in care delivery, for example, if there is evidence that the patient received a blood transfusion, this may indicate there was an episode of patient bleeding during the hospitalization. See Box 12.1 that presents the IHI Global Trigger Tool list of triggers.

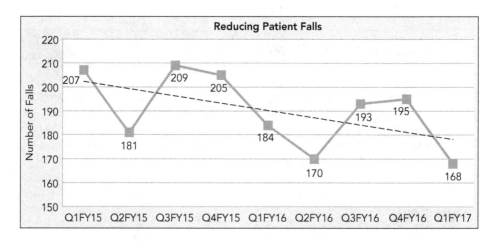

FIGURE 12.1 Example of dashboard displaying the safety measure of patient fall occurrence.

Source: Created by the author based on information from the Department of Veterans Affairs Patient Safety Center of Inquiry (PSCI) on Measurement to Advance Patient Safety (2017).

BOX 12.1 Institute for Healthcare Improvement (IHI) Global Trigger Tool

---

Available at app.ihi.org/webex/gtt/ihiglobaltriggertoolwhitepaper2009.pdf

A. General
- Transfusion of blood or use of blood products
- Code, cardiac or pulmonary arrest, or rapid response team activation
- Acute dialysis
- Positive blood culture
- X-ray or Doppler studies for emboli or deep vein thromboses
- Decrease in hemoglobin or hematocrit of 25% or greater
- Patient fall
- Pressure ulcers
- Readmission within 30 days
- Restraint use
- Healthcare-associated infections
- In-hospital stroke
- Transfer to higher level of care
- Any procedure complication

B. Medication Triggers
- *Clostridium difficile* positive stool if history of antibiotic use
- PTT >100 seconds if on heparin
- INR >6 if on anticoagulants
- Glucose <50 mg/dL if on insulin or oral hypoglycemics
- Rising BUN or serum creatinine two times (2×) over baseline if on meds known to cause renal toxicity
- Vitamin K administration if evidence of bruising, GI bleed, hemorrhagic stroke, or large hematomas
- Diphenhydramine (Benadryl) administration
- Romazicon (flumazenil) administration
- Naloxone (Narcan) administration
- Antiemetic administration for drug
- Oversedation/hypotension
- Abrupt medication stop

C. Surgical Triggers
- Return to surgery
- Change in procedure
- Admission to intensive care postoperatively
- Intubation or reintubation or use of BiPap in PACU
- X-ray intraoperatively or in PACU
- Intra- or postoperative death
- Mechanical ventilation >24 hours postoperatively
- Intraoperative administration of epinephrine, norepinephrine, naloxone, or Romazicon
- Postoperative increase in troponin levels >1.5 ng/mL
- Occurrence of any operative complication

D. Intensive Care Triggers
- Pneumonia onset
- Readmission to the ICU

(continued)

BOX 12.1 Institute for Healthcare Improvement (IHI) Global Trigger Tool (*continued*)

- In-unit procedure
- Intubation/reintubation
- Intubation or reintubation or use of BiPap in postanesthesia care
E. Perinatal Maternal Triggers
  - Terbutaline use
  - 3rd- or 4th-degree lacerations
  - Platelet count <50,000
  - Estimated blood loss >500 mL for vaginal delivery or >1,000 mL for cesarean delivery
  - Specialty consult
  - Administration of oxytocic agents, for example, oxytocin, methylergonovine, and 15-methyl-prostaglandin postpartum
  - Instrumented delivery
  - Administration of general anesthesia
F. ED Triggers
  - Readmission to the ED within 48 hours
  - Time in ED >6 hours

BUN, blood urea nitrogen. INR, international normalized ratio; PACU, postanesthesia care unit; PTT, partial thromboplastin time.

Source: Griffin, F. A., & Resar, R. K. (2009). *IHI global trigger tool for measuring adverse events* (2nd ed.). IHI Innovation Series white paper. Cambridge, MA: Institute for Healthcare Improvement;. Retrieved from http://www.ihi.org/resources/Pages/IHIWhitePapers/IHIGlobalTriggerToolWhitePaper.aspx

Risk Identification and Reduction

Risk identification and reduction, the third component of a culture of safety, studies human error and reduces factors that contribute to human error. Risks are identified both prospectively (looking forward) and retrospectively (looking backward). The examination of any human error associated with these risks analyzes the different factors contributing to the ways that humans make mistakes. Human factors engineering uses what we know about the way humans think, how humans' minds and bodies work, and how humans interact with the environment to make products and processes that are safer to use. Unconscious human safety errors, for example, forgetting to give a medication to a patient or picking up the wrong medication syringe, may derive from a breakdown in an automatic human behavior or a temporary lapse in memory. These breakdowns and lapses leading to unconscious human errors can be influenced by both environmental external factors such as distractions, noise, and time pressure, and by internal factors such as fatigue, expectations about the future, and anxiety. Conscious human safety errors involve a breakdown in a human's decision-making process, for example, a work-around. **Work-arounds** occur when one does not follow the rules and/or works around the rules or correct actions of a patient care process or a work process in order to save time (Table 12.4).

Human beings are prone to making safety errors because we have limited capacity in our short-term memory. Safety improves when we use strategies to reduce reliance on memory. For example, a patient with congestive heart failure (CHF) will be at risk if intake and output amounts are not documented at the time they are measured. It is unlikely that the intake and output amounts can be accurately remembered at the end of a busy shift because human beings have a limited capacity to recall facts. In addition, humans are susceptible to a bias in thinking, which can distort perceptions. For example,

TABLE 12.4 WORK-AROUND EXAMPLES

CORRECT ACTION	WORK-AROUND
Follow up on an alert from an electronic medication administration system about a potentially dangerous drug interaction.	Override an alert from an electronic medication administration record about a potentially dangerous drug interaction.
Read the label of a medication pulled from the drawer in an electronic medication administration system to ensure the "right medication."	Assume that the medication in the drawer is correct and not check the label of a medication pulled from the medication drawer.
Return shared blood pressure cuffs to a central access area when staff has to share the equipment.	Hide the blood pressure cuff so that it is only handy for one clinician.
Bar-code patient medications into an electronic medication administration record at the time the patient takes the medication.	Have another copy of patient wristbands in the nursing station and bar code them all at once, then pass the medications.
Check a patient every 15 minutes as prescribed.	Record all 15-minute patient checks at the beginning of the shift.

if you have been using a specific type of infusion pump on one unit and then you float to another unit, you may assume that the new unit has the same infusion pump. You can use your bias in thinking and make a programming error on the new infusion pump and give the wrong dose of medication if you do not check directions for the new infusion pump. It is probably impossible to eliminate all human errors in healthcare. However, it is possible and very important to work to design a culture of safety that can prevent as many errors as possible before any potential harm caused by errors reaches the patient. For example, white boards used to communicate patient information that are placed on the unit and in patient rooms can reduce the risk of errors that occur through misinterpreted or unclear communication between nurses and physicians.

Teamwork

Teamwork, the fourth component of a culture of safety, must be valued and be evident in healthcare. For safe care to be delivered in today's highly complex healthcare systems, it is critical for clinicians to collaborate in interprofessional teams of nurses, physicians, pharmacists, dieticians, and so on. It is often impossible to safely deliver care, monitor patients, document treatments, and manage changes in the health status of multiple patients while working alone. Interprofessional teams can back each other up, identify potential safety hazards, find solutions to patient safety problems, and provide patient care effectively. For good working teams to exist there must be mutual respect, understanding of respective roles, and trust. For example, when an attending physician asks a student nurse to accompany the medical resident team on morning rounds and provide the nursing assessment about the patient, the physician is showing respect and trust for the student as part of the healthcare team.

Psychological safety is another aspect of teamwork. Psychological safety means one can speak up or ask questions without being afraid of being punished. Staff is more likely to report a mistake when they believe they work in a psychologically safe healthcare organization because there is less fear of reprisal for reporting.

Communication is an essential part of teamwork. One method of communication is called "3Ws©," that is: What I see, What I am concerned about, What I want (Sculli & Sine, 2011).

Nurses can use the 3Ws to avoid suboptimal forms of team communication, and gain timely resolution to clinical concerns and conflicts. For example, the nurse can say to a physician about a surgical patient: "The patient's blood pressure is 90/50; I am concerned that the patient is bleeding internally; I want you to come and evaluate the patient immediately." Using the 3Ws, nurses can convey feedback that is specific, direct, and concise in real time. When the 3Ws are used, there is little doubt on the part of the physician what the nurse's concerns are and what the nurse wants to happen to keep the patient safe.

Teamwork and improved patient safety can also be fostered through programs such as TeamSTEPPS. TeamSTEPPS is an evidence-based system that can enhance individual attitudes about teamwork, increase knowledge about effective team practice, and improve team skills. TeamSTEPPS is discussed more in Chapter 8.

EVIDENCE FROM THE LITERATURE

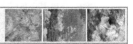

Citation

Marsa, L. (September, 2017). *Take charge of your health care: How to research a surgeon* (p. 20).

Discussion

Here is a four-step process to check a surgeon's background and skills.

1. Confirm state credentials. The Federation of State Medical Boards at www.fsmb.org can tell you if a surgeon is licensed in your state. Click on Consumer Resources, and then click on Learn About Your Physician.
2. Confirm surgical certification. Check with the American Board of Medical Specialties at www.certificationmatters.org, or call 866-ASK-ABMS.
3. Uncover professional reprimands. For a $9 fee, the Federation of State Medical Boards at www.fsmb.org will share the disciplinary history of specific doctors in any state. Click on Credentialing, then click on Physician Data Services on its website. State medical boards also have physician profiles that include board certifications, board actions, criminal convictions and medical malpractice claims. The Federation of State Medical Boards has links to state websites. Go to www.fsmb.org/policy/contacts.
4. Check ratings, procedures and complications. Plug in your ZIP code at www.projects.propublica.org/surgeons. You'll find a directory of local hospitals that perform eight common procedures, along with surgeons on staff who perform them, the number of procedures they've done, and their complication rates. www.surgeonratings.org compares surgeons results for 12 types of surgery performed by 50,000 surgeons.

Implications for Nursing
Information about surgeons is useful in avoiding surgical problems.

THE ROLE OF UTILIZATION MANAGEMENT IN SUPPORTING A CULTURE OF SAFETY

UM is a process of patient case management using evidence-based and standardized criteria such as the McKesson InterQual® reference to evaluate a patient's level of care from hospital admission to discharge. UM supports patient safety by promoting shorter patient lengths of stay and reduced patient readmissions to the hospital through the use of evidence-based decisions about patient care delivery. Prolonged hospital stays are associated with a higher frequency of complications and increased risk of hospital-acquired conditions including infections and skin breakdown. The patient receives the healthcare services and supplies that are no more or less than the patient needs at that particular point in time. Evidence-based criteria are used along with interprofessional team judgment to measure the appropriateness of the patient's level of care.

UM facilitates cooperative teamwork and clear and effective communication among the patient's healthcare providers. For example, an interprofessional team caring for a group of medical–surgical patients meets daily to discuss each patient's readiness for discharge or transfer. The team reviews and, as necessary, revises the care plans to support each patient's progress toward a timely and appropriate discharge. The nurse caring for the patient contributes information about the patient's pain and symptom management and learning needs. The utilization manager reviews objective patient and clinical data, imaging studies, and laboratory findings. UM provides the information needed to know if, given a patient's current status, the patient could receive healthcare services in a different level of care, such as at home (Table 12.5).

The UM comparison helps evaluate whether the service intensity, which is the amount and type of hospital care services provided to the patient, is appropriate for

TABLE 12.5 UTILIZATION MANAGEMENT (UM) PROCESS

DIAGNOSIS	PATIENT INFORMATION FROM MEDICAL RECORD	INTERPROFESSIONAL TEAM DISCUSSION	UM REVIEW
Pneumonia	Day 5 of hospitalization. Chest x-ray shows left lower lobe infiltrate resolving; temperature 98.8° F. Oxygen saturation between 96% and 99%. Patient remains on oral antibiotics.	Physician: There are no medical contraindications to discharge. Nurse: Patient is no longer using oxygen. There have been no instances of labored respirations observed by staff or reported by patient. Physical therapist: Patient is ambulating in corridors at least four times/day and is using a cane appropriately. Social worker/case manager: Home healthcare referral is completed. Patient's wife will drive him home.	Patient no longer meets acute care InterQual Day 5 continuing stay criteria for pneumonia as patient's temperature is below 99.4° F, oxygen saturation is above 92%, and there are no complications or active comorbidities or other problems.

Source: Created with material from McKesson InterQual Evidence-Based Clinical Content (2017)

the particular patient and follows the standards. Evidence-based recommendations are made by UM to the patient's healthcare team and the patient may be transferred to a different level of care as a result. For example, a patient with an exacerbation of chronic obstructive lung disease may be transferred from an ICU to a medical patient care unit as the patient's breathing improves and the need for hourly respiratory therapy interventions and one-to-one nursing care decreases.

The findings from UM reviews are tracked and measured to help leadership determine if patients are consistently admitted to the most appropriate level of care, transitioned to the most appropriate level of care, and discharged in a timely manner to help prevent patient readmission to the hospital. For example, hospital leadership at an acute care hospital approves creation of a substance abuse residential rehabilitation unit after analyzing utilization review data showing that a large number of patients admitted to the medical unit for detoxification are readmitted for another detoxification within 30 days of discharge. Further examination of the utilization review data revealed a lack of available residential substance abuse rehabilitation facilities. Leadership also noted the need for more teaching and follow-up pre- and postdischarge of these patients. The utilization review data enabled hospital leadership to improve the healthcare services provided to people with substance abuse problems. UM review data can also help identify overuse, underuse, and misuse of healthcare services.

OVERUSE, UNDERUSE, AND MISUSE OF HEALTHCARE SERVICES

Overuse, underuse, and misuse of healthcare services undermine efficiency and patient safety. **Overuse of healthcare services** occurs when a healthcare service is provided even though it is not justified by the patient's healthcare needs, for example, a surgical procedure is performed on a patient even though the procedure was not clinically appropriate. Underuse of healthcare services occurs when a healthcare service is not provided even though it would have benefited the patient, for example, a patient who has a heart attack is not prescribed a beta-blocker drug at discharge from the hospital. **Misuse of healthcare services** occurs when incorrect diagnoses, medical errors, and avoidable healthcare complications occur, for example, a patient acquires an infection after a hospitalization for a surgical procedure. Overuse, underuse, and misuse of healthcare services all have the potential to cause harm or an adverse event to a patient.

A PERSON APPROACH VERSUS A SYSTEM APPROACH TO PATIENT CARE SAFETY

When an adverse patient care event occurs, it is possible to analyze what happened in different ways, that is, with a person approach to safety and/or with a system approach to safety. Too often in healthcare, we have taken only a **person approach to safety** in which we blame the person at the end of the long chain of errors for making an error that caused an adverse event from overuse, underuse, or misuse of healthcare services. A **system approach to safety** takes a broader look at an adverse event, looks at the total healthcare system in which the adverse event took place, and considers how to prevent future occurrences through QI of the total healthcare system.

For example, in a culture of safety that uses a system approach to safety, when a nurse gives a wrong dose of a medication, a fishbone diagram is used to do a root cause analysis of the total system of medication administration. The fishbone diagram in Figure 12.2 encourages the healthcare team to consider nurse characteristics, patient characteristics, practice breakdown categories, and system factors as causes of actual or potential harm to a patient in the healthcare system. Nurse characteristics may include how many years one has worked as a nurse, level of education, and years of experience on the particular unit or in the specialty. Patient characteristics may include patient age, level of cognition and mental status, and patient's willingness to participate in self-care. Practice breakdown categories may include safe medication administration, documentation, attentiveness/surveillance, clinical reasoning, prevention, intervention, interpretation of authorized provider's orders, and professional responsibility/patient advocacy. System factors may include communication, leadership/management, backup and support, environment, other health team members, staffing issues, and the healthcare team.

A culture of safety is also referred to as a just culture. A culture of safety does not absolve a nurse from personal responsibility. For example, if a nurse is discovered to be giving patients less injectable opioid analgesics than prescribed and using the drugs herself, there will be consequences for the nurse and her nursing license.

In a culture of safety, healthcare leadership fosters both a person approach and a system approach to safety. Sometimes leadership will examine trends from a large group of similar adverse events, such as falls. Data from fall events for a 3- to 6-month period can be combined and reviewed. The fall events are then separated into subsets of patient injury levels, such as falls causing serious injury and falls causing less serious injury. This separation into injury subsets allows differentiation of the causes of each subset of falls, for example, time, location, medications, environmental conditions, and so on, during

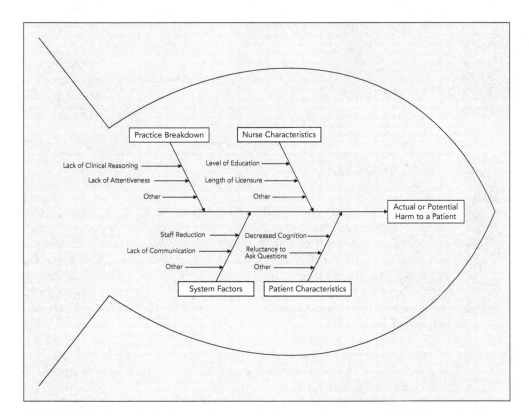

FIGURE 12.2 Use of a fishbone diagram to do a root cause analysis of a medication administration error.

the aggregate review of the falls. An aggregate review is a multistep review process in which critical factors from a group of similar adverse events, for example, falls occurring in a specific time period, are analyzed together. Based on this aggregate review, common root causes of the falls are identified and actions are developed to reduce the causes. The advantage of this aggregate review of falls is that the actions taken to improve care are based on data from multiple adverse events and so are more likely to address problems common to many of them and prevent future falls.

Healthcare leadership often partners with Risk Management (RM) to review adverse events through root cause analysis and to use the aggregated data to decrease safety risk by improving performance. RM protects the assets of the organization by identifying potential threats or actual harm and seeking to prevent and reduce injury to the organization, patients, and employees. Leadership and RM also come together to discuss the results and suggested actions from **Healthcare Failure Mode and Effect Assessments** (HFMEA). An HFMEA is a proactive step-by-step process that examines

REAL-WORLD INTERVIEW

Risk managers rely on staff compliance with patient safety measures—written policies, procedures, documentation, and evidence-based practices—to show that patients are being cared for in a safe and effective manner while meeting accepted standards of care and regulatory requirements. By collaborating with interprofessional staff, including bedside nurses, in gathering, analyzing, aggregating, and reporting patient safety data, today's risk manager is better able to help improve patient safety and to keep nurses with their patients and out of court.

Nancy C. Russell
Hospital Quality, Risk and Health Care Compliance Consultant
Etna, New Hampshire

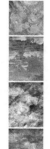

CASE STUDY 12.1

An 81-year-old male is admitted to the hospital for an acute exacerbation of his chronic obstructive pulmonary disease. He also has high blood pressure and is on several medications to control it. He uses a walker to ambulate and becomes confused at night, especially in unfamiliar environments. On his first night of admission, he got up to use the bathroom in his room, began urinating on the way to the bathroom, slipped on his urine, fell, and fractured his right hip. He had a call light and bed alarm, but by the time the staff arrived after hearing the bed alarm, he was already down on the floor.

1. *What role could communication have played in this scenario?*
2. *Are there any individual and/or system actions that would have increased the likelihood of a safe patient outcome?*
3. *Use Table 12.1 and identify a few structures, processes, and outcomes that should be set up and periodically reviewed for this type of patient.*

activities having a high possibility of a negative outcome, such as infrequent administration of an IV chemotherapeutic medication that can cause extravasation, and makes recommendations about what steps could be taken to improve patient and staff safety.

STRATEGIES THAT REDUCE VARIATION AND STANDARDIZE SAFE PATIENT CARE DELIVERY

Reducing variation or differences in care and standardizing safe patient care delivery contribute to creating a culture of safety. One way to reduce variation in patient care delivery is to examine differences in healthcare delivery that cannot be explained by illness, medical needs, or evidence-based healthcare, for example, when a nurse's care varies from the hospital's evidence-based procedure for urinary catheter care and puts the patient at risk for a UTI. Another example of variation in care delivery that negatively affects patient safety is when a nurse caring for a patient with reduced mobility feels she is short of time in her work day and chooses a work-around or short cut. The nurse is varying her patient care from the skin care standards and is not providing quality skin care for this patient. This patient is now at increased risk for decubitus ulcer formation. A nurse who applies restraints to a patient with dementia before using a behavioral intervention is varying her care from the restraints standard and negatively affecting patient safety as the patient can experience self-harm if he or she tries to get out of the restraints. This is also an example of preference-sensitive care, that is, the nurse prefers to apply restraints rather than using nonphysical interventions first. Lastly, variation in healthcare delivery can also be viewed from the point of view of examining supply and utilization concerns. For example, variation from the nurse staffing standards may cause a problem with the delivery of appropriate, adequate, and safe healthcare.

When patterns of patient care delivery vary widely, safety is compromised and patient clinical outcomes suffer. UM, discussed earlier, is one process in a culture of safety that reduces variation in healthcare delivery by using evidence-based criteria to support appropriate hospital length of stay and minimize hospital-acquired infections by shortening a patient's exposure to the many microorganisms found in hospitals. Two other effective ways to reduce variation in patient care delivery are simplification of work processes and standardization of simplified work processes. **Simplification of work processes** is the act of reducing a work process to its basic components and, in so doing, making it easier to complete the work and to understand it. Simplification of work processes requires that only the essential elements of a work process are retained. For example, when you take a patient's vital signs, you take the patient's temperature and monitor pulse and respirations. You then check the patient's blood pressure reading and ask the patient to identify the level of pain on a scale of 1 to 10. Collecting this vital sign data in this format simplifies the work process, decreases the likelihood of variation in the data set of vital signs, and improves the understanding of vital signs among health team members.

Standardization of simplified work processes in an organization facilitates safety, QI, and accurate communication by using a single set of terms, definitions, practices, and/or clinical tools, for example, bundles, routines, checklists, pathways, protocols, and guidelines to reduce variation in patient care delivery (Table 12.6). Standardization of simplified work processes makes it easier to do the right thing to improve healthcare quality and reduce complications.

TABLE 12.6 STANDARDIZED AND SIMPLIFIED WORK PROCESSES USED IN PATIENT CARE

CLINICAL TOOL	DESCRIPTION	EXAMPLE
Bundle	A small set of simple evidence-based practices, which are interventions that have enough scientific support to be considered standards of care	Use of a central line bundle daily to review the necessity of patients' central lines with prompt removal of unnecessary lines, for example, Implement the IHI Central Line Bundle. Available at www.ihi.org/knowledge/Pages/Changes
Routine	A series of actions that ordinarily is followed in a given situation	Use of hourly rounding programs can improve patients' perception of nursing responsiveness and reduce patient falls and call light use. Available at www.ncbi.nlm.nih.gov/pmc/articles/PMC4547690/
Checklist	List of reminders that help reduce healthcare variation by compensating for errors in human memory	Use of a surgical safety checklist by the nurse and anesthetist to confirm the patient's name, procedure, and where the incision will be made before the skin is cut for surgery, for example, Effect of the World Health Organization Checklist on Patient Outcomes. Available at journals.lww.com/annalsofsurgery/Fulltext/2015/05000/Effect_of_the_World_Health_Organization_Checklist.1.aspx
Pathway	Evidence-based algorithm or map that recommends clinical management and decision making based on the patient's status and needs	Use of a total knee arthroscopy pathway that has an interprofessional management plan, timeframes, anticipated clinical milestones, and outcomes, for example, total knee arthroplasty clinical pathway. Available at www.health.q1d.gov.au/_data/assets/pdf_file/0024/433851/pathway_knee.pdf
Protocol	Predetermined steps of care management for a single clinical condition. It can be individualized to a patient's needs	Use of a nurse-driven protocol to evaluate and discontinue unnecessary urinary catheters and to evaluate urinary needs after catheter removal. Available at www.ahrq.gov/professionals/quality-patient-safety/hais/cauti-tools/impl-guide/implementation-guide-appendix-m.html
Guideline	Interprofessional evidence-based recommendations for the diagnosis, management, or prevention of specific diseases or conditions that meet the needs of most patients in most circumstances. A guideline is individualized to the patient	Use of a Management of Diabetes Mellitus in Primary Care guideline to individualize the frequency of self-monitored blood glucose levels based on the frequency of insulin injections, hypoglycemic reactions, level of glycemic control, and patient/provider use of the data to adjust therapy, for example, Management of Diabetes Mellitus in Primary Care (2017). Available at www.healthquality.va.gov/diabetes_mellitus.asp

ORGANIZATIONS THAT SUSTAIN AND SPREAD HEALTHCARE SAFETY

There are many organizations that sustain and spread healthcare safe outcomes by reducing variation in healthcare practices (Table 12.7). They collect, analyze, disseminate, and share evidence-based best practices. These organizations welcome organizational membership and participation by nurses involved in the development and use of standardized clinical practice tools and strategies.

SAFETY INITIATIVES IN HEALTHCARE

Safety initiatives are programs that use standardized clinical practice tools and strategies and focus on reducing healthcare errors and improving patient safety in selected areas of healthcare (Table 12.8). Safety initiatives are often initiated by hospital leadership in a culture of safety. Employees are encouraged to communicate perceived safety issues up and down the power hierarchy of the hospital. This communication can happen in the use of incident reports and during staff meetings with nursing leaders or hospital administration. Effective communication among healthcare professionals in the work setting is essential to patient safety.

Avoidance of Workforce Bullying

One of the most lethal deterrents to effective communication is workforce bullying. **Workforce bullying** refers to both negative behaviors and verbal and nonverbal communications that nurses and other interprofessional team members may inflict on each other, such as rolling their eyes, sighing deeply or turning away every time a team member speaks, not returning phone calls, being reluctant to answer questions, and using a condescending tone of voice. Workforce bullying can go from peer to peer or from supervisor to employee. A new nurse or team member is particularly susceptible to workplace bullying. They may avoid staff interactions necessary for patient care as a means of avoiding workforce bullying. Sometimes they will adopt the behaviors of

TABLE 12.7 ORGANIZATIONS THAT SUSTAIN AND SPREAD HEALTHCARE SAFETY

ORGANIZATION	UNIQUE FEATURE
The Registered Nurses Association of Ontario, www.rnao.org	Provides mobile device downloads of nursing best practice guidelines.
Guidelines International Network (G-I-N), www.g-i-n.net	Provides the world's largest international guidelines library website.
The Cochrane Collaboration, www.cochrane.org	Uses a systematic methodology to assess healthcare research.
U.S. National Library of Medicine National Information Center on Health Services Research and Health Care Technology (NICHSR), www.nlm.nih.gov/hsrinfo/quality.html	Shares information on health services research, clinical practice guidelines, and healthcare technology, including the assessment of such technology.
Joanna Briggs Institute, joannabriggs.org/	Shares evidence-based nursing and healthcare information for nursing, healthcare providers, and consumers.

TABLE 12.8 A SAMPLING OF HEALTHCARE SAFETY INITIATIVES

INITIATIVE	EXAMPLE	SPONSORING ORGANIZATION
Medication safety	Avoid abbreviations that are associated with frequent misinterpretation and medication errors, for example, qd, MS, PCA.	ISMP Error-Prone Abbreviation List. Available at www.ismp.org/tools
Safe patient handling	Prevent falls during patient ambulation by using gait belts with handles.	Association of Safe Patient Handling Professionals Ten Strategies for Reducing Patient Handling Injuries. www.asphp.org/wp-content/uploads/2011/05/Ten_Strategies_for_Reducing_Patient_Handling_Injuries.pdf
Comprehensive unit-based safety program	Partner a senior hospital executive with a medical–surgical unit to improve communication and educate leadership.	Agency for Healthcare and Research and Quality CUSP. Available at ROVINSKI www.ahrq.gov/professionals/education/curriculum-tools/cusptoolkit/index.html
Alarm fatigue	Consider new alarm signal technologies, such as wireless notification devices/pagers, split-screen monitors.	The Johns Hopkins Hospital. Available at www.hopkinsmedicine.org/news/using_data_to_drive_alarm_improvements.html

CUSP, Comprehensive Unit-Based Safety Program; ISMP, Institute for Safe Medication Practice.

workforce bullying, seeing it as the "norm" or as a way to survive in the workplace. Many nurses prefer to quit rather than work in a healthcare system tolerant of workforce bullying. Patient safety is in jeopardy when workforce bullying occurs and is allowed to continue. For instance, staffing patterns may be negatively impacted when the number of nurse aides or healthcare technicians is increased because there are fewer nurses to assign to a unit. Recruitment of new staff may be hard for an organization when team members share their stories about workforce bullying experiences with the healthcare community. Confronting workforce bullying in an organization is difficult, but necessary. The American Psychiatric Nurses Association Task Force on Workplace Violence (www.apna.org) provides strategies for helping nurses deal with workforce bullying and creating a healthy and safe work environment.

CRITICAL THINKING 12.2

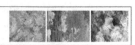

Think about the past several years of your nursing education. Focus on your classroom discussions and clinical debriefing sessions.

1. Were there times when you grew tired of hearing from a particular peer?
2. How did you respond?
3. Were any of your behaviors consistent with workforce bullying?

Comparison of Healthcare Rankings

Comparison of healthcare rankings provides nurses with a broad picture of a hospital's culture of safety. Healthcare rankings are issued by diverse groups of organizations. (These healthcare rankings are listed in another chapter.) The rankings use patient outcome data to measure and compare the safety of different healthcare facilities and organizations, nationally and worldwide. Healthcare rankings provide information on national and international benchmark data. Staff can use the data to focus their efforts and resources to improve safety by reducing risks to patients. For example, Hospital A shows a higher occurrence of hospital-acquired infections than other similar hospitals. Nurses and the interprofessional team investigate and note that the sudden increase in hospital-acquired infections is associated with recent large turnover in staff. They implement an immediate and aggressive hospital-wide education program about how to reduce hospital-acquired infections and the transmission of communicable diseases between patients and healthcare workers.

Comparisons of healthcare outcomes take on different meanings when reviewed with regional, ethnic, and racial variations. It is important to recognize how the comparison information applies to your particular practice setting and patient population. Learn the details that describe your patient population and your healthcare work setting. This information can be obtained from websites such as The American Hospital Directory, (www.ahd.com) and state-specific websites such as the Texas Center for Health Data (healthdata.dshs.texas.gov/HealthFactsProfiles). These websites provide information on the demographics of patient populations and whether these demographics are similar to other healthcare settings in the region.

EVIDENCE FROM THE LITERATURE

Citation

Marsa, L. (September, 2017). *Take charge of your health care: Choose the best hospital* (p. 27).

Discussion

The Centers for Medicare and Medicaid Services has rated 4,000 hospitals nationwide based on 57 quality measures and best practices. Plug in your ZIP code to www.medicare.gov/hospitalcompare to find report cards for hospitals in your area. They contain a large amount of useful data on patient surveys about the quality of care, timeliness and effectiveness of care, surgical complication rates, and hospital readmission and mortality rates. You can also check if the hospital is accredited by The Joint Commission at www.qualitycheck.org. Also find out hospital ratings from independent consumer advocacy groups like the LeapFrog Group at, www.leapfroggroup.org, and media sources like U.S. News & World Report at www.health.usnews.com/best-hospitals, or Consumer Reports at www.consumerreports.org/health/hospitals/ratings.

Implications for Nursing
Nurses can share information with patients about these sources.

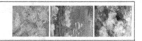

CRITICAL THINKING 12.3

Go to the Centers for Medicare and Medicaid Services (CMS) website, Hospital Compare, at www.medicare.gov/hospitalcompare/search.html. Enter your ZIP code in the designated section, select "general," and click on "find hospital." Click on the "quality of care" tab. Select two hospitals that have checkmarks in the patient safety column, and click on the "compare" button. Review the patient safety findings for each hospital. When you are done, click on the "about the data" tab and review the information there.

1. Is there a difference between the hospitals?
2. How does this information influence your perspective about either of the hospitals?

Safe Nurse Staffing

Safe nurse staffing is associated with better patient care and safe outcomes, especially better outcomes related to patient mortality; failure to rescue a patient from his or her deterioration, death, or permanent disability from a complication of healthcare or an underlying illness; and other patient outcomes sensitive to nursing care (Liu, Sheuan, Pei-Fang, Shu-Ching, & Yu-Chun, 2012).

Nurse staffing plans are guidelines that identify the number of nurses needed to provide safe and adequate care in a given healthcare setting. Fourteen states have enacted legislation or adopted regulations about nurse-to-patient ratios as of September 2015 (Agency for Healthcare Research and Quality, 2016). Nurse staffing plans are associated with patient acuity measurements. **Patient acuity** refers to the degree of healthcare service complexity needed by a patient related to this or her physical or mental status (Table 12.9). For example, patient acuity is higher for a patient who has a central line infusion than for a patient who is receiving oral medications, as the higher acuity patient with a central line infusion will need more nursing resources to provide safe care. Likewise, patients in an ICU have higher acuity and need more clinical attention due to the instability of their conditions than patients on a telemetry unit. Thus, a patient care unit with high patient acuity such as an ICU will require more nursing staff to provide safe care. The lower acuity telemetry patient care unit requires less staffing.

The nursing hours per patient day (NHPPD) calculation, used worldwide, is one of the National Database of Nursing Quality Indicators (NDNQI). The NDNQI computes nurse staffing, that is, RN and/or licensed practical nurse (LPN) staffing. The NHPPD calculation provides a measurement to compare to the desired patient acuity guidelines in the nurse staffing plan. To calculate the NHPPD, multiply the hours worked by each nurse by the number of nurses to equal total nursing hours. Divide the total nursing hours by the number of patients. The result is the nursing hours needed to care for each patient each day on the unit.

For example, 14 nurses worked on Friday on a same-day procedure unit. All nurses worked an 8-hour shift to staff the 35-bed unit that is open 12 hours daily. The unit cared for 40 patients on Friday. The number of NHPPD is 2.8 hours. To calculate the NHPPD, multiply the hours worked by each nurse by the number of nurses (8 multiplied by 14 equals 112 total nursing hours). Divide the total nursing hours by the number of patients cared for (112 divided by 40 equals 2.8 NHPPD). Neither the number of beds on the unit nor the 12 hours that the same-day unit is open are used in the calculation.

TABLE 12.9 PATIENT ACUITY AND NURSE STAFFING RATIOS

UNIT TYPE	TYPE OF PATIENTS	NURSE-TO-PATIENT STAFFING RATIO
Medical–surgical care unit	Patients who require less care than that available in ICUs, step-down units, or telemetry units and receive 24-hour inpatient general medical services, postsurgical services, or both general medical and postsurgical services.	1:5 or fewer
Telemetry unit	Patients who require more care than patients in medical–surgical units and have, or are suspected of having, a cardiac condition or a disease requiring the electronic monitoring, recording, retrieval, and display of cardiac electrical signals.	1:4 or fewer
ICU	Patients who require intensive care and need medical technology to aid, support, or replace a vital function of the body that has been seriously damaged and need specialized equipment and/or personnel providing for invasive monitoring, telemetry, or mechanical ventilation, for the immediate repair or cure of severe pathology.	1:2 or fewer

Source: Compiled from California Code of Regulations (22CCR, 70053.2 and 70217) (2014). Retrieved from https://www.cdph. ca.gov/Programs/CHCQ/LCP/CDPH%20Document%20Library/GACHRLS_Regulations_with_Survey_Procedures.pdf.

NHPPD staffing calculation can provide retrospective information for an aggregate analysis of adverse events, for example, to determine if a relationship exists between the number of patient falls during a shift and the NHPPD. If the number of patient falls increases when nursing staffing is low, this is an unsafe situation. Nurses need to take action to provide safe care for patients. Nurses can bring concerns about unsafe nurse–patient ratios to nursing and hospital leadership. Another importance of NHPPD is that it allows for comparison across hospitals. A larger comparison of data encourages collaboration between healthcare facilities and helps to more strongly justify the safety benefits of appropriate nurse staffing.

CRITICAL THINKING 12.4

You work in a long-term care facility on a 30-bed unit. Most of the patients are elderly and ambulatory with chronic medical conditions and mild-to-moderate cognitive impairment. You arrive for your evening shift and learn that the other nurse scheduled has called in sick. The evening supervisor says that she is unable to find another nurse to work with you but she will send you two extra licensed nursing assistants. This gives you a total of four licensed nursing assistants and yourself for the unit's staffing. The evening supervisor adds that you should call her if you have any problems. She says she is sure you will do fine and she will see you during her regular rounds.

1. If you feel this is an unsafe situation, what actions will you take as an individual nurse and/or as a nurse in a healthcare system?
2. What types of structures or processes should you build into this patient care unit?
3. What outcomes should be monitored on this unit?

Having more nurses does not guarantee better outcomes. However, more nurses with higher levels of basic nursing education such as a bachelor's degree and the use of standardized evidence-based clinical pathways might lead to better patient outcomes (McHugh et al., 2013). Leadership commitment to safe nurse staffing levels and effective nurse retention strategies such as zero tolerance for workforce bullying may also influence the achievement of better and safer patient outcomes due to the stability of clinical staff.

Medication Safety

Improved medication safe outcomes are seen in healthcare facilities that implement prospective and retrospective risk identification and risk reduction activities, such as working with the Institute for Safe Medication Practice (ISMP), to prevent harm to patient or staff. The ISMP (www.ismp.org) is an independent patient safety organization devoted entirely to medication error prevention and safe medication use. The ISMP sponsors a confidential, voluntary medication error reporting program and data bank on the same website, which allow analysis of system causes of medication errors. This analysis facilitates identification and sharing of the best evidence-based practices to improve medication safety. For example, an accidental programming by a pediatric nurse of an infusion pump for 10 times the dose ordered was reported to the ISMP data bank. The ISMP issued evidence-based recommendations on its website for improving patient safety during pediatric administration of IV acetaminophen, including using "smart" IV infusion pump technology when giving maximum dosages of medications and requiring pharmacy preparation of medication doses that are different from the usual strength available commercially.

Nurses With Impairing Conditions

Nurses with impairing conditions are unable to meet the requirements of the Code of Ethics and Standards of Practice of the profession. Impairing conditions are substance use disorders, psychiatric conditions, and physical conditions that can impact a nurse's ability to practice safely. Employers refer nurses with impairing conditions to boards of nursing when they have a concern about a nurse's ability to practice safely. Most state boards of nursing have alternatives-to-discipline programs. An alternatives-to-discipline program ensures patient safety by promoting early identification of nurses with impairing conditions and requiring evidence-based interventions. The benefits to the nurse include the opportunity to demonstrate to the Board of Nursing in a nondisciplinary and nonpublic manner that the nurse can become safe and remain safe while retaining his or her nursing license.

Hand Hygiene

Another risk reduction strategy in a culture of safety is a focus on hand hygiene. Hand hygiene is the single most effective way to prevent the spread of healthcare-associated infections. Hand hygiene is well suited for prospective and retrospective risk identification and risk reduction through direct observation. Although the Centers for Disease Control and Prevention (CDC) and the World Health Organization issued guidelines for hand hygiene that include having the patient remind providers to wash their hands, the compliance of healthcare workers with hand hygiene protocols is frequently low. Nurses may sometimes think that certain types of physical contact with patients are less likely to require hand washing, such as checking blood pressure or straightening bed linens. Staff is often reluctant to correct or remind coworkers to wash their hands. When done with tact and a professional demeanor, communication from one health-care clinician to another about hand hygiene is not only appropriate but can also be effective in improving hand hygiene compliance.

Safe Patient Handling and Mobility

The need for safe manual lifting, moving, and repositioning of patients reminds nurses to use evidence-based recommendations for improving patient and staff safety associated with physical movement. Appropriate safe patient handling equipment, ergonomic training and patient assessment protocols, encouragement of staff participation, and leadership support to obtain necessary resources such as ceiling mounted patient lifts, have been identified as being effective in reducing harm to patients and staff (www.tampavaref.org/safe-patient-handling/index.htm).

Suicide Prevention

Suicide is the 10th leading cause of death in the United States (CDC, www.cdc.gov/nchs/fastats/leading-causes-of-death.htm). Suicide prevention involves prospective and retrospective risk identification and risk reduction for individual patients and high-risk populations such as patients on inpatient mental health units. It is likely that nurses in all areas of the hospital will encounter suicidal patients. Nurses need to understand how to care for these patients and how to avoid an inpatient suicide. Between 2005 and 2016, 67% of suicides occurred in nonbehavioral health units and 5% occurred in EDs of general hospitals (The Joint Commission [TJC], 2017). The primary patient risk factors for suicide include previous suicide attempts and suicidal thoughts; a mental health diagnosis; physical health problems, especially problems with a poor prognosis; and social stressors, such as relationship, financial, or legal problems. In addition, patients who are members of the armed forces or in the lesbian, gay, bisexual, and transgender populations are at higher risk for suicide than the general population (Office of the Surgeon General National & Action Alliance for Suicide Prevention, 2012).

When working with a patient whom you think is suicidal, ask if the patient is thinking about hurting himself or herself or committing suicide. If the patient's answer is yes, ensure that the patient does not have access to sharps, ropes, medications, or other means of self-harm and that the patient is under continuous observation until he or she can be moved to a safe environment. Suicide prevention includes removing clothes hooks and unnecessary doors from a psychiatric unit since these could be used for a suicide by hanging. In the meantime, notify the patient's provider or the psychiatry department per your facility's protocol so that a more thorough patient evaluation can be done. Most often, suicidal patients are only feeling suicidal for a short period of time. It may be a moment of desperation when they are feeling hopeless about the future or devastated by recent losses or overwhelming social stressors. The job for nurses is to get these patients through this time without allowing the patients to hurt or kill themselves.

Environmental Safety

A safe healthcare environment minimizes potential errors and maximizes safe health-care practice. Nursing care units must be accommodating to patient needs. Door alarms alert staff when a patient goes through a door on a healthcare unit that has cognitively impaired inpatients. Pressure-sensitive bed and chair alarms alert staff to patient movement and facilitate interventions to prevent falls when a patient does not call for transfer assistance. A safe healthcare environment controls noise and keeps distractions to a minimum so that staff can focus on patient care. Nurses must be aware of "accidents waiting to happen." For example, if there is an uneven surface in the floor, nurses can report that problem so a patient does not trip and fall. The nurse must speak up. The nurse's perspective is important. Reporting unsafe situations can help change a system and prevent future adverse events.

Safe Patient Handoffs

A healthcare process that requires teamwork and is vulnerable to human errors and adverse events is the patient handoff. A **patient handoff** is the transfer of responsibility for a patient from one clinician to another and it involves sharing current information that is pertinent to the patient's care with time allowed for discussion, questions, and clarification. A patient handoff happens any time a clinician or team taking care of a patient transfers the patient to another clinician or team to continue the patient's care or provide a different type of care. For example, a patient comes into the ED and is seen by the triage nurse. The nurse takes information and does a patient handoff of information to the ED doctor who sees the patient. If the ED doctor decides to admit the patient, another patient handoff takes place between the ED doctor and ED nurse and the doctors and nurses on the patient care unit. If the patient needs surgery, there is another patient handoff from the patient care unit to the surgery team and then a patient handoff from the surgery team back to the patient care unit. At shift change, there is a patient handoff as one nurse transfers the patient's care to another nurse on the oncoming shift. Each time the patient's care is transferred to another clinician, another opportunity for critical information to be lost or misunderstood occurs.

While there are not yet any high-quality research studies to support specific best practices in the area of patient handoffs, standardized checklists are effective tools to help the nurse remember what information is important to share with another nurse. A nurse leaving the unit can use a simplified and standardized patient reporting tool to share information supporting safe patient care and confirm that the information results in the desired action. The **Situation, Background, Assessment, Recommendation, and Response (SBAR) patient reporting tool** is an example of a simplified and standardized work process used by a nurse to ensure patient safety when handing over a patient who has parenteral fluids infusing over to another nurse for continued care (Table 12.10).

Another handoff tool is the "I PASS the BATON" tool, developed by TeamSTEPPS (available at www.ahrq.gov/sites/default/files/wysiwyg/professionals/education/curriculum-tools/teamstepps/instructor/essentials/pocketguide.pdf). An estimated 80% of serious medical errors involve miscommunication between caregivers during the transfer of patients (TJC, 2012). Communication behavior in effective patient handoffs includes giving, asking, and verifying information, and relational behaviors. Relational behaviors include being warm and friendly, using easily understood language, taking steps to make the other nurse feel comfortable and relaxed, being open and honest, and showing compassion. Patient safety during handoffs is supported when both the incoming nursing and the outgoing nurse demonstrate these relational behaviors and use a standardized handoff tool.

TABLE 12.10 SBAR: SITUATION, BACKGROUND, ASSESSMENT, RECOMMENDATION, AND, RESPONSE

What is the situation?	Mr. Jones has normal saline running at 75 mL/hr. I am going to an hour-long safety in-service program.
What is the background?	I hung the normal saline infusion bag an hour ago. Mr. Jones said that his arm was "bothering" him. I put his arm on a pillow.
What is the assessment?	The normal saline infusion is running without a problem; the insertion site in his left arm is not red, swollen, or tender. He has his call bell, is able to use it, and knows that you will be covering for me.
What is the recommendation?	Please assess Mr. Jones and the normal saline infusion site several times during the next hour.
What is the response?	I will make rounds on Mr. Jones in about 10 minutes.

Source: Created with information from SBAR Toolkit, Institute for Health Care Improvement. Retrieved from www.ihi.org/resources/Pages/Tools/sbartoolkit.aspx

Rapid Response Teams

RRTs in a hospital are typically composed of an interprofessional team of critical care nurses, physicians, and respiratory therapists that are called at an early stage of a patient's clinical deterioration in the hopes of preventing a cardiac arrest or an unexpected death (psnet.ahrq.gov/primers/primer/4/rapid-response-systems for more information). A combination of patient assessment changes can also trigger a RRT such as a change in lung sounds with an increase or decrease in respiratory rate. A RRT allows staff to obtain additional assistance when the patient's condition appears to be worsening. Teamwork is the cornerstone to successful use of RRT. RRTs differ from a cardiac arrest team that is called in response to a cardiac or respiratory arrest that has already occurred. While RRTs have been widely implemented and appear to be helpful, there is controversy regarding their measurable effectiveness in reducing hospital mortality. It is hoped that RRTs prevent failure to rescue. **Failure to rescue** occurs when clinicians fail to notice patient symptoms or they fail to respond adequately or quickly enough to clinical signs that may indicate that a patient is dying of preventable complications in a hospital. Timely identification of deteriorating cardiac, neurologic, or respiratory status with prompt and appropriate subsequent action can help avoid serious adverse events in patients.

SAFETY FOR HEALTHCARE STAFF

Safety is an important concern for healthcare staff as well as patients. Healthcare staff face a number of serious safety hazards, including blood-borne pathogens and biological hazards, potential chemical and drug exposures, waste anesthetic gas exposures, respiratory hazards, ergonomic hazards from lifting and repetitive tasks, laser hazards, and workplace violence, as well as hazards associated with laboratories, radioactive material, and x-ray hazards. Safe healthcare environments control the scope and variety of chemicals in the healthcare facility, including those chemicals used for cleaning and those used in treating patients with cancer. Distribution of chemicals in a safe environment is limited to areas that have a facility-approved need to use the particular hazardous chemical. For example, in a safe healthcare environment, only housekeeping would have access to cleansing solutions used to clean rooms where patients with *Clostridium difficile* have stayed. In a culture of safety, all employees know which chemicals are in their work areas, how to use the chemicals appropriately, and how to access the related material safety data sheets (MSDSs) at their facility. MSDSs can also be found at websites such as www.ehso.com/msds.php. MSDSs contain information on the chemical makeup, use, storage, handling, emergency procedures, and potential health effects related to a hazardous material. This is the information that identifies how to reduce the risk of harm caused by chemicals.

In 2015, the healthcare and social services industry reported more work-related injury and illness cases than any other private industry sector—562,000 cases. That is 136,000 more cases than the next industry sector, manufacturing (Bureau of Labor Statistics, www.bls.gov/news.release/pdf/osh.pdf). Between January 2012 and September 2014, nurses accounted for 38% of all identified Occupational Safety and Health Administration (OSHA)-recordable injuries (Gomaa et al., 2015). Rates of patient handling and workplace violence injuries were highest among nurse assistants and nurses. Rates of slips, trips, and falls were also high for these staff. Patient handling injuries and workplace violence injuries clustered in locations providing direct patient care. Nurses are exposed to several musculoskeletal disorder risk factors including caring for overweight and acutely ill patients, long shifts, low nurse–patient ratios, and mobilization of patients almost immediately after healthcare interventions.

The consequences of work-related nursing musculoskeletal injuries, that is, chronic pain, functional disability, absenteeism, and high turnover, are substantial. As many as 20% of nurses who leave direct patient care positions do so because of risks associated with the work. Direct and indirect costs associated with back injuries in the healthcare industry are estimated to be $20 billion annually. Nurses who experience pain and fatigue may be less productive, less attentive, more susceptible to further injury, and may be more likely to affect the safety of others (OSHA, www.osha.gov/SLTC/healthcarefacilities/safepatienthandling.html). The National Public Radio (NPR) series on nurse injuries (available at www.npr.org/series/385540559/injured-nurses) provides many perspectives that relate the typical work of nurses to long-term injuries and how to prevent them

A safe healthcare environment reduces the risk of harm to patients and staff by using assistive patient handling equipment that helps lift, transfer, and reposition patients to reduce the potential for musculoskeletal injuries. A safe healthcare environment also does handling and mobility patient assessments to determine the safest way to lift and move each individual patient. Developing a culture of safety for staff as well as for patients is an important consideration in healthcare organizations today (Table 12.11).

TABLE 12.11 SAFETY RISK REDUCTION FOR HEALTHCARE STAFF

RISK CATEGORY	RISK EXAMPLE	RISK REDUCTION EXAMPLE
Biological	Drug-resistant pathogens	Change gloves and wash hands, especially after contact with body fluids, and even between procedures on the same patient to prevent cross contamination to different body sites.
Chemical	Powdered latex gloves	Use nonpowdered alternatives that do not carry any of the risks associated with glove powder, such a healthcare worker sensitization to natural rubber latex allergens.
Physical	Slips, trips, and falls	Clean spills promptly. Follow safe patient handling guidelines.
Ergonomic	Computer usage and prolonged sitting	Request ergonomic evaluation and workplace accommodation.
Psychological	Shift work and circadian rhythms	Allow sufficient time off to catch up on sleep deficit after working nights.

KEY CONCEPTS

- Safety minimizes the risk of harm to patients through system effectiveness and individual performance.
- Quality structures, processes, and the monitoring of outcomes contribute to a safe healthcare environment.
- A culture of safety has four necessary components: leadership, measurement, risk identification and reduction, and teamwork.
- Utilization management (UM) facilitates patient safety and teamwork.
- Overuse, underuse, and misuse of healthcare services increases the incidence of patient harm.
- A culture of safety is strengthened by a system approach to analysis of adverse events and work processes.
- A culture of safety reduces variation and standardizes the provision of safe patient care.
- Several organizations sustain and spread healthcare safety by sharing evidence-based best practices.
- A culture of safety improves patient care by implementing safety initiatives and programs, for example, prevention of workforce bullying, use of healthcare rankings, safe staffing, medication safety, and programs for nurses with impairing conditions, use of hand hygiene, SPHM, suicide prevention, environmental safety, safe patient handoffs, and RRTs.
- Developing a culture of safety for staff as well as for patients is an important consideration in healthcare organizations today.

KEY TERMS

Adverse event
Culture of safety
Failure to rescue
Healthcare Failure Mode and Effect
   Analysis
Impairing conditions
Misuse of healthcare services
Overuse of healthcare services
Patient acuity
Patient handoff
Person approach to safety
Psychological safety

Rapid response team
Safety
SBAR
Safety initiatives
Simplification of work processes
Standardization of simplified work
   processes
System approach to safety
Underuse of healthcare services
Utilization management
Work-arounds
Workforce bullying

REVIEW QUESTIONS

1. A patient falls and experiences a severe injury. In a culture of safety, what consequences might the assigned nurse, who never had a patient experience an injury before, reasonably anticipate? Select all that apply.

   A. Reeducation about fall risk reduction
   B. Termination of employment

C. Meeting with the risk manager
D. Being the subject of peer review
E. Being reported to the Board of Nursing
F. Being reassigned to a different unit

2. A patient is treated in the ED after a car accident. The patient says to the nurse, "I don't think I would do it but sometimes, like now, I think about ways to kill myself." Of the following, which should be the nurse's priority safety action?

   A. Contact the hospital's psychiatry service.
   B. Remove the patient's access to means of self-harm.
   C. Keep the patient under continuous observation.
   D. Alert other staff members about the patient's statement.

3. The nurse administered the wrong dose of heparin to a patient. This is classified as which of the following?

   A. Deliberate error
   B. Close call
   C. Adverse event
   D. Biased action

4. You are assisting another nurse in providing complex wound care to an alert and attentive patient. The nurse does not wash her hands between her changes of gloves and is in the middle of giving the wound care. Which of the following would be your most appropriate safety action?

   A. Do nothing. The nurse has many years of experience and knows more than you.
   B. Unobtrusively remind the nurse that her hands need to be washed between glove changes.
   C. Do nothing. Report the event to your supervisor immediately after care completion.
   D. Offer the nurse a hand sanitizer at the next glove change in the procedure.

5. The nurse is covering for another nurse who has to attend a committee meeting. During the medication administration process, the nurse notices an alert about a potentially dangerous drug interaction for a patient who has been hospitalized and taking the medication for a week. What is the nurse's safest action?

   A. Override the alert on the electronic medication administration record.
   B. Check with the pharmacy about the alert before giving the medication.
   C. Call the physician and ask for a clarification of the medication order.
   D. Administer the medication since the patient has probably been receiving it for a week.

6. A patient with a known cardiac history tells the nurse that he feels very tired, he can feel his heart beating, and he does not seem to be able to concentrate. The nurse assesses his vital signs and notes that the patient's blood pressure is much higher than usual and he is beginning to complain of chest pain. Which action should the nurse take to ensure the patient's safety?

   A. Call the RRT.
   B. Ask another nurse to assess the patient.
   C. Bring the code cart into the patient's room.
   D. Continue to assess the patient.

7. The nurse is caring for a mobile patient with orthostatic hypotension and mild dementia with some forgetfulness. Which of the following would create a safe environment for this patient? Select all that apply.

   A. Skid-resistant floor mat
   B. Dim lighting in the patient's room
   C. Ceiling-mounted transfer equipment
   D. Bed alarm
   E. Chair alarm
   F. Bright lighting in the patient's room

8. An incoming nurse has many questions about a patient's complex care but is hesitant to ask the offgoing nurse who is sighing heavily and repeatedly looking at the clock. This is an example of which of the following?

   A. Boredom
   B. Workplace bullying
   C. Fatigue
   D. Rudeness

9. The nurse is writing a care plan for a patient who has a sacral pressure ulcer and is at risk for developing several more pressure ulcers due to limited mobility. Which of the following includes standardized clinical patient care and might be useful? Select all that apply.

   A. Routine
   B. Bundle
   C. Protocol
   D. Checklist
   E. Pathway

10. A nurse is concerned about the falls on a medical unit, which have increased over the past 3 months. What actions by the nurse demonstrate individual responsibility and teamwork supporting a culture of safety? Select all that apply.

   A. Discussing her concerns with the nurse manager
   B. Volunteering to do a fall-reduction project
   C. Researching evidence-based fall-reduction programs
   D. Collaborating with RM
   E. Suggesting that the nurses on the unit attend a falls reduction in-service

REVIEW ACTIVITIES

1. You have administered the wrong dose of a medication to a patient, and have been notified that the patient's record is undergoing a peer review. Review the QSEN Competencies Safety table at qsen.org/competencies/pre-licensure-ksas/#safety. Would your feelings about the peer review process depend on whether or not the patient experienced a negative reaction?
2. Watch the video "The Lewis Blackman Story Part 1 & 2" at www.qsen.org/publications/videos/the-lewis-blackman-story/. Describe how a standardized nursing care plan individualized to address potential adverse events would have improved this patient's care.

3. Identify one clinical tool used at your clinical agency that reduces variation in patient care. Ask staff what might occur if the tool was not used or was not used appropriately.
4. Use the SBAR format to give a handoff report on your patients to another nurse at lunch time. Are there differences in the process between your use of the SBAR format compared to other handoffs you have done without the SBAR format?
5. Review the documentation in your assigned patient's medical record against the continuing stay criteria applicable to your patient (obtain criteria from a UM nurse at your clinical agency). Does the documentation in the patient's medical record support continued stay?
6. Find dashboards or graphs related to patient safety posted in your clinical area. Ask staff what safety initiatives were implemented and how work was affected in the clinical area.

CRITICAL DISCUSSION POINTS

1. Think about your clinical experience settings. Where did you feel the safest? Compare that setting to one where you felt less safe. What contributed most to your feeling of safety: the healthcare structures, the processes, or the outcomes in the clinical settings?
2. Consider the components of a culture of safety. Which component do you think is most evident in your current clinical area? Which component is most evident in your nursing practice as a student? How do you think that will change when you graduate?
3. Construct a checklist from memory of a common nursing procedure. Compare it to the written procedure in the procedure reference guide on your assigned unit. Consider the potential negative impact on patient safety if you relied only on your memory for procedures.
4. Think about your assigned clinical area and recall what types of "accidents waiting to happen" were evident. How can you, other nurses, and other staff be motivated to alleviate patient safety risks?
5. Think about a clinical experience on a busy unit. Did you observe interruptions when medications were being administered? What strategies would have supported patient safety? Would the strategies differ depending on who was interrupting, for example, a physician versus a nurse aide?

QSEN ACTIVITIES

1. Go to the QSEN website (www.qsen.org) and search for Safety. Click on Safety and note the OSHA publications, which focus on preventing workplace violence for all nurses who provide care for patients. Review them to improve patient safety.
2. Go to the QSEN website (www.qsen.org) and search for Safety. Click on Safety and note the Patient Safety America Newsletter. Note the monthly newsletters dedicated to educating patients and their care providers about new developments in patient safety. Review them to improve patient safety.

EXPLORING THE WEB

1. Go to the site for The Joint Commission (www.jointcommission.org/standards_information/npsgs.aspx). Find the current year's patient safety goals that are applicable to your assigned healthcare setting. Discuss the collaboration necessary across disciplines and departments in order to achieve these patient safety goals.
2. Go to the National Quality Forum website (www.qualityforum.org/ProjectDescription.aspx?projectID=80757). Search for National Safety Project 2015-2017. Review the measures related to patient safety that can be used for accountability. Choose one that is applicable to your clinical setting and that includes communication between nurses and physicians.
3. Watch the informational video on Florida's Impaired Practitioners Program of Florida (Intervention Project for Nurses [IPN]) at ipnfl.org/informational-videos/. Contrast the change in nurse perceptions from first contact with Intervention Project for Nurses to involvement in the program. How could these changes in perception potentially affect the nurses' interactions with patients, other nurses, and physicians?
4. Search the Cochrane Collaboration site for the abstract "Professions allied to medicine, such as nurses, midwives, and dieticians, can effectively incorporate clinical guidelines to improve patient care guidelines" (www.cochrane.org/CD000349/EPOC_professions-allied-to-medicine-such-as-nurses-midwives-and-dietiticians-can-effectively-incorporate-clinical-guidelines-to-improve-patient-care). Discuss how guidelines can enable a nurse and all practitioners to perform safely.

REFERENCES

Barry, M. E. (2014). Hand-off communication: Assuring the transfer of accurate patient information. *American Nurse Today*, 9(1). Retrieved from https://www.americannursetoday.com/issues-up-close-22/

Department of Veterans Affairs Patient Safety Center of Inquiry (PSCI) on Measurement to Advance Patient Safety. Guiding Patient Safety (GPS) Data Display. Center for Health care Organization and Implementation Research (CHOIR), VA Boston Health care System; 2017.

Gomaa, A. E., Tapp, L. C., Luckhaupt, S. E., Vanoli, K., Sarmienta, R. F., Raudabaugh, W. M., … Sprigg, S. M. (2015). Occupational traumatic injuries among workers in health care facilities—United States, 2012–2014. *Morbidity and Mortality Weekly Report*, 64(15), 405–410, Retrieved from https://www.cdc.gov/mmwr/preview/mmwrhtml/mm6415a2.htm

Griffin, F. A., & Resar, R. K. (2009). *IHI global trigger tool for measuring adverse events* (2nd ed.). IHI Innovation Series white paper. Cambridge, MA: Institute for Healthcare Improvement;. Retrieved from http://www.ihi.org/resources/Pages/IHIWhitePapers/IHIGlobalTriggerToolWhitePaper.aspx

Howard, D. (2017) Office of the Medical Inspector, Veterans Health Administration, Veterans Affairs, personal communications.

Joint Commission Center for Transforming Healthcare Releases Targeted Solutions Tool for Hand-off Communications. (2012). *Joint Commission Perspectives*. 32(8):1-3. Retrieved at https://www.jointcommission.org/assets/1/6/tst_hoc_persp_08_12.pdf

The Joint Commission (TJC). (2017). Summary data of sentinel events reviewed by TJC. Retrieved from https://www.jointcommission.org/assets/1/18/Summary_4Q_2016.pdf

Lagoe, R., Johnson, P., & Murphy, M. P. (2011). Inpatient hospital complications and lengths of stay: A short report. *BMC Research Notes*, 4, 135. doi:10.1186%2F1756-0500-4-135"10.1186/1756-0500-4-135

Liu, L., Sheuan, L., Pei-Fang, C., Shu-Ching, C., & Yu-Chun, Y. (2012). Exploring the association between nurse workload and nurse-sensitive patient safety outcome indicators. *The Journal of Nursing Research, 20*(4), 300–309. doi:10.1097/jnr.0b013e3182736363

Marsa, L. (2017, September). *Take charge of your health care: How to research a surgeon* (pp. 20, 27) Retrieved from https://www.aarp.org/health/conditions-treatments/info-2017/choose-a-surgeon-doctor-surgeries.html

McHugh, M. D., Kelly, L. A., Smith, H. L., Wu, E. S., Vanak, J. M., & Aiken, L. H. (2013). Lower mortality in magnet hospitals. *Medical Care, 51*(5), 382–388. doi:10.1097/MLR.0b013e3182726cc5

National Council of State Boards of Nursing & American Nurses Association. (2015). National guideslines on nursing delegation. Retrieved from https://www.ncsbn.org/NCSBN_Delegation_Guidelines.pdf

Office of the Surgeon General & National Action Alliance for Suicide Prevention. (2012) National strategy for suicide prevention. Retrieved from https://www.ncbi.nlm.nih.gov/books/NBK109917/

QSEN Institute. (2017). Pre-licensure KSAs: Safety. Retrieved from http://qsen.org/competencies/pre-licensure-ksas/

Sculli, G., & Sine, D. M. (2011). *Soaring to success: Taking crew resource management from the cockpit to the nursing unit.* Danvers, MA: HC Pro.

Stone, P. W., Hughes, R. G., & Dailey, M. (2008). Creating a safe and high-quality health care environment. In R. G. Hughes (Ed.), *Patient safety and quality: An evidence-based handbook for nurses* (pp. 594–603). Rockville, MD: Agency for Health care Research and Quality.

von Thaden, T. L., & Gibbons, A. M. (2008). The safety culture indicator scale measurement system (SCISMS). *Technical Report HFD-08–03/FAA-08–02.* Savoy, IL: University of Illinois, Human Factors Division.

SUGGESTED READINGS

American Nurses Association (ANA). (2013). Safe patient handling and mobility. Retrieved from https://www.americannursetoday.com/safe-patient-handling-mobility-journey-continues/

Benner, P. E., Malloch, K., & Sheets, V. (2010). *Nursing pathways for patient safety.* National Council of State Board of Nursing. St. Louis, MO: Mosby Elsevier.

Blouin, A. S., & McDonagh, K. J. (2010). Framework for patient safety. Part 1. *Journal of Nursing Administration, 10*(1), 397–400. doi:10.1097/NNA.0b013e31822edb4d

Blouin, A. S., & McDonagh, K. J. (2011). A framework for patient safety. Part 2. *Journal of Nursing Administration, 41*(11), 450–452. doi:10.1097/NNA.0b013e3182346eae

Institute of Medicine (IOM). (2013). *Keeping patients safe: Transforming the work environment of nurses.* Washington, DC: The National Academies Press.

Reeves, S. A., Denault, D., Huntington, J. T., Ogrinc, G., Southard, D. R., Vebell, R. (2017) Learning to overcome hierarchical pressures to achieve safer patient care: An interprofessional simulation for nursing, medical, and physician assistant students. *Nurse Educator QSEN Supplement, 42*(5), S27–S31. doi:10.1097/NNE.0000000000000427

Robert Wood Johnson Foundation. (2011). Nurses are key to improving patient safety. Retrieved from http://www.rwjf.org/en/library/articles-and-news/2011/04/nurses-are-key-to-improving-patient-safety.html

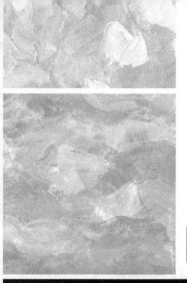

UNIT III.

NURSE LEADERSHIP AND
MANAGEMENT FOR QUALITY
IMPROVEMENT

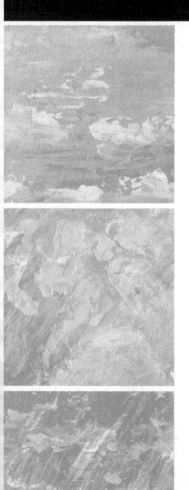

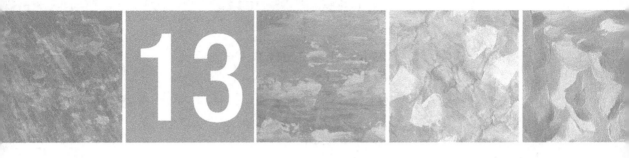

13

ESSENTIALS OF QUALITY IMPROVEMENT

Anthony L. D'Eramo, Melinda Davis, and Joanne Belviso Puckett

Undoubtedly, the most important single requisite is a commitment to quality: an unequivocal desire and determination to dedicate oneself to the best one is capable of, despite every obstacle

—Donabedian, 2003, p. xxix

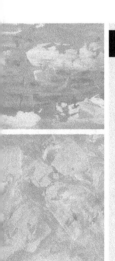

Upon completion of this chapter, the reader should be able to

1. Define quality improvement (QI).
2. Describe the historical evolution of QI.
3. Describe the tracer methodology process employed during a Joint Commission survey.
4. Compare and contrast QI, evidence-based practice, and research.
5. Describe the different QI methodologies, including Plan-Do-Study-Act (PDSA), Lean, and Six Sigma.
6. Describe healthcare failure mode effects analysis as a QI tool.
7. Examine how the root cause analysis process helps understand near miss events or sentinel events.
8. Discuss the impact organizational leadership has on QI activities.

You are a home care nurse admitting a new patient. While conducting medication reconciliation based on the nursing admission policy, the patient hands you a bottle of erythromycin he has been taking for 3 days. However, there is no electronic medical record (EMR) indication that this patient was prescribed erythromycin or any medical history or recent provider notation prescribing erythromycin. You are clearly performing an important assessment and have several questions that needed to be answered. The first question you asked was "Who prescribed erythromycin for you?" The patient responded that he had a cold and decided to go to Urgent Care rather than try to see his provider. The provider at Urgent Care prescribed erythromycin for bronchitis. As the patient explains the situation, you realize this is a consistent problem because the prescribing provider is outside their network, which is why there is no record of this medication or diagnosis in the EMR.

- *From an interprofessional perspective, who would you initially contact based on this observation?*
- *What regulation(s) is the nursing admission assessment policy that stipulates medication reconciliation be conducted on every home visit based on?*
- *Is there opportunity to consider a quality improvement activity based on this scenario?*

INTRODUCTION

Staff nurses who provide direct patient care are best positioned to participate and lead quality improvement (QI) activities, thus affecting the quality of care patients receive. In such manner, it is important that nurses become familiar with the concepts of QI. The purpose of this chapter is to explore QI processes as they promote patient safety and the achievement of the best patient outcomes. QI will be defined and key concepts pertaining to the history of QI will be presented to showcase its interdisciplinary nature. Research and evidence-based practice (EBP) will be differentiated from the process of QI. The Donabedian model for change and Deming's Plan-Do-Study-Act (PDSA) process will be introduced as models commonly used in QI activities. Improvement methodologies such as Six Sigma and Lean will be explored. A proactive tool, namely the healthcare failure mode effects analysis (HFMEA™), is presented. Reactive tools such as the root cause analysis (RCA) process are discussed as evaluation tools used to determine the root cause of a significant near miss, an error, or sentinel event. Implementing and sustaining a culture of safety through the delivery of evidence-based high-quality healthcare using an interdisciplinary approach supported by leadership are key to continuous QI.

DEFINING QI

Quality improvement (QI) is defined the same for both prelicensure and graduate nursing education by the Quality and Safety Education for Nurses (QSEN) as "Use data to monitor the outcomes of care processes and use improvement methods to design and test changes to continuously improve the quality and safety of healthcare systems" (QSEN, 2017a; 2017b). The knowledge, skills, and attitudes (KSAs) differ, however, in that the prelicensure expectations focus on preparing the new nurse to participate in or lead small-scale QI activities while graduate students are expected to take a greater role and facilitate QI activities across the organization. QI is the process of collecting and analyzing data to determine the extent to which quality healthcare is being delivered according to a set standard. Standards may be internal, such as those created by the organization, or external, such as those created by regulatory bodies. QI can be considered as both an art and a science (McLaughlin, Houston, & Harder-Mattson, 2012). Indeed, the art of QI involves asking questions and coming up with creative ideas and visionary innovations of how to approach and consider improvement interventions. The science of QI involves the ongoing process of testing improvement interventions to measure if improvements lead to the intended outcomes.

A key aspect of QI includes the actions taken to decrease inconsistent patient outcomes, poor patient outcomes, patient outcomes that do not meet expectations related to EBP or regulatory standards, or do not meet the patient's needs and expectations. Such outcomes may be specific to a patient (e.g., a medication error), groups of patients (e.g., hospital-acquired pressure ulcer rates), or may identify a process that needs improving (e.g., transition from acute care to home care). Generally speaking, QI is a continuous process that includes elements of prevention (risk reduction), recognition, and alleviation of harm as well as the ongoing search for performance excellence.

QI is a structured series of events that involves planning, implementing, and evaluating healthcare outcomes (Hughes, 2008a). In addition, the National Academy of Medicine, formerly the Institute of Medicine (IOM, 2001), identified six aims for care delivery: that care delivery is safe, effective, patient-centered, efficient, equitable, and timely. Each aim provides an avenue for data collection and analysis that may trigger evidence that improvement is required or desired.

There are several key steps to formal QI projects, including assembling a team, understanding the organization as a complex system, accessing and interpreting data, implementing interventions to improve outcomes, and taking actions based on performance outcomes. Certainly, it is safe to say QI focuses on improving processes and outcomes, including those that result from practice decisions, and measuring or evaluating such outcomes compared to an established, evidenced-based standard, goal, or industry benchmark. Many organizations exist to provide resources and expertise to individuals, teams, and organizations working to improve. Examples of such organizations are listed in Table 13.1. It is also well recognized that there are cultural factors of the organization that influence improvement activities such as engaged and supportive senior leadership, interdisciplinary teams, staff buy-in, technology support, and direct supervisory commitment for time to work on improvements (Mitchell et al., 2015). A just culture, or a culture where reporting errors or risks is welcome because such reporting leads to improvements, is another cultural factor that distinguished organizations that strive and meet performance excellence.

TABLE 13.1 EXAMPLES OF ORGANIZATIONS ASSOCIATED WITH HEALTHCARE QUALITY

ORGANIZATION AND WEB ADDRESS
Agency for Healthcare Research and Quality (AHRQ), ahrq.gov
American Society for Quality (ASQ), asq.index.aspx
Centers for Medicare and Medicaid Services (CMS), cms.hhs.gov
Hospital Compare, medicare.gov/hospitalcompare/search.html
Institute for Healthcare Improvement (IHI), ihi.org/Pages/default.aspx
Institute for Safe Medication Practice (ISMP), www.ismp.org
National Center for Nursing Quality (NCNQ), www.nursingworld.org/ncnq
National Association for Healthcare Quality (NAHQ), www.nahq.org
National Quality Forum, www.qualityforum.org/Home.aspx
Quality and Safety Education for Nurses (QSEN), qsen.org
The Joint Commission (TJC), jointcommission.org
The Leapfrog Group, www.leapfroggroup.org

As nurses care for patients or communities, it is our professional responsibility to obtain and apply the KSAs of QI into our daily practice. The American Nurses Association (ANA) Code of Ethics, specifically Provision 3, speaks to nurses as patient advocates, protecting patient rights and safety (nursingworld.org/DocumentVault/Ethics-1/Code-of-Ethics-for-Nurses.html). This provides an ethical basis for nurses taking part in QI activities. Organizations do not ONLY hold nurses accountable to recognize and mitigate risk, but also to analyze patient outcomes to determine if improvement is warranted. In addition, nurses must have skills to evaluate organizational processes and report those processes that impede care delivery. Analyzing patient outcomes and evaluating complex processes requires the QI KSAs outlined by QSEN. These QI actions should sound familiar as they mimic the nursing process. It is truly an exciting time to be a nurse! Nurses have the ability to not only impact the well-being of patients, groups, and communities, but also the ethical responsibility and accountability to impact continual improvement that leads to improved patient and organizational outcomes, and potentially care delivery systems. It is no wonder why the public consistently ranks nurses as the most trusted, ethical, and honest profession 16 out of the last 17 Gallup polls (www.nationalnursesunited.org/press/entry/the-most-trusted-profession-nurses-once-again-top-poll/). Sometimes, the most challenging aspect of QI activities is getting started. Take a look at Real World Interview 13.1, how a newly graduated nurse describes her first QI project.

REAL-WORLD INTERVIEW

After graduating with my Bachelor of Science in Nursing in 2015, I started a position in a nurse residency program, a yearlong program at a VA Medical Center that provided a well-supported transition into the nursing profession. One of the requirements of the program was the opportunity to pursue an evidence-based quality improvement (QI) project. The thought of starting and implementing an improvement project was both intimidating and exciting. In the beginning, I felt concerned that my inexperience as a registered nurse would stand in the way of the positive impact that I was aspiring to achieve through QI.

Multiple ideas for improvement projects ran through my mind, and, not wanting to bite off more than I could chew, I found it at first difficult to narrow down a specific process to improve. During my senior practicum, I completed an evidence-based QI project. This project, however, due to time constraints, did not come to fruition or make it to the implementation phase, and was actually much too broad of a project for just one person to implement. I reflected on this experience when initiating my project and learned from my previous mistakes.

The idea for my project came to me one day during my medical–surgical rotation. I had just discharged a patient who would be going home with a central line for IV antibiotics. I reached out to my colleagues to find out what educational tools they used prior to discharging a patient home with a central line in place, and found that they did not have any education or a protocol in place for this. Realizing that this puts patients at risk for air emboli and central line infections, I chose this process as an improvement project. At this point, I was very excited to have chosen a project, and looked forward to moving forward with the process.

While receiving guidance from my mentor and input from many nurses and interdisciplinary team members, I created a chart audit tool, reviewed the charts of patients going home with central lines in place, and was able to narrow down

(continued)

REAL-WORLD INTERVIEW (continued)

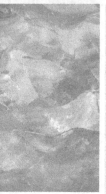

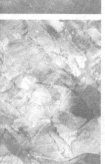

the specifics of my project. I created evidence-based patient education for patients discharging with central lines, and also provided in-services to inpatient nurses. The input I received from nurses and various members of the interdisciplinary team was invaluable in helping guide the direction and aims of the project. I reviewed results and found that the rates of clotting and infection had decreased during the period of time following implementation of the education.

As time went on, I began to realize the importance of utilizing the many resources I had at my fingertips. It was inspiring to me that so many of my colleagues wanted to be a part of my efforts. This was empowering to me; I was enlightened that in the future, I too would be able to help others with their various improvement projects. This gave me more hope for the success of my own project. One year later, I am happy to say that the professional connections I was able to make during my own project have provided me the opportunity to assist with multiple other improvement projects both on my unit and throughout the facility. As a result, I am afforded the opportunity to make positive changes that impact the veterans whom I am honored and privileged to care for. This was truly a well-supported journey!

Cristina Varney, BSN, RN
Staff Nurse, VA Medical Center White River Junction, VT

Getting started also includes gathering support for a project, soliciting staff to participate on the QI team, and getting time to conduct the QI project. Watch the video in Critical Thinking 13.1. You will see there are tips to gather team support that you can apply to any QI activity.

CRITICAL THINKING 13.1

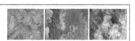

View the short video "A Good First Step to Any Improvement Project" at www.
youtube.com/watch?v=c1IQ81J70rk.
How can you apply the concept discussed in this video to your improvement activities?

HISTORY AND EVOLUTION OF QI IN HEALTHCARE

Prior to the 20th century, there was no such thing as a standard of care for physicians or hospitals let alone nursing care standards of practice. Patient outcomes were not tracked or reported. With little to no emphasis on measuring patient-care outcomes, it is not surprising that improvement, let alone quality, was not a consideration.

The establishment of the American Medical Association (AMA) started in the early 20th century from the efforts of Dr. Ernest Codman. The AMA set out to create standards of care and expectations for physicians, improve medical education, and improve public health. Dr. Codman began to push for patient case review and the tracking of patients posthospitalization to ensure the care they received was effective. It was through Codman's efforts to track patient outcomes, morbidity, and mortality following hospital stays and surgical procedures that the American College of Surgeons (ACS) was born. The primary responsibility of the ACS was to act as an oversight organization to physicians and hospitals. In the early 20th century, the ACS developed five minimum standards for hospital care. To be certified by the ACS, a hospital had to:

1. Organize the physicians practicing at the hospital into a medical staff.
2. Limit staff membership to well-educated, competent, licensed physicians and surgeons.
3. Have rules and regulations governing regular staff meetings and clinical review.
4. Keep medical records that included the history, physical exam, and results of diagnostic testing.
5. Supervise diagnostic and treatment facilities such as laboratory and radiology departments (Luce, Bindman, & Lee, 1994).

For the next 40 years, meeting minimum standards for hospital care was considered a satisfactory means to demonstrate quality care. By the 1960s there was a shift from meeting the minimum standards to identifying outcomes outside those that were expected, often referred to as outliers. Identifying and improving physician outliers became the impetus to achieving quality care. To identify physician outliers, a common QI tool used was a peer review of patient charts. Individual physician care data were collected from patient charts and analyzed. Patient care characteristics such as readmission rates, transfers to the ICU, needs for transfusion, and antibiotic use were reviewed in an attempt to identify poorly performing physicians. Efforts could then be made to educate and support QI in physician practice through mentoring. The results of this peer-review process were eventually used by hospitals in credentialing physicians. Physicians not performing up to standards or failing to correct practice deficiencies could potentially lose their privileges to practice at that institution.

As physicians were being peer reviewed, there remained little to no attention to nursing care quality at this time. However, that was not the case in the manufacturing sector. The work of many experts including Deming and the PDSA model became intriguing to businesses that could demonstrate improved production by employing principles of continuous improvement. As part of this revolution, industrial leaders began welcoming frontline staff participation and evaluation of processes since they were involved with the day-to-day operations. Frontline staff could easily and often quickly identify opportunities for improvement that could impact production. This belief and even the PDSA described later in this chapter eventually influences healthcare quality methodologies.

There were numerous historical events that have brought light to healthcare quality. For the purpose of this chapter, several will be highlighted including Title XVIII of the Social Security Act that signed Medicare into law; regulatory oversight of healthcare, such as The Joint Commission (TJC); and several IOM publications.

In 1966, Medicare was signed into law providing healthcare for Americans 65 years and older followed by Medicaid that provided healthcare resources to low-income Americans. Today, both programs are combined into the Centers for Medicare and Medicaid Services (CMS). These programs have gone through revisions over the years including identifying quality indicators. For example, the Experimental Medical Care Review Organizations were established in 1972 to review quality and appropriateness of care delivered (Owens & Koch, 2015). In 2001, CMS instituted the Hospital Quality Initiative making aggregated healthcare quality data publicly accessible. The National

Quality Foundation identified "never events" in 2001 as sentinel events or preventable errors that should never occur. In 2007, the CMS restructured reimbursement of never events holding organizations more financially accountable for the cost associated with never events. The **Hospital Value-Based Purchasing** (HVBP) Program introduced by the CMS in 2011 is a payment model with roots in the Affordable Care Act (ACA). Traditionally, reimbursement for healthcare has mainly been and remains a fee-for-service model where the patient or the paitent's insurer, if an insurer exists, is billed directly. The HVBP model shifts payment from fee-for-service to value based. This shift equates to insurers such as Medicare to reward or penalize hospitals based on patient-care and process outcomes. The HVBP recognizes providers who deliver better outcomes at lower costs (Aroh, Colella, Douglas, & Eddings, 2015; Figueroa, Tsugawa, Zheng, Orav, & Jha, 2016; VanLare & Conway, 2012). With HVBP, hospital performance is based on four quality domains: patient experience (30%), clinical processes of care (20%), outcomes (30%), and efficiency (20%). Because reimbursement is tied to meeting established outcomes, the belief is that HVBP would result in cost containment. In 2015, while HVBP provided bonus payments to 1,713 hospitals for their outcomes and cost saving, it reduced reimbursement for 1,371 hospitals who did not meet expectations (Fos, 2017).

TJC on Accreditation of Healthcare Organizations (JCAHO) was founded in 1951 through the collaborative efforts of the American College of Physicians, the American Hospital Association, the AMA, and the Canadian Medical Association. JCAHO was initially charged with regulatory oversight of hospital quality (www.jointcommission. org/about_us/history.aspx). JCAHO, currently called TJC, also assumes regulatory oversight of nursing homes and laboratory facilities among other duties. Access to TJC specific regulatory requirements is available with payment of a fee by those organizations seeking TJC accreditation. By meeting a set of widely recognized standards and elements of performance, a healthcare organization demonstrates achievement of quality measure sets. One example of a TJC requirement, specifically a National Patient Safety Goal, is medication reconciliation that was discussed in the chapter scenario.

In the 1970s and 1980s, the focus on quality care transitioned from a peer review of patient charts to identifying "problem physicians" to improving the performance of a group of physicians and hospitals through implementing practice guidelines. The goal of practice guidelines was to standardize care decision making. Practice guidelines would apply up-to-date evidence that would inform clinical decision making resulting in improved patient outcomes, and a reduction in morbidity and mortality.

As TJC matured, the focus moved from quality of care being a physician responsibility to an intraprofessional responsibility. All healthcare workers were now responsible and accountable to ensure quality and safety within their practice. The scope of responsibility not only included patients, but staff and visitors who were also in the healthcare environment and could be subject to safety risks. The environment of care, for example, has many TJC requirements to protect patients, visitors, and employees. A simple spill of ice chips on a floor can lead to falls for anyone in that area, not just patients.

In 2002, TJC initiated the requirement that all hospitals seeking their accreditation begin reporting their performance on core patient quality measures. These core patient quality measures are a listing of standardized evidence-based care that should be delivered to certain patient groups, for example, all patients with pneumonia should receive an antibiotic before they leave the ED or all patients with a myocardial infarction should be prescribed a beta-blocker. Since hospital payers (e.g., insurance companies, CMS) often require proof of accreditation before they will reimburse health services, hospitals became motivated to participate in improving their performance given the financial implications. TJC patient quality measures change based on evidence or outcome trends. To learn more about TJC quality measures, visit www.jointcommission.org.

TJC also changed its approach to how it assessed an organization's compliance to the standards by shifting from a scheduled to an unannounced site visit. In addition, TJC implemented the **tracer methodology** that traces an individual patient through their transitions of care across the organization, and also included "system tracers," such as medication management and infection control, tracing those complex processes across the entire organization. Consider a patient with congestive heart failure (CHF) on an acute care medical unit who has had multiple admissions for CHF. This patient is improving but previously on arrival to the ED, was intubated and admitted to the medical ICU (MICU). Prior to a tracer activity, a TJC surveyor will request a complex patient, such as the patient with CHF, be identified who has been admitted across several care settings during this admission. The surveyor will request to meet with the intraprofessional team starting with the current team on the medical unit, and then will trace the care delivery backward to previous settings and request to meet with those intraprofessional teams. During the time with the medical unit team, all staff involved, including the nurse caring for the patient that day, will be asked to meet with the surveyor. The surveyor will ask the team about their care delivery to determine if the team is following their policies and procedures, which are often created based on TJC regulatory requirements. The surveyor may also request to speak to the patient and the family to assess if patient education has occurred and if they are satisfied with the care and services they have received. Once the surveyor has completed this discussion, which may take hours, the surveyor traces care and services backward to meet with the previous care team. In this example, the surveyor would go to talk with the MICU followed by the ED team. The patient's electronic medical record (EMR) is discussed, as well as documentation and any other aspects of care and services that the surveyor chooses to look into. During the team discussions, the surveyor is making notes, perhaps policy questions to look up after the discussion, and will include visits to other departments that were involved in the care delivery for this patient. Since the patient was previously intubated, you would expect respiratory care services and the radiology department to both receive visits from this surveyor. The intent of tracers is to determine if staff is following their policies and procedures based on TJC requirements for accreditation. This level of review adds value to the accreditation and ultimately to patients because it goes beyond compliance (yes–no type questions) to more of a process approach ("talk to me about your admission assessment"). For nurses, a tracer is nothing more than explaining what you did for the patient and/or family that is based on the scope of your practice. As nurses, our contribution to the patient's plan of care is crucial and necessary. There is no need to fear taking part in the tracer, only to fear not following your organization's policies and procedures! You should expect questions about process related to medication administration, assessment/reassessment, documentation, patient education, discharge planning, and care coordination across settings. Read a nurse's experience whenparticipating in a tracer in the Real World Interview 13.2. Also appreciate that TJC surveyors are well versed in all TJC requirements. Although they may be on the unit conducting a tracer, they will be assessing the environment, looking in storage areas, and watching staff in action, including hand hygiene (HH) compliance. Read more about tracers at www.jointcommission.org/facts_about_the_tracer_methodology/.

A greater emphasis on risk reduction can be seen in TJC standards and process. In 2017, TJC changed their approach to how deficiencies are identified and scored during surveys. Now, deficiencies are reported based on risk of harm and scope of the deficiency. This change allows the organization to mitigate or take corrective action on the highest risk deficiencies first by prioritizing them for immediate action (TJC, 2016). As seen in the new scoring methodology called Survey Analysis for Evaluating Risk (SAFER) Matrix, deficiencies are categorized by the likelihood of harm and the scope

REAL-WORLD INTERVIEW

Despite, my high level of experience and confidence as a homecare nurse, I always feel anxious if I am the nurse in a tracer. I think no matter how well you prepare, you always worry that they will find something and it is your fault. I do feel the best way to prepare is to try and do what is right every day, and then you are always ready. During my visit, the patient had a free-standing oxygen tank—because I immediately saw it and knowing home oxygen is a safety risk, I quickly placed the tank into a storage cylinder where it belonged and re-educated the patient that oxygen tanks cannot be left freestanding, which pleased the surveyor. The patient also had an OTC med not on the medication list. I was able to address that as part of the routine medication reconciliation we do and ensured it was documented before the surveyor could even make it back to the office! Our electronic record allowed me quick communication and documentation that the demonstrated medication reconciliation process worked! We are well informed as home care nurses that handwashing and bag technique will be closely watched by the surveyor and should not cause anxiety, but errors happen even though you know the right techniques because you are being watched. The process of preparing for a survey or tracer can be challenging because one never really knows what they will ask. When I was a newer nurse, I used to be much more anxious but experience has taught me to do my job to the best of my ability, be able to adjust along the way, and know your procedures and follow them and talking with a surveyor is not as stressful. I also have found if I do not know an answer, the surveyor helps to coach me. There is also sharing of best practices the surveyor may have seen at other organizations that our team can benefit from. All in all, it can be stressful but also educational!

Carol A. Mello, MSN, RN
Staff Nurse, Hospital in Home Program
Providence VA Medical Center
Providence, RI

of the deficiency. This new approach allows the surveyor who identified the deficiency to analyze the deficiency based on the likelihood of harm (high, moderate, and low) as well as the scope of the deficiency (widespread, pattern, and limited). As seen in the SAFER Matrix in Figure 13.1, the deficiency is evaluated and inserted into the matrix based on the surveyor's analysis. This provides the organization a risk-based prioritized list of deficiencies to correct. Regardless of risk (except for identification of immediate risk to life or safety), the organization will have 60 days for corrective action. However, for those high-risk deficiencies, TJC will request additional information and evidence of corrective actions and sustainment (TJC, 2016).

Several publications by the IOM highlighted the continued quality challenges facing the healthcare system. *To Error Is Human: Building a Safer Health System* (2000) recognized the grim reality of patient deaths associated with medical errors. The publication, *Crossing the Quality Chasm: A New Health System for the 21st Century* (2001), addressed healthcare system failures emphasizing it was not the fault of the employees but poor care delivery processes, or systems, that needed improvement. In response, many organizations have taken improvement actions to address these issues utilizing the QI tools discussed later in this chapter.

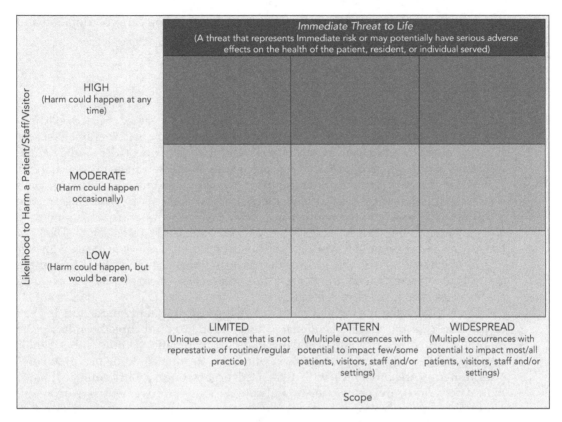

FIGURE 13.1 The Joint Commission SAFER (Survey Analysis for Evaluating Risk) matrix.

Source: From The Joint Commission. (2016). The SAFER matrix: A new scoring methodology. *The Joint Commission Perspectives®, 36*(5), 1, 3. Reprinted with permission.

As the public became better informed about the mounting problems within the healthcare industry, the staggering cost of healthcare continued and continues to rise today at alarming rates. In fact, for every $5.00 spent by the federal government, $1.00 (20%) goes toward healthcare (CMS, 2014). Despite significant funding, continued evidence of less than optimal healthcare outcomes are realized. Patients complain of long wait times for appointments and access to care challenges. Care coordination gaps exist as do healthcare disparities with the focus on episodic care rather than preventive care (Salmond & Echevarria, 2017). There are many examples that contribute to increased healthcare costs, such as the demand for greater, sophisticated technology, prescription medications (Squires & Anderson, 2015), waste, excessive administrative costs, unnecessary services, and preventive failures (Berwick & HackBerth, 2012).

With increased healthcare costs, Americans often find healthcare unaffordable with 50 million American uninsured and another 40 million underinsured (Salmond, 2015). For years, consumers of healthcare asked for healthcare reform for affordable healthcare coverage. In response, the ACA (2010) was passed by the Congress. The ACA went beyond healthcare coverage; it supported many programs and reimbursement models aimed at "fixing" the healthcare system. An example is the Patient-Centered Medical Home program to provide a team-based approach to primary care in the patient's home. Patients with chronic disease are prime candidates for the medical home program because the focus is to improve the patient's self-management of their chronic conditions while providing care coordination and evidenced-based care.

QI in Nursing

Traditionally, the practice of nursing has been perceived as a valued, trusted contribution to patient care. Because nurses are members of teams and often carry out interventions identified by other team members, consider the complexity of identifying unique indicators of nursing practice that are specific to nursing. There are many questions as to how the unique practice of nursing equates to quality care outcome measures. How does nursing judgment impact patient outcomes? How is efficiency of nursing practice measured? As these and many other questions have been raised regarding nursing and patient outcomes, the IOM, QSEN, ANA, and others have taken action. The IOM has called for a stronger body of EBP for all healthcare disciplines to create a greater empirical evidence-based care delivery by that discipline. Through the KSAs of the QSEN competencies, nurses are being better prepared to question practice, evaluate the literature, and take active roles in QI.

The ANA funded the development of nurse-sensitive quality indicators in 1998 to provide data on specific acute-care outcomes that could directly indicate the quality of nursing care delivery. Participating organizations could submit their outcomes for trending and comparison purposes. Results could be useful to compare nursing care outcomes with like-sized organizations with either evidence that expectations are being met or indications that improvement is warranted. These data in the National Database of Nursing Quality Indicators (NDNQI®), now managed by Press Ganey (accessible at www.pressganey.com/solutions/clinical-quality/nursing-quality), continue to evolve and are likely to change as new empirical evidence substantiates new, specific, nurse-sensitive indicators on patient outcomes. Other organizations have created nurse-sensitive indicators, such as the National Quality Forum (NQF) that include many of the NDNQI indicators (accessible at www.qualityforum.org/Home.aspx). The bottom line is that capturing nurse-sensitive indicators that effectively and accurately capture nursing care is challenging. Other sources have identified indicators that are used and are useful but further research is needed that demonstrate unique, empirical relationships between such indicators to specific patient outcomes. In addition, indicators for all practice settings are needed as most of the current nurse-sensitive measures focus on acute care settings.

Today's healthcare organizations are highly complex systems that are often multisite and provide various levels of care. Perhaps one of the most important aspects of QI is the organization's culture and expectations regarding quality care delivery and outcomes. To continually improve successfully, leadership expectations should foster innovative system thinking of all staff and serve as role models by participating with staff in QI activities. Read the Real-World Interview 13.3 that demonstrates how one Department of Defense organization created an innovative way to support both civilian and enlisted staff's attention to improving their system. This interview demonstrates success by both leadership and employee engagement, all toward making improvement. Leadership support is more though: It includes educating employees on QI methods, providing time for QI activities, recognizing staff for identifying opportunities for improvement, ensuring that patients' and families' feedback is used toward improvement, and sustaining those QI outcomes that have met the improvement aim(s).

REAL-WORLD INTERVIEW

In rolling out the U.S. Air Force's Continuous Process Improvement (CPI) model, our hospital, the 48th Medical Group's leadership, wanted everyone involved and responsible for the hospital's success. To ensure that success, methods used would be systematic, replicable, and sustainable in a highly mobile workforce. That meant a culture where quality improvement (QI) was embraced at every level from senior management to frontline staff. To create this environment, two key cultural components were needed: making the process easier and recognizing those who did the improvement work.

All members of the Air Force understand that time is a limited resource, so QI means that those daily process irritants or obstacles, within their capability to change, are primary targets. In addition to our Lean Six Sigma Green Belt projects, our facility also chose to focus heavily on the Lean concept of "Just Do Its"—a strong process improvement tool that typically does not involve a formal team. It does require an aptitude to be innovative and quickly put actions into place that yield timely results. The acronym JEDI—"Just *Easy* Do Its" was created by our hospital Quality Office to promote interest and a sense of fun among our predominantly young military staff. An Airman[a] who identifies a problem has an opportunity under the JEDI initiative to provide simple data to show the extent of the problem, identify the desired performance target and most likely root cause, and take action to make the process better. If the new performance target is achieved, the redesigned process could be standardized across the enterprise as appropriate. Two commonly used tools to accomplish these improvements are an abbreviated Air Force CPI Practical Problem Solving Method, and a "Five Whys Analysis." These tools led to new and innovate ways of doing business by all levels of staff from management to frontline to volunteers. Giving them easy tools jump started the process. Delivering meaningful change with easy-to-understand tools creates and supports a culture where Airmen are innovative. They clearly recognize the improvements brought about by change. This commitment is celebrated by the hospital as the improvements are published and shared. A certificate of recognition is given to each JEDI Leader by the Medical Group's commander, which further enhances staff satisfaction and engagement. When these everyday improvements are incorporated into hospital policy, the effects are far-reaching. The CPI is no longer "person-dependent," but a systematic, replicable, sustainable event that continues a focus on innovation and improvement hospital wide. Interestingly, while these innovations are sustained, many are further improved when another Airman determines an even better way to improve the original process improvement.

Innovation and process improvement have become a part of our daily performance at the 48th Medical Group. Sustaining that required a cultural shift to encourage ownership by all staff for hospital success. Since JEDI's introduction, more than 65 improvements have spread throughout the entire organization resulting in savings of time and money; increased staff and/or patient satisfaction; and reduction of risk. That is what real CPI is about . . . *Every Airman, Every Day, A Problem Solver*.

Colonel Michael H. Ross, RN, MSN, CNS, APRN
Chief Nurse Executive, USAF 48th Medical Group RAF
Lakenheath, United Kingdom

[a]*Airman*—when used with a capital A, "Airman" is the term used by the USAF to refer to all USAF employees—male, female, active duty, government civilian employees, and contractors.

Is QI EBP or Research?

It is important to be able to differentiate QI from EBP and research. QI projects incorporate a data-driven systematic process in which individuals collaborate to improve specific internal processes within an organization. One key aim of QI is the analysis of data into decision-making information to determine if improvement is warranted. As you will see, this aim is different from EBP and research.

EBP does not analyze information, data, or seek to problem solve, but rather it critically appraises all relevant evidence to answer a clinical, educational, or administrative question. The aim of EBP is to determine if evidence supports clinical, educational, or administrative practice. If evidence exists, it validates practice. If evidence does not exist, the need for research to provide new evidence may be supported. One similarity between QI and EBP involves a review of literature. Reviewing the literature is a basic aspect of EBP but there is merit in assessing the literature when conducting QI. The literature may provide relevant interventions that a team may wish to employ. For nurses, as you gain clinical experience, both QI and EBP are fundamental expectations of practice. We must apply basic QI principles for continued improvement and question practice to determine if practice is based on sound evidence.

Research is a scientific process of generating new knowledge. The aim of research is to test hypotheses that may be generalizable beyond the research setting. Reducing bias is crucial to generalize research outcomes. Quantitative research often includes an intervention group (those who received the study intervention) and a control group (those not receiving the intervention) allowing to test for statistical differences between groups. Conducting research is neither a basic skill nor an expectation of nursing practice. Advanced degrees are necessary for nurses who may wish to become researchers, but nurse in general should be able to participate in a research project if they are interested and have the related competencies to do so. When conducting research, approval and oversight by an institutional review board (IRB) is required to ensure the safety of human subjects who will be participating in the research study. Although the aims of research and QI are different, we will soon see that differences can be vague, especially if patients are included in a QI project.

As you are learning in this chapter, QI can be a simple, individual act such as reorganizing a utility room making it easier and quicker to find supplies, to a unit-based team working to improve unit outcomes, to a system-wide initiative that includes intraprofessionals all involved in the process that needs improvement. With QI, there are two distinct types of data. There are data that support the need for improvement (baseline data) and data generated from the QI project that are used to compare the baseline to the improvement to determine if the improvement worked. Outcome data, often referred to as accountability data or performance measure outcomes, represent the outcomes of healthcare delivery processes. These outcomes are not based on QI interventions or projects but are inherent to practice and systems. For example, patient falls can be measured as one outcome indicator of nursing care. The total time it takes from a CT scan order, to scan, to read, and to communicate results, is a process that can be measured. Patient or process outcomes relate to accountability of employees and the organization. These outcomes are frequently public and reported to regulatory bodies as an indication of organizational performance. Analysis of outcome data serves as a basis for decision making, regarding whether improvement is warranted or not.

Implementing a QI intervention for improvement also results in data from the QI activity, or the postintervention measurement outcome. For example, if an indicator such as HH was measured on a nursing unit for 1 month and was found to be 70% compliant with Centers for Disease Control and Prevention (CDC) HH requirements,

70% represents an outcome measure and would serve as the baseline if a project was planned to improve HH compliance. Analysis of this outcome, including unit trends of HH compliance over time, is necessary to determine if improvement is warranted. If improvement of HH compliance is determined necessary, a QI activity could occur. The QI activity would involve implementing an intervention to improve the baseline outcome measure of 70%. The measurement obtained to evaluate the effect of the intervention is the postintervention measure. In this example, if an intervention was introduced and resulted in HH compliance of 88%, that result represents the postintervention measure, which is an improvement from the baseline measure of 70%. If an intervention to improve HH was introduced but the goal was not obtained, an additional intervention may be needed. If the intervention had no effect, the team would need to identify a new intervention or consider reevaluating how the original intervention was implemented, which may be the contributing factor to not meeting the goal.

So far, EBP, research, and QI seem to be very distinct approaches to measurement. As patient care and process outcomes have greater influence on reimbursement, the need for measurement and sophisticated QI interventions will become more important. In addition, the study of QI interventions has become a relevant area of research. In fact, the literature has numerous examples of QI research where the focus of the research hypothesis is on the intervention itself and how the intervention was deployed. Confusing, right? But consider a QI project with the aim to reduce falls on a nursing unit. The intervention consists of one group of patients assessed with Fall Risk Scale A, another group with Fall Risk Scale B, and a third group who did not have a risk assessment performed. Although there would be unit-level baseline outcome data on falls and the scope of the project is within one unit with no intent to generalize outcomes, the fact is patients are being randomized. Randomization is a research methodology, thus this QI project is now moving into a QI research realm. As described in the example, the QI activity is now QI research because patients were randomized with a control group. If the project aim had been to reduce falls by trialing one fall risk assessment that all patients received, without randomizing patients, there would be no research methodologies underway. Traditionally, we have used the terms "QI," "research," and "data" with confidence that employees could easily differentiate them. That confidence may be risky. Understanding the difference among QI Nonresearch, QI Research, and Accountability data that represent Patient/Process outcome can increase confidence that, as a staff nurse, you can take improvement actions appropriately and safely, and are not including research methodologies as a member of a QI team. The distinction among QI Nonresearch, QI Research, and Accountability data, as they relate to performance measurement, is important because each has different value, aim, and specific processes associated with it. O'Rourke and Fraser (2016) differentiate QI as both a research and practice activity. Lloyd (2010) identified three faces of performance measurements. Table 13.2 is useful in differentiating the characteristics of all three measurement approaches. Notice the aim statements clearly provide key differences as they relate to context. In summary, the aim of a QI research project is to understand why and how improvement interventions work in different contexts to determine if they are generalizable. The focus of QI research is therefore to study and understand the intervention itself. The aim of QI-Nonresearch is to improve processes and outcomes within a local context, not to imply the outcome has implications across settings, although that may well be the case when sharing/standardizing successful projects. Patient and process outcomes are not a project at all, but the measures from care and service delivery serve as baseline and require analysis for QI decision making.

TABLE 13.2 THREE APPROACHES TO PERFORMANCE MEASUREMENT

ELEMENTS OF EACH APPROACH	PERFORMANCE MEASUREMENT APPROACH		
	QI NONRESEARCH	QI RESEARCH	ACCOUNTABILITY-PATIENT/PROCESS OUTCOME DATA
Aim	Improve patient care within a local context	New knowledge as to why and how QI interventions work in different contexts	Benchmark Evidence of meeting or not meeting a measurable expectation Provides opportunities for improvement
Intervention	Identified, applied, revised based on local context	Tested, explored, often a control group to compare impact of intervention(s)	No intervention, evaluate current performance
Project lead	Expert in local context	Expert in research methods	No project
Bias	Accept bias	Designed to eliminate bias for greater generalizability	Measure and adjust to reduce bias
Sample size	Small sample is usually adequate	Statistically calculated	Utilize 100% of available data
Flexibility of hypothesis	Hypothesis is flexible to allow for changes during intervention	Fixed, unchangeable	No hypothesis
Testing and time frame	Sequential tests with goal to complete quickly; rapid cycles	One large test that is time intensive	No testing; technological systems are frequently instituted for review of aggregate data analysis and decision making
Project approval	IRB not required	IRB required	Not a project
Determining if outcome is an improvement	Commonly run or control charts	Hypothesis statistical testing	No testing
Confidentiality of data	Data used only by QI intervention team	Participant data are protected	Data available to stakeholders and usually public

IRB, institutional review board; QI, quality improvement.

Source: Adapted from Lloyd, R. C. (2010). Navigating in the turbulent sea of data: The quality measurement journey. *Clinics in Perinatology, 37*, 101–122. doi:10.1016/j.clp.2010.01.006; O'Rourke, H. M., & Fraser, K. D. (2016). How quality improvement practice evidence can advance the knowledge base. *Journal for Healthcare Quality, 38*(5), 264–274. doi:10.1097/JHQ.0000000000000067

QI MODELS AND METHODOLOGIES

There are various QI models that provide a comprehensive framework for evaluating healthcare quality. Some of the most common are Donabedian's Structure, Process, Outcomes Model, and methodologies such as Deming's PDSA, Six Sigma, and Lean. It is important to familiarize yourself with the types and workings of the models, as you will encounter them in your professional nursing practice.

Donabedian's Model

Over 50 years ago, Avedis Donabedian proposed a model of quality assurance that is still used today: structure, process, and outcomes of care (Donabedian, 2003). **Structure** refers to "the conditions under which care is provided" such as nursing staff ratios, supplies available to provide patient care, and so on (Donabedian, 2003, p. 46). **Process** refers to "the activities that constitute healthcare" such as healthcare policies and standards of care (Donabedian, 2003, p. 46). **Outcomes** refer to the "changes (desirable or undesirable) in individuals and populations that can be attributed to healthcare" (Donabedian, 2003, p. 46). Outcomes may be clinical (urinary tract infections), functional (mobility), patient safety (medication errors), or patient/family satisfaction measures. It is important to understand that structure, process, and outcomes are not isolated. In fact, structures, processes, and outcomes are interdependent, meaning "specific attributes of one influence another according to the strength of the relationship" (Hughes, 2008b). When evaluating outcomes, it is important to consider both the structural and process impacts on the outcomes. You will read in Chapter 14 that outcome data are used to determine if outcomes meet, exceed, or fail to meet expectations. When outcome data do not meet expectations, improvement interventions may be warranted. The structural and process elements associated with the outcome provide ideal opportunities for improvement interventions.

Donabedian's model was applied by the ANA's development of the NDNQI®. The ANA's aim was to identify nurse-sensitive measures that could demonstrate the impact of nursing care on patient outcomes (Jones, 2016). Table 13.3 provides structure, process, and outcomes examples that support the delivery of patient care. This table will serve as a resource as you work through Case Study 13.1.

TABLE 13.3 EXAMPLES OF STRUCTURES, PROCESSES, AND OUTCOMES

STRUCTURES	PROCESSES	OUTCOMES
Staffing (nurses, physicians, nursing assistants, advanced practice nurses)	Evidence-based guidelines Nursing process Standards of care Pathways	Hospital-acquired infections (e.g., catheter-associated urinary tract infections, central line–associated
Infection control Skill mix Education level of staff Resources (e.g., computers, library databases) Supplies Technology Budget Leadership commitment/ engagement	Policies Motivated, engaged staff Core measures Care routines (e.g., hourly rounding)	blood stream infections, ventilator-associated pneumonia) Hospital-acquired pressure ulcers Fall rates Patient satisfaction Medication errors Infection rates Sentinel events/never events

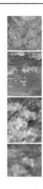

CASE STUDY 13.1

In looking at the list of nurse-sensitive indicators and their outcomes, classify them into Donabedian's model of structure, process, and outcomes.

Nurse-sensitive indicator results:

1. *Unit fall rate of 0.0 for the last 3 months.*
2. *Fifty percent of unit staff have completed specialty certification.*
3. *Monthly pain reassessment (30 minutes) post-IV narcotics was at 44%.*
4. *Patient nursing satisfaction has been greater than 90% overall the last 6 months.*
5. *Unit vacancy is at 5% for the last month.*
6. *Staff mix for a long-term care dementia unit: RN, 75%; LPN, 20%; and NA, 5%.*
7. *The unit utilizes the Braden Scale for skin assessment.*
8. *Patient satisfaction with discharge education has decreased from 92% to 90% over the last month.*
9. *Restraint prevalence was found to be 0.0 for the last 12 months.*
10. *The unit adopted a standardized tool to conduct handoff communication.*

In analyzing these outcomes, what outcome would you consider most concerning that may need an improvement team to further assess?

Plan-Do-Study-Act

Quality experts often use Dr. W. Edwards Deming's **Plan-Do-Study-Act** model to implement QI projects. Deming incorporated knowledge of engineering, operations, and management with the goal of improving accuracy, reducing costs, and increasing efficiency and safety, all leading to satisfied customers. Deming described his philosophy as "a system of profound knowledge" composed of four parts: (a) appreciation for a system, (b) understanding process variation, (c) applying theory of knowledge, and (d) using psychology (Evans, 2008). The PDSA model and the actions within each step can be seen in Figure 13.2. Although some refer to the cycle as Plan-Do-Check-Act (PDCA), as originally developed by Walter Shewhart, Deming had strong beliefs that the terminology, PDCA, and PDSA, were very different and he only used the "PDSA cycle" to describe process improvement (Moen & Norman, 2009). Deming argued that "study" implied more of a rigorous scientific approach to QI measurement and outcomes analysis where "check" did not have the same connotation.

The advantage of using the PDSA cycle is that it is easy to understand, can be used cyclically on a smaller scale to perform small tests of change, or used when implementing large, system-wide improvements. The following questions can be used during the PDSA process (Langley, Nolan, Nolan, Norman, & Provost, 2009).

1. What is the goal of the project?
2. How can it be determined that the goal of the project was reached?
3. What needs to be done in order to reach the goal?

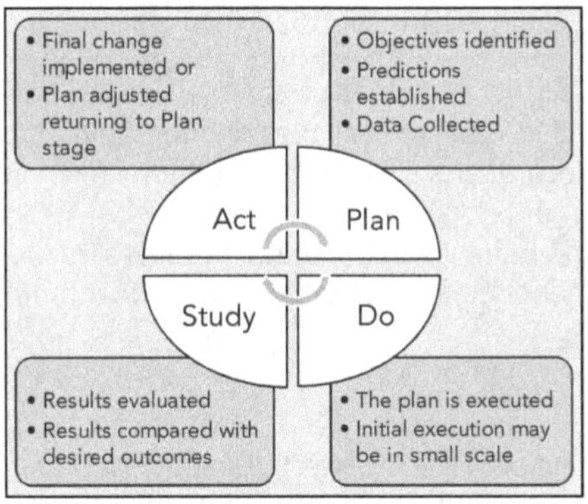

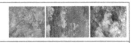

Figure content:

- Final change implemented or
- Plan adjusted returning to Plan stage

- Objectives identified
- Predictions established
- Data Collected

Act | Plan

Study | Do

- Results evaluated
- Results compared with desired outcomes

- The plan is executed
- Initial execution may be in small scale

FIGURE 13.2 Plan-Do-Study-Act model.

In the "Plan" stage, a plan to improve quality is developed. The plan's actual execution is evaluated during the "Study" stage, and either the plan is finally implemented during the "Act" stage or the plan is adjusted for further improvements. Then, the PDSA cycle restarts back to the "Plan" stage again as needed. The PDSA cycles continue until a solution is reached and implemented (Langley et al., 2009). Table 13.4 provides an example of how the PDSA model works in an organization. As nurses, we have an advantage in applying the PDSA because the PDSA model is closely replicated in the nursing process of assessment (plan), diagnosis (plan), planning (plan), implementation (do), and evaluation (study and act).

Even when methodologies are frequently used, such as PDSA, frequency and ease of use do not imply the QI process will always succeed. Marshall et al. (2016) spoke about their experience conducting an improvement and identified six risks to be aware of that may contribute to QI process failures:

1. The problem may be defined too vaguely or lack clarity.
2. There may be a lack of a clearly defined methodology, such as PDSA.
3. Interventions involve people who function in a social context. Social context may not be considered in the identification or deployment of the intervention.
4. What the intervention is, how it is deployed, and the organizational context are interdependent.
5. Evaluation and actions based on evaluation may occur too rapidly.
6. QI teams may lack a necessary level of expertise. Service users, improvement specialist, clinicians, and potentially academic partners can all contribute.

CRITICAL THINKING 13.2

You have learned about Plan-Do-Study-Act (PDSA). View the brief video "Plan Do Study Act (PDSA)" at www.youtube.com/watch?v=STXZHfINZGk.

1. How does the presenter address PDSA as it relates to Value-Based Purchasing?
2. The presenter states "All improvements result in change but not all change results in improvement." How does that quote come to light in the PDSA cycle?

TABLE 13.4 EXAMPLE OF PDSA

Problem: Patients do not appear to understand health education provided in the hospital as evidenced by high rates of readmissions for the same diagnosis, patients not understanding medications and not taking them as directed, and missing appointments with the physician after discharge.

Solution: Assess the patient's understanding of health information by using the Health Literacy Assessment using the REALM Short-Form Tool.

PLAN

We plan to
- Train nurses to use the REALM Health Literacy Assessment tool to identify those patients with low health literacy. Patients identified as having low health literacy will have education provided at an easier-to-understand level.
- Implement the REALM tool for 1 week on one unit for all patient admissions to assess health literacy.
- Create an area in the computerized charting system to document the results.

DO

We found that
- Not all patients are directly admitted to the unit; therefore, they did not have a health literacy assessment.
- Completing the REALM tool was time consuming until the nurses became used to the tool.
- The findings from the use of the REALM tool were not used to individualize health education materials.

STUDY

We learned that
- The tool accurately identified those patients with a low health literacy level.
- We need to create a way to use the REALM tool findings to individualized health education materials.

ACT

We concluded that
- The REALM tool does identify those patients with low health literacy.
- We need to look at what we do with the information from the REALM health literacy assessment.
- We need to look at ways to meet the patient's individual health education needs by creating an online repository of health education materials designed for low health literacy education.

PDSA, Plan-Do-Study-Act; REALM, Rapid Estimate of Adult Literacy in Medicine.

Lean

The principles of **Lean** thinking strive to eliminate forms of waste within a process to increase efficiency while enhancing effectiveness (Shankar, 2009). According to a Health Affairs publication, *Health Policy Brief: Reducing Waste in Health Care*, accessible at www. healthaffairs.org, it is estimated that there is between 20% and 30% waste in U.S. healthcare today and forward-thinking, high-performing healthcare organizations are moving more and more toward Lean thinking and environments. There are eight identified sources of waste in organizations: unnecessary services/overproduction, mistakes/defects, delays in waiting, unnecessary motion, over processing, excessive inventory, excessive transport, and unused human potential (Hadfield, Holmes, Kozlowski, & Sperl, 2009). When these sources of waste occur, employees may figure out work-arounds rather than considering new processes to improve efficiency. A work-around is a non-approved process created to accomplish a task due to all the waste associated with the approved process. For example, the nursing assistant is tasked with changing bed linens for each patient every day. To make the process quicker, the midnight shift nursing assistant collects the linens and places them in each patient's room. This action saves the day shift nursing assistant time in having to gather linens. Although a seemingly innocent and kind gesture, a problem arises when the original patient is discharged before the linens are used. The linens are then sent back to laundry for cleaning causing an increase in workload for the laundry workers. Even worse, the linens might be used for the newly admitted patient causing an increased risk of the spread of infection.

The danger of a workaround is the error that may result from creating and applying nonapproved processes. Lean interventions center on improving efficiency, reducing waste, and streamlining processes that are patient and employee centered. Lean thinking builds on the belief that it is the sum or cumulative effect of many small improvements that create the greatest impact in performance (Evans, 2008). Small, low-cost, and low-risk improvements are easily implemented with the goal to keep the project simple over a short duration of time. Lean addresses visible problems. For example, you can see that items in a clean utility room are orderly or in disarray. Color-coding shelves to hold specific types of equipment or supplies helps to quickly identify an item. Placing items together that are typically needed at the same time such as an indwelling urinary catheter kit next to a clean specimen collection kit is an example of Lean. A nurse searching for supplies is wasted time that can be much better spent. Simple Lean tools, such as the 5S process, can be quickly and easily applied to ensure the work environment is clean and organized, which will reduce that nonvalue-added activity that wastes the nurse's time. The improvement process of 5S also impacts patient safety by standardizing the environment, allowing staff to consistently locate the products used to deliver patient care. The 5S process includes the following:

1. **Sorting** the necessary from the unnecessary; discard unnecessary items.
2. **Set** items in order; everything has a place and keep everything where it belongs.
3. **Shine**: keep the area clean, neat, and organized.
4. **Standardize** the area.
5. **Sustain** the first four Ss (Hadfield et al., 2009).

Lean is easily taught, intuitive, and easy to apply in practice. One aspect of Lean that is sometimes overshadowed by the larger, more complex QI projects is the concept of "Just-Do-Its (JDIs)," a simplified methodology that anyone can use to fix a problem with a known or simple solution. An example of a Just-Do-It from one organization can be seen in Figure 13.3.

This example demonstrates how this organization developed JIDs using a creative abbreviation, such as "JEDI," that is fun, easy to remember, and helps to remind staff that their contributions working on JEDIs are significant for the organization's continual improvement. Not every "improvement" requires a formal, full team to be successful! As a new nurse, you bring a great advantage to your work area as you will see opportunities for small changes and daily improvements that other staff may not recognize. Every organization has problems big and small and every process has at least some irritant. It is the staff doing the work every day that is most knowledgeable about what those irritants are, how they affect the workflow, and what the best possible fixes may be. When you have every staff member making "seemingly small" improvements every day, what you end up with is a fully engaged workforce committed to improvement and together over time that can add up to significant organizational improvements in patient care and outcomes. By encouraging and recognizing those

"Trusted Care": Every Airman, Every Day, A Problem Solver

Completed JEDI ("Just Easy Do Its") Improvement

Flight: Pediatric Clinic	Improvement supports which MDG Strategic Priorities?	
JEDI Leaders: Maj ---- & SSgt ----	**Readiness** ___	**People _X__**
Completion Date: Feb 2017	Access **_X__**	Quality and Safety ___

* What was the problem or opportunity for improvement? * Provide the DATA that showed the extent of the problem * What was your new desired performance target?	• Over the past year, the Pediatric Clinic No-Show rate had reached a high of 9.5% as of Jan. 2016. In addition to the inefficiencies, and wasted appointments and staff resources, it also caused an increase of approximately 3 days in wait times for access to care, with an average of 11 days to the 3rd next available routine appt. • New desired target was to meet/exceed the Air Force Medical Service goal of less than 5% No-Show rate.
* What was the main root cause? * What actions did you take to address the root cause and change the PROCESS for the better?	• Routine well-child appointments were booked up to 3 months in advance. Why? That was the process in place to help improve the HEDIS measure for well-child appointments • First cycle of improvement in July 2016 was initiation of a new process to "mail-out" appointment reminders to patients 2 weeks in advance. • Second cycle of improvement was to call each patient/parent who "no-showed" to follow-up, reschedule, and remind them to cancel if unable to come in. • Also posted the number of no-shows from previous month on the waiting room TV display, and on the *Trusted Care Board* inviting patients to make suggestions for improvement.
* Provide measureable outcome DATA that showed you achieved your desired performance target.	• By Nov 2016 the No-show rate dropped to ~7%. • By Feb 2017 the No-show rate dropped to ~5.5% • A subsequent improvement was an increase of ~30% in our HEDIS Well-Child Measure!
* How did you standardize the process and share successes and lessons learned? (e.g., new policy/procedure; share at flight and squadron meetings, and with SGHQ)	• New processes were added to the clinic's Continuity Binder to assure spread and sustainability • Most recent improvement and lesson learned: the "auto-reminder" phone call system was turned-on for the Peds clinic appointments. It was previously assumed this could not be used since we were overseas. • Improvements shared with Quality office for posting on the Med Group webpage and for presentation and recognition at Executive Staff.

FIGURE 13.3 Example of Just-Do-It.

daily improvements, leaders evidence respect for the knowledge, skills, and commitment already existing at the work-unit level. Staff is empowered and sees the value of doing "what is possible today." New staffs that are sometimes overwhelmed by the complexity, length, and breadth of large formal QI projects that can go on for months or more, can appreciate and enjoy the small successes that come from the JDIs. Those successes can then be the impetus for involvement in bigger and better QI projects.

A common standardized report called an A3 (based on the ISO A3-sized traditional sheet of paper) is most often used to document and share the work done for formal Lean projects and was first employed by the Toyota Corporation. The A3 generally consists of eight steps and is often referred to as a Practical Problem Solving Method. The eight steps include the following:

1. Clarify the Problem
2. Breakdown the Problem
3. Set the Target
4. Analyze the Root Cause
5. Develop Countermeasures
6. See Countermeasures Through
7. Monitor the Process and Results
8. Standardize Successful Processes

An example of a completed A3 can be seen in Figure 13.4.

Technological advances have provided resources in documenting Lean and other QI activities, as seen in Case Study 13.2.

48th Fighter Wing AFSO21 | **AIR FORCE 8-STEP IMPROVEMENT PROCESS** **48 Medical Group (MDG)** "Order-to-Door"

CHAMPION: Colonel --- (48 MDG/SGH)
PROCESS OWNER: Capt --- (MSU), Maj ----(MSU) **FACILITATORS:** Mr. ---
(48 CES), Capt --- (48 AMDS) **OBSERVERS:** SSgt ---, MSgt ---

TEAM MEMBERS (Function):
Capt--(MSU), Maj---(MSU), Maj --- (ENT), Maj--(Pediatrics), Maj---(Surgery),Maj
---(Pharmacy),Capt--(Lab), Ms--- (Tri-Care),Capt--- (Internal Med), SSgt---
(Mental Health),SSgt--(Pt Admin),Mr---(Systems),andMs---(Medical Records)

1. Clarify & Validate the Problem

The MSU's ability to manage bed availability and effectively utilize staff and other resources is reliant on prompt and consistent discharge (D/C) times. However, between January and March 2015, the average processing time for patients discharged from the 48 FW/MDG Multi-Service Unit (MSU) was 102 minutes (slow) with times ranging from 31 to 240 minutes.

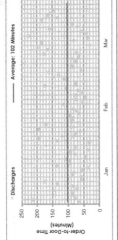

2. Break down the Problem/Identify Performance Gaps

The D/C process begins when an admitted patient's care is completed and they no longer require hospital support. However, certain criteria must be met, which the doctor identifies on a D/C Order. Once an IT system generates the D/C Order, MSU staff are then prompted to review the D/C Order and perform necessary actions to satisfy D/C criteria. Once achieved, the patient is able to depart the MSU, ending the D/C process. Gemba workshops captured 11 D/C's, revealing common voice-of-customer themes and waste hot-spots to target.

VOICE OF CUSTOMER:
Patient: "I was told I was being discharged, but I wasn't able to leave for another 3 hours."
MSU Staff: "I'm constantly stopping the process to fix an error or clarify something with the Dr."
Doctor: "The only way I see this process going faster would be to predict when a patient will be discharged, which is impossible."

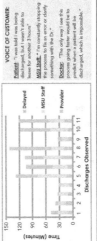

3. Set Improvement Target

Based on the data collected, the 48 MDG Commander determined that eliminating waste in their processes would allow the MSU to achieve an average patient discharge time of less than 60 minutes by the end of the year.

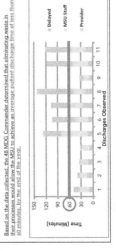

4. Determine Root Cause

Team brainstormed and prioritized issues according to perceived impact. Team identified three common root causes using, "5-Why's" analysis.

ISSUES	IMPACT
Discharge Process initiated late/inconsistently	11
Not managing patient expectations	6
Double brief of post-op care	4
Timing/over-processing of ORYX measure reviews	4
D/C Summary form connected to D/C Instructions form	6
Nurses interpreting Essentris orders for input into CHCS	1
Lack of role-pute communication between IT systems	2
	1

5-WHYS ANALYSIS

RC1	FUNCTIONALLY SILOED COMMUNICATION
RC2	POORLY INTEGRATED IT SYSTEM
RC3	UNESTABLISHED PROCESSES

5. Develop Countermeasures

Team brainstormed & summarized countermeasures, and evaluated their potential impact in relation to ease of implementation using a "PICK" Chart.

CM1	IMPROVE COMMUNICATION & VISUAL MANAGEMENT
CM2	MODIFY EHR SYSTEM
CM3	DEVELOP STANDARDIZED PROCESSES

Each countermeasure was deemed feasible for implementation. The team then developed an action plan in support of each. The action plan was then approved by

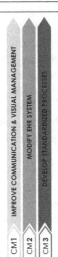

POSSIBLE — IMPLEMENT / CHALLENGE — KILL
PERCEIVED EFFORT / PERCEIVED IMPACT

6. See Countermeasures Through

TASK	POC (FUNCTION)	STATUS
Develop agenda (checklist) for nightly rounds	Maj--(MSU)	Complete
Develop Patient Discharge Brochure	Capt-- (MSU)	Complete
Con-leave template	Capt--- (IM)	Complete
Designate Provider AM Schedule for rounds	Capt--- (IM)	Complete
Huddle tracking board	Capt--- (MSU)	Complete
Manage huddles	Maj---(Surgery)	Complete
Display functional capabilities to all MSU personnel	Capt--- (MSU)	Complete
ESSENTRIS Screen "save"	Mr--(Systems)	Complete
Separate D/C Summary from D/C Instructions	Mr--- (Systems)	Complete
Designated D/C Computer	Mr--- (Systems)	Complete

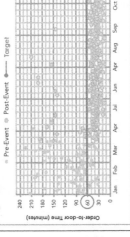

7. Confirm Results & Process

Since implementation, order-to-door process times have been reduced to now reflect an average of 46 minutes.

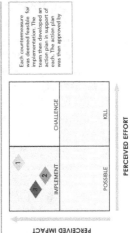

Collateral Victories:
- Relationships between multi-functional staff improved due to huddles.
- Training employees is easier due to standard process and visual aids.
- Hospital currently making headway with "24-hour Observation Status" after idea was proposed during event.

8. Standardize Successful Processes

- MSU implemented long-term visual management tools, such as affixing huddle boards to walls and adding documents such as meeting agendas, checklists, and brochures to file plan.
- Project details uploaded to CPI-MT and USAFE Capturing Innovations site to provide best-practice adoption opportunities.

FIGURE 13.4 Example of an A3.

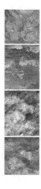

CASE STUDY 13.2

During your hospital's monthly review of patient satisfaction data, you see that there has been no significant movement in the performance over the past 4 months. It is pretty much flat lined. Although your performance has been slightly above average compared to national patient satisfaction data, your team agrees that they would like to be seen as one of the *best* healthcare facilities nationally, in support of your organization's **Vision** "To be a world-class healthcare delivery system."

Your team decides to initiate a vigorous improvement project using a version of the Lean model for improvement that a U.S. Air Force (USAF) friend recently told you about. In fact, he shared with you information about a free mobile app from Griffin Mobile for your iPhone or Android called AFCPI (Air Force Continuous Process Improvement). The AFCPI mobile app quickly and easily demonstrates the tools and methodologies used for a continuous process improvement project. While some of the tools specifically reference the Air Force, you notice the majority of terms, descriptions, and use of the tools and methodologies are broadly used in Lean and Six Sigma. Comparison to define, measure, analyze, improve, and control (DMAIC) and PDC(S)A is also included. Detailed content thoroughly addresses the applicability and content of the USAF 8-Step A3 Certification Rubric, and interactive use of each individual step. While many healthcare organizations have Lean Six Sigma Green or Black Belt practitioners to facilitate big projects, you now recognize that resources such as this app make it absolutely possible for anyone with in-depth knowledge of their own work processes, and a strong interest in improvement, to work successfully with these tools.

You think this may be a helpful framework as your organization launches a patient satisfaction improvement project, so you decide to give it a look. Load the AFCPI app to your phone.

Following are the eight Lean Steps previously discussed in this chapter. Check out the tools and descriptions under each step in the app and select one tool for each step that you think might be helpful for your team.

1. *Clarify the Problem*
2. *Breakdown the Problem*
3. *Set the Target*
4. *Analyze the Root Cause*
5. *Develop Countermeasures*
6. *See Countermeasures Through*
7. *Monitor the Process and Results*
8. *Standardize Successful Processes*

Six Sigma and DMAIC

Six Sigma, one of the more advanced methodologies adopted from the business sector, encompasses interventions with the goal to reduce variation in existing processes. In doing so, it often leads to new process design or redesign. When a process is carried out inconsistently, the outcomes of that process vary over time leading to process variation. The goal is to reduce variation by standardizing the process so that it is consistently performed over time. Consider you are nursing on a surgical unit with a common nursing intervention of pain reassessment postpain medication. Because the pain reassessment policy would stipulate the reassessment and documentation postmedication administration, we can measure how consistently that is being accomplished. If the policy used 30 minutes as the time frame from administration to reassessment, outcomes hovering around that 30-minute time frame would demonstrate a stable process. If the average time were found to be 45 minutes with a range of 33 to 48 minutes, the process demonstrates variation. Not only does this example show if staff are following their policy, but also speaks the risk that patients may continue to experience pain because they are not consistently being reassessed.

Why is the reduction of process variation referred to as Six Sigma? In the discussion in Chapter 14 on standard deviation, you will learn that the upper control limits are commonly set at three standard deviations (SDs) above the mean while the lower control limits are set at three SDs below the mean. Common cause variation exists when the data points fall within the upper and lower control limits, which when added together represent six SDs, or Six Sigma.

Six Sigma incorporates several problem-solving steps to reduce variation in a healthcare process (Evans, 2008). The steps are known as: define, measure, analyze, improve, and control, or DMAIC, as defined in Table 13.5.

Although similar, there are appreciable differences between Lean and Six Sigma. Lean focuses on reducing waste while Six Sigma is more focused on variation in performance, and requires specialized skills and statistical tools making it a more sophisticated improvement approach. There are QI professionals who believe it is first necessary to make a process more efficient before attempting to reduce variation, thus combining the two methodologies within QI activities, as seen in the Current Thoughts From the Literature 13.1.

TABLE 13.5 DEFINE, MEASURE, ANALYZE, IMPROVE, AND CONTROL (DMAIC)

Define	Identifies the QI focus.
	Defines the team, operational definition of the variable, baseline data, and improvement aim or expected level of performance when variability is reduced, and the project timeline.
	Tools such as fishbone diagrams and process maps are used to define the problem.
Measure	Includes identifying the current process, validating the variable to measure, assessing baseline performance, and selecting who will conduct measurement procedures.
	Tools such as Pareto charts and process control charts are often useful in this step (see Chapter 14).
Analyze	Rigorous analysis to understand top causes of why errors are occurring.
	Tools such as statistical measurements, control charts, fishbone diagrams, and hypothesis testing are often useful in this step (see Chapter 14 and the fishbone diagram in this chapter).
Improve	Brainstorming what solutions may be useful in reducing variation and conducting small-scale trials of possible solutions.
Control	Methods to sustain improvements, such as employee education, and the process for ongoing measurement to ensure the new and improved processes are sustained over time.

QI, quality improvement.

EVIDENCE FROM THE LITERATURE

Citation

Pocha, C. (2010). Lean Six Sigma in healthcare and the challenge of implementation of Six Sigma methodologies at a Veterans Affairs medical center. *Quality Management in Health Care, 19*(4), 312–318.

Discussion

The purpose of this improvement team was to reduce the number of portable chest x-rays in an ED. Many patients who present to an ED receive a portable chest x-ray, which may be difficult to interpret compared to the more specific posterior/anterior and lateral (PAL) x-ray. To address the problem, the team used define, measure, analyze, improve, and control (DMAIC) to work through the problem.

Define

The team hypothesized that 30% of portable chest x-rays completed in the ED would be repeated within 24 to 48 hours of admission as PAL views for improved interpretation, leading to duplication of service and increased costs. A team was gathered of experts, including a Six-Sigma consultant who served as educator and team facilitator. The team used Lean concepts of efficiency and the Six-Sigma approach to reduce variability of those patients receiving both a portable and postadmission repeated PAL x-ray.

Measure

The team collected baseline data for 6 months that demonstrated 254 patients who were admitted to medicine service through the ED had a portable chest x-ray while in the ED. Of the 254 patients, 79 (32%) received a postadmission PAL chest film.

Analysis

Many variables were assessed, for example, the cost of one portable chest x-ray was $147.98. A reduction of 30% would equate to an annual savings of $23,380, not to mention less radiation exposure, radiology technician time, and patient satisfaction.

Improve

Strict criteria for portable chest x-rays were established related to diagnosis groups, including acute coronary ischemia, pulmonary emboli, and for those patients unable to stand. After implementing these new criteria, there was a reduction in portable chest x-rays, from 32% to 23% over a 1-month period.

(continued)

EVIDENCE FROM THE LITERATURE

(*continued*)

Control

The team will continue to monitor the percent of patients who receive both a portable and postadmission chest x-ray.

Implications for Practice

Lean Six Sigma tools can successfully be used for the systematic implementation of an improvement process. In addition, these tools can be taught and applied by teams, leading to a high degree of success. The author describes the value of utilizing both Six Sigma and Lean within a single project. In summary, Lean incorporates a systems approach to decrease inefficiencies but does not provide the scientific rigor of Six Sigma while Six Sigma does not offer standard solutions from a systems perspective. Interestingly, the author concludes with the criticality of the teams' buy-in and willingness to change practice. Furthermore, despite an improvement project application, adoption of new criteria by some providers did not occur. The author confirms the reality of all projects that, although there may be evidence of a need to improve and a clear intervention that may be agreed upon, it does not guarantee those expected to carry out the intervention will comply. Identifying barriers and rationale for such decisions is a valuable process when analyzing outcomes.

Take a moment to watch the video in Critical Thinking 13.3. In the video, there is more discussion about Six Sigma and how it compares to a continual improvement philosophy known as *Kaizen*.

CRITICAL THINKING 13.3

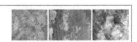

According to the Kaizen Institute (www.kaizen.com/about-us/definition-of-kaizen. html), Kaizen is a continual improvement philosophy with a notable feature that states "big results come from many small changes accumulated over time." The Kaizen philosophy is that everyone in the organization is making improvements. As you have learned, the Plan-Do-Study-Act (PDSA) cycle is an improvement method for small tests of change and is an important Kaizen tool. You have also learned that Six Sigma is another methodology to reduce defects within a process by systematizing the process or changing the process to reduce defects. View the brief video "Process Improvement: Six Sigma & Kaizen" at www.youtube.com/watch?v=ilDAYBR5sQU.
What are the key differences and similarities between Kaizen and Six Sigma?

APPROACHES TO QI PROBLEMS

The QI process is often a critical response to an adverse event, near miss, or sentinel event. To identify the actual cause of a problem and implement improvement strategies, it is important to know how the problems are identified and resulting specific actions by a QI team. Uncovering the problem can be more difficult than one might expect. Reactive strategies are those actions that occur after an event has taken place, such as peer review (discussed earlier in the chapter) and RCA. Healthcare Failure Modes and Effects Analysis (HFMEA™) is a proactive method to identify risks before they result in errors, allowing the team to prevent problems in high-risk processes before a near miss or adverse event occurs.

Retroactive Approach: RCA

A **root cause analysis** is an investigation of what caused a problem and why the problem occurred. TJC, in their sentinel event policies and procedures (accessible at www.jointcommission.org/sentinel_event_policy_and_procedures/), stipulates that an investigation such as an RCA be conducted whenever a sentinel event occurs (TJC, 2017). The top reported root causes of sentinel events to TJC from 2005 to 2016 can be viewed at www.jointcommission.org/assets/1/18/Summary_4Q_2016.pdf.

The RCA process is also a valuable tool that can be used in any instance where the need to know the underlying root cause of a problem exists. Based on the findings from an RCA, an action plan can be developed and implemented in order to reduce risk of a future similar adverse or sentinel event. To understand how an RCA works, we will use an example to walk through the steps. A patient with insulin-dependent diabetes is given the wrong dose of insulin. Although the patient did not experience any detrimental effects, the medication error is considered an adverse event. The staff determined that an RCA can help determine the contributing factors to the medication error and how to prevent similar errors from occurring. An interprofessional team is gathered to investigate the problem consisting of nurses, physicians, nursing assistants, quality department representative, central supply representative, and clinical educator. To conduct an RCA, the following steps occur:

1. Identify what happened.
2. Review what should have happened.
3. Determine causes.
4. Develop causal statements.
5. Generate a list of recommended changes.
6. Share findings with those who affect or are affected by the outcome.
7. Ensure actions are taken and sustained to prevent or reduce the risk of future recurrence.

The first step, identify what happened, occurs through a dialogue among all team members. The team starts with the statement that a medication error occurred resulting in 10 times the ordered dose of insulin given to the patient. The clear statement brings all team members to the same starting point to examine the problem.

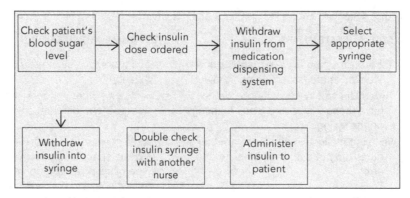

FIGURE 13.5 Flow chart of insulin preparation.

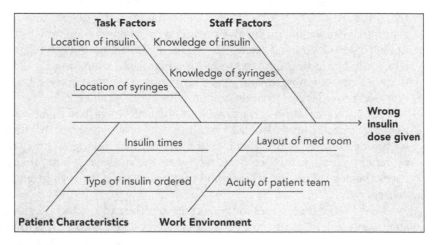

FIGURE 13.6 Fishbone diagram.

To understand what happened, the team develops a flow chart (Figure 13.5) of the insulin preparation process. Team members use the flow chart to identify and examine factors in the process that may have contributed to the near miss or sentinel event. The process is mapped out to show each of the steps involved with insulin preparation process.

Those team members directly involved with the medication error provide information about steps that can highlight process problems. It is important to note here that the RCA looks at process breakdowns rather than individual person's error. In this scenario, the nurse is not viewed as causing the error, rather a breakdown in the process allowed the error to occur. This encourages all participants to fully engage in identifying contributing factors.

The next step is to determine causes. A cause-effect diagram, or fishbone diagram, helps participants understand the contributing factors to the medication error. The "bones" of the fish, as seen in Figure 13.6, represent the common areas that might contribute to the problem and include, at minimum, task factors, patient characteristics, work environment, and staff factors (IHI, 2017). It is important to note that the categories, or bones of the fish, may have different labels depending on what template is used.

Each area is discussed by team members and examined in terms of what happened during the near miss or sentinel event that contributed to the outcome. During this

TABLE 13.6 CAUSAL STATEMENTS AND RECOMMENDED CHANGES

CAUSAL STATEMENTS	RECOMMENDED CHANGES
Tuberculin syringes were inappropriately stocked in the insulin syringe drawer	Move tuberculin syringes to a different location
Tuberculin and insulin syringes both have orange caps and black markings on the syringe	Check with other vendors about the availability of different colored syringes
Verifying the insulin dose with another nurse did not catch the medication error	Double checks with another nurse need to include specific steps such as looking at the type of syringe, the amount of medication in the syringe, and the dose ordered

process, an effective method to get at the core causes of the problem is to ask "why" five times. Asking "why" five times helps the team dig deeper into the actual process issues that caused the problem. Consider a problem you are now facing or have faced in the past. Ask yourself "why" five times. Be honest with your responses. Your problem could be finding time to study for a big exam, preparing for clinical, or needing to give a presentation to your class. Write down your responses. Did the fifth "why" question provides information on the root of your problem?

During the creation of the flowchart, the team identified that the nurse reached for a syringe from a drawer labeled "insulin syringes" but instead, the drawer was stocked with tuberculin syringes. This resulted in the nurse giving 10 times the ordered dose of insulin. Another misstep occurred when the nurse asked another nurse to double check the dose of insulin. The second nurse glanced at the syringe and agreed the dose was correct.

Based on findings from the flow chart and the cause-effect diagram, a list of causal statements and recommended changes is created (Table 13.6). It is important to appreciate that.

RCAs are intended to focus on system problems rather than placing individual blame for any problems or sentinel events. Now that you have learned about the RCA process, see if you can apply it to the situation in Case Study 13.3.

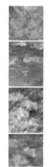

CASE STUDY 13.3

A patient arrives in the ED at 6:30 a.m. (0600), nearing the end of the night shift, complaining of chest pain. The ECG shows an acute myocardial infarction in progress and morphine sulfate 2 mg, nitroglycerin drip IV, and oxygen are ordered. The nurse goes to the medication dispensing unit, removes a syringe of morphine sulfate 2 mg, and administers the medication IV push as ordered. Within 3 minutes the patient stops breathing, going into anaphylatic shock. The nurse calls a code. The patient survives despite being allergic to morphine sulfate. The nurse feels terrible about this human error, which resulted in a sentinel event. The nurse fills out an incident report and also alerts the nursing supervisor.

- *Name the factors that contributed to this medication error.*
- *How could this sentinel event have been prevented?*
- *Name safety guards that can be implemented to prevent future similar sentinel events.*

Proactive Approach: HFMEA™

Healthcare Failure Mode and Effects Analysis (HFMEA™) is a prospective risk analysis system to identify, assess, and address vulnerabilities in high-risk processes. Failure Mode and Effects Analysis (FMEA) has its roots in the U.S. military, engineering, and aerospace industries, where steps are taken to minimize or eliminate the risk that an accident or failure will occur. In 2001, the U.S. Department of Veterans Affairs, National Center for Patient Safety, developed a hybrid model specific to, and ideal for, the healthcare environment (DeRosier, Stalhandske, Bagian, & Nudell, 2002). At the same time, TJC introduced a new Leadership Standard, still in effect today, that requires hospital leaders to include a proactive risk assessment of at least one high-risk process every 18 months (TJC, 2017). Healthcare organizations soon widely adopted these approaches. Three basic questions are the focus of any proactive failure mode/risk analysis:

1. What could go wrong?
2. Why would the failures occur?
3. What would be the consequences of each failure?

The goal of the team is to improve the safety of known, complex, high-risk healthcare processes before they result in adverse events by identifying, minimizing, or eliminating high-risk aspects and other vulnerabilities of the process. Both flow mapping and fishbone diagrams are commonly used tools by HFMEA teams. For example, the administration of a heparin infusion, a high-risk medication, involves many complex steps including calculating the patient's weight in kilograms, ensuring the correct amount of heparin is in the solution, changing doses, and administering boluses based on laboratory studies. Consider the role of the provider who must order the heparin correctly, the pharmacist who may prepare or deliver the heparin, both of which are processes that may lead to errors. HFMEA™ allows the team to assess potential risks of each step. Teams prioritize actions based on a severity of risk rating scale. The VA National Center for Patient Safety (accessible at www.patientsafety.va.gov/professionals/onthejob/hfmea.asp) identifies five steps to be completed during a HFMEA:

1. Define the HFMEA topic.
2. Assemble the team.
3. Graphically describe the process.
4. Conduct a hazard analysis.
5. Actions and outcome measures.

HFMEA improvement strategies commonly involve redesigning processes to minimize or eliminate identified risks. Of consideration, nurses should maintain an ongoing awareness of those high-risk processes that may serve well for an HFMEA. Nurses should also be encouraged to participate or lead teams, as many high-risk processes involve nursing judgment and oversight, and will therefore benefit from that nursing expertise.

Teams conducting an HFMEA will identify many actions believed to reduce the risk of error from occurring. To better understand how actions are prioritized, complete the activities outlined in Critical Thinking 13.4.

Now that you have learned some of the basics of QI, including models and improvement methods, you can appreciate the added value of nursing participation and leading QI activities. As you begin your nursing career, you want to take charge, make improvements, and get involved as a valued team member. Being new and wanting to make change can be challenging. Work through Case Study 13.4. This exercise may help!

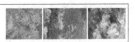

CRITICAL THINKING 13.4

Go to app.ihi.org/Workspace/tools/fmea/AllTools.aspx and select a tool that interests you from the list. Select one of the topics and view the report. Explore the failure mode, causes, and effects listed.

1. How do the actions listed in the right column affect the failure mode, cause, and effect listed?
2. What factors contribute to the Risk Profile Number (RPN) and how is the RPN used?

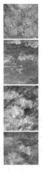

CASE STUDY 13.4

You are interested in quality improvement (QI) and ask your manager if you could attend further training on QI processes and methods. Your manager acknowledges your interest to learn but is not familiar with QI educational resources. In speaking with a new colleague, he shares that the last organization he worked for brought in some team of experts to help get them "Up to speed in the quality stuff." He calls it "TCAB" but cannot recall what it stands for. You conduct a search and discover TCAB refers to "Transforming Care at the Bedside." Go to the Robert Wood Johnson Foundation website at www.rwjf.org/.

1. *In the search box, type in "TCAB outcomes."*
2. *Several pages of references discussing TCAB are listed. Select and read the article "Transforming Care at the Bedside by Empowering Nurses" (June 28, 2012) and answer the following questions:*
   a. *In the first paragraph, what improvement methodology is described?*
   b. *What organizations teamed to create TCAB?*
   c. *What is the overall goal of TCAB?*
   d. *You see that the Institute for Healthcare Improvement (IHI) has an educational resource; what is it?*
   e. *What key factor was required by the 13 facilities participating in the second phase of TCAB?*
   f. *In the sixth paragraph, open the link "major initiatives." Scroll down and view the short TCAB story from Eastern Maine Medical Center. What was the Red Zone project? Describe the Provider/Nurse Rounding intervention?*

THE ROLE OF THE NURSE IN QI

Traditionally, nurses are taught to collect and analyze patient data early in their student experiences, which is an important aspect of nursing and QI. This analysis leads to prioritizing nursing interventions that are implemented and evaluated over time. Nurses must assess the impact of their interventions and determine the need to eliminate or implement new interventions based on observed patient outcomes.

In today's complex healthcare organizations, it is the responsibility of both novice and expert nurses to improve practice (Painter, 2010). It is intuitive to nurses to want to improve and focus on enhanced patient outcomes (Berwick, 2011). In fact, the optimal goal of nurses caring for patients is to improve health, improve the processes and systems that contribute to positive outcomes, and reduce harm. And, increasingly, nurses are taking the lead in QI initiatives.

Asking questions is an important aspect of QI. Nurses approach the processes and systems of care they use every day as variables that constantly need evaluation; they identify processes that may enhance care or lead to errors, and determine how such processes can be improved to promote patient safety and performance excellence. Nurses are expected to have the KSAs to assess, analyze, intervene, and evaluate not just patient outcomes, but outcomes that reflect individual and interdisciplinary practice.

Nurses can assume a variety of roles when conducting QI activities. As a novice nurse committed to improving care, you can help collect data or assist with literature reviews for more complex improvement interventions; therefore, it is important to know what sources of data and information are available, how to access them, and who your QI resources are. You can also accomplish simpler "Just Do It" improvement projects quickly and easily within your area of control.

Nurses, consistently making improvements at any level, contribute significantly to the organization, service, unit, and patients. Advanced practice and experienced nurses are expected to lead QI teams for more complex issues, and serve as a resource to team members.

Leadership Support

A supportive and empowering hospital culture and effective leadership are necessary for optimal QI. Given the ramifications of quality outcome performance for hospital reimbursement and patient care, it is imperative that the hospital, nursing, and medical staff have leadership's full support for improving hospital processes. Leaders who round on patient care units and directly talk to staff about quality and safety concerns tend to be more effective in identifying areas of improvement and involving staff in the pursuit of solutions. Effective leaders partner with their employees by empowering them to ask questions, seek new ways of doing business, remove fear of failure, and provide the resources needed to try new ideas that may improve organizational performance. Lindberg and Kimberlain (2008) note that if the intent of every healthcare worker is to provide quality care, then the responsibility of executives is to create a culture for that to occur.

Hospital leaders support QI activities by providing a set of clear expectations and ongoing and meaningful feedback. When hospital leadership is involved with QI projects from the top down, it sends the message that quality is a shared team responsibility. By the same token, nurses, physicians, and the entire interdisciplinary healthcare team must actively engage in QI efforts by bringing issues to leadership's attention from the ground up, and by actively participating in the improvements that are then more likely to be meaningful and sustained.

Feedback and dissemination of the results of QI projects are essential for improvement. Hospitals use a variety of mechanisms including newsletters, new employee orientation, email communication, staff training, staff meetings, and unit-based communication boards. One method of sharing QI data is to use scorecards or dashboards that use a quick-look approach to show where the current standing is on a quality issue in relation to benchmarks.

Quality information tends to be most effectively disseminated at the microsystem level, in other words where direct patient care is given, so frontline staff can readily implement changes. Nurse managers and leaders must use caution, however, on the amount of raw data and information shared, as large quantities of unanalyzed data and information can become difficult to understand and less meaningful for staff. It is best to share concise analyses that highlight how a process was improved or how a quality benchmark was met (Lindberg & Kimberlain, 2008).

Overcoming Barriers

Although it is the goal of many healthcare facilities to engage the healthcare team in QI initiatives, some barriers to QI exist. One significant barrier is adequate time for nursing and support staff to participate in improvement projects. Additionally, nurses may want to, or feel obligated to, participate in QI initiatives but may lack the knowledge and skills necessary to comfortably and actively participate. Leadership needs to provide QI education and training for nurses, in addition to allocated time to work on QI initiatives. Moreover, many of these challenges can be overcome with a style of leadership called shared governance.

Shared governance is a professional practice model founded on the principles of partnership, equity, accountability, and ownership that form a culturally sensitive and empowering framework, enabling sustainable- and accountability-based decisions to support an interdisciplinary design for excellent patient care (Anthony, 2004; Cox-Sullivan, Norris, Brown, & Scott, 2017). It is the shared control over nursing practice and clinical decision making that empowers staff nurses and managers to work together for successful QI projects. When frontline staff nurses actively participate in QI and take control over their practice, the expected result is a better work environment, better staff satisfaction, improved staff retention, and better patient outcomes.

Leaders at all levels of the organization are responsible for the creation and oversight of a quality culture, safe environment, and high-quality patient outcomes. QI education and training is clearly necessary for this process as is the leadership commitment to both patients and staff.

Academic challenges remain in not only preparing students to apply QI methodologies but in developing student interest and motivation to value their role in QI as professional nurses. A small study conducted by Peterson-Graziose and Bryer (2017) supports the existence of this academic-practice gap regarding QI. The researchers asked 73 undergraduate nursing students their perceptions to the extent they acquired the knowledge, skills, and attitudes of the six QSEN competencies. Regarding QI, students reported that QI content was taught the least in the curriculum, the lowest skill set they felt prepared for, and rated QI the least important of all six QSEN competencies. These results are concerning because as students transition to practice, this gap has impact. Organizations desperately seek nurses with the QI KSAs to recognize processes needing improvement, to take action, implement improvement interventions, evaluate the outcomes of actions, and determine if the outcome meets the expectation or not. Faculty must utilize clinical settings as a rich environment to teach principles of QI. Additionally, organizations have many experts and staff who participate in QI. Such staff can serve as resources to faculty to help teach QI, engage students, and share their QI experiences. Learning principles of QI in a classroom is necessary but applying principles of QI in clinical settings is critical for students to appreciate the value and role of the nurse in QI.

It is truly an exciting time for nurses and those participating in and leading QI activities. Empowering and preparing nurses to be active participants in QI activities encourage them to make decisions that impact the quality and safety of their patients' care. To successfully contribute to QI efforts, nurses must be able to understand and utilize a broad array of QI tools. Identifying new, improved ways to provide care and services is only one part of the QI equation. Disseminating outcomes from QI projects to other colleagues helps others to improve their own practices. Once the QI KSAs are obtained, the ability to improve patient outcomes and organizational processes is limitless. Are you prepared and ready?

KEY CONCEPTS

1. Quality improvement (QI) is defined as to "use data to monitor the outcomes of care processes and use improvement methods to design and test changes to continuously improve the quality and safety of healthcare systems" (Cronenwett, et al., 2007).
2. QI began with the work of the American Medical Association in the early 1900s. Over time, QI changed from standardizing care to include measurements of the process of care and healthcare outcomes in response to accreditation standards of The Joint Commission. The current focus of QI continues to evolve in response to the Centers for Medicare and Medicaid Services (CMS) programs such as Value-Based Purchasing.
3. QI is the incorporation of existing information and data into QI activities. Evidence-based practice (EBP) focuses on translating evidence into clinical, educational, or administrative practice. The aim of research is to generate new knowledge by testing theories or interventions.
4. Donabedian's model looks at three areas for QI: structure, process, and outcomes. Deming's model prescribes how QI takes place in a cyclical manner using Plan-Do-Study-Act (PDSA). Six Sigma prescribes five steps for QI to reduce variation in performance: define, measure, analyze, improve, and control (DMAIC). Lean interventions focus on improving efficiency, reducing waste, and streamlining processes through the cumulative effect of small improvements.
5. Patient satisfaction data are collected and reported to the CMS. CMS makes the patient satisfaction data publicly available on their website. The data allow consumers to make an informed decision about where to seek healthcare.
6. A root cause analysis (RCA) is conducted after a near miss or sentinel event has occurred. An RCA is an investigation of what caused a problem and why the problem occurred. The Joint Commission requires that an RCA take place whenever a sentinel event occurs.
7. Examine how the RCA process helps understand near miss events or sentinel events.
8. Healthcare Failure Mode Effects Analysis (HFMEA™) is a QI tool that looks at a healthcare process to determine the potential for risk. The goal of an HFMEA is to improve the safety of a complex, high-risk healthcare process before an adverse event occurs by identifying and eliminating high-risk aspects of the process.
9. Nurses, both experienced and novice, are expected to have the knowledge, skills, and attitudes to assess, analyze, intervene, and evaluate not just patient outcomes, but outcomes that reflect individual and interdisciplinary practice. Nurses

approach the processes and systems of care they use every day as variables that constantly need evaluation; recognizing processes that may enhance care or lead to errors, and recognizing how such processes can be improved to promote patient safety and performance excellence.

KEY TERMS

Health Failure Mode and Effects
    Analysis (HFMEA™)
Hospital Value-Based Purchasing
Lean
Outcomes
Plan-Do-Study-Act

Process
Quality improvement
Root cause analysis
Six Sigma
Structure
Tracer methodology

REVIEW QUESTIONS

1. You are a staff nurse caring for a patient that The Joint Commission (TJC) surveyor has selected for a tracer. This is the first day you are caring for this patient. Because you are not familiar with this patient, what action would be best for you and the organization?

   A. Explain to the surveyor that this is your first day caring for the patient.
   B. Request another patient.
   C. Review the electronic medical record (EMR) to ensure all provider documentation is up to date.
   D. Transfer the patient to another unit.
   E. Request the nurse from the previous shift stay to talk with TJC surveyor.

2. Which of the following is a *primary* goal of quality improvement (QI)?

   A. Improve patient outcomes.
   B. Improve data reported to external regulatory agencies.
   C. Improve cost-effectiveness of care delivery.
   D. Improve reimbursement rates by insurers.

3. Which improvement methodology emphasizes risk reduction before an error occurs?

   A. Six Sigma
   B. Lean
   C. Healthcare Failure Modes and Effects Analysis (HFMEA™)
   D. Root cause analysis (RCA)

4. A group of nurses on a medical–surgical unit noted their readmission rates were higher than other units. With further investigation, the nurses identify that patients were readmitted to the hospital based on a lack of understanding of discharge instructions. As a team, they decide to look at how they could assess every patient's health literacy level (i.e., understanding of health information) because health literacy was identified as a contributing factor to increased readmissions. The team identifies three tools commonly found in the literature. They decide on one tool that is appropriate for their medical–surgical population of patients. To implement the tool, they teach the staff how to use it, document the patient's

literacy level score in the electronic medical record (EMR), and brief the rest of the patient's care team on use of that health literacy information during interactions with the patient. Readmissions are reduced from 15% to 8% at the end of a 4-month trial period. Is this considered research, quality improvement (QI), or evidence-based practice (EBP)?

A. It is research since the nurses research each tool to find evidence.
B. It is QI since the nurses used data and identified an intervention to improve their readmission outcome.
C. It is EBP since the nurses evaluated three tools and selected the most appropriate tool for their patient population.
D. It is none of the above since the nurses only wanted to find out the patient's literacy level.

5. Which of the following processes using Deming's Plan-Do-Study-Act (PDSA) method for quality improvement (QI) is correct?

A. Collect baseline data, evaluate the improvement, measure outcomes, redesign the plan.
B. Collect baseline data, use small-scale trials for change, collect data and compare against desired outcomes, adjust the plan.
C. Implement small-scale change, collect data, disseminate the data, and sustain the improvement.
D. Implement changes, evaluate effects from change, identify data, and readjust the plan.

6. Many organizations are combining Lean and Six Sigma concepts within their quality improvement (QI) efforts. What option below best explains why this combination may be successful?

A. Lean focuses on optimizing existing processes (e.g., removing nonvalue added activities) for cost reduction and efficiency while Six Sigma focuses on minimizing variability to eliminate defects.
B. Lean focuses on variability reduction over time while Six Sigma focuses on efficiency in the current existing process.
C. Lean, emphasizing efficiency, and Six Sigma, emphasizing increasing variability, are seldom combined as they both focus on separate improvement methods.
D. Lean focuses on eliminating existing processes to reduce costs while Six Sigma focuses on eliminating defects to increase variability over time.

7. Which option below is true about a fishbone diagram?

A. It is a useful data analysis tool in determining variability over time.
B. It visually represents a process, from beginning to end.
C. It is commonly used to determine definitive cause and effect relationships.
D. It is a quality improvement (QI) tool to identify relationships among possible factors.

8. Healthcare Failure Mode and Effects Analysis (HFMEA™) is different from a Root Cause Analysis (RCA) because of which of the following?

A. HFMEA is a proactive process to assess, eliminate, or reduce the risks related to complex, high-risk processes before they result in adverse events. RCA is a retrospective analysis of an event that has already occurred.

B. HFMEA is a proactive process of an event that has already occurred. RCA is a retrospective process to identify the most appropriate intervention when developing a Plan-Do-Study-Act (PDSA).

C. HFMEA is an adverse events documentation system commonly employed by organizations to track sentinel events. RCA is an improvement tool that must be done annually on one significant event that occurred within the organization.

D. HFMEA is one single process used to enhance the quality culture within the organization. RCA is a part of every PDSA and is documented as part of the D ("Do") phase.

9. Which of the following types of problems would likely prompt the initiation of a root cause analysis (RCA)? Select all that apply.

A. A suicidal patient signs out of the ED against medical advice.

B. An adult dose of heparin is given to an infant.

C. Surgery was performed on the wrong leg.

D. Failure to resuscitate a patient after an inadvertent morphine overdose in the hospital.

E. Two different hemostats, one reusable, one disposable, are stocked in the clean utility room within the same bin.

10. A new nurse can participate in quality improvement (QI) activities by (select all that apply)?

A. Conducting data collection and sharing information with others.

B. Assembling a unit team to address a quality problem within his or her control, or fix a simple process irritant, by completing a "Just Do It" improvement.

C. Conducting reviews of the literature to identify possible improvement interventions.

D. Educating staff on how to implement an intervention.

REVIEW ACTIVITIES

1. Go to the Institute for Healthcare Improvement (IHI) website at www.ihi.org. Select EDUCATION followed by IHI Open School. Select Take a Course. Select course number PS 201 (Root Cause & Systems Analysis) and complete the course.

2. Consider the following situation: The headlines of your school's daily newspaper reads "Food Services to Increase Prices." The article explains revenue from sales has decreased by 20% leaving no other option but to increase prices. Now, go to the IHI website at ihi.org. Select TOPICS. Under TOOLS AND RESOURCES, select the Plan-Do-Study-Act (PDSA) Worksheet. Scroll down to DOCUMENTS, where the PDSA worksheet is available in PDF. Divide into groups of four to five students. Use the PDSA worksheet to develop a small scale of change that could reduce the cost increase incurred by students and faculty. Create an AIM and PLAN. Identify an Intervention you would DO. Create a measurement plan to STUDY. If your intervention was successful or not, describe how you would next ACT. Compare student group ideas for improvement.

3. Go to the Baldrige Performance Excellence Program at www.nist.gov/baldrige. Select Award Recipients. Select 2011 as your year option and in the Search section,

select 2011 as the year and Health Care for the sector. Three healthcare award recipients will be available. Select the Award Application Summary for Henry Ford Health System (HFHS).

A. Identify examples of innovations that demonstrate performance excellence.
B. Would you want to be employed by this organization; why or why not?
C. View the YouTube video from HFHS: www.youtube.com/watch?v=rw380n6JhW4. How does this performance by senior leadership speak to performance excellence?
D. Is there evidence of Lean/Six Sigma?

4. Access the American Society for Quality website at asq.org. Select Learn About Quality. Many quality topics are listed that were discussed in this chapter. As you learned, preventive actions are taken when a risk for error is identified. From the Quality Topics A to Z list, select Mistake-proofing. Read through this brief explanation including the accompanying flow chart.

A. Can you apply the restaurant example to an outpatient clinic? What questions could be asked?
B. Can you think of an operating room procedure that was created using mistake-proofing principles?

CLINICAL DISCUSSION POINTS

1. Although Quality and Safety Education for Nurses (QSEN) nicely defines quality improvement, would consumers of healthcare define it the same?
2. Why did quality of care delivery evolve slowly? What factors may have influenced expanded attention to quality of care delivery?
3. What rationale might explain The Joint Commission's decision to conduct unannounced surveys?
4. What advantage does Six Sigma have over Lean improvement methodology?
5. How can Plan-Do-Study-Act (PDSA) be applied to struggling career goals?
6. What is one of the greatest benefits of conducting a Healthcare Failures Mode and Effects Analysis (HFMEA™)?
7. Although processes may include risk-reduction interventions, such as a surgical time out to prevent wrong site surgery, why do failures still occur including incidence of wrong site surgery?

EXPLORING THE WEB

1. Agency for Healthcare Research and Quality: ahrq.gov
2. Magnet Recognition Model: www.nursecredentialing.org/Magnet/Program Overview/New-Magnet-Model
3. National Committee for Quality Assurance (NCQA): www.ncqa.org/tabid/142/ Default.aspx
4. Patient Safety Measures Tools & Resources (Agency for Healthcare Research and Quality): www.ahrq.gov/professionals/quality-patient-safety/patient-safety-resources/index. html
5. Quality Improvement Methodology: www.integration.samhsa.gov/pbhci -learning-community/toolkit-evaluation-quality-improvement

REFERENCES

Anthony, M., (2004). "Shared Governance Models: The Theory, Practice, and Evidence." *Online Journal of Issues in Nursing. Vol. 9* No. 1, Manuscript 4. Available: www.nursingworld.org/MainMenuCategories/ANAMarketplace/ANAPeriodicals/OJIN/TableofContents/Volume92004/No1Jan04/SharedGovernanceModels.aspx

Aroh, D., Colella, J., Douglas, C., & Eddings, A. (2015). An example of translating value-based purchasing into value-based care. *Urologic Nursing, 35*(2), 61–75.

Berwick, D. M. (2011). Preparing nurses for participation in and leadership of continual improvement. *Journal of Nursing Education, 50*(6), 322–327. doi:10.3928/0148483420110519-05

Berwick, D. M., & Hackbarth, A. D. (2012). Eliminating waste in us health care. *Journal of the American Medical Association, 307*(14), 1513–1516. doi:10.1001/jama.2012.362

Centers for Medicare & Medicaid Services (CMS). (2014). *National health expenditures 2014 highlights.* Retrieved from https://www.cms.gov/Research-Statistics-Data-and-Systems/Statistics-Trends-and-Reports/CMSProgramStatistics/2014/2014_NATL.html

Cox-Sullivan, S., Norris, M. R., Brown, L.M., & Scott, K.J. (2017). Nurse manager perspective of staff participation in unit level shared governance. *Journal of Nurisng Management, 25*(8), 624-631. doi: 10.1111/jonm.12500.

Cronenwett, L., Sherwood, G., Barnsteiner J., Disch, J., Johnson, J., Mitchell, P., . . . Warren, J. (2007). Quality and safety education for nurses. *Nursing Outlook, 55*(3), 122–131. doi:10.1016/j.outlook.2007.02.006

DeRosier, J., Stalhandske, E., Bagian, J. P., & Nudell, T. (2002). Using health care failure mode and effect analysis™: The VA national center for patient safety's prospective risk analysis system. *The Joint Commission Journal on Quality Improvement, 28*(5), 248–267. doi:10.1016/S1070-3241(02)28025-6

Donabedian, A. (2003). *An introduction to quality assurance in health care.* New York, NY: Oxford University Press.

Evans, J. R. (2008). *Quality & performance excellence: Management, organization, and strategy* (5th ed.). Mason, OH: Thompson South-Western.

Figueroa, J. F., Tsugawa, Y., Zheng, J., Orav, E. J., & Jha, A. K. (2016). Associations between the value-based purchasing pay for performance program and patient mortality in us hospitals: Observational study. *British Medical Journal, 353*(i2214), 1–7. doi:10.1136/bmj.i2214

Fos, E. B. (2017). The unintended consequences of the Centers for Medicare and Medicaid Services pay-for-performance structures on safety-net hospitals and the low-income, medically vulnerable population. *Health Services Management Research, 30*(1), 10–15. doi:10.1 11177/095148816678011

Hadfield, D., Holmes, S., Kozlowski, S., & Sperl, T. (2009). *The new lean healthcare pocket guide: 5S in healthcare-why you need it.* Chelsea, MI: MCS Media.

Hughes, R. G. (2008a). Tools and strategies for quality improvement and patient safety. In R. Hughes (Ed.), Patient safety and quality: *An evidence-based handbook for nurses* (chap. 44). AHRQ Publication No. 08-0043. Rockville, MD: Agency for Healthcare Research and Quality. Retrieved from http://www.ahrq.gov/qual/nurseshdbk

Hughes, R. G. (2008b). Nurses at the "sharp end" of patient care. In R. Hughes (Ed.), Patient safety and quality: *An evidence-based handbook for nurses* (chap.2). AHRQ Publication No. 08-0043. Rockville, MD: Agency for Healthcare Research and Quality. Retrieved from http://www.ahrq.gov/qual/nurseshdbk

Institute for Healthcare Improvement (IHI). (2017). *Cause and effect diagram.* Retrieved from http://www.ihi.org/resources/Pages/Tools/CauseandEffectDiagram.aspx

Institute of Medicine (IOM). (2000). *To err is human: Building a safer health system.* Washington, DC: National Academies Press.

Institute of Medicine (IOM). (2001). *Crossing the quality chasm: A new health system for the 21st century.* Washington, DC: National Academies Press.

Jones, T. L. (2016). Outcome measurement in nursing: Imperatives, ideals, history, and challenges. *The Online Journal of Issues in Nursing, 21*(2), 1. Manuscript 1. doi:10.3912/OJIN.Vol21No2MAN01

Langley, G. L., Nolan, K. M., Nolan, T. W., Norman, C. L., & Provost, L. P. (2009). *The improvement guide: A practical approach to enhancing organizational performance* (2nd ed.). San Francisco, CA: Jossey Bass. Retrieved from https://www.cdc.gov/std/foa/aapps/api-model-improvement-and-change-concepts.pdf

Lindberg, L., & Kimberlain, J. (2008). Quality update: Engage employees to improve staff and patient satisfaction. *Hospitals & Health Networks, 82*(1), 28-29.

Lloyd, R. C. (2010). Navigating in the turbulent sea of data: The quality measurement journey. *Clinics in Perinatology, 37*, 101–122. doi:10.1016/j.clp.2010.01.006

Luce, J. M., Bindman, A., & Lee, P. R. (1994). A brief history of health care quality assessment and improvement in the United States. *The Western Journal of Medicine, 160*, 263–268. Retrieved from http://www.ncbi.nlm.nih.gov/pmc/articles/PMC1022402

Marshall, M., De Silva, D., Cruickshank, L., Shand, J., Wei, L., & Anderson, J. (2016). What we know about designing an effective improvement intervention (but too often fail to put into practice). *BMJ Quality & Safety 26*, 572-577. doi:10.1136/bmjqs-2016-006245

McLaughlin, M., Houston, K., & Harder-Mattson, E. (2012). Managing outcomes using an organizational quality improvement model. In P. Kelly (Ed.), *Nursing leadership & management* (3rd ed., pp. 474–496). Clifton Park, NY: Delmar.

Mitchell, S. E., Martin, J., Holmes, S., Van Deusen-Lukas, C., Cancino, R., Paasche-Orlow, M., . . . Jack, B. (2015). How hospitals reengineer their discharge processes to reduce readmissions. *Journal for Healthcare Quality, 38*(2), 116–126.

Moen, R., & Norman, C. (2009). *Evolution of the PDCA cycle. Associates in process improvement.* Retrieved from http://cissp.tjscott.net/standards/moen.norman.pdca.origins.pdf

O'Rourke, H. M., & Fraser, K. D. (2016). How quality improvement practice evidence can advance the knowledge base. *Journal for Healthcare Quality, 38*(5), 264–274. doi:10.1097/JHQ.0000000000000067

Owens, L. D., & Koch, R. W. (2015). Understanding quality patient care and the role of the practicing nurse. *Nursing Clinics of North America, 50*, 33–34. doi:10.1016/j.cnur.2014.10.003

Painter, D. R. (2010). Nurse's responsibility to improve practice (editorial). *Nephrology Nursing Journal, 37*(3), 227.

Peterson-Graziose, V., & Bryer, J. (2017). Assessing student perceptions of quality and safety education for nurses competencies in a baccalaureate curriculum. *Journal of Nursing Education, 56*(7), 435–438. doi:10.3928/01484834-20170619-09

Pocha, C. (2010). Lean six sigma in health care and the challenge of implementation of six sigma methodologies at a veterans affairs medical center. *Quality Management in Health Care, 19*(4), 312–318. doi:10.1097/QMH.0b013e3181fa0783

QSEN Institute. (2017a). *Graduate KSAs : Quality improvement.* Retrieved from https://qsen.org/competencies/graduate-ksas/#quality_improvement

QSEN Institute. (2017b). *Pre-licensure KSAs: Quality improvement.* Retrieved from https://qsen.org/competencies/pre-licensnure-ksas/#quality_improvement

Salmond, S. (2015). Nurses leading charge: The time is now! In D. A. Forrester (Ed.), *Nursing's greatest leaders: A history of activism* (chap. 12). New York, NY: Springer.

Salmond, S. W., & Echevarria, M. (2017). Healthcare transformation and changing roles for nursing. *Orthopedic Nursing, 36*(1), 12–25. doi:10.1097/NOR.0000000000000308

Shankar, R. (2009). *Process improvement using Six Sigma.* Milwaukee, WI: ASQ Quality Press.

Squires, D., & Anderson, C. (2015). US health care from a global perspective: Spending, use of services, process, and health in 13 countries. *The Commonwealth Fund, 1819*(15), 1–15. Retrieved from http://www.commonwealthfund.org/publications/issue-briefs/2015/oct/us-health-care-from-a-global-perspective

The Joint Commission. (2016). The SAFER Matrix: A new scoring methodology. *The Joint Commission Perspectives®, 36*(5), 1–3.

The Joint Commission. (2017). Hospital Standard (Leadership), Edition: Standard LD 04.04.05, element of performance 10.

VanLare, J. M., & Conway, P. H. (2012). Value-based purchasing—National programs to move from volume to value. *New England Journal of Medicine, 367*(4), 292–295. doi:10.1056/NEJMp1204939

SUGGESTED READINGS

Almoosa, K. F., Luther, K., Resar, R., & Patel, B. (2016). Applying the new Institute for Healthcare Improvement inpatient waste tool to identify "waste" in the intensive care unit. *Journal for Healthcare Quality*, 38(5), e29–e38. doi:10.1097/JHQ.0000000000000040

Anderson-Elverson, C., & Samra, H. A. (2012). Overview of structure, process, and outcome indicators of quality in neonatal care. *Newborn & Infant Nursing Reviews*, 12(3), 154–161. doi:10.1053/j.nainr.2012.06.002

Blackmore, C. C., Williams, B. L., Ching, J. M., Chafetz, L. A., & Kaplan, G. S. (2016). Using lean to advance quality improvement research. *Journal for Healthcare Quality*, 38(5), 275–282. doi:10.1097/01.JHQ.0000462684.78253.a1

Brown, D. S., Donaldson, N., Burnes-Bolton, L., & Aydin, C. E. (2010). Nursing-sensitive benchmarks for hospitals to gauge high-reliability performance. *Journal for Healthcare Quality*, 32(6), 9–17. doi:10.1111/j.1945-1474.2010.00083.x

Burhans, L. M., & Alligood, M. R. (2010). Quality nursing care in the words of nurses. *Journal of Advanced Nursing*, 66(8), 1689–1697. doi:10.1111/j.1365-2648.2010.05344.x

Crawford, B., Skeath, M., & Whippy, A. (2015). Multifocal clinical performance improvement across 21 hospitals. *Journal for Healthcare Quality*, 37(2), 117–125. doi:10.1111%2Fjhq.12039"10.1111/jhq.12039

Crespy, S. D., Van Haitsma, K., Kleban, M., & Hann, C. J. (2016). Reducing depressive symptoms in nursing home residents: Evaluation of the Pennsylvania depression collaborative quality improvement program. *Journal for Healthcare Quality*, 38(6), e76–e88. doi:10.1097/JHQ.0000000000000009

Denny, D. S., Allen, D. K., Worthington, N., & Gupta, D. (2012). The use of failure mode and effect analysis in a radiation oncology setting: The cancer treatment centers of America experience. *Journal for Healthcare Quality*, 36(1), 18–28. doi:10.1111/j.1945-1474.2011.00199.x

Draper, D. A., Felland, L. E., Liebhaber, A., & Melichar, L. (2008, March). *The role of nurses in hospital quality improvement*. Research Brief Number 3. Center for Studying Health System Brief. Retrieved from http://www.rwjf.org/pr/product.jsp?id=27532

Farrokhi, F. R., Gunther, M., Williams, B., & Blackmore, C. C. (2015). Application of lean methodology for improving quality and efficiency in operating room instrument availability. *Journal for Healthcare Quality*, 37(5), 277–286. doi:10.1111/jhq.12053

Grazier, K. L., Quanbeck, A. R., Oruungo, J., Robinson, J., Ford, J. H., McCarty, D., . . . Gustafson, D. H. (2015). What influences participation in QI? A randomized trial of addiction treatment organizations. *Journal of Healthcare Quality*, 37(6), 342–353. doi:10.1111/jhq.12064

Institute of Medicine. (2015). *Vital signs: Core metrics for health and health care progress*. Washington, DC: The National Academies Press.

Joynt, K. E., DeLew, N., Sheingold, S. H., Conway, P. H., Goodrich, K., & Epstein, A. M. (2017). Should medicare value-based purchasing take social risk into account? *New England Journal of Medicine*, 376(6), 510–513. doi:10.1056/NEJMp1616278

Makai, P., Cramm, J. M., Van Grotel, M., & Nieboer, A. P. (2012). Labor productivity, perceived effectiveness, and sustainability of innovative projects. *Journal for Healthcare Quality*, 36(2), 14–24. doi:10.1111/j.1945-1474.2012.00209.x

Momani, A., Hirzallah, M., & Mumani, A. (2016). Improving employees' safety awareness in healthcare organizations using DMAIC quality improvement approach. *Journal for Healthcare Quality*, 39(1), 54–63. doi:10.1097/JHQ.0000000000000049

Moore, L., Lavoie, A., Bourgeois, G., & Lapointe, J. (2015). Donabedian's structure-process-outcome quality of care model: Validation in an integrated trauma system. *Journal of Trauma and Acute Care Surgery*, 78(6), 1168–1174. doi:10.1097/TA.0000000000000663

Palleschi, M. T., Sirianni, S., O'Connor, N., Dunn, D., & Hasenau, S. M. (2014). An interprofessional process to improve early identification and treatment for sepsis. *Journal for Healthcare Quality*, 36(4), 23–31. doi:10.1111/jhq.12006

Pearson, M. L., Needleman, J., Beckman, R., & Han, B. (2016). Facilitating nurses' engagement in hospital quality improvement: The New Jersey hospital association's implementation of transforming care at the bedside. *Journal for Healthcare Quality*, 38(6), e64–e75. doi:10.1097/JHQ.0000000000000007

Rodriguez-Cerrillo, M., Fernandez-Diaz, E., Inurrieta-Romero, A., & Poza-Montoro, A. (2012). Implementation of a quality management system according to 9001 standard in a hospital in the home unit: Changes and achievements. *International Journal of Health Care Quality Assurance, 25*(6), 498–508. doi:10.1108/09526861211246458

Stevens, K. R., & Ferrer, R. L. (2016). Real-time reporting of small operational failures in nursing care. *Nursing Research and Practice, 2016,* 1–7. doi:10.1155/2016/8416158

Tucker, A. L., Edmondson, A. C., & Spear, S. (2002). When problem solving prevents organizational learning. *Journal of Organizational Change Management, 15*(2), 122–137. doi:10.1108/09534810210423008

Van den Heuvel, J., Koning, L., Bogers, A. J., Berg, M., & Van Dijen, M. E. (2005). An ISO 9001 quality management system in a hospital: Bureaucracy or just benefits? *International Journal of Health Care Quality Assurance Incorporating Leadership in Health Services, 18*(4–5), 361–369. doi:10.1108/09526860510612216

West, B. (2012). Rapid cycle improvement: Avoid the pitfalls. *Nursing Management, 43*(11), 50–53. doi:10.1097/01.NUMA.0000421673.95475.80

Wojciechowski, E., Pearsall, T., Murphy, P., & French, E. (2016). A case review: Integrating Lewin's theory with lean's system approach for change. *Online Journal of Issues in Nursing, 21*(2), 1–17. doi:10.3912/OJIN.Vol21No2Man04

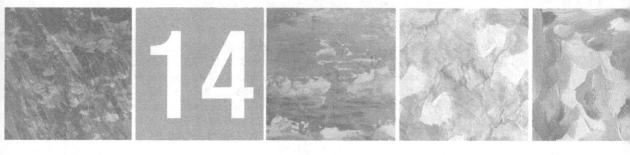

14

TOOLS OF QUALITY IMPROVEMENT

Anthony L. D'Eramo and Joanne Belviso Puckett

Modern health care demands continual system improvement to better meet social needs for safety, effectiveness, patient centeredness, timeliness, efficiency, and equity. Nurses, like all other health professionals, need skills and support to participate effectively in that endeavor, and, often, to lead it.

Donald M. Berwick, 2011

Upon completion of this chapter, the reader will be able to

1. Define data, including the various types of data and methods used to display data.
2. Identify the value of using basic statistics in quality improvement work.
3. Differentiate three commonly used methods to display data.
4. Differentiate common cause variation from special cause variation.
5. Discuss the tools used by quality improvement teams.

As a day shift nurse on a patient-care unit, you perform assessments on your patients at the beginning of the shift. The first patient that you assess is an 85-year-old man admitted yesterday with pneumonia. During shift report, the night nurse stated the patient had a fever on admission but that the patient's temperature was normal during the night shift. The patient had an elevated white blood cell count of 12.4 K/cmm on admission and received three doses of IV antibiotics since admission. As you assess the patient's vital signs, you find the patient has a temperature of 101.1°F (38.4°C). The patient offered no complaints other than shortness of breath. You noted the patient is flushed with a respiratory rate of 20 and a pulse oximeter reading of 95% on 1.5L of oxygen delivered through a nasal cannula. His repeat white blood cell count on the morning of your care is 13.2 K/cmm. Prior to your assessment, the healthcare team enters the patient's room. The physician asks, "Is he improving?"

- *How will you respond to the physician?*
- *What questions should you have asked during the handoff shift report when it was reported that the patient had a normal temperature during the night shift?*
- *Is a temperature finding of 101.1°F or a white blood cell count of 13.2 K/cmm an improvement?*

Quality is whatever patients and family members define it to be. Beyond the prevention, reduction, or elimination of harm is the search for innovations and breakthrough improvements that contribute to quality outcomes. With innovative improvements come the opportunity to advance good performance to excellence in performance. Such innovations occur with visionary thinking of what can be, what healthcare processes can be changed to enhance patient and staff satisfaction, and by understanding and applying quality improvement (QI) methods into our daily clinical practice. This chapter focuses on the science and process of QI.

For nurses to obtain the necessary knowledge, skills, and attitudes to continuously improve healthcare quality, safety, and systems used to delivery healthcare, the Quality and Safety Education for Nurses project (QSEN Institute, 2017; www.qsen.org,) defines **QI** as to "Use data to monitor the outcomes of care processes and use improvement methods to design and test changes to continuously improve the quality and safety of health care systems."

This chapter includes defining data and commonly used descriptive statistics applied in QI activities. We explore the types and uses of data for QI including how data are displayed for analysis and how data are analyzed to identify both the need for improvement or if improvement occurred. Statistical process control (SPC) is introduced to include the run and **control charts**. When indicated, interprofessional teams may conduct QI activities. The teams have a variety of improvement tools and methods they can employ. The most basic and effective processes used by teams are described.

WHAT ARE DATA

Nursing practice decisions and organizational healthcare processes all produce outcome data that can be measured, displayed, and compared. So what are data? **Data** are the raw numbers or results collected to measure processes and outcomes. Data can also be results provided by external sources, such as the number of acute-care Joint Commission survey findings for an organization. Data are used to determine if healthcare performance meets the expected goal (e.g., the number of patients with blood pressure in control). Data are used to measure performance quality that is valued by purchasers of care, accreditation agencies, governing bodies, the general public, and providers of healthcare (Carey, 2003). A clear understanding of the context or goal related to data measurement is necessary for interpretation. For example: What is the measureable goal? Why was that goal selected? Are we striving to meet a defined requirement; a minimum standard, or a long-term goal?

By itself, data do not require a nurse to take action. Consider the following: A heart rate of 60 is an isolated piece of data from one assessment finding. By itself, the heart rate data point of 60 looks good. As healthcare workers, we do not usually base any changes on one piece of data, unless it indicates a critical change or value. If we look at heart rate readings over time (e.g., the heart rate is taken twice a shift for 1 day providing six pieces of data), we can see if a trend exists. A trend looks at changes in data over time. If the six heart rate readings were 110, 100, 90, 80, 70, and 60, we would have information. **Information** is analysis of collected data that is used to make decisions. As nurses, information is used to make nursing care decisions. In the heart rate example, the trend provides information that the heart rate has steadily fallen over three shifts. The nurse needs to decide if action is needed, such as informing the provider of the trend, reviewing medications or changes in medications over the past three shifts, or monitoring the patient more closely to watch for any other assessment changes.

Patients can provide both subjective and objective data. **Subjective (patient) data** are reported by the patient. For example, a patient may state pain status as "5" on a scale of 1 to 10. **Objective (patient) data** may include what the healthcare worker can see or measure, such as the patient's blood pressure or blood glucose results. Both subjective and objective data are collected, analyzed, and interpreted as information. This information is used to make clinical decisions about whether the patient is getting better, worse, or if the information requires provider notification.

Sources of Objective Data for QI

Nurses are inundated with data, representing patient, unit, or organization performance outcomes. **Internal data** are those found within a healthcare organization and are generated by staff, such as falls and medication errors. **External data** are data provided from outside sources (e.g., state quality review organizations) that evaluate and report on the organization's internal processes and outcomes. **Baseline data** are the preintervention data measurements that are used to identify a problem needing improvement. **Postintervention data** are the changes from baseline data after an improvement intervention and confirm the success or failure of the intervention. For example, a team is working to decrease the number of hospital-acquired pressure ulcers (HAPUs). The average number of HAPUs was six per month for the last 3 months. Six HAPUs represent baseline data. Because six HAPUs were unacceptable, a QI intervention to reduce HAPUs was instituted. After the QI intervention, the average number of HAPUs was three per month, or a reduction of 50% in HAPUs over a 3-month period. Three HAPUs represent the postintervention data. Although a 50% reduction occurred, the team must analyze the postintervention data into information and decide if three HAPUs is acceptable or if further improvement is needed.

When data are collected internally, it is important to distinguish between incidence and prevalence data. Incidence and prevalence data both typically use a quarterly or 3-month time frame. A quarter is 3 months. **Incidence** data are the actual counts of every event that occurred during a specific time frame. For example, counting the number of falls that occurred on a medical–surgical unit for one quarter. **Prevalence** data are a snapshot of event under measure during one day. For example, counting the number of falls that occurred on one specific day during the quarter. To illustrate further, suppose the prevalence rate was measured on one specific day and no fall occurred on the specific date of measurement. The prevalence rate would be zero. Now suppose over the same 3-month period, the actual incidence of falls was 11. Based on how the data were collected, either incidence or prevalence, it can result in dramatically different outcomes. It is important to understand the difference between incidence and prevalence data as organizations may report either

420

TABLE 14.1 PERCENT COMPLIANCE WITH CDC HAND HYGIENE GUIDELINES USING OBSERVATIONS (THREE MEDICAL/SURGICAL UNITS)

	JANUARY (%)	FEBRUARY (%)	MARCH (%)	APRIL (%)	MAY (%)	JUNE (%)	JULY (%)	AUGUST (%)	SEPTEMBER (%)
Unit A	**91**	80	87	86	73	69	80	77	79
Unit B	40	45	44	54	79	59	50	50	61
Unit C	87	88	84	88	90	93	90	79	89

Compliance goal is set at 90%. Bolded = Meeting 90% compliance goal; shaded = Not meeting 90% compliance goal.

depending on their preference or on external reporting requirements. For example, the National Database of Nursing Quality Indicators™ (NDNQI®) requires reporting of pressure ulcers as prevalence data (Hart, Bergquist, Gajewski, & Dunton, 2006). In the example regarding HAPUs, because both the baseline and postintervention data were actual numbers of HAPUs over a 3-month period, both data points represent incidence data. If the number of HAPUs was a snapshot on a given day, that would have represented prevalence data. Appreciate that regardless of the type of data, incidence or prevalence, analysis of the data into information for clinical decision making must occur for data to be useful.

Aggregate Data

When subjective and/or objective data are collected for process improvements or to assess care delivery, such as HAPUs, it is necessary to ensure that no patient identifiers are captured linking outcomes to specific patients, families, or staff. This will help to protect privacy and confidentiality of data. QI projects generally use **aggregate data**, which are large, grouped data without patient identifiers. These aggregate data, often listed in a table format, may be grouped by time, cause, diagnosis, or the variable being studied. An example of a study variable can include the staff's adherence to hand hygiene practices, as seen in Table 14.1. In Table 14.1, nursing hand hygiene compliance data are reported in aggregate form that compares three units over a 9-month period. Notice that there is no ability to identify which staff was in or out of compliance during measurement based on the aggregate data.

In Table 14.1, the use of bolding (met the target) and shading (did not meet the target) helps to quickly identify areas needing improvement when looking at large numbers of aggregate data.

Operational Definitions

An essential part of looking at any data is to have a clear definition of what is being measured to ensure that everyone is measuring the same thing. An **operational definition** describes in detail what is being specifically measured, how it is being measured, who will measure it, and when measurement should occur.

It is important to know how the data for QI activities are defined, collected, including who can collect the data and when using clearly defined operational definitions. Because many staff may be collecting the data at different time points, having one clear operational definition ensures that the data are collected and measured the same way, regardless of where the data are collected or who collects the data. For example, in Table 14.1, we looked at aggregated data on hand hygiene compliance from three different medical–surgical units. To make sure these data are collected and measured the same way on all units, we would need to state the following in the operational definition: the definition for hand hygiene, who is to collect the data, when the data are to be collected, the number of hand hygiene observations expected, and when the results are to be reported and to whom. Once these variables are known, a numerator and denominator can also be defined. An example of an operational definition and the numerator and denominator is provided as follows:

> Hand hygiene, a required organizational measure related to patient safety, is defined as compliance with the Centers for Disease Control and Prevention

(CDC) hand hygiene guidelines accessible at www.cdc.gov/handhygiene/providers/guideline.htm. Each unit will identify a "secret" observer on each shift who will monitor hand hygiene compliance for that unit on the first day of each month. Each observer will assess at least 10 interprofessional staff on the unit by observing their hand hygiene during interactions with patients. Results of compliance with CDC hand hygiene guidelines will be reported to the infection control staff within 48 hours of observation. Infection control staff will aggregate the observations as follows:

Numerator: Total number of hand hygiene observations, for example, 45
Denominator: Total number of observations that followed CDC hand hygiene guidelines correctly, for example, 39
Example Answer: 39 hand hygiene observations were correct out of 45 hand hygiene observations (87% compliance)

In this example, there is a clear numerator and denominator for reliable measurement. It can be challenging to develop a clear operational definition to guide a sustainable, consistent process for data collection among the observers.

CRITICAL THINKING 14.1

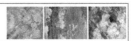

Select the best operational definition for a fall and explain why you selected the option.

1. A "fall" is defined as the number of patients who fall and for which an incident report is completed. The patient safety officer will collect the data and report them to the Unit Practice Council annually using a control chart.
2. A "fall" is defined as the number of patients admitted to the unit who fall and who suffer no injuries, whether minor (e.g., a laceration) or major (e.g., fractured hip). All such incidents will be reported using electronic incident reporting procedures per policy 101-5.
3. A "fall" is defined as any patient who falls that results in no injury, a fall that results in a minor injury (laceration), or a fall that results in a major injury (fractured hip). All such incidents will be reported using electronic incident reporting procedures per policy 101-5. The fall numerator is the number of falls and the fall denominator is the total number of patients on the unit during the measurement period.

Data Collection

Data are only useful when collected rigorously, meaning that data collection tools must be valid (measures what it is supposed to measure) and reliable (consistently measuring what it is supposed to measure). To illustrate, in the hand hygiene compliance example, although all staff are expected and taught to follow hand hygiene compliance, every "secret" observer should complete additional training on the

CDC guidelines and demonstrate competency in hand hygiene compliance before monitoring and observing other staff. The additional training can secure validity by helping the observer accurately measure if hand hygiene compliance occurred according to the CDC guidelines (validity). A second trained observer can observe the first observer to compare both observers, concluding the results comply with the CDC guidelines. By doing this, the second observer is helping to establish reliability of data collected by the first observer on hand hygiene compliance. **Interrater reliability** (IRR) is a process that provides evidence that those collecting data are applying the CDC guidelines correctly to determine if the staff is following the guidelines correctly or not. When IRR exists, the data are considered reliable because data are collected consistently. Conducting IRR may identify observers who need additional education in the interpretation and application of the CDC hand hygiene guidelines, a lesson to learn before hygiene compliance data are reported. One type of data collection error is identifying that a problem exists when in fact there is not a problem. For example, hand hygiene compliance may include using both a hand sanitizer and when indicated soap and water. If the trained observer misunderstood the definition of hand hygiene compliance and only counted the instances where the healthcare worker used soap and water, the findings would be inaccurate. In this case, the number of healthcare workers that used the waterless hand sanitizer was not counted causing a decrease in the percent of hand hygiene compliance. When the trained observer reports the observations, one could easily be concerned that hand hygiene compliance needs improvement when in reality it may not!

Another interpretation of error can also occur. Let us say the trained observer misunderstood the hand hygiene guidelines and interpreted them to say that the only time the healthcare worker had to use the hand sanitizer or wash his or her hands was if the worker touched the patient. The trained observer would then only count compliance when the patient was touched and hand hygiene was completed, missing the fact that hand hygiene should be completed every time the healthcare worker enters and leaves the room. The hand hygiene compliance rates would not clearly identify if any hand hygiene practices need improvement.

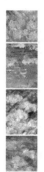

CASE STUDY 14.1

Two nurses have agreed to collect data on a QI project to decrease the number of patients who cancel their clinic appointments at two different surgical clinics. These patients are called clinic no-shows. The nurse manager over both clinics asks the two nurses to ensure IRR. Not being familiar with the concept of IRR, the nurses look to the literature and discover that this term inidcates that those collecting data should be following the same data collection procedures. The nurse manager requests a written plan to ensure IRR between both nurses at the two clinics. How would you write this plan and ensure both nurses are measuring their clinic no-shows consistently?

DESCRIPTIVE STATISTICS

Descriptive statistics are tools used to analyze and summarize relationships among variables. Statistics can identify significance within the data and relationships between variables (Nelson, Batalden, & Godfrey, 2004). **Descriptive statistics** are used to define and describe a set of data. For aggregate data, descriptive statistics are commonly calculated and include the mean, median, mode, range, and standard deviation (SD) of a set of data. Review the data displayed in Table 14.2. Note how the mean, median, mode, and range are calculated given a set of data. Determine the **mean** or average of a set of numbers by adding all the numbers together and then dividing by the total number of observations. In looking at hand hygiene compliance for Unit A, note that there are 9 months of hand hygiene compliance percentages reported. The mean compliance for Unit A is calculated by adding all findings and dividing by 9, the number of months. Table 14.2 demonstrates the calculation of mean for Unit A.

An example of a mean that you may be familiar with is your grade point average (GPA). A common GPA scale: A = 4 points, B = 3 points, C = 2 points, D = 1 points, and F = 0 points. If you took all of your grades earned in one semester over the time spent in college and converted the grades to point values as described, you could calculate your GPA using the illustration from Table 14.2. For example, if you took five courses and received one A, two Bs, and 2 Cs, your GPA would be calculated as 4 + 3 + 3 + 2 + 2 = 14/5 = 2.8 GPA.

The **median** of a set of data is determined by listing the hand hygiene findings from lowest to highest values. Once listed, the median is the value at the separation point, where half of the data is above and the other half below the data point that falls within the middle of the set of data. To illustrate, here are five data points arranged from lowest to highest: 4, 6, 11, 13, and 15. The median is 11 or the middle number of the set as there are two data points before and after 11. When there is an even number of results, the median is the average of the two middle results. For example, if the values were 4, 6, 7, 11, 13, and 15, the median would be 9, the average of 7 and 11, or 18/2 = 9. Table 14.2 illustrates the median, or 80%, for hand hygiene compliance on Unit A. The median statistic is used less frequently than the mean in statistical QI work.

In QI activities, the mode is of less use compared to the other descriptive statistics but it may be included in analyses, therefore it is useful to define. The **mode** is simply the value that is repeated most frequently in a set of data or the "typical" value observed. To illustrate this, refer to Table 14.2. Note the value 80 is repeated.

TABLE 14.2 UNIT A DESCRIPTIVE STATISTICS

SUMMARY STATISTIC	ILLUSTRATION
Mean	91 + 80 + 87 + 86 + 73 + 69 + 80 + 77 + 79 = 722 722 divided by 9 (months) = 80.22
Median	91, 87, 86, 80, **80**, 79, 77, 73, 69 80 is the middle point
Mode	91, **80**, 87, 86, 73, 69, **80**, 77, 79 80 is repeated
Range	91, 80, 87, 86, 73, 69, 80, 77, 79 69 (lowest value) to 91 (highest value)

The **range** represents the lowest and highest values in the data. Reviewing the range of data is a quick measure of **variability**. Variability refers to the differences between the numbers in a data set. A simple measure of variability can be determined by observing the range of a data set.

Table 14.2 illustrates the range of values for Unit A from 69 to 91. Knowing data variability helps you to identify just how far apart the data are. Consider this: You are working on a QI project to reduce falls. Over 12 months, one unit had a high of 13 falls and a low of zero falls. The variability shows you that the unit is not consistent in reducing falls, unless, of course, it went from 13 to 0 over time as the result of continuous improvement.

The most common method used to describe the variability of a data set is **SD**, which reflects how "tightly" the data points cluster around the mean as seen in Figure 14.1. SD is often abbreviated as the Greek letter sigma (σ). In a "normal" distribution of a data set, most measures hover around the mean while a few measures tend to be at opposite extremes from the mean. In a SD curve, the mean is located at the center of the graph and is represented as 0 in Figure 14.1. In a normal distribution, it is expected that 68.3% of outcomes will fall within one SD above or below the mean (+1/-1). Another 27.1% of outcomes should fall within two SD from the mean (+2/-2) accounting for 95.4% of all expected outcomes. An additional 4.2% of outcomes should fall within 3 SD from the mean (+3/-3), which accounts for 99.8% of all outcomes.

Note that, if 20 students completed a test with a mean score of 80%, it is expected that most of those students (68.3%) would hover around an 80% score. More, or 95.4%, of students would be expected to fall within two SD of 80%, and even more (98.8%) of students would fall within three SD from the mean. SD of a set of data can be easily calculated using software such as Microsoft Excel®.

As seen in Figure 14.1, outcomes (99.8%) are expected to fall within three SD of the mean. Variability in a data set is an important concept in QI activities and are further examined with SPC later in the chapter. For practice calculating basic descriptive statistics refer to Case Study 14.2.

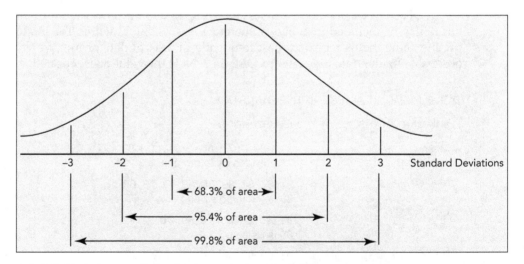

FIGURE 14.1 A normal distribution standard deviation curve.

Source: Fowler Byers, J., & Rosati, R. J. (2008). Foundation, techniques, and tools. In L. R. Pelletier & C. L. Beaudin (Eds.), *Q solutions: Essential resources for the healthcare quality professional* (p. 47). Glenview, IL: National Association for Healthcare Quality. Copyright © 2008 by the National Association for Healthcare Quality, Reprinted with permission.

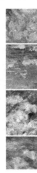

CASE STUDY 14.2

You have just completed data collection on a QI project to reduce calloffs on your unit. To obtain calloff baseline data, you have been asked to document the number of calloffs over a 3 week period to identify the number of calloffs more prominently for each shift. Your results are listed as follows:

Week 1: (Days) 3 (Evenings) 1 (Nights) 1
Week 2: (Days) 4 (Evenings) 2 (Nights) 2
Week 3: (Days) 1 (Evenings) 3 (Nights) 1

Now that you have your outcomes, calculate the mean, median, mode, and range of these results.

DATA DISPLAY

Data are visible in all healthcare settings. It is difficult to walk onto an inpatient or outpatient area without seeing data. It is necessary, however, to analyze and interpret data into usable information. **Data display** refers to a visual picture or graphing of data that best depicts the story you want that data to exhibit. Data should be displayed in ways that staff, patients, and families can understand. Figures, graphs, and tables are acceptable methods of displaying data. Whatever the format, data must include a clear title of what is being presented, including the use of footnotes to clarify aspects of the table or figure (Nelson, Batalden, & Godfrey, 2004). For example, footnotes may be useful to define a column title, or to refer the reader to the operational definition of a specific value. Recall Table 14.1, hand hygiene compliance for three nursing units. For easier interpretation, those months meeting the targeted goal of 90% were highlighted while those not meeting the goal were shaded.

Data alone do not always offer guidance regarding improvement priorities. For example, looking at Table 14.1, Unit B lists outcomes for May (79%) and June (59%). Does this decrease in compliance require immediate attention? A "yes" response may be premature. In fact, the answer to that question should not be determined by comparing two results alone as two results may not provide enough data for analysis and decision making. Fortunately, more sophisticated methods are available to better inform improvement decisions. As you will learn, visually displaying data over time is useful when assessing outcomes to better inform if interventions are needed, if improvement occurred, or if improvement was sustained.

When data are generated, they must be interpreted as meaningful information. For example, in Table 14.1, if Unit B wanted to improve its hand hygiene compliance rate (mean = 53.5% over 9 months), some change or intervention must be implemented. Recall that 53.5% or the baseline measure will be compared to the postintervention percent compliance to determine if the intervention worked. At this point, we have only discussed data. We now look at how data are displayed in various graphical formats. Our discussion focuses on commonly used formats including a histogram, scatter plot diagram, and Pareto charts, as well as run and control charts. Note that when data are plotted within a graph, the horizontal axis of the graph is referred to as the x-axis and the vertical axis of the graph as the y-axis.

Histograms

A **histogram**, as seen in Figure 14.2, is a bar graph that displays the data. Data displayed using a histogram allows for easier visualization of large, aggregate data that may originate from a table. To understand a histogram, it is important to know the y-axis and x-axis. The y-axis is the vertical line and is easily remembered as "y to the sky." The x-axis is the horizontal line and can be remembered as "x to the left." Histograms are useful in determining patterns within historical data or displaying baseline data. In Figure 14.2, the histogram uses a bar to display the lengths of stay for the last 50 admissions.

The number of admissions is located on the vertical y-axis. The variable along the horizontal x-axis (lengths of stay in days) is sequential starting with the shortest to the longest length of stay. The most frequent average length of stay (14 observations) is between 3 and 4 days. Histograms are easily made with or without software and quickly depict the distribution of a set of data or outcomes.

Scatter Plot Diagrams

Scatter plot diagrams display relationships between two variables by providing a visual means to test the strength of the relationship between the two variables. The design of the dots within the scatter plot diagram is used for interpretation. Several designs can be depicted when observing the scatter plot diagram, a positive, negative, or no relationship design. Examples of each scatter plot design are depicted in Figure 14.3. The scatter plot looks at two variables, or issues, that you want to look at. A relationship between the two variables does not indicate that one variable caused the other. The scatter plot assists in determining if a relationship exists.

Consider the length of stay data displayed in the histogram in Figure 14.2. The relationship between the variable of length of stay could be compared to another variable, such as patient satisfaction using a scatter plot (Figure 14.3).

The scatter plot diagram in Figure 14.4 illustrates the relationship between lengths of stay (in days) and patient satisfaction scores using a Likert scale ranging from 5 to 1, where 5 is most satisfied, 3 is neutral, and 1 is least satisfied. In Figure 14.4, the design of the scatter plots indicates there is no relationship between length of stay and patient satisfaction for the 50 patients in this sample.

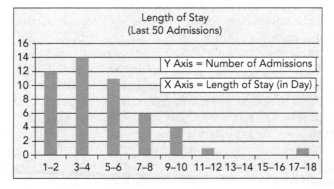

FIGURE 14.2 The histogram.

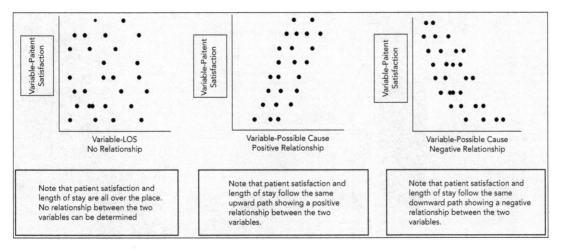

FIGURE 14.3 Basic scatter plot patterns.

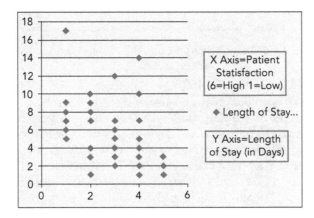

FIGURE 14.4 Scatter plot diagram (variables patient satisfaction and length of stay).

Pareto Charts

The Pareto chart is another type of bar graph. It is similar to the histogram because it depicts how often data represent a particular value. The difference between a histogram and a Pareto chart is that the **Pareto chart** orders findings in a descending order from high to low with the most frequent issue contributing to the results furthest to the left on the x-axis. Visualizing results from high to low allows prioritizing, or identifying what data most impact the variable in question. One benefit of the Pareto chart is in demonstrating the Pareto principle that 80% of the problem comes from 20% of the causes. When the causes of problems are ranked in order of effect on the QI problem, you can clearly identify those causes having the greatest effect. The Pareto chart in Figure 14.5 illustrates that tardiness of the oncoming shift, furthest to the left, is the most common cause of unit overtime during a 1 month period.

In Figure 14.5, the four most common causes of overtime, that is, tardiness, turbulence, hand off delays, and staffing pattern, are ranked from high to low as you read from left to right. These four causes represent 81% of the problems leading to overtime. You can look above the column labeled "staffing patterns" and see where the line marks 81% of the problems. These four causes will serve as target problems needing improvement to reduce overtime costs. The manager can easily visualize, prioritize causes, and plan improvement interventions to reduce overtime usage based on review of the Pareto chart. Appreciate that the leading cause of a problem may not

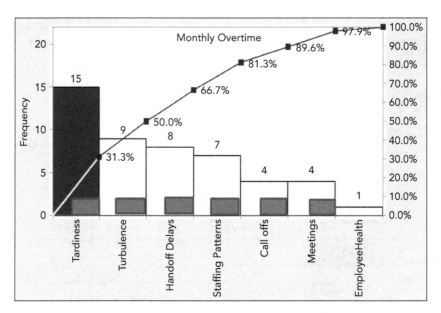

FIGURE 14.5 Pareto chart on causes of overtime for 1 month.

be the focus of improvement. In this example, if meeting with the Employee Health Department has been the greatest cause of overtime, it may not be feasible to address since the manager of the unit may have little control over employees appropriately seeking Employee Health services. Or, looking at that scenario from another perspective, if meeting with Employee Health services was the greatest cause of the overtime, you may want to do a root cause analysis (RCA), fishbone diagram, or ask the five Whys discussed in Chapter 13 to determine why there is so many more staff than usual seeking Employee Health services and driving up overtime usage.

STATISTICAL PROCESS CONTROL

Thus far, we have illustrated figures and tables commonly used to analyze and represent data. In the Pareto chart depicted in Figure 14.5, tardiness is the most significant cause of overtime. However, the chart does not illustrate any change from previous months. Perhaps calloffs were once the most frequent cause of overtime but are now reduced? Perhaps these causes of overtime are changing month to month? The Pareto chart categorizes factors leading to specific outcomes, however, these data are mainly a snapshot of what existed at the time the data were collected (Grube, 2008). Other approaches exist that depict data trends over time that allow for improved decision making and prioritization. SPC is an approach for analyzing data adding science to QI decision making (Nelson, Batalden, & Godfrey, 2004). SPC uses statistical methods to monitor and control quality processes to reduce or eliminate waste. This chapter will only introduce you to and cover the basics of SPC as they apply to QI projects.

SPC adds the ability to identify variation within a process (Evans, 2008). **SPC** is a type of statistic that, when applied, demonstrates a statistical approach to QI decision making. SPC is used to monitor a process over time (time-series design) but adds the ability to identify variation within that process by plotting data points within a run chart or control chart.

In Figure 14.5, after identifying tardiness as the major contributing factor to overtime, it would be valuable to apply principles of SPC to assess variability in the causes of overtime and identify the need for change. For example, 15 causes of overtime in Figure 14.5 were from tardiness. Is this a new outcome? Was tardiness noted only twice last month and suddenly increased? Is tardiness a priority to improve or are there other competing processes needing attention first? SPC depicts process variability, the degree to which the process is stable or unstable over time. Think about the hand hygiene data in Table 14.1. Any change in the percent of hand hygiene compliance from one month to the next month is variability. In Table 14.1 data are presented in a time series, from January through September. However, data displayed in tables do not allow for analysis beyond descriptive statistics. Could the hand hygiene data represent an unstable hand hygiene process, meaning the data fluctuate unpredictably over time? These are important questions answered by applying SPC when analyzing data. In order to answer these questions, the concepts of common cause and special cause variation must be understood.

On any given day, your lunchtime may vary anytime between 11 a.m. and 1 p.m. This is an expected variation, referred to as **common cause variation** or "noise," the inherent variability seen in a stable "in control" process (Carey, 2003). If one day an emergency prevented you from eating lunch until 3 p.m. that time point is very different from your expected lunchtime. Lunch occurring between 11 a.m. and 1 p.m. is expected. When a data point varies significantly in an unpredictable or unexpected manner, it is referred to as **special cause variation**, which signals that something happened (an emergency occurred) that changed the process for better or worse and that the process is "out of control" (Carey, 2003). Because all processes have inherent variation, such as lunch between 11 a.m. and 1 p.m., determining common cause from special cause variation is important. The risk of not knowing if common cause or special cause variation exists is that common cause variation may be prioritized for improvement when improvement is not warranted. Additionally, when special cause variation is identified, that raises a red flag that the process is no longer in control, which may need immediate attention.

Assessing for common cause and special cause variability captures the essence of SPC, or being able to look at data over time to determine the type of variability that exists. Both common cause and special cause variation require further interpretation. When special cause variation is found, efforts should focus on identifying an explanation of what occurred that resulted in the process being out of control. If the process exhibits common cause variation, it may not need improvement. When common cause variation exits, the analysis must include answering the question if the process is performing at an acceptable or desired level. Just because the process is under control (common cause variation) does not mean the process could not be improved to a higher level of performance. For example, say hand hygiene data that illustrate compliance to the CDC hand hygiene guidelines was measured monthly for a home healthcare team. The annual mean of compliance was reported as 65%, within common cause variation. Although 65% is within common cause variability, the question remains if 65% is acceptable. If it is not, an improvement could be recommended. If it is not but other priorities for improvement take precedence, working to increase hand hygiene compliance may need to wait.

In SPC, assessing variability requires use of formats such as the run chart (Figure 14.6) or Shewhart control chart (Figure 14.8). Because the goal is to reduce variation within processes and to sustain that over time, there is considerable movement in healthcare to use SPC as a QI methodology when analyzing outcome data (Mohammed, Worthington, & Woodall, 2008). Both the run chart and the Shewhart control chart are tools used to assess process variation.

The Run Chart

The run chart depicts data in a time series format where an outcome variable, for example, compliance to hand hygiene CDC guidelines on the y-axis, is plotted on a graph over a period along the x-axis. Recall that a time series format refers to the

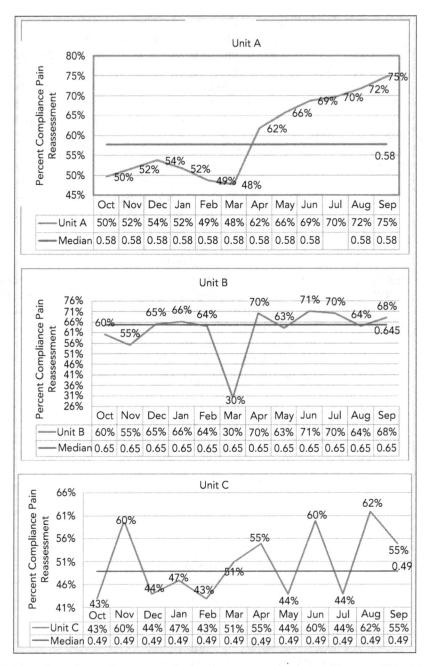

FIGURE 14.6 Run charts demonstrating pain reassessment compliance within 60 minutes of IV pain medication administration for three units.

representation of data over consecutive time points. It can be used for any type of data, including measurement and count data created by hand or using software. Characteristic of all time series charts, the x-axis (horizontal) represents the period and the y-axis (l vertical) represents the variable being measured (Figure 14.6).

The purpose of a **run chart** is to identify trends in a process or movement away from a central point, such as the median. The run chart allows teams to assess how a process is working. The process can be routine, such as assessing pain reassessment post IV pain administration or assessing a new process implemented for improvement. Simply stated, the run chart is a visual display of a process performance.

The run charts depicted in Figure 14.6 show how the data are organized. The time frame being shown is 12 months (*x*-axis) in chronological order. The outcome variable, percent compliance of pain reassessment, is seen on the *y*-axis. When using SPC, the range of percent will vary by unit based on each unit's outcomes. This is illustrated in Figure 14.6, where Unit A has a range between 48% and 75% (lowest point and highest point) and Unit B has a range between 30% and 71% (lowest point and highest point). You may choose to include a table of the raw data within the run chart for additional detail. Expert opinions vary, but generally 12 to 16 time points are adequate for statistical differentiation. In addition, more than 25 time points will not increase the statistical power (Carey, 2003). The median or middle point of the data set is used as the centerline on run charts because it is not sensitive to **outliers**, like the mean may be. As seen in Figure 14.6, the mean compliance of pain reassessment post IV pain medication administration for Unit A is 58%. Recall that the median is calculated by first arranging the data from low to high (48, 49, 50, 52, 52, 54, 62, 66, 69, 70, 72, 75). Because the median is the middle point and there are 12 time points on the graph (October to September), the sixth (54%) and seventh (62%) data points are added and divided (54% + 62% = 116/2 = 58%). In assessing the run chart, first consider if the data are hovering close to the median line or if the data are spread inconsistently from the median. If the data points hover close to the median, the process variation is minimal. If the data are inconsistently away from the median line, that represents greater process variation. When data points fall significantly above or below the median line, an outlier or an unusual finding exits. Now, look at Unit C in Figure 14.6. The median center line is at 49%, which was determined by the raw compliance percent in chronological order from low to high: 43, 43, 44, 44, 44, 47, 51, 55, 55, 60, 60, and 62. Because we have an even number of data points, the two middle points (47 and 51) are averaged (47 + 51 = 98/2 = 49%).

The run chart is useful in determining QI potential. When using a run chart, there is no true statistical analysis occurring in comparison to the control chart discussed in the following section. However, the run chart allows for quick analysis and visual review of how a process is performing. Looking back at Figure 14.6, does any unit's data demonstrate an outlier or finding different from the others? If you said Unit B, you would be correct. With a median of 65% compliance, the 30% compliance seen in March is an outlier. In general, Unit B is relatively stable with most compliance scores hovering around the median line, except for March, which was a drastic drop from February (64%). Unit B should ask, what happened in March? Is there an explanation for this change? Perhaps Unit B was orienting new nurses who were not yet familiar with the pain policy. Also notice the improvement in April (70%). Is this improvement based on a QI intervention or did the new nurses become familiar with the pain policy? Before mobilizing resources to improve an outlier representing special cause variation, first determine if there is an explanation. If so, monitor the unit for the next few months to determine if that outlier was incidental or if there actually is a problem needing QI intervention. If one special cause data point cannot be explained that might place patients at risk, further QI intervention is needed.

How would you compare the three units in Figure 14.6 regarding their compliance with pain reassessment? Unit A was below the median for the first 6 months then steadily improved over the last 6 months. What is not known is if the unit implemented a QI intervention in March with the following 6 months demonstrating positive improvement. If an intervention was implemented it should be sustained and celebrated. Also unknown is if the change from April (48%) to May (62%) was special cause variation. With the additionalsubsequent data points in June and September, it appears that the pain reassessment process changed for the better and that improved performance is being sustained. One challenge when interpreting a run chart for outliers or determining at what point on the chart the data represent the outlier is that this is subjective. You will see subjectivity is eliminated by using the control chart, described in the following section. Unit B's process has been in control except for that one special cause finding in March. Unit C demonstrates lots of variability in outcomes. There is little consistency month to month. Although no special cause can be clearly defined, a QI intervention may be needed to reduce or explain the process variation that is illustrated.

When comparing units or process outcomes, establishing the goal or target that demonstrates a success process not needing improvement is necessary, as discussed as part of the operational definitions earlier in this chapter. If the goal is 90% compliance, no unit in Figure 14.6 is meeting the goal. It may be helpful to include the goal on the run chart. Additionally, relative internal and external comparisons can provide benchmarking opportunities. For example, organizations may wish to compare their outcomes to other organizations and such comparisons could be used to determine if one organization is performing at a different level than another. Table 14.3 summarizes types of variation, analysis considerations, and potential QI actions. Prioritization is based on the volume and criticality of the outcomes and should include the consensus of QI experts and staff involved in the process. The run chart is helpful to determine improvement priorities and actions to be taken based on analysis. Additionally, although Unit C might like to reduce its variation, the reality is other more critical problems may require attention first.

One advantage of using a run chart is its ease in interpretation; run charts are commonly used by healthcare organizations. One disadvantage is that it is not as statistically sensitive as other tools with more specificity (Lloyd, 2010). There is another type of chart, the Shewhart control chart, commonly referred to as the control chart, described in the following section that adds a statistical advantage to the run chart that clearly detects outliers or unusual findings and eliminates the need for guessing. It takes time and practice to interpret run charts. For a closer look at interpreting a run chart, refer to Case Study 14.3.

TABLE 14.3 VARIATION INTERPRETATIONS, ANALYSIS, AND QI ACTIONS

TYPE OF VARIATION	ANALYSIS	QI ACTIONS
Common cause variation (process in-control)	Is the process demonstrating acceptable variation/acceptable level of performance?	No QI actions is required
	Is the process in control but a wide range of or unacceptable variation exists?	QI actions may be required based on QI priorities
Special cause variation (process out-of-control)	Is the process statistically demonstrating a problem, a change that is not desirable?	Action is required
	Is the process statistically demonstrating improvement based on QI efforts?	Continue to monitor to determine if efforts are sustained over time; if so, spread the lessons learned

QI, quality improvement.

CASE STUDY 14.3

Use the data from Figure 14.6. At a Unit C QI meeting, a nurse asks for assistance interpreting if the unit improved their pain reassessment compliance. The nurse notes that the first 3 months' results are October: 52%, November: 45%, and December: 50% (Figure 14.6, Unit C). How would you respond as to whether the pain reassessment compliance improved or did not?

The Shewhart Control Chart

The Shewhart control chart, often referred to as simply a control chart, is the same as the run chart but it adds statistical control limits to the run chart using SD. Because SD is used, the centerline is represented by the mean of the data set rather than the median that is seen on the run chart. The x- and y-axis are set up the same on both charts, with the x-axis being the time points and the y-axis being the variable or process under study. The Shewhart control chart has the same purpose as the run chart, that is, to distinguish common cause from special cause variation.

Recall the discussion about SD and that "sigma" is another term used for SD. The Shewhart control chart, created by software such as QI Macros®, will set SD control limits at 1, 2, and 3 SD above and below the mean of the data set. The advantage of the Shewhart control chart is the addition of SD because there is no guessing if an outlier or abnormal data point is present, which will be demonstrated shortly. When analyzing a Shewhart control chart, the **upper control limit** (UCL) is defined as the line 3 SD above the mean while the **lower control limit** (LCL) is the line 3 SD below the mean. A process that is considered to be in control or demonstrating common cause variability will have all data points between the UCL (+3 SD from the mean) and LCL (-3 SD from the mean). Together, the upper and lower control limits represent Six Sigma. When a data point falls above or below the UCL or LCL, the process is said to have a statistically significant outcome, referred to as special cause variation, or abnormal finding.

Before examining the Shewhart control chart, it is a good time to think about what we have already learned. Data can be displayed using a variety of formats, including histograms, Pareto charts, run charts, and Shewhart control charts. Each format has a purpose and a value within QI. Consider the Pareto chart in Figure 14.7. These data represent the annual incident reports of a large multisite organization. Medication errors are the leading cause of incident reports over a 12-month period. That outcome could trigger a QI activity. However, we now know there are more sophisticated SPC methods available to better analyze these incident report data.

In Figure 14.8, aggregate medication errors are shown on a Shewhart control chart using a time series design over 12 months. A range of outcomes, in this case from eight to 37 medication errors, is depicted, which represents significant variation. In analyzing aggregate medication errors in Figure 14.8. What do you notice different in the control chart as opposed to a run chart? The major difference includes the addition of the UCL and LCL, which can be used to analyze the process range. Because nearly 100% (specifically 99.8%) of outcomes are expected to fall within three SD from the mean, as seen in Figure 14.1, using three SD is generally considered acceptable when analyzing for special cause variation. In Figure 14.8, the UCL was established at 22.2 and the LCL at 4.5 automatically using the QI Macros software.

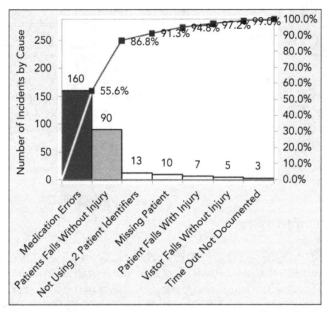

FIGURE 14.7 Incident report data over 12 months using a Pareto chart.

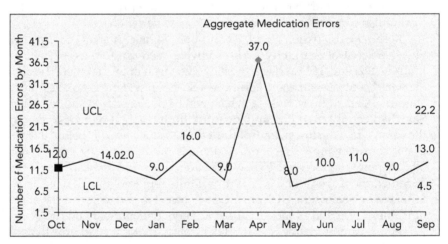

FIGURE 14.8 Aggregate incident report data over 12 months using a Shewhart control chart.

Evaluating the UCL and LCL is valuable because these limits specify the process range. As illustrated in Figure 14.8, the mean of aggregated medication errors over the 12-month period was 13. The UCL or 3 SD above the mean is 22 while the LCL or 3 SD below the mean is 4.5. The significance of this is that anywhere between 22 and 4.5 medication errors could occur each month and be considered in control, or within Six Sigma of the mean. In this case, that alone might trigger a QI activity as 22 medication errors a month while being considered in control would be concerning from a patient safety perspective. Also note in Figure 14.8 the centerline is the mean of the data points in a Shewhart control chart, whereas the centerline on a run chart is the median of the data set.

There are several different types of Shewhart control charts and their interpretation rules. At this point, it is important to apply the same rule used with the run chart, that is, identifying if an outlier or unusual data point exists. With the Shewhart control chart, your job is made easier in this analysis as special cause is evident when a data point appears either above or below the control limits. Analysis and QI actions taken based on the interpretation of the run chart outlined in Table 14.3 also apply to the Shewhart control chart: 37 incidents in April is nicely depicted significantly above the UCL in Figure 14.8. There is no guessing required if the data point represents special cause variation as it is above the UCL of 22. The Shewhart control chart reduces interpretation errors and the risk of not implementing QI activities when necessary or implementing QI activities when not necessary, leading to inappropriate resource utilization. In addition, notice that the number of medication errors was significantly reduced in the month of May to eight and remained hovering around the mean of 13 through September. This is a good example that when an unusual outcome occurs, such as 37 medication errors in April, it may be advantageous not to react and implement a QI activity but rather to acknowledge the outcome, continue to assess it, and follow the trends to determine if the number of medication errors continue to rise over time that would demonstrate statistical significance by being above the UCL.

Stratification

Stratification is the process of breaking the data down into subsets to better interpret what is happening and where (Fowler Byers & Rosati, 2008). Suppose the Patient Safety Officer is studying Figure 14.8 and prioritizes medication errors for a QI project. Before moving forward, stratification of the 160 aggregated medication errors could help target where QI efforts should focus. To do so, the 160 medication errors could be stratified into outpatient and inpatient areas. Data could be further stratified among inpatient or outpatient units to better determine if one particular unit is contributing to the abnormal finding. Additional questions should be considered: Were there truly so few errors, except in April? Does all staff understand the reporting process? Is the operational definition of medication errors clear? Does the organization's culture support reporting medication errors?

CRITICAL THINKING 14.2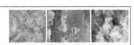

You are a nurse in a women's health clinic assigned to an improvement team with the aim to reduce the rate of the clinic breast cancer deaths. The clinic, located in Boston, Massachusetts, has a breast cancer rate of 10 per 100,000 female patients. Your first assignment is to research how the clinic's rate compares to the entire state breast cancer death rate. In addition, you have been asked to identify the top five states with the lowest breast cancer death rates as the actions these states may have implemented may be a valuable source of interventions for the project. Go to the AHRQ website: statesnapshots.ahrq.gov/snaps10/index.jsp. Select "State Rankings for Selected Measures". When clicking on each state, their 2010 National Healthcare Quality Report will open that includes the state's breast cancer death rate and state rank. Determine how the clinic's rate compares to the state's rate. Review each state and determine which states have the lowest breast cancer death rates.

OTHER QI TEAM TOOLS

Interprofessional teams are often created to bring experts and or process owners together to address problems and make improvements. QI tools, such as those described by Scholtes, Joiner, & Streibel, (2003), Gantt charts, parking lots, and flow maps help teams work through projects. These team tools as well as those discussed in Chapter 13, such as cause and effect or Fishbone diagrams, LEAN thinking, Six Sigma, Plan-Do-Study-Act (PDSA), Health Failure Modes Effect Analysis (HFMEA), and RCA are all QI tools used by teams.

Gantt Chart

A **Gantt chart** is a graph depicting the phases of a project over the project's time line and is used to keep the team on schedule (Figure 14.9). All known project tasks are included in the Gantt chart, from beginning to end. Because QI takes time and effort, line 16 of the Gantt chart in Figure 14.9 nicely reminds us to celebrate and share success, something all teams should include in their planning.

Flow Map

QI is focused on improving healthcare process; therefore, understanding each step within the process must be considered before interventions are identified. A **flow map**, or process flowchart, is a visual depiction of a process from the beginning of the process to the conclusion or end of the process and allows the QI team to diagram the actual sequence of activities and decisions within the process. Clarifying the sequence of a process reduces redundancy, unnecessary steps, and may illustrate overly complex processes that can be eliminated. Because healthcare processes are often complex, reducing the number of steps or decisions within a process is not only more efficient but may enhance patient safety. In addition to identifying inefficient steps in a process, flow maps also provide a visual step-by-step flow of a process that may not need to be more efficient but rather to provide a visual tool outlining the steps of a task or procedure. For example, although a nursing procedure such as blood administration will outline a written step-by-step process that the nurse must follow when administering blood, it is not uncommon to include a visual flow map of that process within the procedure.

ID	Task Name	Start	Finish
1	Defined Global aim of the project	1/29/2010	2/21/2010
2	Defined Specific Aim of the project	3/15/2010	3/24/2010
3	Created ED flow Log	3/15/2010	3/19/2010
4	Team coaching regarding the tool	3/24/2010	3/24/2010
5	Data Collection (Pre)	4/9/2010	4/29/2010
6	Study and Evaluate ED tools	3/25/2010	4/8/2010
7	Satisfaction survey (Pre) for Patients and ED Staff	4/26/2010	4/30/2010
8	Created Share Point access to data and satisfaction survey	4/26/2010	4/29/2010
9	Made Changes to Computerized Triage Template	5/7/2010	5/7/2010
10	Team coaching regarding the Triage tool	5/7/2010	5/12/2010
11	Data Collection (Post)	5/8/2010	6/9/2010
12	Analyzed the data	6/10/2010	6/14/2010
13	Satisfaction survey (Post) for Patients and ED Staff	6/23/2010	6/30/2010
14	Displayed the results to the team	7/7/2010	7/7/2010
15	Report to management in PDSA format	7/1/2010	7/30/2010
16	Celebrate and Share success	7/14/2010	7/14/2010

Timeline columns: Feb 2010, Mar 2010, Apr 2010, May 2010, Jun 2010, Jul 2010 (weeks: 1/24, 1/31, 2/7, 2/14, 2/21, 2/28, 3/7, 3/14, 3/21, 3/28, 4/4, 4/11, 4/18, 4/25, 5/2, 5/9, 5/16, 5/23, 5/30, 6/6, 6/13, 6/20, 6/27, 7/4, 7/11, 7/18, 7/25)

FIGURE 14.9 The Gantt chart.

(Courtesy of Providence VA Medical Center, Providence, RI.)

Different steps or actions within a healthcare process are represented by specific symbols in a flow map, such as ovals to depict the beginning and end points. Squares are used to identify steps in the healthcare process. Diamonds identify decision points, and arrows identify directional flow of the process. Figure 14.10 shows a patient flow map through an ED.

We have examined what data are and how data can be displayed for QI decision making and monitoring. Tools, such as those described in the SPC section earlier, provide the QI team with the most efficient, systematic means of determining what healthcare process needs improvement or if a QI was sustained over time. Given the advantages of SPC, these methods should be applied to healthcare decision making whenever possible. Creating and analyzing data using run or control charts require time and practice. Collaborating with QI experts for assistance is recommended. The next step in the QI journey is to empower a team who utilizes appropriate QI tools for data-driven QIs.

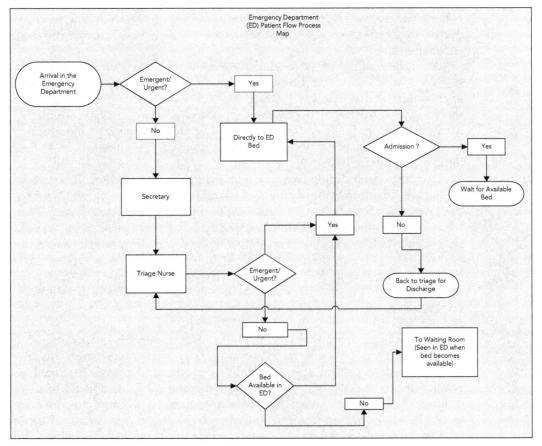

FIGURE 14.10 Emergency department patient flow map.

REAL-WORLD INTERVIEW

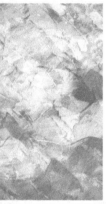
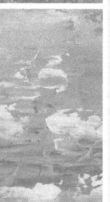

I was asked to participate in Lean training. A group from our unit went to the training not knowing what LEAN really referred to. None of us were sure what this LEAN was or what it involved. Content was presented using lots of new terminology. We heard about PDSA but process mapping? Fishbone diagrams? As the program progressed, it became clear that the expectation of the participants was to complete a LEAN project. Although nervous and wondering what did we commit to, we all were intrigued and believed we had lots of ways of making our unit more efficient.

We focused on brainstorming, process mapping, flow diagrams, and creating a PDSA. This was enlightening. Here we were flow mapping healthcare processes! What was most exciting was how we might use some of these tools on our unit. We were always so busy just responding to the many demands of patient-care that we seldom took the time to discuss our unit and how we could make things better. We gained insight how to creatively make change. It was an amazing feeling!

After the training we were all energized and eager to continue our discussion on a project and to get others on the unit involved. We were successful in creating our first Systems Redesign project using LEAN principles. We all shared similar frustrations with inefficiency in delivering patient care, particularly in our supply areas. Supplies were scattered instead of being grouped together. If a nasogastric tube needed to be inserted, it required travel to four different supply locations.

Our large clean supply area was changed due to construction. This gave us the impetus to improve the supply area layout for efficiency using LEAN principles. We tagged unnecessary or duplicate supplies and eliminated them. We collaborated with other departments; had quality experts take pictures so we could compare the before and after changes; we worked with supply staff to consider how we might change the utility room layout, added photos of supplies, and logically arranged supplies together (e.g., oxygen administration supplies were all reorganized to the same bin area; patient-care supplies, pajamas, toothbrushes, urinals, and any personal care items were all relocated in one spot, saving us time and frustration!)

What was amazing was our collaboration and success in working with other departments. We interacted with laundry, carpenters, infectious disease, pharmacy, central supply, quality experts, and housekeeping. Our group was on fire. We had actually implemented tools introduced to us in training. None of us ever collected data or worked through an improvement process from beginning to end. Yet we did it and had fun at the same time because we created a positive change for our unit. It has been exciting, overwhelming, and frustrating at times to be involved in such a project. I started off completely unprepared for such an activity. After all, I am just a staff nurse, right? Never would I have imagined taking a lead role in the redesign project and now I can say I contributed to a successful change on my unit. What a journey!

Annette M Phillips, BSN, CCRC
Research Nurse, Boston VA Healthcare System, Boston, Massachusetts

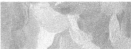

KEY CONCEPTS

- Quality improvement (QI) is a continuous process used to prevent, recognize, and reduce harm. It includes the ongoing search for performance excellence.
- QI is defined using the Quality and Safety Education for Nurses (QSEN) definition, to "Use data to monitor the outcomes of care processes and use improvement methods to design and test changes to continuously improve the quality and safety of health care systems."
- Quality initiatives are data driven and patient centered.
- Many sources of data exist, including internal, external, baseline, postintervention, incidence, prevalence, and aggregate.
- Data can be displayed using a variety of formats, including Histograms, Pareto charts, Scatter plot diagrams, and run and control charts).
- The science of quality improvement, mainly statistical process control, is concerned with minimizing variability within healthcare processes.
- Teams, often interprofessional, bring expertise and innovation to improving outcomes.
- Teams can use a variety of tools (Flow maps, Parking lot, and Gantt chart) during the improvement process.

KEY TERMS

Aggregate data
Baseline data
Common cause variation
Control chart
Data
Data display
Descriptive statistics
External data
Flow map
Gantt chart
Histogram
Incidence
Information
Internal data
Inter-rater reliability
Lower control limit
Mean
Median
Mode
Objective data
Operational definition
Outliers

Pareto chart
Postintervention data
Prevalence
Quality improvement
Range
Run chart
Scatter plot diagram
Special cause variation
Standard deviation
Statistical process control
Stratification
Subjective (patient) data
Upper control limit
Variability

REVIEW QUESTIONS

1. You are reviewing a control chart that depicts the number of falls over a 24-month period. You note a special cause variation occurred at month six. Which characteristic below is indicative of a special cause variation?

   A. The 6th month data point is between the upper and lower control limits.
   B. The 6th month data point is two standard deviation (SD) below the mean.
   C. The 6th month data point is one SD above the mean.
   D. The 6th month data point is above the mean at three SDs.

2. At a staff meeting, your nurse manager reports patient satisfaction has declined on your unit. In analysis of the patient comments, 30% of the 100 discharged patients surveyed over the last month complained about the noise at night. You are asked to be a participant in an improvement team to increase patient satisfaction. Which of the following questions are most appropriate to ask your manager before the team begins their quality improvement (QI) project (select all that apply)?

   A. How many staff will be invited to participate in the team?
   B. Is there evidence this finding is a special cause variation?
   C. What time frame is permitted to complete the project?
   D. Will there be overtime to attend meetings?
   E. How will trends be measured?
   F. How will participation affect my performance?

3. One of the key concepts of quality improvement (QI) is how a need for change does actually become an improvement. Which of the following is not an appropriate option for launching a QI project:

   A. High priority findings from a proactive risk assessment such as the Healthcare Failure Mode and Effects Analysis recently completed on your Mental Health unit.
   B. A fellow staff nurse's poor performance which is negatively affecting patient care.
   C. Ongoing concerns identified in the Medication Usage Review Committee.
   D. Need for innovation to close the gap between your organization's restraint usage and that of the identified benchmark or best practice.

4. Tardiness of evening-shift staff has been a problem on your unit. This has led to excessive overtime to ensure that patient shift handoffs are conducted in a timely manner. Your manager invites you to monitor evening-shift tardiness for 1 week. There are eight evening nurses. You just completed data collection and are preparing a spread sheet to share with your manager. Using the findings below in the Table 14.4, what is the mean time for tardiness and range of minutes that evening staff were tardy over this 7 day period?

   A. Mean = 8.0 minutes   Range = 3.0–20.0
   B. Mean = 5.0 minutes   Range = 3.0–20.0
   C. Mean = 5.0 minutes   Range = 123
   D. Mean = 8.2 minutes   Range = 3.0–20.0

TABLE 14.4 TARDINESS OF EVENING SHIFT

NURSE	SUNDAY	MONDAY	TUEDAY	WEDDAY	THUDAY	FRIDAY	SATDAY
A	OFF	OFF	OT	3 min	OT	OFF	OT
B	OT[a]	12 min	5 min	OFF	13 min	11 min	OFF
C	OT	OFF	OT	5 min	OT	12 min	OFF
D	OT	OT	OFF	OT	OT	OT	OFF
E	OFF	3 min	OT	OT	3 min	OFF	5 min
F	OFF	OT	ILL	5 min	OFF	OT	15 min
G	OT	OFF	20 min	OT	OT	OT	OFF
H	OFF	OT	4 min	OFF	7 min	OT	OT

[a] OT, on time.

5. When considering data display options, which order of display, from least scientific to most scientific exists when examining process variation?

   A. Range-Run Chart-Control Chart
   B. Run Chart-Pareto Chart-Control Chart
   C. Range-Control Chart-Run Chart
   D. Only a control chart allows for analysis of variability

6. The most distinguishing characteristic of a Pareto chart includes which one of the following?

   A. Upper and lower control limits.
   B. Depicts 80% of the problem comes from 20% of the causes.
   C. Displays data using a time series format.
   D. Is used when determining if special cause variation exists.
   E. Provides information about primary causes of a problem.

7. Statistical process control (SPC) is defined as which of the following options?

   A. Assessed using a run or control chart.
   B. Assessed only when data are presented in a control chart.
   C. A sophisticated measurement using the data range as the centerline.
   D. Easily assessed using a run chart (no, can make interpretation errors, many guesses).

8. Stratification of data refers to

   A. averaging the number of data points.
   B. identifying the lowest and highest data point.
   C. three standard deviation above or below the mean.
   D. segmenting the data from aggregate to more specific sub-sets.

9. When a quality improvement (QI) team wants to document a process from beginning to end, which of the following tools is most helpful?

   A. Flow map diagram
   B. Fishbone diagram
   C. Scatter plot diagram
   D. Pareto chart

10. Why is baseline data useful in quality improvement (QI) activities?

   A. It is used to differentiate common from special cause variation.
   B. It is used as the operational definition.
   C. It is used to demonstrate a sustained improvement outcome.
   D. It is used to compare preintervention to postintervention outcomes.

11. Of the following options, which is the most important requirement when creating an operational definition?

   A. Using the dictionary as a reference.
   B. Creating a numerator/denominator for measurement purposes.
   C. Listing the team member names.
   D. Have the approval of the organization's director before defining the variable.

REVIEW ACTIVITIES

1. National Association for Healthcare Quality (NAHQ) nahq.org. Read about NAHQ's history and code of ethics. Explore how healthcare professionals, including nurses, can become certified in healthcare quality.
2. The Joint Commission (TJC) www.jointcomission.org. Select the "Sentinel Event" tab then select the listings of "Sentinel Events." Select one of the alerts. Consider the impact of this alert. What data is presented on the sentinel alert? Conduct a web search on the sentinel alert to identify the prevalence of the problem in healthcare. Consider quality improvement (QI) ideas that might eliminate this occurrence from happening? How would you approach preventing this incident in your organization?
3. The Institute for Healthcare Improvement (IHI) www.ihi.org. Create an account to access IHI content. Select the "Resources" tab. Select the "How to Improve" tab. Notice the Plan-Do-Study-Act (PDSA) cycle is presented with many resources that improvement team can access. Explore how IHI speaks about "Forming the Team" and examples of effective teams.

CRITICAL DISCUSSION POINTS

1. Data comes in various types and there are various methods to display the data. During your next clinical experience, ask a nurse about what data are shared with them. Ask to see the data. Where are the data shared? In what format are the data shared?
2. Provide an example of what common cause variation and special cause variation might look like from your daily life or from your clinical experiences. Explain how the example meets the common cause or special cause variation rules.
3. Review the tools commonly used by quality improvement teams. Develop a case study that demonstrates how one of the tools is used by a quality improvement team. Explain how the tool was used and what other tools might also be considered for your example. Defend your selection of tool.

EXPLORING THE WEB

1. Robert Wood Johnson Foundation: rwjf.org
2. Agency for Healthcare Research and Quality; Data Sources: www.ahrq.gov/research/data/dataresources/index.html
3. The Healthcare Effectiveness Data and Information Set (HEDIS): www.ncqa.org/hedis-quality-measurement
4. Health-Related Datasets: www.healthdata.gov

REFERENCES

Berwick, D. M. (2011). Preparing nurses for participation in and leadership of continual improvement. *Journal of Nursing Education, 50*(6), 322–327. doi:10.3928/01484834-20110519-05

Carey, R. G. (2003). *Improving healthcare with control charts*. Milwaukee, WI: ASQ Quality Press.

Evans, J. R. (2008). *Quality & performance excellence: Management, organization, and strategy* (5th ed.). Mason, OH: Thompson South-Western.

Fowler Byers, J., & Rosati, R. J. (2008). Foundation, techniques, and tools. In Pelletier L. R. & Beaudin C. L. (Eds.), *Q solutions: Essential resources for the healthcare quality professional* (p. 66). Glenview, IL: National Association for Healthcare Quality.

Grube, J. A. (2008). Strategy and leadership. In Pelletier L. R. & Beaudin C. L. (Eds.), *Q solutions: Essential resources for the healthcare quality professional* (p. 79). Glenview, IL: National Association for Healthcare Quality.

Hart, S., Bergquist, S., Gajewski, B., & Dunton, N. (2006). Reliability testing of the national database of nursing quality indicators pressure ulcer indicator. *Journal of Nursing Care Quality, 21*(3), 256–265. doi:10.1097/NCQ.0b013e3182169452

Lloyd, R. C. (2010). Navigating in the turbulent sea of data: The quality measurement journey. *Clinics in Perinatology, 37*, 101–122. doi:10.1016/j.clp.2010.01.006

Mohammed, M. A., Worthington, P., & Woodall, W. H. (2008). Plotting basic control charts: Tutorial notes for healthcare practitioners. *Quality and Safety in Healthcare, 17*, 137–145. doi:10.1136/qshc.2004.012047

Nelson, E. C., Batalden, P. B., & Godfrey, M. M. (2004). The model for improvement: PDSA SDSA. In Nelson, E. C. Batalden, P. B. & GodfreyM. M. (Eds.), *Quality by design: A clinical microsystems approach* (pp. 271–283). San Francisco, CA: Jossey-Bass.

QSEN Institute. (2017). *Pre-licensure KSAs: Quality improvement*. Retrieved from http://qsen.org/competencies/pre-licensure-ksas/#quality_improvement

Scholtes, P. R., Joiner, B. L., & Streibel, B. J. (2003). *The team handbook* (3rd ed.). Madison, WI: Oriel Incorporated.

SUGGESTED READINGS

Ashley, L., Dexter, R., Marshall, F., McKenzie, B., Ryan, M., & Armitage, G. (2011). Improving the safety of chemotherapy administration: An oncology nurse-led failure mode and effects analysis. *Oncology Nursing Forum, 38*(6), E436–E444. doi:10.1188/11.ONF.E436-E444

Berwick, D. M. (1991). Controling variation in health care: A consultation from Walter Shewhart. *Medical Care, 29*(12), 1212–1225.

Berwick, D. M., Nolan, T. W., & Whittington, J. (2008). The triple aim: Care, health, and cost. *Health Affairs, 27*(3), 757–769. doi:10.1377/hlthaff.27.3.759

Donaldson, M. S. (2008). An overview of to err is human: Re-emphasizing the message of patient safety. In Hughes R. G. (Ed.), *Patient safety and quality: An evidenced-based handbook for nurses* (pp. 1–9). Rockville, MD: Agency for Healthcare Research and Quality.

Duclos, A., & Voirin, N. (2010). The p-control chart: A tool for care improvement. *International Journal for Quality in Health Care, 22*(5), 402–407. doi.10.1093/intqhc/mzq037

Goldmann, D. (2011). Ten tips for incorporating scientific quality improvement into everyday work. *British Medical Journal of Quality and Safety, 20*(Suppl. 1), i69–i72. doi:10:1136/bmjqs.2010.046359

Hall, L., Moore, S., & Barnsteiner, J. (2008). Quality and nursing: Moving from a concept to a core competency. *Urologic Nursing, 28*(6), 417–425. Retrieved from http://www.unet.univie.ac.at/~a0400309/MyFiles/DropBox/Alex/quality%20in%20nursing.pdf

Kimsey, D. B. (2010). Lean methodology in health care. *American Journal of Perioperative Room Nurses, 92*(1), 53–60. doi:10.1016/j.aorn.2010.01.015

Oman, K. S., Flynn-Makic, M. B., Fink, R., Schraeder, N., Hulett, T., Keech, T., . . . Wald, H. (2011). Nurse-directed interventions to reduce catheter-associated urinary tract infections. *American Journal of Infection Control, 30*, 1–6. doi:10.1016/j.ajic.2011.07.018

vretveit, J. (2011). Understanding the conditions for improvement: Research to discover which context influences affect improvement success. *British Medical Journal of Quality and Safety, 20*(Suppl. 1), i18–i23. doi:10:1136/bmjqs.2010.045955

Pocha, C. (2010). Lean six sigma in health care and the challenge of implementation of six sigma methodologies at a veterans affairs medical center. *Quality Management in Health Care, 19*(4), 312–318. doi:10.1097/QMH.0b013e3181fa0783

Shewhart, W. A., & Deming, W. E. (1939). *Statistical method from the viewpoint of quality control.* Washington, DC: Department of Agriculture.

Vest, J. R., & Gamm, L. D. (2009). A critical review of the research literature on six sigma, lean, and studer-group's hardwiring excellence in the United States: The need to demonstrate and communicate the effectiveness of transformation strategies in healthcare. *Implementation Science, 4*(35), 1–9. doi:10.1186/1748-5908-4-35

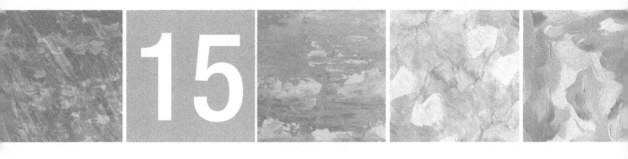

15

QUALITY IMPROVEMENT AND PROJECT MANAGEMENT

Jamie L. Vargo-Warran

Trying to manage a project without a project manager is like trying to play a football game without a game plan.

—K. Tate

Upon completion of this chapter, the reader should be able to

1. Explore quality improvement using a project management (PM) approach.
2. Explain the role of the nurse as a leader in quality improvement projects.
3. Describe systematic approaches used by nurse leaders for PM.
4. Apply the systematic steps of PM to a healthcare problem.
5. Describe the skills needed by nurses to manage a project.
6. Understand the benefits and limitations of PM.

You are the department director of an ED. You recently received the monthly report on your department's satisfaction score showing you ranked in the fourth percentile due to the volume of dissatisfied patients waiting more than 2 hours to be seen by a doctor and almost 8 hours to be admitted. You see that a sister hospital previously had the same issues and used a project management approach to help with delays resulting in increased patient satisfaction. You will need to decide which project management approach to apply. You have questions that you want to find answers to, for example:

- *How can I define the scope of the project?*
- *How will I identify and prioritize the project methodology?*
- *How can I identify the team members needed for the project?*

There is an increased need for healthcare organizations to achieve greater operational efficiency in care processes, improve patient safety and clinical outcomes, reduce costs, and increase patient satisfaction.

This chapter provides an overview of how PM is used in healthcare with definitions and practical applications to address these needs. The role of the nurse as a project leader is explored. PM is presented as a quality improvement (QI) tool using a systematic approach. An examination of the benefits and limitations of PM as well as the purpose and value of PM is detailed. The chapter presents the skills needed by practicing nurses to lead and manage projects. Applying PM to nursing practice is explored, including actions taken to improve healthcare processes.

▰▰▰ QI AND PROJECT MANAGEMENT

In the current healthcare setting, costs associated with providing care have exceeded expectations and continue to rise. The Centers for Medicare and Medicaid Services (CMS) stated the National Health Expenditure (NHE) grew 5.8% to $3.2 trillion in 2015, or $9,990 per person (CMS, 2017). The projected NHE for 2016 to 2025 will grow at an average of 5.6% annually (AHA, 2017). Additionally, there is a growing consumption of healthcare services and associated costs imperative to providing safe, high-quality patient care. A critical need has emerged for healthcare organizations to manage costs while maintaining a focus on quality patient-care outcomes. To contain costs while maintaining quality patient-care outcomes, hospitals must carefully examine and measure current patient-care processes and outcomes, then select appropriate projects for QI using PM approaches (Figure 15.1).

The 2015 National Healthcare Quality and Disparities Report stated a 17% decrease in hospital-acquired conditions in response to QI projects (Agency for Healthcare Research and Quality [AHRQ], 2015). **PM**, as defined by the Project Management Institute (PMI, 2017), is "the application of knowledge, skills, tools, and techniques to project activities to meet the project requirements" (PMI, 2017). PM involves an interprofessional team approach to address a problem with a defined beginning and end point. Projects are typically unique and temporary, requiring input from multiple perspectives. PM approaches can help save time, costs, and eliminate wasteful processes by standardizing and optimizing current work processes. PM involves a variety of methods, techniques, skills, and processes that are designed to manage quality initiatives to solve patient-care problems. Each quality initiative is different, therefore, PM methods will vary depending on the type of QI initiative.

QI is the use of data to monitor the outcomes of care processes and use improvement methods to design and test changes to continuously improve the quality and safety of healthcare systems (QSEN, 2007). In contrast, PM is a structured approach to examining the efficiency of processes. By using a PM approach, nurse leaders can see where there are opportunities for improvement or redesign of a current process. PM, whether in healthcare or another industry, is determining the desired end product, which is typically implementing a specific change to affect the efficiency and effectiveness of patient care. The outcome is dependent on how it is explained, what the perception of the explanation was by all parties, and a clear understanding of desired outcomes.

REAL-WORLD INTERVIEW

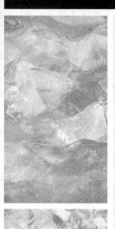

Quality improvement (QI) initiatives are required of all bedside nurses to increase positive patient outcomes. QI initiatives are decided by hospital nursing leadership and conveyed to staff in departmental meetings, informal conversations, or emails. It is usually leadership that plays vital roles in the project management (PM) side of QI initiatives by deciding what initiative to take on and then planning the roll out. However, it is crucial for nurses to understand the ramifications and the outcome or goal so initiatives are successful. As bedside nurses it is best for us to have a grasp on what the evidence-based practice shows so there is a basis for the initiative.

Daxtyn Lampa, BSN, RN
Emergency Room Charge Nurse
Valley Hospital
Las Vegas, Nevada

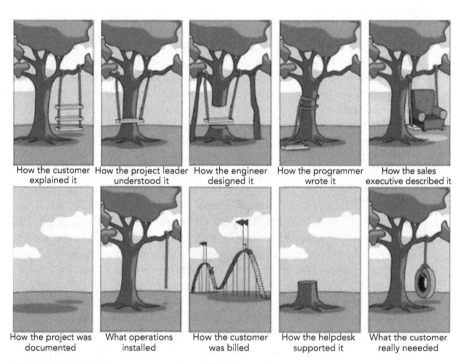

FIGURE 15.1 Project management tree.

ROLE OF NURSES AS LEADERS OF QI PROJECTS

We learned in Chapters 11 and 13 that QI applies the best available evidence to a clinical problem. How we approach the clinical problem is the PM aspect of QI. The role of nursing in QI includes carrying out interprofessional processes to meet organizational goals by using evidence-based practice to achieve better patient outcomes. No matter what level of nursing or title, from the Chief Nursing Officer to the direct care nurse, every nurse plays a part in QI. The demand for hospitals to report quality measures, meet value-based purchasing requirements, and achieve benchmarks for quality care have all impacted the role of the direct care nurse in QI projects. Nurses are at the frontline of patient care and as such, they are in the best position to identify patient-care process problems and affect the implementation and sustainability of QI projects. While the involvement of nursing leadership is crucial in QI, bedside nurses play a more direct role in QI activities.

For example, Mary is a direct care nurse on a medical–surgical nursing unit. Mary noticed that many times she has to order compression stockings for her postoperative patients from the storeroom when the patient is a same-day admission for surgery. Mary discusses the problem of postoperative patients arriving to the unit without having compression stockings on at the monthly unit meeting. The Unit Manager assumed all patients arrived with the required compression stockings from surgery as it was part of their postoperative protocol and no one raised this problem previously. Because Mary provides direct patient care to this population of patients she is able to identify a problem and call attention to her concerns about the quality of patient-care processes.

In the example, Mary identified a problem in the patient-care process that could detrimentally affect patient-care outcomes. Direct care nurses have a unique perspective on patient care and can identify problems in providing quality patient care. As discussed in Chapter 11, nurses have an obligation to question current nursing practices when something does not seem right or a process does not have the expected outcomes.

SYSTEMATIC APPROACH TO PM FOR NURSE LEADERS

Nursing leadership and multidisciplinary teams use PM approaches to achieve QI initiatives. PM approaches help the nurse leader to consider key issues with the identified problem and ensures that steps of PM are not missed.

PM is similar to the nursing process in that each uses a systematic approach to problem solving. PM is the overall process of initiating, planning, executing, monitoring and controlling, and closing to achieve a specific goal. To understand each stage of PM, including tools to facilitate it, the phase and the nurses' role are detailed.

CRITICAL THINKING 15.1

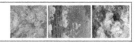

You are a managing director for a surgery center in your community. A new state-of-the art surgery center is being developed and it has determined current processes to deliver care will not work in order to deliver the quality of care envisioned. Leadership has determined new processes need to be designed that deliver the cutting-edge patient care as promised to the community. As a managing director and having PM experience, you are asked to be the project lead for determining process improvement.

1. How do you identify an appropriate project leader?
2. How do you determine what processes need improvement?
3. How would you explain the need for new process operations to your colleagues?

Initiating

There are some key steps during the initiating phase that can influence the success of any project. The first step is to identify the key individuals that must be included on a PM team. The key individuals are important since they either affect or are affected by the problem. These individuals are called **stakeholders** and can include persons, groups, or organizations who have an interest in, are affected by, or can affect a practice change (Registered Nurses' Association of Ontario [RNAO], 2012). While seemingly easy, this step requires careful thought and planning to ensure that the right individuals are brought in to participate on the team. It is important to note that on any team that works on a project involving any aspect of patient care that a direct care nurse is involved. Stakeholders should be engaged in the PM team based on their influence on the success of the project. Those stakeholders with high influence and high support should be engaged first. Table 15.1 demonstrates how to identify stakeholders with strategies to engage them in the project.

Prior to initiating a project, the project goals must be clearly stated in a way that is both attainable and measureable. Clarifying the goals of the project helps all members of the team to understand the rationale for the project and the expected outcomes. When assigning responsibilities for tasks, two roles need to be identified at the beginning of any project: project lead and project manager. Although these two terms are similar, they are not the same. The project lead is responsible for the overall delivery of the project plan and is the main point of contact for problems with the project. The project manager is the person responsible for producing, updating, and maintaining the project plan.

The next step is to come to a consensus as a team on the **scope** of a project or the work to be completed in order to achieve the goal (PMI, 2017). Current processes involved with the problem are detailed using a flow chart. The flow chart simply illustrates the steps of the current process including decision points. Chapter 13 illustrates a flow chart for insulin preparation. Once the team completes these steps they are ready to begin the planning phase.

Planning

To deliver a successful project, a project plan is essential. A project plan lists all the tasks and activities to be completed to achieve the goal of the project. Each task is given a start date and an end date that is within the project timeline. Once tasks are determined they are assigned by the project manager to groups or individual people to be completed. Tasks are typically assigned based on an assessment of strengths for each team member. Project setup and structure can include listing meeting schedules, identifying key components, designing detailed project plans, defining priorities, identifying risks, and defining clear measurable outcomes. The need for a project is identified through an assessment of the problem and the tasks needed for completion of the project. Figure 15.2 is an example of a project plan task list with a project time line that illustrates where tasks should be completed and anticipated achievement of milestones. A project plan can help keep the team stay on time for completing specific tasks.

When applying any template or form to a project plan, checkpoints are built in for deadlines. Building checkpoints in the timeline occurs in the planning phase. The planning phase and initiating phase are often considered to occur at the same time as they are seamless in nature. During the planning phase, everyone should know what is expected of him or her, including assigned due dates as outlined in the timeline.

Stakeholder Influence & Support Grid (with generic strategies for engagement)		
	High **Influence** **Low**	
High **Support**	• Will positively affect dissemination and adoption • Need a great deal of attention and information to maintain buy-in **Strategies:** • Collaborate • Involve &/or provide opportunities where they can be supportive • Support and nurture • Encourage feedback • Prepare for change management • Empower High Support High Influence	• Can positively affect dissemination and adoption if given attention • Need attention to maintain buy-in and prevent development of neutrality **Strategies:** • Collaborate • Encourage feedback • Empower with professional status • Encourage participation • Prepare for change management • Involve at some level High Support Low Influence
Low	Low Support High Influence • Can negatively affect dissemination and adoption in a big way • Need great amount of attention to obtain support &/or neutrality • Work towards buy-in **Strategies:** • Consensus • Build relationships • Recognize needs • Use external stakeholders & consultants • Involve at some level • Stress how BPG are developed • Don't provoke into action • Monitor	Low Support Low Influence • Least able to influence dissemination and adoption • Could have negative impact on plans • Some attention to obtain support &/or neutrality • Work towards project buy-in **Strategies:** • Consensus • Guild relationships • Recognize needs • Use external stakeholders and consultants • Involve at some level • Monitor

RNAO, 2012

TABLE 15.1 STAKEHOLDER SUPPORT, INFLUENCE, AND STRATEGIES FOR ENGAGEMENT.

CRITICAL THINKING 15.2

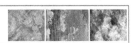

In your current course, you are required to submit your assignments to the professor as a hard copy in class. Your classmates would like to submit the papers electronically so that there is documentation of the submission. Use the information in Table 15.1 to identify stakeholders, including their level of influence and support on the problem. Determine appropriate strategies to engage the stakeholders in your project.

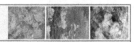

EVIDENCE FROM THE LITERATURE

Citation

Norris, J. M., While, D. E., Nowell, L., Mrklas, K., & Stelfox, H. T. (2017). How do stakeholders from multiple hierarchical levels of a large provincial health system define engagement? A qualitative study. *Implementation Science, 12*(98). Retrieved from https://implementationscience.biomedcentral.com/articles/10.1186/s13012-017-0625-5

Discussion

Stakeholder engagement is widely accepted as important for the success of any project. What is not known are the strategies that are most effective for engaging stakeholders. Engagement is difficult to achieve and even harder to measure across diverse healthcare settings. While known to be important, the meaning of stakeholder engagement is not consistently defined. The aim of this study was to understand how stakeholders of healthcare improvement initiatives defined engagement.

Three interrelated themes arose from the study:

1. Engagement is active participation from stakeholders who are willing and committed, and ranged from sharing information to vested decision making.
2. Engagement involves a shared decision-making focus for meaningful change for all participants, typically those who are impacted the most by the change.
3. Engagement involves respectful two-way interactions where all felt heard and understood.

When stakeholders feel heard and understood they tend to be more engaged in the success of a project.

Implications for Practice

The findings provide a guide for engaging stakeholders when working on a project. Understanding the characteristics of "engagement" allows project leaders to create a team culture that fosters meaningful engagement of all stakeholders.

Executing

The next phase in PM is executing, also described as the implementation phase. In the executing phase, every individual involved with the project should have a clear understanding of the project goal. Tasks in this phase include understanding the current ways of working or the current process and agreeing on priority areas. One way to achieve executing or implementing a project is through methods such as Lean, Six Sigma, or five-step (5S) methodology as shown in Table 15.2. Chapter 13. introduces and explains each of these methods in depth.

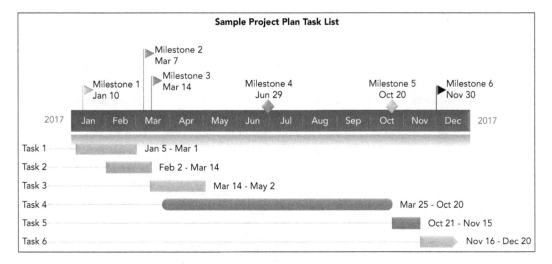

FIGURE 15.2 Sample project plan task list.

Source: Registered Nurses' Association of Ontario (RNAO) (2012). *Toolkit: Implementation of best practice guidelines* (2nd ed.). Toronto, ON: Registered Nurses' Association of Ontario.

CRITICAL THINKING 15.3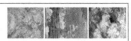

PMI created free templates for project management. Included are templates for project initiation, project planning, project execution, project monitoring and controlling, project closure, and project documents. These are all free to download and use. Go to www.projectmanagementdocs.com and select "project initiation" on the middle menu bar. Select a template listed. Pay special attention to the section in each template titled "executive summaries." Note how they differ from template to template.

1. Notice the different project initiations to choose from. How can you determine which template works best for your project?
2. How do the executive summaries differ from template to template?

CASE STUDY 15.1

You are a unit director at a hospital that has an unacceptable number of mislabeled lab specimens. As the unit director you decide to apply PM techniques to decrease the number of mislabeled specimens and have assigned this as one of your unit's quality initiative goals. The first step in PM is initiation. It is clear that the overall goal of the project is to decrease mislabeled specimens, but the PM method needs to be determined.

Based on the information provided:

1. *Identify two PM methods that could be used to guide this project.*
2. *How will you decide which will be the most effective method?*
3. *Create one measurable goal for the project.*

TABLE 15.2 TYPES OF PROJECT MANAGEMENT METHODS

METHOD	PROCESS USE	OUTCOME
• Lean	• Makes processes more efficient by streamlining them	• Eliminated waste in processes
• Six Sigma	• Improves the quality and efficiency of processes by streamlining them using statistical methods	• Optimized process
• 5S	• Reorganizes the workplace	• Standardized workplace organization process.

5S, five step.

The selection of PM methods is based on the type of project, the context or setting for the project, and the goals of the project. Understanding types of PM approaches important to the successful implementation of any project. The three methods commonly used in healthcare for executing or implementing a project are presented.

Lean Method for PM

Lean has been around for at least 100 years and while Henry Ford first applied this method of thinking to Ford manufacturing, it was Taiichi Ohno from Toyota who perfected the Lean methodology. Simply put, Lean streamlines processes making them more effective. The goal of Lean is to systematically eliminate waste and make processes less cumbersome. In Lean, waste is considered any task or step that does not add value to a service or product. The project manager should concentrate on making the workflow as smooth as possible by concentrating on dependencies of that process. In other words, what outside processes are necessary to effectively streamline the process? The project manager also carries the load of facilitating creativity and recognizing talent. By adding the Pareto principle, or the 80/20 rule, unnecessary processes can be determined. In Chapter 14, the Pareto principle is explained with a Pareto chart illustrating how roughly 80% of the problems arose from 20% of the causes.

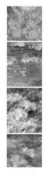

CASE STUDY 15.2

Based on Case Study 15.1 you are the unit director at the hospital that has an unacceptable number of mislabeled lab specimens. As the unit director you decide to apply PM to decrease the number of mislabeled specimens and have assigned this as one of your unit's QI goals.
The first step in PM is initiating, the next step in PM is executing.
Based on the information provided and the project method chosen in Case Study 15.1:

1. *How would you apply the Pareto principle to determine waste?*
2. *Once waste was determined, as project manager, how would you carry out the PM through initiating and execution?*

Six Sigma

Six Sigma strives for optimizing processes, performance, and ultimately supporting QI efforts. Six Sigma achieves QI goals by eliminating defects and variations from within a process (Shankar, 2009). Statistical analysis is done on data collected from defined measures on processes and outcomes. Six Sigma differs from Lean with the application of statistical analysis to identify variations in practice, uncovering root causes of problems. Six Sigma is taught using levels of "belts" to signify completion of training that is similar to martial arts. Varying degrees of expertise are awarded belt levels starting with Green and finishing with the Master Black Belt. Master Black Belts serve as coaches for others in Six Sigma methodologies, as project leaders, and work on QI projects. Green Belts take on the responsibilities of PM as assigned by the Master Black Belt. A complete explanation of Six Sigma, including techniques and methodologies, can be found in Chapter 13.

5-Step Methodology

The 5S methodology was also developed in Japan to assist in optimizing processes found in the workplace. It is referred to as 5S because it has five steps: Seiri, Seiton, Seiso, Seiketsu, and Shitsuke. Translated into English the steps are Sort, Set in Order, Shine, Standardize, and Sustain. Sort refers to sorting out what is needed and not needed in a work area. Set in Order is arranging items so they are easily accessible and ready to use. Shine is cleaning the workspace on a regular basis. Standardize is simply revisiting the first three steps of the 5S methodology frequently to ensure they are consistently followed. Sustain is keeping to the rules to maintain standards. Ideally, when the 5S methodology is implemented correctly, efficiency and effectiveness in reorganizing the workplace and eliminating waste are achieved. Chapter 13 explains the 5S methodology in detail. During the executing phase, workshops may be organized, meetings to discuss process design may occur, and drafting new procedures may occur simultaneously among teams.

Monitoring and Controlling

Monitoring in PM is a dynamic and continuous process. Gathering data on the process and outcomes from a QI project provide valuable information about the effectiveness of the QI project. Feedback from those involved with the change also helps to identify how well or poorly the new processes are working. The continuous collection of data and feedback allows rapid identification of problems. Typically, the project manager or leader may assign a particular group of team members the duty of monitoring and controlling phases of the project.

For example, Jane is part of the medical-surgical unitís QI team. They are currently working on a project to reduce patient falls. To determine if their interventions have the desired effect, the QI team implements the changes on one unit. By using one unit, the team can test their new interventions and make changes before initiating the change throughout the hospital. The QI team wants to measure two things: adherence to evidence-based interventions and the effect that their project had on reducing falls. In the beginning of any new project, frequent monitoring helps identify a problem before it becomes a major problem. The team measures process indicators such as audits for compliance with the interventions to reduce falls for high-risk patients such as colored socks, signage on the door, call light within reach, and hourly rounding implemented for any patient identified as high risk. The team would also measure the outcomes of number of falls reported on the unit every week. Chapter 14 explores audit measures for both process and outcomes indicators. Weekly audits provide data to see if the interventions were adhered to appropriately. Theoretically, adherence to the interventions should reduce the number of falls. Closely monitoring both the process and outcome of a QI project helps improve awareness of any problems with the process, unintentional outcomes, or other variables not yet considered and is essential to PM.

Once the changes are in place and determined to have both the process and outcomes desired, the team begins to implement the plan for spreading the change throughout all patient-care areas. Assigning specific individuals to continue the same audit on each unit ensures that data are tracked and collected using identical procedures. Standardizing data collection is essential for monitoring the effectiveness of the new interventions, processes, or change.

Closing

The final step in PM is closing. The closing of a project is vital because it ensures the project is complete and the results are sustainable. Reflection on how the project went and what changes may need to occur in future projects is documented. The entire PM team gathers to consider sustainability of the project and to build in triggers that would provide a warning that a process broke down. For example, for the falls example mentioned earlier, triggers could be built in such as monthly quality audits for compliance with the steps of the process. The audits could be done by a nurse on the unit and reported to the Unit Director. Another trigger could be a reporting threshold. If the total number of falls rises above a set amount then it could trigger the QI team to reassemble to look at the process. The closing of a project also allows time for team members to reflect and refine their PM skills. Leadership can use this time to mentor and guide new team members.

APPLICATION OF SYSTEMATIC APPROACH TO PM

To understand how PM can support quality healthcare, an example of a current healthcare quality issue provides the framework for discussion. A problem exists with the nursing shift change process. Hospital leadership has identified labor costs averaging 50% of total hospital revenue and wasteful practices must be contained and controlled while not sacrificing quality of care. One area for opportunity is the shift change report given between the nursing staff. It has been identified that nurses are staying past their shift completion time due to lengthy shift reports, causing an increase in overtime. The goal of this project is to improve the efficiency of the nursing shift change report. Leadership has decided to use the Six Sigma methodology following the Define, Measure, Assess, Implement, and Control (DMAIC) QI approach (Chapter 13 explains Six Sigma and DMAIC). Leadership assigned a Black Belt as the team mentor, the nurse manager as project manager, and a medical-surgical nurse as the project lead. The team is composed of the following stakeholders: three medical-surgical nurses, two nursing assistants from the medical-surgical unit, a nursing supervisor, and representatives from lab, respiratory, and physical therapy departments. The following shows how a PM approach is used to explore QI methods to address a problem.

Define

The first step in the DMAIC approach is to define the problem. The shift change report, as defined by nursing management, is a tool to ensure continuity of care as patient-care staff changes shift. The report contains patient information that is essential to patient care and is given from the nurse completing the shift to the nurse coming on duty and taking the assignment. Charge nurses are responsible for making assignments, which can be subjective in nature. Typically the nurses coming onto the day shift may have to interact with more than one night shift nurse who will have to wait until the day shift nurses are available. If nurses coming on duty could spend less time waiting for report they could spend more time interacting with their patients. Patient interaction can have a positive impact on the hospital consumer assessment of healthcare provider and systems or Hospital Consumer Assessment of Health Plans Survey (HCAHPS), which is a method by which patients can rate their experience. HCAHPS scores can affect hospital reimbursement from Medicare/Medicaid, making the financial aspect of the problem an important consideration. As directed by the hospital leadership, the shift change report should take no more than 30 minutes to complete. Anything longer than 30 minutes is considered too long. During any shift change, there is the opportunity for increased efficiency depending on the number of shift change reports given.

Measure

Measure is the next step in the DMAIC approach. In order to measure improvement, the current time it took to complete a shift change report needs to be documented to establish a baseline. The project lead nurse observed 30 reports being given at random without the staff nurses' knowledge. The stopwatch function on the smartphone was used to keep the time measurement accurate and consistent. Nurses were timed at a distance so they did not feel the pressure of being timed and the observation could happen in an unhampered state. Both the morning and evening shifts were timed. Based on the 30 observed shift change reports that were measured, the average report time was 43 minutes.

The next step is to determine how much of the 43 minutes accounted for nonvalue added (NVA) steps. NVA steps are those parts of the report process that were unnecessary to perform the task. The team decided if the nurses were waiting and not delivering the report or listening to the report, the time could be considered NVA. To identify the NVA time during reports, the team mapped out the report process from beginning to end. The mapping, which is similar to concept mapping, revealed 23 minutes was NVA and was associated with oncoming nurses waiting for report from the previous shift. It was noted that one oncoming nurse waited for report from three different nurses leaving their shift before she could start her work.

Analyze

The next step in the DMAIC approach is to analyze the data. In order to begin addressing potential solutions for NVA time, it is appropriate for a health failure mode and effects analysis or HFMEA™ chart to be done. The Joint Commission requires healthcare providers to select a minimum of one process per 18 months that can be considered high risk and perform a proactive risk assessment, or HFMEA, on the process. A HFMEA provides a mechanism to evaluate for the risk of patient injury and provide a proactive and preventive technique to gauge the severity of the risk before it happens. Conducting a HFMEA helps a PM team identify and prioritize problems.

For the problem concerning shift report, a HFMEA is conducted with input from all committee members. There are 5Ss involved in a HFMEA discussed in Chapter 13 that are applied to the shift change reporting problem:

1. Define the HFMEA topic.
2. Assemble the team.
3. Graphically describe the process.
4. Conduct a hazard analysis.
5. Identify actions and outcome measures.

Conducting a complete HFMEA involves specific training and expertise in QI methodology. As a new nurse, knowing the basic steps of a HFMEA, why it is conducted, and understanding the goal of a HFMEA are appropriate.

Improve

Improve is the next step in the DMAIC process. After the team defines and measures the data, the key area for most effectively eliminating waste was identified. The most controllable source of unnecessary costs exists in the NVA wait times of nurses to get report. To fully understand the problem, the team looked at other organizations, at the literature, and talked with others about best practices in restructuring the unit layout to improve nurses' efficient use of time. The team decided to redesign the layout so assignments are created in clusters based on geographical location on the unit as well as bed assignments based on patient acuity level.

Control

The final step in the DMAIC process is the control step. During a 30-day pilot phase, the new assignments based on clusters were trialed and nurses were surveyed. The results were highly favorable of the new assignments. Under the new assignment layout, any given nurse would have no more than two nurses to provide shift change report to. To

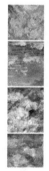

CASE STUDY 15.3

A local hospital is in the process of moving to a new location and will need to review all the current processes in the hospital's daily operations. A Master Black Belt in Lean Six Sigma was brought in to oversee the project and asks all leadership to participate in a HFMEA event. By using HFMEA, the goal is to maintain patient safety in the transition to a new facility. One process identified in conducting the HFMEA was that the movement of materials such as food, pharmaceuticals, linen, and waste were crossing paths with patient transfers. As a result of the HFMEA, a need was identified to bring the service to the patient whenever possible rather than bringing the patient to the service.

1. *Based on information in the case study, go to www.queri.research.va.gov/implement ation/quality_improvement/tool.cfm and complete the questionnaire.*
2. *Which tool would be best suited for organizational restructuring as mentioned in the case study? Explain your selection.*

further the process change, communication was delivered via unit meetings, emails, and informal discussion. The sigma level increased from 0.7 to 3.3, indicating the process increased in efficiency (the higher the score the more efficient the process).

LEADERSHIP SKILLS FOR PM

Recall that the project lead facilitates leading the project and incorporates all levels of nursing. To do so, the project lead must possess skills in both leadership and management for the success of a project. Chapter 3 details the characteristics of effective leaders, which are adapted to leading PM initiatives.

1. Creating a shared vision for the team and goal for the project.
2. Dealing effectively with conflict.
3. Fostering motivation and commitment of the team.
4. Managing priorities and tasks.
5. Facilitating team cohesiveness.
6. Accepting responsibility for understanding vision and goals by the team in relation to their roles in the project.
7. Serving as a role model.
8. Advocating for the team.
9. Maintaining momentum for the project (Gardner, 1993).

As a direct care nurse, you may find yourself serving in a project lead role as you obtain training and grow in your experiences working on QI projects. Your role may be as an informal leader who is charged with coordinating and managing a project. In this role, you will be required to possess effective communication skills and work between varying hierarchal layers. The project lead must work and collaborate with senior leadership as well as nursing leadership so nurses at the bedside will feel empowered as the project progresses.

The project lead must have a thorough understanding of the organization. This is accomplished by first assessing the organizational culture to ensure the existing culture is open and flexible based on evidence and quality outcomes (Lavin, 2013).

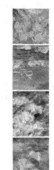

CASE STUDY 15.4

As a direct care nurse, you are asked to lead a project to address compliance with hourly rounding. You are part of a team that includes administration such as the Chief Nursing Officer, Supervisor, and Unit Manager as well as a Quality Nurse, two direct care nurses (one from your unit and one from another unit in the hospital), and one Certified Nursing Assistant (CNA). The nurses and CNA describe problems adhering to hourly rounding when the unit becomes busy with new admissions, discharges, and changes in patient acuity. Administration wants 100% compliance with hourly rounding.

1. *As the project lead, what are your priorities for managing the team?*
2. *How will you employ the characteristics of effective leaders to reconcile the team's differing perspectives?*

The project lead must be able to connect with nurses delivering bedside care as well as any other members from interdisciplinary teams that are affected by the project. A project lead must be able to ascertain what skills each team member brings to the project and capitalize on these strengths and mentor others in developing skills. By supporting and growing an individual's skills, buy-in to a project is higher and satisfaction is increased. The project lead must empower team members and be a strong agent for change by supporting their work and championing the project. The project lead should be cognizant of project budget constraints and adhere to the project plan. However, the project lead needs to know when it is time to end a project and be able to justify why.

CRITICAL THINKING 15.4

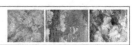

Go to the website: www.mindtools.com/pages/article/newPPM_60.htm. Complete the PM Skills Self-Assessment located on the website. Use the "Calculate My Total" at the bottom to see your score and determine your score interpretation. Look at the bottom of the page for information about your results. Compare your findings to others in your class. What are your PM strengths? What areas are your opportunities for improvement? Based on findings from the class, who would be the best leader of a project?

BENEFITS AND LIMITATIONS FOR PM

While PM in healthcare can help lessen risks and improve the chances of achieving goals, there are other clearly defined benefits. PM can help clarify not only what you are doing but why you are doing it. The initiating/planning phase of PM helps define not only immediate goals, but also future goals. There are times you may discover that there is no clear reason for the project. Effective PM forces team leaders to ask two important questions: are we doing the right things and are we doing things right? The "right things" refers to the sequence of activities or tasks to accomplish a goal. On the other hand, "doing things right" looks at the quality of the work. Other benefits of PM include awareness of costs, allocating resources, and budget management. Teamwork is a critical component of PM as collaborating with others who have differing perspectives of a problem is essential to understanding the issue. Capitalizing on the strengths of each team member and using PM as a learning process help each member grow. Successful PM gets the most out of each worker and fosters a sense of belonging. The tangible benefit of teamwork leads to an intangible benefit of a productive workforce, which is fundamental to a successful organizational culture.

Limitations of PM

Limitations can exist with any methodology and a project manager needs to be aware of these limits. There are limitations that arise from unexpected changes during the project such as changes to team composition or participant's jobs, available resources, commitment level, or leadership. These changes may require recentering the team by bringing everyone back together and reviewing the mission and goals for the project. Team members disagreeing can affect a project's control and the project manager should set expected standards for performance. Specification limits are harder to handle and are usually stakeholder related. A stakeholder may show some dissatisfaction with the project and ultimately try to sway or undermine the project. The project manager should clearly define the limits with the stakeholder prior to onset of the project.

Another limitation is the human element limitation. Team members are individuals and some variability in performance, commitment, and conflicts in personalities do happen. These limitations can be avoided by good communication skills, including both open communication as well as good listening skills. Limitations may also include the inability to stick to the project scope, unable to complete the project with proposed budget and/or schedule, or even following one exclusive methodology. Taking a step back and continually reviewing the project plan can help mitigate limitations.

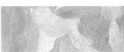

KEY CONCEPTS

- The use of project management (PM) in healthcare provides professionals with a way to improve the quality of care at a healthcare organization through projects.
- Effective PM requires individuals involved in a project to contribute through distinct roles, each with their own responsibilities.
- Project management consists of five main phases: initiating, planning, executing, monitoring and controlling, and closing.
- There are many project methodologies with the three most common being Lean, Six Sigma, and 5-step (5S) methodology.
- Benefits of project management include lessening risks while increasing organizational success, decreasing expenditures, and streamlining processes.
- Limitations of project management include control limits, specification limits, human element limits, and methodology limitations.

KEY TERMS

Project management   Scope
Quality improvement   Stakeholders

REVIEW QUESTIONS

1. A key element of project management is to do which of the following?

   A. Provide the organization with a method for improvement.
   B. Measure and compare the results of key work processes with those of the best performers in evaluating organizational performance.
   C. Identify clinical areas running seamlessly within the organization.
   D. Facilitate quality improvement initiatives by providing a methodology to plan, organize, lead, and control resources to achieve specific goals.

2. Which is the correct order for project management phases or steps?

   A. Initiating, planning, executing, monitoring and controlling, and closing
   B. Planning, executing, diagnosing, monitoring and controlling, and closing
   C. Assessing, diagnosing, planning, implementing, and evaluation
   D. Define, measure, analyze, improve, and control

3. Which of the following would not be considered a process for project management?

   A. Patient wait time to be seen in the ED by a physician is below the national norm.
   B. Patient satisfaction scores as provided by Hospital Consumer Assessment of Health Plans Survey (HCAHPS) are above the national average.
   C. Patient supply room inventory is needed to be restocked more than once a day.
   D. Patient dietary request are being fulfilled correctly 100% of the time.

4. A Failure Modes and Effect Analysis (FMEA) may be done to detect errors in a process before they have a chance of occurring. When looking at the FMEA process, all are included except:

   A. Failure causes
   B. Failure frequency
   C. Failure effects
   D. Steps in the process

5. As a clinic manager you have discovered patient scheduling has become a nightmare due to the high volume of patients. Some patients have to wait up to 6 months for routine appointments. You realize you need to realign the scheduling process and decide to utilize your project management skills to complete the task. Which of the following would be best suited to realign the scheduling process?

   A. Failure Modes and Effect Analysis (FMEA)
   B. 5-Step (5S) methodology
   C. Six Sigma
   D. Lean

6. During what phase of project management does the need for a project become identified?

   A. Initiating
   B. Closing
   C. Planning
   D. Evaluation

7. The U.S. Department of Veterans Affairs Quality Enhancement Research Initiative (QUERI) was created to improve the healthcare of veterans and is a free site for healthcare providers to access. Which of the below is not a function of this website?

   A. Providing treatment plans
   B. Provides a mechanism to help identify what quality improvement method is recommended
   C. Provides a QUERI implementation guide
   D. Provides a Heart Failure toolkit

8. The Joint Commission requires healthcare facilities to apply Failure Modes and Effect Analysis (FMEA) to processes to be proactive in identifying possible areas of error. How many FMEAs are required yearly?

    A. 1
    B. 2
    C. 3
    D. 4

9. When utilizing the Six Sigma methodology for project management, DMAIC is applied. The "A" in DMAIC stands for?

    A. Association
    B. Analyze
    C. Agency
    D. Aquired

10. Limitations in project management can affect the entire quality improvement (QI) process. Which of the following is an example of a limitation in project management?

    A. When there is no human element concern
    B. Differences in the types of methodologies available to organizations
    C. When a project leader has a clear understanding of the methodology chosen
    D. When a stakeholder sways a project

REVIEW ACTIVITIES

1. Explore the National Library of Medicine/National Institute of Health's Health Services Research Information Central website at www.nlm.nih.gov/hsrinfo/quality.html. The website is a repository of quality information, resources, and research related to all aspects of healthcare quality.
2. Practice using project management skills by streamlining everyday processes you currently do. Go to www.queri.research.va.gov/tools/default.cfm and choose different method tools to gain practice in implementing the tools.
3. The Institute for Healthcare Improvement at www.ihi.org provides resources on healthcare improvement. Search for Health Care Failure Mode and Effect Assessment (HFMEA) in the search box and the tool will come up. Download the tool and practice doing a Failure Modes and Effect Analysis (FMEA) on an upcoming event you will be participating in.
4. The Project Management Institute at www.pmi.org offers the PMBOK® Guide and Standards. Register for a free account to become familiar with project management standards.
5. The American Society for Quality (ASQ) at asq.org provides a library of quality resources. Register for a free account to access the many tools and library of information.
6. Use the Health Resources and Services Administration's (HRSA) quality improvement (QI) toolkit available on their website (www.hrsa.gov/quality/toolbox/methodology/index.html to work through the modules on developing and implementing a QI plan.

CRITICAL DISCUSSION POINTS

1. Review the quality improvement content in Chapter 13. Identify a quality improvement initiative in a clinical setting, either during a clinical experience or, if you work in the clinical setting, then one with which you are familiar. Describe how you would apply a project management approach to address the problem.
2. As a new nurse you may be involved with a quality improvement project. Describe the role you might play as a new nurse. How does this role evolve as you gain experience?
3. Project management requires leadership skills as described in the chapter. How might you gain these leadership skills? What resources do you need to help you gain these skills?

EXPLORING THE WEB

1. Agency for Healthcare Research and Quality (AHRQ; www.ahrq.gov)
2. National Database of Nursing Quality Indicators (NDNQI; www.ndnqi.org)
3. Centers for Medicare and Medicaid Services (CMS; www.cms.gov/Research-Statistics-Data-and-Systems/Statistics-Trends-and-Reports/NationalHealth ExpendData/downloads/highlights.pdf)
4. Quality Enhancement Research Initiative (QUERI)—U.S. Department of Veterans Affairs QUERI (www.queri.research.va.gov/default.cfm)
5. Project Management Institute (PMI)—Project management documents (www.projectmanagementdocs.com)

REFERENCES

Agency for Healthcare Research and Quality (AHRQ). (2015). *2015 National healthcare quality and disparities reports*. Retrieved from https://www.ahrq.gov/sites/default/files/wysiwyg/ research/findings/nhqrdr/nhqdr15/2015nhqdr.pdf

American Hospital Association (AHA). (2017). *TrendWatch: Chartbook 2017*. Retrieved from http://www.aha.org/content/17/costofcaringfactsheet.pdf

Centers for Medicare and Medicaid Services (CMS). (2017). *National health expenditures 2015 highlights*. Retrieved from https://www.cms.gov/Research-Statistics-Data-and-Systems/Statistics-Trends-and-Reports/NationalHealthExpendData/downloads/ highlights.pdf

Cronenwett, L., Sherwood, G., Barnsteiner J., Disch, J., Johnson, J., Mitchell, P., Sullivan, D., Warren, J. (2007). Quality and safety education for nurses. *Nursing Outlook, 55*(3)122–131. doi:10.1016/j.outlook.2007.02.006

Gardner, J. (1993). *On leadership*. New York, NY: The Free Press.

Lavin, P. (2013). Boots on the ground: The role of the Magnet® project director. *Nursing Management, 44*(2), 50–52. doi:10.1097/01.NUMA.0000426140.60785.0d

Project Management Institute, Inc. (PMI). (2017). *PMBOK guide* (5th ed.). Newtown Square, PA: PMI. Retrieved from https://www.pmi.org/pmbok-guide-standards/foundational/ pmbok

Registered Nurses' Association of Ontario (RNAO) (2012). *Toolkit: Implementation of best practice guidelines* (2nd ed.). Toronto, ON: RNAO.

Shankar, R. (2009). *Process improvement using Six Sigma*. Milwaukee, WI: ASQ Quality Press.

▉▉▉ SUGGESTED READINGS

Arthur, J. (2016). *Lean six sigma for hospitals: Improving patient safety, patient flow and the Bottom Line* (2nd ed.). New York, NY: McGraw-Hill Education.

Berwick, D. M., & Hackbarth, A. D. (2012). Eliminating waste in US health care. *JAMA, 307*(14), 1513–1516. doi:10.1001jama.2012.362

Daudelin, D. H., Selker, H. P., & Leslie, L. K. (2015). Applying process improvement methods to clinical and translational research: Conceptual framework and case examples. *CTS Clinical and Translational Science, 8*(6), 779–786. doi:10.1111/cts.12326

The Joint Commission. (2016). *Patient safety systems (PS)*. Retrieved from https://www.jointcommission.org/assets/1/18/PSC_for_Web.pdf

National Database of Nursing Quality Indicators (NDNQI). (2012). *Frequently asked questions*. Retrieved from http://www.nursingquality.org/FAQs

Shirley, D. (2011). *Project management for healthcare*, Boca Raton, FL: Taylor and Francis Group, LLC.

Stanley, D., Malone, L., & Shields, L. (2016). Process management supports the change process. *Nursing Management, 47*(6), 52–55. doi:10.1097/01.MUMA.0000483130.35813.d9

Toussaint, J. S., & Berry, L. L. (2014). The promise of Lean in healthcare. *Mayo Clinic Proceedings, 88*(1), 74–82. doi:10.1016/j.mayocp.2012.07.025

Visich, J. K., Wicks, A. M., & Zalila, F. (2010). Practitioner perceptions of the A3 method for process improvement in health care. *Decision Sciences Journal of Innovative Education, 8*(1), 191–213. doi:10.1111/j.1540-4609.2009.00251.x

Ward, J. (2010, July 08). *The Project management tree swing cartoon, past and present [the Project Management Tree Swing Cartoon, Past and Present]*. Retrieved from http://www.tamingdata.com/2010/07/08/the-project-management-tree-swing-cartoon-past-and-present/

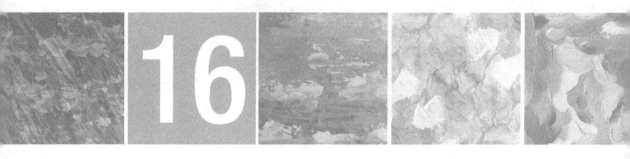

16

THE FUTURE ROLE OF THE REGISTERED NURSE IN PATIENT SAFETY AND QUALITY

Jerry A. Mansfield, Danielle Scheurer, and Kay Burke

This nation built the highways it decided to build. Its journey to the moon began with the decision to get there, and in no other way. It will prove the same for the health and care this nation seeks. (Berwick, 2017)

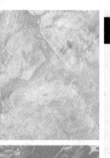

Upon completion of this chapter, the reader should be able to

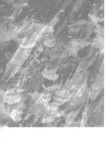

1. Discuss movement toward the future of healthcare.
2. Discuss the future of patient-centered care.
3. Support the role of the RN as a full member of the interprofessional team in the delivery of high-quality and safe patient care in the future.
4. Review the future of evidence-based practice (EBP).
5. Discuss the future of quality improvement (QI) and patient safety.
6. Review the importance of informatics use by the healthcare team of the future.
7. Describe the future leadership and management role of the nurse in attaining quality and safety in healthcare.
8. Explore leadership commitment to listening to the voice of the nurse.

Y ou recently accepted a job as a medical–surgical nurse in a 350-bed community-based hospital about 200 miles from where you graduated from nursing school. In your nursing leadership course, you learned a great deal about how healthcare needs to change and transform from a focus on treatment of disease to keeping patients, families, and communities well. You recently learned during a staff meeting that the number of patients who fell and were injured on your unit has increased over the past year. You have been asked to participate in a group to reduce patient harm from falls.

1. *What is important to know from the literature about preventing patient falls from the best available evidence?*
2. *What best practice evidence from the literature is already in use to prevent patient falls on your unit?*
3. *What actions could you take to facilitate future changes to patient care delivery within your own nursing unit?*

The current RN workforce (3.9 million) is large and thereby influential in terms of health-care delivery (NCSBN, 2017). Based on nurses' regular contact with patients and their families and their proximity to patients across the continuum of patient care, the nurse is in a unique position to partner with other health professionals in creating a preferred future for healthcare in the United States (Institute of Medicine [IOM], 2011c).

Healthcare is an industry that continues to evolve through many changes. These changes will affect nursing and nursing education in the future. For example, the increased growth in the number of patients older than 65 years means that people are living longer with increasing numbers of chronic illnesses and difficulties with managing activities of daily living. The increasing diversity of patient populations signals a need to ensure that patients' ethnic background, primary spoken language, and health literacy are required considerations in meeting patients' personal healthcare needs. There is exponential growth in advanced technological and informatics applications to manage patient care populations across the patient care continuum. New programs to manage population-based healthcare will impact future roles of healthcare providers, offering new ways to manage patient populations outside of traditional hospital and clinic-based settings. **Population health** is an approach to healthcare that aims to improve the health of an entire human population, not just individual patients. Increasing costs to provide healthcare in the United States will continue to drive demand for changes in health policy and regulation. The evolving need for interprofessional collaboration and education will change how future nurses and other healthcare providers provide collaborative team care in the future. Increasing demand for nurses in the workforce will challenge schools and colleges of nursing to keep up with a sufficient supply of new graduates to offset the increasing number of nurses retiring from the workforce. With all of these changes, the eyes, ears, and voices of over 3 million nurses are well positioned to improve the quality and safety of patient care in the future. Nurses have a responsibility to lead and manage the care of patients in current and new care delivery settings.

This chapter discusses movements toward the future of healthcare and the role of every nurse to lead change and improvements in healthcare delivery. The chapter also discusses the future of patient-centered care and the role of the nurse as a full contributing member of the interprofessional team in delivering high-quality and safe patient care. It will review future considerations for the use of evidence-based practice (EBP) and discuss the future of quality improvement and safety. The chapter also describes future developments in informatics and implications for those anticipated changes in patient care delivery. In addition to emphasizing the importance of a leadership commitment to listen to the voice of the nurse, the chapter also describes the role of every nurse as a leader in improving patient care delivery in their own practice setting.

HEALTHCARE FUTURE

A recent initiative (Dzau et al., 2017) combined the voices of more than 150 researchers, scientists, and policy makers from across the United States, to outline future priority issues for health policy. These priorities are the following:

- Call for a new paradigm of healthcare delivery and financing.
- Embrace the centrality of population and community health.
- Increase focus on individual and family engagement.
- Increase use of biomedical innovation, precision medicine, and new diagnostic capabilities.
- Increase use of advances in digital technology and telemedicine.
- Promote the use of "big data" to drive scientific progress (Dzau et al., 2017, pp. 5–6).

The experts involved in outlining the priorities mentioned earlier described the overall future vision of the U.S. healthcare system as, "A health system that performs optimally in promoting, protecting, and restoring the health of individuals and populations and helps each person reach their full potential for health and well-being" (Dzau et al., 2017, p. 7). "Nursing is the protection, promotion, and optimization of health and abilities, prevention of illness and injury, facilitation of healing, alleviation of suffering through the diagnosis and treatment of human response, and advocacy in the care of individuals, families, groups, communities, and populations" (American Nurses Association, 2015, p. 7). Nurses in the future, by embracing population health, by engaging patients and families in their care, and by using new tools and technology along with data to drive EBP, can lead change in healthcare that will enhance patient and population health outcomes. Throughout this chapter, each section describes how the healthcare industry is changing and the role of the nurse in transforming that future.

PATIENT-CENTERED CARE

Patient-centered care is built on the principle that the individual patient should be the ultimate decision maker when it comes to choices regarding the type of treatment and care he or she receives (IOM, 2011c). Some definitions of patient-centered care include the patient's family as part of patient-centered care. The Institute for Patient- and Family-Centered Care states that **patient- and family-centered care** is an approach to the planning, delivery, and evaluation of healthcare that is grounded in mutually beneficial partnerships among healthcare providers, patients, and families (IPFCC, 2017). Individualizing the patient's plan of care to coordinate goals, interventions, and outcome measurements that are shared by all members of the interprofessional team can enhance the achievement of outcomes. The IOM report describes what patients should expect from their healthcare (Table 16.1).

Patient-centered care in the future will increasingly be delivered in a growing number of nontraditional settings, such as patient-centered medical homes. **Patient-centered medical homes** are a team-based care delivery model whereby patient treatment is led by a healthcare provider and provides comprehensive patient care with the goal of achieving maximal health outcomes in the patient's home, a hospice or other ambulatory setting, or by telehealth. Transitions for patients among these settings should be easy and seamless, communication should flow freely, and patients should always know where to go with questions or concerns (Picker

TABLE 16.1 WHAT PATIENTS SHOULD EXPECT FROM THEIR HEALTHCARE

- "You will have the care you need when you need it . . . whenever you need it."
- "You will be known and respected as an individual."
- "Your medical record is yours to keep, to read, and to understand." The rule is: 'Nothing about you without you.'"
- "The system promises you excellence as its standard."
- "You will be safe in the care system."
- "You will experience proactive help, not just reactions."
- "Your care will not waste your time or money."
- "The walls between professions and institutions will crumble, so that your experiences will become seamless."
- "You will never feel lost."

Source: Institute of Medicine (IOM). (2011c). *The future of nursing: Leading change, advancing health*. Washington, DC: National Academies Press.

Institute, 2013). There will be expanding roles for nurses who help patients and their families navigate the healthcare system and coordinate their care. In addition, nursing can help to ensure people stay healthy in their daily lives, rather than focusing on patients who only interact with care providers in healthcare settings (Picker Institute, 2013). Complexity in patient care will grow with advances in biotechnology, human genome mapping, and an ever-increasing capacity to predict disease and prevent illness.

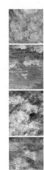

CASE STUDY 16.1

You recently went on patient rounds with the interprofessional team. You are aware that the patient has concerns that the patient did not mention during rounds.

1. *How can you advocate for the patient to ensure that the patient's values, preferences, and needs are expressed to the interprofessional team?*
2. *What could be the reasons why the patient is not actively involved in their care on rounds?*
3. *What resources could a nurse use to ensure patient needs and wishes are considered in rounds and the plan of care?*

CRITICAL THINKING 16.1

Nurses should increasingly involve patients and families in their care.

1. What are best practices in relation to involving patients and families in their care?
2. How can patients and families be involved in settings other than hospitals?
3. What other resources are available from other healthcare systems on how to involve patients and their families?

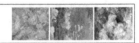

CRITICAL THINKING 16.2

The Institute of Medicine (2011c) described what patients and families should expect from healthcare delivery (e.g., " . . . care you need when you need it"; " . . . be known and respected as an individual"; and "you will be safe").

1. As a nurse, what actions can you take to meet patients' expectations?
2. How can the nurse influence the interprofessional team in meeting the expectations of patients in the healthcare setting?
3. What resources are available to help the nurse improve his or her practice in this expectation?

Predictive, Preventive, Personalized, and Participatory (P4) Medicine

P4 Medicine (i.e., medicine that is predictive, preventive, personalized, and participatory) is emerging out of the convergence of systems biology, the increasing activation of networked consumers, and the digital revolution in communications and information technology (IT; P4 Medicine Institute, 2012). For example, "predictive" medicine may include using the results from a genetic test to determine the risk a patient may have for a particular health problem. "Preventive" medicine could include encouraging patients and families to get an annual influenza vaccination during flu season. Hood, Balling, and Auffray (2012) envision a future where each patient will be associated with a virtual data cloud of billions of data points (e.g., height, weight, medications, diseases, lab values, hospitalizations, vital signs). As a result, examining the patients' "personalized" needs and patterns compared with others can generate hypotheses about health and/or disease for each individual patient. While care coordination has always been a part of nursing practice, the complexity of patient care in the future will increasingly require the nurse to solicit patient "participation." The nurse should assertively manage the coordination of the patient's care and serve as a patient/family advocate. Evidence shows that when patients are engaged in managing their healthcare, they have better outcomes (Doyle, Lennox, & Bell, 2013; Hibbard & Greene, 2013). In the future, the nurse and the patient, as well as the healthcare team, will have access to much more information about each individual patient. This ultimately enhances continuity of care and communication among the interprofessional team.

Future Marketing and Nursing

Future nurses can contribute to patient-centered care by reflecting on their unique contribution to the patient's experience. Consider if you, as a hospitalized patient, were to personally pay each day for direct nursing care, what would you "value"? Do patients want what nurses' offer? Do patients really know what nurses offer in the provision of high-quality, safe nursing care? Do nurses know what patients want and need? How can nurses more effectively market themselves or their nursing services? Product, placement, promotion, and price are four classic elements of marketing (The Times 100, 1995–2013).

Upon introducing oneself to a patient, the nurse shares with the patient that the nurse will monitor the patient's vital signs, listen to the lungs, check circulation in the legs and arms, watch for any unexpected complications, and ensure the highest level of quality and safe care for the shift (product). This will help the patient recover from a surgical procedure on a medical–surgical floor (placement). Through this introduction, and answering the patient's questions and concerns, the nurse is "promoting" the service being provided to the patient. The price is the amount the patient pays for the product. Currently, the nursing "price" in many hospital settings is part of the room charge billed to patients.

Nurses of the future will consider if each nursing unit or department addresses the product needs of a different market or group of patients. What do nurses know about their patients/customers product needs regarding demographic differences, conditions, or responses to actual or potential health problems? Where and how should these needs and differences be addressed? How could the practice of nursing and other healthcare services in the future be paid for by patients? Answers to these and other questions have implications for expanded nursing roles in the future (Table 16.2).

Finally, patient engagement in healthcare remains a challenge. Most healthcare systems today still do things "to" or "for" patients instead of "with" patients. In the future, nurses and interprofessional teams will develop true partnerships with patients. The ultimate goal of patient-centered care is to get people invested in their own care as active participants by establishing reciprocal partnerships—relationships built on mutual trust and respect between the patient and his or her nurse and the interprofessional team.

TABLE 16.2 IMPLICATIONS FOR FUTURE EXPANDED NURSING ROLES

FUTURE GROWTH AREA	IMPLICATIONS FOR NURSING
Telemedicine and ambulatory care nursing	• Telemedicine: Telemedicine is currently used by hospitals to extend their outreach to underserved patient populations and hospitals that lack a sufficient supply of specialists (e.g., neurology, cardiology, mental health). Healthcare teams can remotely connect with specialist providers in order to efficiently and effectively diagnose and evaluate patients for earlier treatment and intervention. In some cases, patients can be treated without unnecessary transportation to a higher level of hospital care. Nurses working in such settings that either offer or receive telemedicine services will learn new ways of interacting with interprofessional teams and provide patient-centered care. • In the future, nurses will increasingly use telemedicine technology to help patients manage chronic illnesses (e.g., heart failure, diabetes) in their homes; ongoing patient interventions by the nurse may reduce hospitalizations and prevent unnecessary visits to urgent care or emergency departments. • Ambulatory care nursing: There is a growing trend to expand roles for nurses in ambulatory settings such as clinics, schools, surgery and diagnostic procedure centers, freestanding community facilities, care coordination organizations, and other community health and wellness programs. Nurses in these settings help patients and families access acute care and other community services to meet their health and illness needs.

(continued)

TABLE 16.2 IMPLICATIONS FOR FUTURE EXPANDED NURSING ROLES *(continued)*

FUTURE GROWTH AREA	IMPLICATIONS FOR NURSING
Biotechnology and big data	• Nurses will be needed in expanded roles for biotechnology research in order to determine new ways of treating debilitating and/or rare diseases (e.g., cardiovascular disease, HIV, and hepatitis C). Nurses are needed to ensure patient safety and provide care to patients undergoing treatment and research-based clinical trials for new medical devices, equipment, and pharmaceuticals. • **Precision medicine (PM)** is a term for a medical model that proposes the customization of healthcare, with medical decisions, practices, or products being tailored to the individual patient (Lu, Goldstein, Angrist, & Cavalleri, 2014); in this model, molecular diagnostics, imaging, and analytics are often employed for selecting appropriate and optimal therapies based on the patient's genetic content. Nurses will be needed to help patients manage their response to actual and potential health problems as healthcare becomes even more individualized for each patient. • **Big Data** is a term for data sets that are so large or complex that traditional data processing application software is inadequate to deal with them. Analysis of big data can find new correlations to spot business trends, prevent diseases, combat crime, and so on (*The Economist*, 2010). In the future, nurses will have access to more and more information, that is, big data, which will change how nursing care is delivered. Imagine the use of information, collected and analyzed on a large number of patients, in order to target interventions to improve population health!
Human genome mapping	• In the future, nurses need to be experts at obtaining comprehensive family histories in order to facilitate the identification of family members at risk of developing disease, reduce the potential for genomic-influenced drug reactions, helping patients understand genetic tests and results, as well as referring patients and families to experts in genetics for assessment, treatment, or follow-up.

TEAMWORK AND COLLABORATION

It is vital that the nurse of the future be adept and comfortable working within interprofessional teams. Because of this, nurses and other healthcare disciplines are being educated to execute positive working relationships within these interprofessional teams (Poston, Haney, Kott, & Rutledge, 2017). Often, the nurse serves as the team "quarterback" and coordinates care among many team members, and serves as the ultimate patient advocate in the process. Because of this, it is important for the nurse of the future to be educated and trained as a full partner in interprofessional teamwork, and to learn and understand the basic concepts of good team communication skills and practices. One example of such a skill toolkit is **TeamSTEPPS**, which is a teamwork system designed to improve communication skills among healthcare professionals (AHRQ, 2017). Some examples of commonly utilized TeamSTEPPS tools are outlined in Table 16.3. The nurse of the future will utilize or encourage the use of these tools, based on the practice setting, to improve team performance and patient outcomes.

TABLE 16.3 EXAMPLES OF COMMONLY UTILIZED TEAMSTEPPS TOOLS

TEAMSTEPPS TOOL	BASIC CONCEPTS
Read back	A tool designed to teach healthcare professionals to state, out loud, what they just heard from another team member; used primarily in situations where critical information is being verbally transferred between healthcare providers, such as when reporting a critical lab value or a medication request during a code
Huddle	A structured tool designed to gather a team together to plan for a future event or set of events (such as a prereview of an operating room day); it ensures a common understanding of the work to be accomplished and potential risks to be aware of, such as a high-volume day or the high acuity of certain patients
Debriefing	A structured tool designed to standardize the gathering, analysis, and learning of information on a team, usually after an unanticipated event such as a fall or medication error
SBAR	An acronym designed to standardize the transfer of patient information among team members; SBAR stands for "Situation, Background, Assessment, Recommendation"

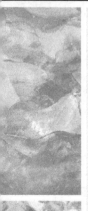

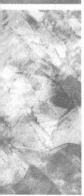

REAL-WORLD INTERVIEW

Pharmacists and nurses collaborate to achieve drug therapy outcome goals that include:

- Administering the right drug and the right dose at the prescribed time
- Ensuring proper quality controls for medications
- Accurately recording patient medication lists
- Providing appropriate education on risky medications to prevent side effects or possible complications that lead to harm

Pharmacy and nursing also collaborate on making sure that patients' medication lists are accurate and that patients understand the use and side effects of their medications. This involves a collaborative team of pharmacists and nurses to observe and map out the medication workflow process and coordinate efforts to get a patient's medication history, along with ensuring that patients have access to medications at discharge. Pharmacists and nurses also participate in follow-up discharge phone calls to patients that help to reinforce valuable information about medications and prevent an adverse drug event.

Robert J. Weber, PharmD, MS, BCPS, FASHP, FNAP
Senior Director, Pharmaceutical Services
The Ohio State University Medical Center
Columbus, Ohio

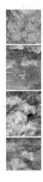

CASE STUDY 16.2

John is a nurse on a cardiovascular unit in a large academic healthcare center working on an interprofessional team that cares for patients with congestive heart failure (CHF). John heard in a staff meeting that the readmission rate for patients with CHF at the hospital was higher than the national benchmark. An interprofessional team is to be formed to examine the care of previously discharged patients with CHF from the hospital who were readmitted within 30 days of discharge posthospitalization.

1. *What is the role of the nurse in participating on an interprofessional team to reduce readmissions for patients with CHF?*
2. *What other interprofessional team members could be involved in the work group?*
3. *What current healthcare processes are in place to improve the care of patients with CHF across the continuum of care?*

EVIDENCE-BASED PRACTICE (EBP)

As more research is conducted, the amount of information available for development and implementation of evidence-based clinical care guidelines and protocols to ensure high-quality patient care in every setting increases. The interprofessional team of clinicians must review the literature and together develop clinical practices to ensure that patients receive the most current and safe care possible. Nurses and all interprofessional team members must continue to review the evidence that challenges or supports the current approach to care. This holds the interprofessional team accountable to evidence-based care practices and associated patient care outcomes.

The nurse of the future may encounter barriers in practicing evidence-based care. For example, nurses may experience resistance from other nurse colleagues, nurse leaders, and managers; in addition, the hospital or health system may not provide sufficient budgetary support or resources (*American Journal of Nursing*, 2017; Melnyk, Fineout-Overholt, Gallaher-Ford, & Kaplan, 2012; Melnyk et al., 2016). Belonging to professional organizations that support EBP, including ongoing education, resources and guidelines, continuing formal education at the undergraduate and/or graduate level, and supportive cultures that promote informed clinical practice are all examples of current ways for nurses to engage in EBP. The future will ideally support the nurse in questioning nursing practice and providing access to up-to-date and reliable evidence.

In the future, RNs will contribute to the evidence in the management of specific diseases or disease impacts on certain underserved populations. This begins with the collection of thousands of patient-specific data via electronic medical records (EMRs). By using this patient-specific data and analyzing nursing interventions and associated patient outcomes, new knowledge will help guide future nursing practice. Imagine embedding evidence in all clinical documentation systems that support patient interventions, making EBP seamlessly integrated into clinical practice. In the future, all nurses will understand that EBP is part of their social obligation for nursing care and the expectation will be that all nurses demonstrate competency in evidence-based nursing care at all times for all patient care.

CASE STUDY 16.3

During your orientation, you are asked to complete a procedure on a patient. When you review the policy and procedure to refresh your memory on best practices, your preceptor says, "We don't follow those polices on this unit!"

1. *Review the Nurse Practice Act in the state for which you are licensed. Who is accountable for the delivery of nursing care?*
2. *How does a new nurse know standards of care and practice?*
3. *What resources should a nurse use to ensure that he or she is practicing according to the best evidence?*
4. *What is your response to your preceptor?*

QUALITY IMPROVEMENT

The QI era in healthcare significantly gained traction in the early 2000s when the IOM published two landmark reports, entitled *To Err Is Human* (2000) and *Crossing the Quality Chasm* (2001). The former report described the prevalence and impact of low quality on the current and future state of healthcare; the latter report provided a framework for moving forward and improving patient quality on a large scale. In the latter report, the IOM defined six domains of quality, which are still very relevant today, and are aligned with what patients expect out of healthcare, that is, healthcare that is Safe, Timely, Effective, Efficient, Equitable, and Patient-centered (STEEEP). Most national, regional, and local quality efforts and measurements are still framed according to these six domains.

In the future, quality efforts and measurements will need to add the domain of healthcare value. The most widely adopted definition of **healthcare value** is achieving the best health outcomes (quality + experience) at the lowest cost (Scheurer, Crabtree, & Cawley, 2016). This definition assumes a patient-centered model of care, where value is in the eye of the beholder. Based on the definition, in order to provide high healthcare value, one either needs to increase quality and experience or decrease cost for both. It is no longer acceptable to raise cost without raising an equivalent amount of quality or experience. The healthcare value equation is extremely relevant in healthcare finance as well, with the advent of a growing number of government and private payers that reimburse healthcare systems according to the healthcare value provided to the patient. Three of the most common and financially impactful healthcare pay-for-value programs for hospitals from the Centers for Medicare and Medicaid Services (CMS) are outlined in Table 16.4.

A major reason that the healthcare industry has needed to evolve from quality to value is the cost of healthcare in the United States. Although the United States spends more per capita on healthcare than any other nation in the world, healthcare outcomes lag far behind most developed countries, including preventable morbidity and mortality outcomes. For example, the United States is projected to spend $2.8 trillion on healthcare this year alone, which comprises approximately 18% of the entire U.S. gross domestic product (GDP). This is more than what Australia, Canada, Brazil, China, France, Germany, Italy, Japan, and the United Kingdom combined spend on healthcare. The more the United States spends on healthcare, the less money there is to invest in other public programs, for example, infrastructure, education, and so forth. In the words of Donald Berwick, former Administrator for the CMS: "What healthcare takes, others lose" (Berwick, 2013). With this in mind, it becomes clearer that the U.S. healthcare

TABLE 16.4 PAY-FOR-VALUE PROGRAMS FOR HOSPITALS

PROGRAM	DESCRIPTION	IMPACT ON HOSPITAL
Value-based purchasing program	Measures care in four domains: • Clinical care • Safety • Efficiency-cost • Patient-centeredness	Up to 2% decrease in hospital reimbursements based on performance relative to other hospitals
Readmission reduction program	Measures overall and disease-specific readmission rates	Up to 3% decrease in hospital reimbursements based on actual performance compared to expected performance
HAC penalty	Measures potentially preventable hospital-acquired conditions	Up to 1% decrease in hospital reimbursements based on performance relative to other hospitals (CMS, 2017)

CMS, Centers for Medicare and Medicaid Services; HAC, hospital-acquired condition.

system must not only focus on quality, but it also has an obligation to reduce the cost of healthcare, as our economy and future healthcare system depend on it.

There are many other drivers to propel the U.S. healthcare system to improve the value of care provided to patients. The biggest driver, as mentioned in Table 16.4, is the rapid evolution in how payers reimburse for healthcare from an old model of fee for service to a new model of payment for healthcare value, that is, a value-based purchasing program. An example of a value-based purchasing program is the emerging model of bundled payments for care improvement, which links the CMS payments for the multiple services patients receive during an episode of care. Under bundled payments for care improvement, hospitals enter into payment agreements that include financial and performance accountability for episodes of care. The CMS has declared that it simply will not continue to pay hospitals and providers for low healthcare value. Simply put, healthcare systems that provide low healthcare value will not be viable in the future.

Another driver for a healthcare system to enhance its value is that its reputation and market share depend on value due to the explosive growth in public transparency and the volume of value measures that are reported on public websites, such as CMS Hospital Compare. Public information drives increasing competition among healthcare systems to outperform each other, as most public reporting shows relative rankings of performance. For example, the CMS website, Hospital Compare, (www.medicare.gov/hospitalcompare/search.html) houses more than 100 quality measures that allow patients to compare and contrast performance among hospitals. The website displays performance using a star rating on a 1 to 5 scale (Medicare.gov, 2017). Another website example is a non-for-profit company, Leapfrog, (www.leapfroggroup.org/) which compares hospitals' performance and displays it in a letter grading system (The Leapfrog Group, 2017). Although these websites have been criticized for oversimplifying quality performance, they are very easy to access and to understand by patients, and therefore have increased the pressure on healthcare organizations to rapidly improve their performance.

Another driver of the need to provide high-value care is the expectations of patients and families that they deserve and expect high-quality care and a good experience at the lowest possible cost. Increasing patient and family responsibility for healthcare cost has also driven them to demand lower cost services.

With respect to quality and value reporting, there are also major changes likely in the future, to include the following:

- More refined attempts to risk-stratify patients and populations, to even out the playing field of comparing populations. For example, comparing patient deaths among hospitals, taking into account how ill the patient is when he or she arrives. One of the biggest ongoing criticisms of publicly reported measures is their inability to risk-stratify the patients, and therefore their tendency to penalize healthcare systems that take care of sicker patients.
- Increased attempts to study and predict any unintended consequences of publicly reported quality measures. For example, for many years, hospitals had to publicly report their patient's pain control and hospitals received higher ratings and higher reimbursements if patients rated better pain control. There are critics that now blame the opiate epidemic to the overemphasis on patient pain control. As a result, pain control questions are being removed from pay-for-value programs, and the questions are being reworded to reflect how well pain was discussed, not controlled. This is an example of an unintended consequence of a well-intended measure. In the future, there needs to be more emphasis on predicting and mitigating or reducing these unintended consequences before quality measures are publicly reported.
- More attempts to measure quality across the spectrum of care of a patient. For example, most quality measures currently reflect the care provided at a single patient encounter or phase of care for a patient. Few quality measures reflect a holistic approach to the longitudinal care of a patient. In the previous example, measuring a patient's pain control during a single inpatient encounter gives little information about the patient's overall longitudinal pain care over time.
- More measurements of things that matter to patients, not providers. For example, for knee replacement surgery, most healthcare systems measure outcomes such as patient infections or complications. While these are understandably important to patients, there needs to be more emphasis on how the knee replacement impacted the patient's well-being or functional status. These measures are referred to as patient-reported outcomes and they better reflect what really matters to patients in their daily life over time rather than at a single point in time. For example, how does the patient function immediately postoperatively, 1 month later, 1 year later, and so on?

In summary, the nurses of the future will play a critical role in the future of quality improvement, which will focus much more on the healthcare value provided to the patient, that is, quality care plus patient experience divided by cost. Nurses have a huge impact on the quality of patient care, the patient experience, and the cost of care delivery. There are a number of patient, provider, payer, and healthcare system factors

CRITICAL THINKING 16.3

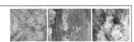

Patients and families are increasingly seeking online information about how healthcare systems treat patients and the experiences of those patients.

1. What online information is available to current and future patients about healthcare?
2. What are some of the pros and cons of considering online resources about healthcare?
3. Explore CMS Hospital Compare, Star Ratings: www.medicare.gov/hospital-compare/Data/HCAHPS-Star-Ratings.html. What did you see at the site?

EVIDENCE FROM THE LITERATURE

Citation

Rayo, M. F., Mansfield, J., Eiferman, D., Mignery, T., White, S., & Moffatt-Bruce, S. D. (2016). Implementing an institution-wide quality improvement policy to ensure appropriate use of continuous cardiac monitoring: A mixed-methods retrospective data analysis and direct observation study, *British Medical Journal, 25,* 796–802.

Discussion

Nurses at a large academic healthcare center were concerned due to the frequency with which RNs were required to accompany patients off the unit for tests and procedures due to continuous cardiac monitoring. Too often, when multiple patients left the unit, the remaining staff had to care for ever-increasing numbers of patients, well beyond the budgeted workload requirement. An interprofessional team examined the evidence and developed a new cardiac monitoring policy. Cardiac monitoring rates decreased, the need for nurse-accompanied transport decreased, and there were no untoward effects on length of stay or patient mortality.

Implications for Practice

Interprofessional teams can effectively create practice change, and improve patient outcomes by using the evidence to transform patient care delivery.

that are driving the need to increase the healthcare value provided to patients. Major future changes will include adjusting risk stratification, reducing unanticipated consequences of quality measurement and reporting, and enhancing quality measures that more reflect patient longitudinal care and patient outcomes over time.

SAFETY

The growth in the patient safety movement closely mirrors that of the QI movement. In 2000, the first IOM report made it glaringly obvious that healthcare systems were not equipped to keep patients safe " . . . as many as 98,000 people die in hospitals each year as a result of medical errors that could have been prevented . . . " (IOM, 2000). Although the U.S. healthcare system has made some progress in patient safety, patients still frequently experience preventable and unnecessary harm on a daily basis. This is likely because many healthcare systems continue to approach patient safety on a project-by-project basis, reacting to individual issues or events in a disjointed or isolated approach. The future of patient safety, however, will depend on the ability of healthcare systems to adopt a framework of a high reliability organization, discussed in Chapter 4, to improve patient care reliability across the healthcare system. Figure 16.1 is adapted from a discussion of high reliability by The Joint Commission (TJC, 2017a). High reliability in healthcare consists of a healthcare system with a culture of safety, a just culture, a learning culture, a reporting culture, leadership engagement, commitment to zero harm, and robust process improvement.

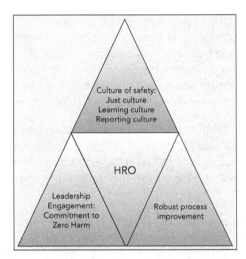

FIGURE 16.1 The Joint Commission depiction of high reliability.

Source: Adapted from The Joint Commission (2017). Retrieved from https://www.jointcommission.org/assets/1/6/Chassin_and_Loeb_0913_final.pdf

- A culture of safety is a fundamental element of building a healthcare system that can safely and reliably deliver care to all patients across the spectrum of their care. There are several components to a culture of safety (see Chapter 12: Patient Safety).
- **A just culture**, where all healthcare team members will be treated equally and fairly for their actions, is based on the situation they are placed in and the behavioral choices they make in that situation. A just culture takes into account that all humans make mistakes, and that safe healthcare systems must be built around a just culture to ensure that no single human error can result in patient harm. It also recognizes that humans may drift into unsafe behavior unknowingly, and that leaders have to recognize and coach them back into safe behaviors. Finally, a just culture recognizes that while recklessly unsafe behavior is rare, there must be swift disciplinary action for members of the interprofessional team that exhibit unsafe behavior, even if patient harm does not result because of unsafe behavior. The interprofessional team and hospital leadership have a vital role in upholding the tenets of a just culture, ensuring that they treat each other's behaviors within the framework of a just culture, including consoling other members of the interprofessional team for making a mistake, and helping understand how the mistake happened to prevent it from happening again.
- A **learning culture,** where all team members recognize that they have a duty to continuously learn and change, for the betterment of themselves, their patients, and the healthcare system in which they work. In a learning culture, team members are not resistant to change; instead, they are willing and eager to continuously improve the healthcare system in which they work. As the largest segment of the healthcare workforce, nurses can have a huge impact on identifying and improving healthcare system deficiencies that increase the risk of patient harm.
- A **reporting culture**, where all care team members know how to report and feel comfortable reporting all harm, near misses, and unsafe conditions. This requires a reporting system that is easy to use and that results in positive change (not punitive action). In most healthcare systems, the majority of reporting occurs by nurses.
- Leadership engagement requires a belief system that harm is preventable and that the leadership will be perpetually dissatisfied with any patient harm. It is also a leadership responsibility to create and improve a culture of safety to achieve this.

- **Commitment to zero harm** means that the healthcare system has leaders that believe and commit to eliminating all patient harm, referred to as zero harm.
- The final element of a high reliability organization is having an easy, reproducible, flexible, and understandable mechanism for strong and robust process improvement. Examples of some tools used for this include Lean, Six Sigma, and change management further detailed in Table 16.5.

With this high reliability framework for a patient safety program in place, a healthcare system should then implement project-based improvements for specific high-risk components. These should include, but should not be limited to, the following high-risk areas that continue to cause patient harm across many healthcare systems in the United States:

- *Medication administration:* Develop a program that includes as many safe medication administration elements as feasible, such as identifying look-alike/sound-alike drugs, for example, prednisone and prednisolone; robust strong allergy alerts; medication ordering in an electronic order entry system; pharmacy order double checks; bar code scanning medication administration; and smart pump use for IV medications.
- *Patient fall prevention:* Develop a program that includes the core elements of identifying high-risk patients and implementing patient risk reduction factors, such as medication review, delirium prevention efforts, implementation of skid-proof footwear and bed-chair alarms, and evaluating and safely mobilizing patients at least daily.
- *Alarm fatigue reduction:* Develop a program that endeavors to measure and reduce the amount of noise caused by alarms, for example, bedside monitors or call bells; and mitigate or reduce the risk of alarms being ignored by team members.
- *Establishment of good patient handoffs:* Implement and conduct good patient hand-offs among interprofessional teams, between units and between shifts, preferably with the patient and family; use a structured handoff template that allows for questions to be answered by the receiver of the information.
- *Clear patient identification (ID):* Implement a patient ID program that ensures all patients have at least one reliable form of visible identification, usually an arm-band that is used by all team members to confirm the correct patient before any patient contact, for example, blood draws, procedures, medication administration.

TABLE 16.5 ROBUST PROCESS IMPROVEMENT TOOLS

PROCESS IMPROVEMENT TOOL	BASIC CONCEPTS
Lean	Systematic method for waste minimization; maximize customer value while minimizing waste, thus creating more value with fewer resources. For example, having computers on wheels to improve documentation near the patient.
Six Sigma	Set of techniques to improve work processes by reducing the probability of errors or defects. For example, reducing the rate of patient blood specimens being labeled with another patient's information, that is, mislabeled specimens.
Change management	Approach to transitioning work teams into seamlessly changing or reshaping their operations or processes. For example, using techniques to ease the transition and adoption of a new electronic health record.

Many of these high-risk areas are in The Joint Commission National Patient Safety Goals Program (NPSG) as well as in the Institute for Healthcare Improvement framework for safety and reliability (Institute for Healthcare Improvement, 2017; TJC, 2017b). Most of these high-risk areas come up in daily work for nurses and have a much greater impact on nursing workflow when compared to other healthcare disciplines. Therefore, nurses can have the greatest impact on ensuring these patient safety programs are functioning well.

The future of patient safety in healthcare needs to move from a project-by-project focus, to one that is built on a framework of high reliability. With this framework in place, a healthcare system can improve upon individual high-risk issues, such as medication administration, safety, falls, alarm fatigue, patient handoffs, and patient identification.

INFORMATICS

The scope of nursing informatics focuses on a data, information, knowledge, wisdom (DIKW) information management model that translates data to information, information to knowledge, and knowledge to wisdom (American Nurses Association [ANA], 2015; Figure 16.2). During the course of any nursing shift, large amounts of data are collected. Informatics provides tools to help process, manage, and analyze the data collected for improved patient information and subsequent development of knowledge and wisdom to improve patient care. The scope of nursing will continue to expand as further technology innovations are developed to enhance future healthcare delivery. Current demands for safer, cost-effective, quality care require evidence of best practices in the transformation from data to wisdom. Nurses need to be adept at using patient-centered IT tools to achieve this.

Data, Information, Knowledge, and Wisdom

DIKW are central to safe and effective healthcare delivery. In the DIKW information management model, each level increases in complexity and requires greater application of human intellect. EBP, decision support, and maturing electronic health records (EHRs) enable the evolution of this transformation.

Data can be collected in multiple ways, both manually and by way of automation. Table 16.6 describes how data can be used to make decisions in caring for patients. For example, discrete numbers (i.e., data) become information when organized as a patient's "vital signs." The nurse, using knowledge, interprets the patient's vital signs as normal or abnormal. If the nurse makes a decision to act on the patients vital sign results, the data have been transformed to wisdom. Examining the pattern of vital signs over time, across a variety of illnesses and conditions, and in response to patient care interventions can lead to new knowledge and wisdom that guide future patient care. Informatics provides tools to help process, manage, and analyze the data collected and this may guide the development of new treatment protocols for future patients. While knowledge focuses on what is known, wisdom focuses on the appropriate application of that knowledge and the development of a keen understanding of the consequences of selected actions. This truly is the cornerstone of how technology and informatics affect the current and future delivery of quality and safe patient care.

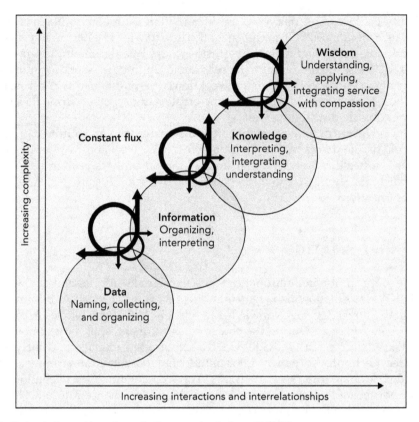

FIGURE 16.2 Data, information, knowledge, and wisdom (DIKW).

Source: American Nurses Association (ANA). (2015). *Nursing informatics: Scope and standards of practice* (2nd ed.). Silver Spring, MD: Author; Revised Nelson Data information Knowledge Wisdom (DIKW) Model Version 3, © 2013. Ramona Nelson, Ramona Nelson Consulting. All rights reserved. Reprinted with permission.

Future of Informatics

Effective interaction with and utilization of IT tools is the standard for nurses today. The move from paper-based healthcare documentation to computer-based records has catapulted the healthcare industry's capabilities to transform data into wisdom. The future of informatics will require that nurses are adept at navigating more advanced technologies and being responsive to more mature EHRs.

Given the paradigm shift from fee-for-service to value-based healthcare delivery, the reliance on accurate data to target coordinated care efforts to manage the overall health of populations is of paramount importance. **Accountable Care Organizations (ACOs)** are a group of care providers who assume risk in order to manage the full continuum of care and are accountable for overall costs and quality of care for a defined group of patients. In this digital era of healthcare, managing population health requires advanced nursing informatics skills. Digital health technologies that support population health include but are not limited to the following:

- **Telehealth**: Expands access to quality healthcare by remotely connecting patients with their care providers using telecommunications technology.
- **eHealth (electronic health):** Health services and information delivered through communication technologies to improve the quality of healthcare thus empowering patients to take an active role in their care management.

TABLE 16.6 LEVELS, DEFINITIONS, AND EXAMPLES OF THE DIKW MODEL

LEVEL	DEFINITION	EXAMPLES
Data	A collection of numbers, characters, or facts that are named, collected, and organized according to a perceived need for analysis; discrete entities that are described objectively without interpretation	98.6 68 120 60 20
Information	Data that have been interpreted, organized, or structured	98.6°F temperature, 68 pulse, 120/60 blood pressure, 20 respirations
Knowledge	Information that is synthesized so that relationships are identified and formalized based on a logical process of analysis and provides order to thoughts and ideas	The nurse's awareness that vital signs, such as those listed, are within normal limits for an adult
Wisdom	The use of data, information, and knowledge in making decisions and implementing appropriate interprofessional team actions	Abnormal vital signs for patients in certain situations that lead to a nursing intervention

Source: Developed with information from American Nurses Association (ANA). (2015). *Nursing informatics: Scope and standards of practice* (2nd ed.). Silver Spring, MD: Author.

- **mHealth (mobile health)**: The use of smartphones and tablets to collect data, provide health services, and educate patients about preventive healthcare. mHealth is part of eHealth.
- **Wearables**: Mobile electronic devices that can be worn by patients as part of clothing or as an accessory; collects biometric variables that communicate with a patient's EHR.

These examples of digital health technologies will continue to be a critical focus for nursing informatics and interprofessional caregivers as we aim to improve population health. Patients can use digital health to better manage their own health and wellness activities. This supports our increasingly consumer-driven healthcare industry. Implantable pacemakers, smart pillboxes, Bluetooth-enabled scales, and wearable fitness bands that integrate with EHRs are all examples of digital health solutions. According to the Food and Drug Administration (FDA), "Together these advancements are leading to a convergence of people, information, technology, and connectivity to improve health care and health outcomes" (FDA, 2017).

Predictive analytics (PA) at the point of care has also grown in importance for nursing informatics. **PA** uses technology and statistical methods to search through massive amounts of information, analyzing it to predict outcomes for individual patients (Winters-Miner, 2014). As data collection practices mature, so should nurses' abilities to detect poor outcomes before they actually occur. Early intervention healthcare practices using PA have improved with the advancement of EHRs. As nurses document throughout the day, algorithms can be enabled to detect changes in a patient's condition, alerting nurses that the patient is at risk for clinical deterioration, readmission, or sepsis.

There are many widely used example of PA tools used by nurses, all based on the notion that patient deterioration can be seen through changes in their physiological measurements and biometric variables. Often PA scores are calibrated based on patient populations, such as Early Warning Score (EWS), which are specifically developed in response to the needs of certain patients. For example, Pediatric Early Warning Score (PEWS), Modified Early Warning Score (MEWS), Children's Hospital Early Warning Score (CHEWS), and Modified Early Obstetric Warning Score (MEOWS), to name a few. More and more PA models are being developed and integrated into EHRs, resulting in higher quality care delivery and improved patient outcomes.

Communication and Information Management

Nursing informatics enables the professional nurse to truly coordinate patient care, leveraging communication technology to drive interprofessional care delivery. Now more than ever before, nurses are able to manage all information related to the nursing process and patient care delivery. Accurate documentation collection, evidence-based clinical pathways, and standardized workflows all lead to optimal coordination of care delivery. Communication is a major factor in healthcare delivery, which is replete with complexities and requires critical wisdom that is supported by informatics. Managing data for quality improvement, including enabling healthcare system capabilities to collect and report patient safety errors, is a critical component of informatics.

EHRs provide essential information to nurses at the point of patient care, providing advanced capabilities to integrate pertinent patient information into one patient record. In addition to advanced data collection, other functions of EHRs include electronic prescribing and medication refills, automatic pharmacy formulary checking, electronic lab and imaging ordering, interoffice clinical messaging, remote access to the patient chart, results trending, clinical alerts, patient education, and disease management.

Electronic Clinical Decision Support Tools

Nurses make decisions from their unique perspectives based on their education, experience, and specialty. Decision making, the process of choosing among alternatives, is guided by their critical thinking. **Electronic clinical decision support (CDS) tools or systems** provide nurses with knowledge and patient-specific information, intelligently filtered and presented at appropriate times. CDS encompasses a variety of tools that affect decision making in the clinical workflow, and include alerts, reminders, recommended guidelines or order sets, and relevant reference information. These CDS tools are particularly effective in increasing quality of care and enhanced patient outcomes, avoiding errors and adverse events, and improving efficiencies. CDS tools continue to mature, factoring in more and more patient-specific data, and advancing logic that presents helpful information to nurses at the point of care. Information must be filtered, organized, and presented in a way that supports the current workflow, allowing the user to make an informed decision quickly and take action. Different types of CDS may be ideal for different processes of care in different settings, and provide platforms for integrating evidence-based knowledge into safe care delivery.

Benefits and Limitations of Informatics

The driving forces for the rapid development of the EHR are patient safety and the need to restructure the healthcare delivery system to improve the quality of care delivery while containing increasing costs. The power of EHRs is their ability to collect, present, and communicate patient data, resulting in time and financial savings for those who participate in the patient's care. The development of data exchange standards that ensure uniform data capture and encoding so that the same patient data are collected from all EHRs allows the ability to analyze data from multiple patients over time, referred to as longitudinal analysis. An example of a data exchange standard for patient care includes the following: (a) what is collected (e.g., document patient weight on all patients on admission); (b) how it is presented (e.g., always document weight in pounds or kilograms); and (c) how it is encoded (e.g., a patient weight of 210 pounds may be encoded or converted to "210%20pounds"). Overarching benefits of the EHR include but are not limited to the following:

- Improved data integrity (e.g., readability, discrete data entry standardizes input)
- Increased productivity (e.g., ability to share patient information between and among the interprofessional team)
- Improved quality of care (e.g., electronic alerts to documented food, drug allergies)

While the standardized utilization of integrated EHRs has promised many benefits including higher quality care delivery and decreased healthcare costs, there have been serious unintended consequences from the implementation of these EHR systems. Suboptimal EHR system design and improper use can cause EHR-related errors that not only jeopardize data integrity, but also can lead to poor patient safety outcomes. For example, if an RN fails to document that a pain medication was given to a particular patient, another nurse may give a duplicate dose of pain medication to the same patient. Such unintended consequences might also incur financial penalties, result in significant legal problems, and/or cause irrevocable damage to patients.

Large scale use of data, information, knowledge, and wisdom relies on accessibility. Historically, patient data and information were handwritten in an unstructured format on paper and placed in various versions of a patient record. Naturally, this made it more difficult to compare data sets like vital signs, interpret and synthesize them, and utilize the data to make appropriate clinical decisions. Nurses must be active participants in the design of automated EHR systems to ensure that the information is recorded easily and accurately and in a format that is easily accessible to all healthcare providers. Current, accurate information is the key to safe, high-quality, patient-centered care.

Successful implementation of EHRs require thoughtful and intuitive design that supports standardized nursing workflows. Often, the pace at which EHRs have been implemented has not allowed time for their optimal design, thus challenging nurses at the bedside. Table 16.7 is a list of common indicators of a successful EHR implementation.

Education and Roles

Nurses are expected to use clinical information systems in order to carry out their daily patient care responsibilities. In order to do so effectively, nursing informatics competencies are increasingly being incorporated into standard interprofessional team education requirements. Informatics competencies are deemed essential as a means to facilitate the delivery of safer, more efficient care, to add to the knowledge

TABLE 16.7 COMMON INDICATORS OF A SUCCESSFUL ELECTRONIC HEALTH RECORD (EHR) IMPLEMENTATION

INDICATOR	EXAMPLE
Fast documentation	Allows user to quickly enter and retrieve data
Familiar	Follows familiar graphical user interface (GUI) conventions that provide visual ways for people to interact with computers using icons, menus, and windows
Flexible documentation style	Allows personalization of documentation style, enabling the EHR to meet the information needs of many types and categories of users
Workflow enhancement	Improves work efficiency and effectiveness
Documentation improvement	Improves the process of documentation
Regulatory requirements	Supports regulatory requirements related to data content and information security measures

base for the interprofessional team and transition toward EBP. There is also an increasing presence of formalized informatics roles across the healthcare industry, as these roles are seen as valuable contributors to how organizations achieve positive patient outcomes.

Nursing Informatics Competencies

The Healthcare Information and Management Systems Society (HIMSS) conceived an important informatics initiative known as TIGER (Technology Informatics Guiding Education Reform). TIGER addresses informatics education reform across the interprofessional community, focusing on leadership development, usability and clinical application design, education and faculty development, competencies, national IT agenda, and interoperability. The objective of the TIGER initiative was to maximize the integration of technology and informatics into seamless healthcare practices, education, and research resource development. Ultimately, the TIGER group created a vision for the future of nursing to provide safer, higher quality patient care through informatics. Informatics competencies will vary based on nurse tenure (beginner or more experienced) as well as becoming nurse specialists in informatics (Table 16.8).

As we continue to see more mature healthcare technologies evolve and more examples of digital health emerge, nursing informatics competencies will need to expand to meet these advancements.

Nursing Informatics Roles

Nurses who dedicate their careers to informatics are often called informatics nurses (INs) or informatics nurse specialists (INSs). These individuals are experts in utilizing the nursing process using critical thinking skills to analyze and support the utilization of technology by nurses. INs understand patient care delivery workflow and integration touchpoints, seizing opportunities for automation and for decreasing the patient care documentation task burden. Often, INs are board certified in Nursing Informatics by the American Nurses Credentialing Center (ANCC).

TABLE 16.8 NURSING INFORMATICS COMPETENCIES

BEGINNING NURSE COMPETENCIES	EXPERIENCED NURSE COMPETENCIES
• Has basic computer skills • Uses computer applications • Uses sources of data • Uses technology for care delivery, communication, and decision support • Respects and protects patients' rights to privacy and confidentiality of information	• Understands the value of data and information • Uses technology to trend and aggregate individual and population-based patient information for decision support and communication • Evaluates quality of information sources • Advocates for technology solutions that improve care delivery
INFORMATICS NURSE COMPETENCIES	**INFORMATICS NURSE SPECIALIST COMPETENCIES**
• Uses advanced computer systems and tools to manage, evaluate, integrate, and communicate data, information, knowledge, and wisdom • Assesses current capabilities and limitations of technology and their impact on users and organizations • Actively seeks to improve the data, information, knowledge, and wisdom available for clinical decision making	• Conducts research related to nursing informatics • Influences top-level decisions and policy design that impact clinical information management • Builds theoretical models of nursing informatics • Evaluates system level informatics initiatives, such as workflow improvement projects or standardized electronic health record bundles to reduce practice variability and improve patient outcomes

Sources: Developed from Technology Informatics Guiding Education Reform (TIGER). (2009). Informatics competencies for every practicing nurse: Recommendations from the TIGER collaborative. Retrieved from http://www.himss.org/collaborating-integrate-evidence-and-informatics-nursing-practice-and-education-executive-summary; American Nurses Association (ANA). (2015). Nursing informatics: Scope and standards of practice (2nd ed.). Silver Spring, MD: Author.

Leaders in nursing informatics, often identified as Chief Nursing Information Officers, Chief Nursing Informatics Officers, or Directors of Nursing Informatics, offer strategic and operational nursing leadership in the development, deployment, reengineering, optimization, and integration of EHRs to support interprofessional patient care. These leaders facilitate the utilization of information systems and evidence-based content, consistent with the goals and objectives of organizations' clinical and strategic initiatives. Ultimately, they lead technology-enabled process change that maximizes patient safety, quality of care, and operational efficiency.

Considerations for the Future

In today's increasingly digital and networked society, the volume of data captured electronically continues to grow. Digital health innovations, while critically important to support population health initiatives, raise grave concerns about information security. Wearables, for example, fitness trackers, smart watches, portable heart rate monitors, and so forth, collect tremendous amounts of data that can be collected and analyzed in a variety of ways. Concerns surrounding privacy, compliance, and security have skyrocketed, as wearables are prone to cybersecurity attacks. As national laws advocating for the protection of health information become more stringent, nurses must ensure the ethical use of data, and must prioritize data integrity, security, and confidentiality of protected information.

NURSE LEADER AND MANAGER

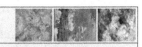

Susie Walking Bear Yellowtail, RN, was instrumental in modernizing the Indian Health Service and eliminating abuses in care, for example, forced sterilization of Native American women. She went on to serve on the Council on Indian Health, Education and Welfare and the Federal Indian Health Advisory Committee. She founded the first professional association of Native American nurses and in 2002, was inducted into the American Nurses Association Hall of Fame. Read more about her at www.nursingworld.org.

Social media also poses significant information security considerations. Like digital health solutions, social media provides a consumer-driven outlet to collect, analyze, and share healthcare data, allowing patients to benefit from self-management tools. Social media applications open the door for privacy concerns, as new information about health is transmitted often in an insecure manner. While the increased availability of data and information can be beneficial for both the patient and the interprofessional healthcare team, the abuse of data must be eliminated and the privacy of information must be preserved.

FUTURE TRANSFORMATIONAL LEADERSHIP ROLE OF THE NURSE

Porter-O'Grady and Malloch (2011) identify tomorrow's transformational nursing leaders as those who "create a new and improved system that allows individuals to contribute to their fullest potential to deliver the most effective health care possible" (p. 375). Transformational nursing leaders in the future will facilitate the development of highly reliable organizations. They will further develop skills of improved communication, rapport, dialogue, conflict resolution, and consensus building to positively change the patient care delivery process of the future and ensure that all six Quality and Safety Education for Nurses (QSEN) elements of quality and safety—quality improvement, safety, informatics, patient-centered care, teamwork and collaboration, and EBP (QSEN, 2012)—are delivered (Table 16.9).

Healthcare leaders in the future are nurses, administrators, physicians, pharmacists, dieticians, respiratory therapists, rehabilitation specialists, and other healthcare professionals. All have a personal responsibility to work together as a team to ensure the quality and safety of patient care. The sheer number of nurses in the workforce, the amount of time spent with each patient, and the proximity of nurses in the delivery of patient care across the healthcare continuum positions nurses to use firsthand knowledge and experience gained from observing actual or potential errors and unsafe conditions at the unit or department level to improve patient safety. However, knowledge and experience alone will not provide the greatest improvement in patient safety. It is only by changing patient care work processes and monitoring outcomes of patient care that nurses and other members of the healthcare team will impact today's complex healthcare environment. Nurses at all levels of an organization must be actively involved, not only in providing and monitoring the daily delivery of patient care, but also in sharing information to set up an environment for high-quality care delivery and preventing errors from occurring in and

TABLE 16.9 FUTURE TRANSFORMATIONAL NURSING LEADERSHIP ROLE IN SUPPORTING QSEN QUALITY AND SAFETY ELEMENTS

QSEN QUALITY AND SAFETY ELEMENT	FUTURE TRANSFORMATIONAL LEADERSHIP ROLE
Quality improvement	• Monitor clinical, patient satisfaction, financial, and other outcomes to improve quality • Review healthcare rating systems. Strive to be number 1! • Benchmark with other high-performing healthcare organizations to improve patient care • Transfer knowledge and best practices from patient care departments that have shown positive health outcomes for patients and families to other patient care departments
Safety	• Structure the design of healthcare work space to reduce error • Create and sustain healthcare processes to develop a culture of safety • Build flexibility into staffing models to ensure that appropriate care providers are on hand to respond quickly to both scheduled and unscheduled events • Accept that errors do occur and shift from a culture of blame to a just culture in which error is perceived as an opportunity for improvement by both individuals and by the total healthcare system • Monitor patient and staff outcomes
Patient-centered care	• Develop a policy to enhance transparency (e.g., in both clinical practice and patient care outcomes) in patient care delivery • Develop more opportunities to involve patients in their care, that is, more education programs, patient satisfaction surveys, bedside hand-offs/rounds, mutual goal setting, and so on • Reframe the work of healthcare to enhance partnerships among patients, families, and providers • Teach and encourage all staff and patients to manage their own health effectively • Monitor patient outcomes for satisfaction, safety, respect, access, clinical outcomes, and so on
Evidence-based practice (EBP)	• Support EBP • Adopt evidence-based management and leadership practices • Review EBP guidelines from professional organizations
Teamwork and collaboration	• Develop rapport with all team members and maximize the capability of the interprofessional team • Adopt TeamSTEPPS and/or SBAR practices to build interprofessional teamwork • Utilize safe patient handoff communication • Build opportunities for teams to interact and develop rapport into organization design and interprofessional meetings • Incorporate high-quality expectations into job descriptions and peer and annual evaluations • Develop reward and recognition systems for high-quality care

(continued)

TABLE 16.9 FUTURE TRANSFORMATIONAL NURSING LEADERSHIP ROLE IN SUPPORTING QSEN QUALITY AND SAFETY ELEMENTS *(continued)*

QSEN QUALITY AND SAFETY ELEMENT	FUTURE TRANSFORMATIONAL LEADERSHIP ROLE
Informatics	• Create an environment for informatics and EBP that includes increased access to computers, librarians, continuing education programs, quality improvement and safety information, and so on • Utilize EHRs and other computer tools to improve documentation, monitor patient outcomes, and improve clinical decision making

Sources: Developed with information from Institute of Medicine (IOM). (2004). *Keeping patients safe: Transforming the work environment of nurses.* Washington, DC: National Academies Press; Porter-O'Grady, T., & Malloch, K. (2011). *Quantum leadership: Advancing innovation, transforming health care* (3rd ed.). Sudbury, MA: Jones & Bartlett Learning; Quality and Safety Education for Nurses (QSEN). (2012). Retrieved from http://www.qsen.org.

beyond their home unit or department. This information can be shared at the local, state, and national level. Errors that happen in one clinical unit along with the steps implemented to reduce future occurrences may be useful information to share with other units in a hospital or clinic. Failure to share best practices and lessons learned across all clinical care areas may reduce the possibility of catching or preventing a repeat error. This results in patient harm that could have been prevented.

THE VOICE OF THE NURSE

The voice of the nurse is critically important in current healthcare practice to inform healthcare changes that will prevent errors in the future (Aiken, 2012). The voice of the nurse, heard when nurses participate in patient care, hospital committees, and other hospital decision-making bodies, as well as when nurses monitor and improve care based on data about patients and their outcomes, will guide future patient care. A key component of the Magnet® journey is structural empowerment. Structural empowerment describes hospital environments that include structures and processes for shared governance and decision making by RNs. In a study of nurses working in hospitals recently designated Magnet®, nurses describe "voice" as a key thematic change: " . . . the nurses felt very empowered . . . that was one of the things that changed the most, that the decision making happened at the lowest level possible and the people doing the work have a say in how they were doing the work" (Urden, Ecoff, Bacliq & Gerber, 2013, p. 406). In the future, nurses leading patient care conferences, actively participating as members of the interprofessional patient care rounds, leading meetings, reviewing and presenting EBP findings to hospital system committees will improve patient care and nurse engagement. In addition, accurate assessment of patients by nurses and other healthcare providers along with accurate and timely data entry into EMRs will help build wisdom and the evidence of what works to improve patient care delivery and patient outcomes. Ensuring that nursing assessment and patient data are documented timely and accurately are foundational steps in developing information, knowledge, and wisdom to inform future clinical decision making as technology continues to advance in hospitals and clinics. The IOM has set a goal that by 2020, 90% of clinical decisions will be supported by accurate, timely, up-to-date information and will reflect the best available evidence (IOM, 2011a).

CONCLUSION

There has never been a more exciting and transitional time in healthcare than now. In a series of white papers, the National Academy of Medicine reminds all healthcare providers of the challenges ahead: (a) persistent inequities in health; (b) rapidly aging population; (c) new and emerging health threats; (d) persisting care fragmentation and discontinuity; and (e) constrained innovation due to outmoded approaches (Dzau et al., 2017). Yet nurses and the interprofessional team, by actively participating in all settings in every organization to improve quality, enhance safety, provide patient-centered care, use the best available evidence, work through excellent teamwork and collaboration, and utilize informatics, will facilitate change. By facilitating change, nurses and the interprofessional team will also use lessons learned in the process to enhance future improvements in healthcare delivery. By experiencing these changes firsthand, nurses will advocate for better healthcare, not only within their organizations and health systems but also by sharing best practices and advocating for policy change at the local, state, and federal level. The future is developing as we speak! Seize the moment!

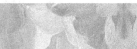

KEY CONCEPTS

- Patient-centered care can improve outcomes by engaging patients in decisions that impact their health. Nurses and the interprofessional team can engage patients in decision making regarding choices about interventions and treatments and/or by mutually setting outcome goals.
- Nursing and the interprofessional team, supported by a culture of safety where all are encouraged to learn from mistakes, are in a good position to facilitate the journey toward a future healthcare system.
- The nurse is a full member of the interprofessional team in the delivery of high-quality and safe patient care now and in future patient-centered care initiatives.
- Consistent use of teamwork tools, for example, Read back, Huddle, Debrief, and SBAR, can enhance team outcomes and improve patient safety.
- Evidence-based practice (EBP), which is the key to improving care in all settings, must be fully supported by nursing, the interprofessional team, and hospital leadership to enhance its effectiveness in transforming patient care.
- There are multiple national initiatives geared toward improving future patient safety, patient-centered care, EBP, teamwork and collaboration, informatics, and quality improvement.
- The healthcare system in the United States is transforming from one based on quantity and volume of care provided to a healthcare system based on value (i.e., low cost, high quality, and best patient experience).
- High reliability organizations improve the delivery of patient care by establishing a system of a culture of safety, a just culture, a learning culture, a reporting culture, leadership engagement, commitment to zero harm, and robust process improvement.
- Data, information, knowledge, and wisdom are central to safe and effective healthcare delivery. By collecting data through electronic health records and other devices, analyzing information across patient populations, and transforming that information into knowledge and wisdom to enhance our ability to predict care outcomes, we can design more effective interventions to improve quality and safety outcomes for patients.

- Transformational leadership helps promote quality and safety in healthcare delivery systems.
- The voice of the nurse can inform healthcare changes that will prevent errors in the future.

KEY TERMS

Accountable Care Organizations
   (ACOs)
Big data
Commitment to zero harm
Data
Debriefing
eHealth (electronic health)
Electronic clinical decision support
   (CDS) tools or systems
Healthcare value
Huddle
Information
Just culture
Knowledge
Learning culture

mHealth (mobile health)
P4 Medicine
Patient-centered medical homes
Patient- and family-centered care
Population health
Precision medicine
Predictive analytics (PA)
Read back
Reporting culture
SBAR
TeamSTEPPS
Telehealth
Wearables
Wisdom

REVIEW QUESTIONS

1. Transformational leadership is an essential component to drive positive change in future healthcare delivery. Select the best example of the use of transformational leadership to support safety.

   A. Discuss patient safety issues at staff meetings.
   B. Accept that errors do occur and shift from a culture of blame to a just culture in which error is perceived as an opportunity for improvement.
   C. Notify all staff members when a safety event occurs.
   D. Let the nurse manager know when you witness any staff member providing unsafe patient care.

2. In healthcare settings that are creating new models of patient-centered care delivery, who should be the ultimate decision maker regarding the care of the patient?

   A. The patient
   B. The RN
   C. The physician
   D. The patient's attorney

3. RNs should take an active role in the development and implementation of evidence-based clinical practice guidelines. What are the best resources that the nurse can use to ensure future care is based on the best available evidence? Select all that apply.

   A. Unit-based staff meeting minutes
   B. The Internet

    C. Professional nursing organizations; for example, Oncology Nursing Society, American Academy of Ambulatory Care Nursing.

    D. Members of the interprofessional team

    E. Literature searches

4. Healthcare organizations around the country are investing in electronic health records (EHRs). Which of the following are the common ways that an EHR promotes safe patient care? Select all that apply.

    A. It allows users to quickly enter and retrieve data.

    B. It improves work efficiency and effectiveness.

    C. It always notifies management when a nurse forgets to document patient care.

    D. It supports regulatory requirements related to information security.

    E. EHRs prevent spelling errors in documentation.

5. If patient data are recorded in an EHR and stored in a clinical data repository, the data can later be analyzed to improve information about quality and safety of care for other patients in the future. Select the best term that describes the electronic aggregation of accurate, relevant, and timely clinical data.

    A. Root cause analysis

    B. Data, information, knowledge, and wisdom

    C. Evidence-based practice

    D. Quality improvement

6. Preventing hospital readmissions is a healthcare reform opportunity for future nurses. How can nurses best prevent unnecessary hospital readmissions?

    A. Screen patients "at risk" for readmission, for example, older patients, patients with a higher number of medications, and so on, and work with case managers and social workers on the discharge plan of care.

    B. Document that the patient states understanding of any discharge teaching.

    C. Provide medication information handouts to the patient's family members.

    D. Give the patient/family the nursing unit phone number so that the patient can call with any questions after discharge.

7. Acknowledging that all humans make mistakes, a just culture environment ensures that all patient care team members are treated equally and fairly for their actions. What statement is not illustrative of a just culture environment?

    A. Supporting the nurse for an error the nurse did not intend to make.

    B. Discussing and blaming interprofessional team member's mistakes in a staff meeting.

    C. Reporting unsafe practices using private confidential intranet online systems.

    D. Holding oneself accountable for personal clinical practice.

8. Mary, a new nurse, has been asked to participate on an interprofessional workgroup to reduce central line-associated bloodstream infections (CLABSI). To best prepare and contribute to the team's work, she prioritizes the following activities. Which activity will Mary do first?

    A. Review current data on CLABSI on her unit and the other hospital units.

    B. Compare her own practice with the current policy and procedure for caring for central lines.

C. With the help of a hospital librarian, conduct a literature review on best practices for preventing CLABSI

D. Refuse to participate in the workgroup as she believes she is too new to participate.

9. Reimbursement models for healthcare are changing in the United States. Which are examples of programs intended to enhance value in healthcare? Select all that apply.

   A. Fee-for-service payments
   B. Hospital-acquired condition penalties
   C. Readmission reduction program
   D. Clinical decision support
   E. Value-based purchasing program

10. A culture of safety is a foundational element of building healthcare systems that deliver safe and reliable patient care. Which of the following is not an example of a culture of safety?

   A. A reporting culture
   B. A just culture
   C. A learning culture
   D. An accountability culture

REVIEW ACTIVITIES

1. Learn about incivility in clinical practice and recommendations by front line nurses in practice to positively impact the work environment at www.qsen.org/faculty-resources/incivility/.
2. Explore this website and learn how interprofessional teamwork can impact patients with chronic conditions: www.hhs.gov/ash/about-ash/multiple-chronic-conditions/education-and-training/curriculum/module-4-interprofessional-collaboration/index.html.
3. A key tenet in patient-centered care is actively involving patients in decision making, particularly engaging their willingness to take independent actions to manage their health and illness. What can nurses do to increase patient involvement in their healthcare?
4. Nurses document the care they provide for patients. Documentation describes what was done for the patient. How can patient data in an electronic medical record improve care and contribute to information, knowledge, and wisdom for other patients in the future?
5. Interprofessional team communication improves patient outcomes. What tools/best practices are available to team members to improve their collaborative communication?
6. You recently found evidence in the literature that a current practice in your clinical area could be improved. What are your next steps in using the evidence-based findings to improve healthcare delivery on your unit or within your nursing department?
7. Access to evidence-based resources is important to improve patient care. Describe resources available to you to improve your nursing practice.

CRITICAL DISCUSSION POINTS

1. During your last clinical experience, what quality improvement initiatives were underway on your nursing unit or within the department of nursing?
2. What evidence-based practice resources are available to nurses within the nursing unit or department of nursing where you have your clinical rotation?
3. Have quality outcomes improved for patients and families in your clinical site? If so, how?
4. What information from the electronic health record helps you safely care for patients in your clinical site?
5. Does your healthcare system employ a just culture system of care? How do the nurses feel about the culture of safety within their work environment?
6. How are nurses involved in decision making in a healthcare system that you are familiar with?
7. How are patients included in daily interprofessional rounds at your clinical site? What is the role of the nurse during these rounds?
8. If a nurse has an idea that will improve the quality and safety of patient care delivery, where would the nurse take that idea in a healthcare system that you are familiar with?

QSEN ACTIVITIES

1. Go to the QSEN website (www.qsen.org) and search for the teaching strategy, Using Evidence to Address Clinical Problems (www.qsen.org/USING-EVIDENCE-TOADDRESS-CLINICAL-PROBLEMS/). Follow the directions on the teaching strategy page to help students identify how to use evidence during clinical rotations.
2. Locate "Nurse as the leader of the team huddle. An unfolding oncology case study" on the QSEN website (www.qsen.org/nurse-as-the-leader-of-the-team-huddle-anunfolding-oncology-case-study/). Focus on the identification of evidence-based interventions for the patient in the case study as well as the patient's preferences. PowerPoint and YouTube videos accompany the unfolding case study.

EXPLORING THE WEB

1. Explore the Agency for Healthcare Research and Quality website at www.ahrq.gov/chsp/index.html. See how research on health systems is advancing new knowledge to improve quality and safety outcomes for patients.
2. Consider taking quality improvement courses through the Institute for Healthcare Improvement (IHI Open School) at www.ihi.org/education/ihiopenschool/Pages/default.aspx.
3. Gain familiarity with the Leapfrog Group. Consider how you and/or your patients and families compare healthcare systems when choosing where they will seek healthcare in the future (www.leapfroggroup.org/).

REFERENCES

Agency for Healthcare Research and Quality (AHRQ). (2017). *TeamSTEPPS*. Retrieved from https://www.ahrq.gov/teamstepps/index.html
Aiken, L. (2012). Improving health care outcomes through research (part one). *Reflections on Nursing Leadership, 38*(1), 5.

American Journal of Nursing (AJN). (2017). The top nursing stories of 2016. *American Journal of Nursing, 117*(1), 15.

American Nurses Association (2015). *Nursing: Scope and Standards of Practice* (3rd ed.). Silver Spring, MD: Author.

Berwick, D. M. (2013). On transitioning to value-based health care. *Health Care Financial Management, 67*(5), 56–59.

Berwick, D. M. (2017). Vital directions and national will. JAMA, 317(14), 1420–1421. doi:10.1001/jama.2017.2962

Centers for Medicare and Medicaid Services (CMS). (2017). *Hospital-acquired condition (hac) reduction program.* Retrieved from https://www.cms.gov/Medicare/Quality-Initiatives-Patient-Assessment-Instruments/Value-Based-Programs/HAC/Hospital-Acquired-Conditions.html

Doyle, C., Lennox, L., & Bell, D. (2013). A systematic review of evidence on the links between patient experience and clinical safety and effectiveness. *BMJ Open, 3*(1), 1–18. doi:10.1136/bmjopen-2012-001570

Dzau, V. J., McClellan, M., Burke, S., Coye, M. J., Daschle, T. A., & Diaz, A. (2017). Vital directions for health and health care. *National Academy of Medicine.* Retrieved from https://nam.edu/wp-content/uploads/2017/03/Vital-Directions-for-Health-Health-Care-Priorities-from-a-National-Academy-of-Medicine-Initiative.pdf

Fowler, M. D. (2015). *Guide to nursing's social policy statement.* Silver Spring, MD: American Nurses Association.

Hibbard, J. H., & Greene, J. (2013). What the evidence shows about patient activation: Better health outcomes and care experiences; few data on costs. *Health Affairs, 32*(2), 207–214.doi: 10.1377/hlthaff.2012.1061

Hood, L., Balling, R., & Auffray, C. (2012). Revolutionizing medicine in the 21st century through systems approaches. *Biotechnology Journal, 7*(8), 992–1001. doi:10.1002/biot.201100306

Institute for Healthcare Improvement (IHI). (2017). *IHI framework.* Retrieved from http://www.ihi.org/resources/Pages/IHIWhitePapers/Framework-Safe-Reliable-Effective-Care.aspx?utm_campaign=Database+Re-engagement&utm_source=hs_automation&utm_medium=email&utm_content=42606587&_hsenc=p2ANqtz-_FFUq4X7Or9tz8a9b-35A6_5ygL6fEObk6ukdL9QmcMTjZVYiWfvi7w8dkBTGoPLd89OZNfGuiTpSOqPs71R_YM3N70Jw&_hsmi=42606587

Institute of Medicine (IOM). (2000). *To err is human.* Washington, DC: National Academies Press.

Institute of Medicine (IOM). (2001). *Crossing the quality chasm.* Washington, DC: National Academies Press.

Institute of Medicine (IOM). (2004). *Keeping patients safe: Transforming the work environment of nurses.* Washington, DC: National Academies Press.

Institute of Medicine (IOM). (2011a). *The learning health system and its innovation collaborative.* Washington, DC: National Academies Press.

Institute of Medicine (IOM). (2011c). *The future of nursing: Leading change, advancing health.* Washington, DC: National Academies Press.

Institute for Patient- and Family-Centered Care (IPFCC). (2017). *Defined.* Retrieved from http://www.ipfcc.org/about/pfcc.html

Lu, Y. F., Goldstein, D. B., Angrist, M., & Cavalleri, G. (2014). Personalized medicine and human genetic diversity. *Cold Spring Harbor Perspectives in Medicine, 4*(9), a008581–a008581. PMC 4143101. doi:10.1101/CSHPERSPECT.A008581

Medicare.gov. (2017). Hospital Compare. Retrieved from https://www.medicare.gov

Melnyk, B., Fineout-Overholt, E., Gallagher-Ford, L., & Kaplan, L. (2012). The state of evidence based practice in US Nurses: Critical implications for nurse leaders and educators. *The Journal of Nursing Administration (JONA), 42*(9), 410–417. doi:10.1097/NNA.0b013e3182664e0a

Melnyk, B., Gallagher-Ford, L., Thomas, B. K., Troseth, M., Wyngarden, K., & Szalacha, L. (2016). A study of chief nurse executives indicates low prioritization of evidence-based practice and shortcomings in hospital performance metrics across the United States. *Worldviews on Evidence-Based Nursing, 13*(1), 6–14. doi: 10.1111/wvn.12133

National Council State Boards of Nursing (NCSBN). (2017). *Active RN licenses.* Retrieved from https://www.ncsbn.org/6161.htm

Picker Institute. (2013). *Patient-centered care: The road ahead*. Retrieved from http://www.ipfcc. org/resources/Patient-Centered%20Care%20The%20Road%20Ahead.pdf

P4 Medicine Institute. (2012). *P4Medicine*. Retrieved from http://p4mi.org/p4medicine

Porter-O'Grady, T., & Malloch, K. (2011). *Quantum leadership: Advancing innovation, transforming health care* (3rd ed.). Sudbury, MA: Jones & Bartlett Learning.

Quality and Safety Education for Nurses (QSEN). (2012). Retrieved from http://www.qsen.org

Rayo, M. F., Mansfield, J., Eiferman, D., Mignery, T., White, S., & Moffatt-Bruce, S. D. (2016). Implementing an institution-wide quality improvement policy to ensure appropriate use of continuous cardiac monitoring: A mixed-methods retrospective data analysis and direct observation study. *British Medical Journal, 25*, 796–802. doi:10.1136/bmjqs-2015-004137

Technology Infomratics Guiding Education Reform (TIGER). (2009). *Informatics competencies for every practicing nurse: Recommendations from the TIGER collaborative*. Retrieved from http://www.himss.org/collaborating-integrate-evidence-and-informatics-nursing-practice-and-education-executive-summary

The Economist. (2010). *Data, data everywhere*. Retrieved from http://www.economist.com/node/15557443#

The Joint Commission (TJC). (2017a). *High-reliability health care: Getting there*. Retrieved from https://www.jointcommission.org/assets/1/6/Chassin_and_Loeb_0913_final.pdf

The Joint Commission (TJC). (2017b). *Hospital: 2018 national patient safety goals*. Retrieved from https://www.jointcommission.org/hap_2017_npsgs/

The Leapfrog Group. (2017). Compare Hospitals. Retrieved from www.leapfroggroup.org.

The Times 100. (1995–2013). *Business case studies, marketing mix (price, place, promotion, product)*. Retrieved from http://businesscasestudies.co.uk/business-theory/marketing/marketing-mix-price-place-promotion-product.html#axzz2ZqHdqGJg

Urden, L.D., Ecoff, L.K., Bacliq, J. & Gerber, C.S. (2013). Staff nurse perceptions of the Magnet® journey. *Journal of Nursing Administration, 43*(7/8), 403–408. doi:10.1097/NNA.0b013d31829d61aa

U.S. Food and Drug Administration. (2017). *Digital health*. Retrieved from https://www.fda.gov/medicaldevices/digitalhealth/

Winters-Miner, L. (2014). Seven ways predictive analytics can improve healthcare. Retrieved from https://www.elsevier.com/connect/seven-ways-predictive-analytics-can-improve-healthcare

SUGGESTED READINGS

Berwick, D. M. (2017). Vital directions and national will. *JAMA, 317*(14), 1420–1421. doi:10.1001/jama.2017.2962

Bittner, N. P., Gravlin, G., Hansten, R., & Kalisch, B. J. (2011). Unraveling care omissions. *Journal of Nursing Administration, 41*(12), 510–512. doi:10.1097/NNA.0b013e3182378b65

Clancy, C., & Berwick, D. (2011). The science of safety improvement: Learning while doing. *Annals of Internal Medicine, 154*(10), 699–701. doi:10.1059/0003-4819-154-10-201105170-00013

Donabedian, A. (1966). Evaluating the quality of medical care. *Milbank Memorial Fund Quarterly, 44*, 166–206. doi: 10.1111/j.1468-0009.2005.00397.x

Kelly, L., McHugh, M., & Aiken, L. (2011). Nurse outcomes in Magnet® and non-magnet hospitals. *The Journal of Nursing Administration (JONA), 41*(10), 428–433. doi:10.1097/NNA.0b013e31822eddbc

Kendall-Gallagher, D., Aiken, L., Sloane, D., & Cimiotti, J. (2011). Nurse specialty certification, inpatient mortality, and failure to rescue. *Journal of Nursing Scholarship: An Official Publication of Sigma Theta Tau International Honor Society of Nursing/Sigma Theta Tau, 43*(2), 188–194. doi:10.1111/j.1547–5069.2011.01391.x

Kendall-Gallagher, D., & Blegen, M. (2010). Competence and certification of registered nurses and safety of patients in intensive care units. *The Journal of Nursing Administration (JONA), 40*(Suppl. 10), S68–S77. doi:10.1097/NNA.0b013e3181f37edb

McHugh, M., & Lake, E. (2010). Understanding clinical expertise: Nurse education, experience, and the hospital context. *Research in Nursing & Health, 33*(4), 276–287. doi:10.1002/nur.20388

Needleman, J., Buerhaus, P., Pankratz, V., Leibson, C., Stevens, S., & Harris, M. (2011). Nurse staffing and inpatient hospital mortality. *New England Journal of Medicine, 364*(11), 1037–1045. doi:10.1056/NEJMsa1001025

O'Neill, S., Jones, T., Bennett, D., & Lewis, M. (2011). Nursing works, the application of lean thinking to nursing processes. *Journal of Nursing Administration, 41*(12), 546–552. doi:10.1097/NNA.0b013e3182378d37

Poston, R., Haney, T., Kott, K., & Rutledge. (2017). Interprofessional team performance, optimized. *Nursing Management, 48*(7), 36–43.

Rees, S., Leahy-Gross, K., & Mack, V. (2011). Moving data to nursing quality excellence. *Journal of Nursing Care Quality, 26*(3), 260–264. doi:10.1097/NCQ.0b013e31820e0e8c

Scheurer, D., Crabtree, E., & Cawley, P. J. (2016). The value equation: Enhancing patient outcomes while constraining costs. *American Journal of the Medical Sciences, 351*(1), 44–51. doi:10.1016/j.amjms.2015.10.013

Schluter, J., Seaton, P., & Chaboyer, W. (2011). Understanding nursing scope of practice: A qualitative study. *International Journal of Nursing Studies, 48*(10), 1211–1222. doi:10.1016/j.ijnurstu.2011.03.004

Titler, M., Shever, L., Kanak, M., Picone, D., & Qin, R. (2011). Factors associated with falls during hospitalization in an older adult population. *Research & Theory for Nursing Practice, 25*(2), 127–148.

Vogus, T., & Sutcliffe, K. (2011). The impact of safety organizing, trusted leadership, and care pathways on reported medication errors in hospital nursing units. *The Journal of Nursing Administration (JONA), 41*(Suppl. 7–8), S25–S30. doi:10.1097/NNA.0b013e318221c368

White, S. V. (2011). Interview with a quality leader: Carol Wagner on Washington State Hospital Association (WSHA) and their statewide improvement. *Journal for Health care Quality: Promoting Excellence in Health care, 34*(1), 62–64. doi:10.1111/j.1945-1474.2011.00161.x

Yee, T., Needleman, J., Pearson, M., & Parkerton, P. (2011). Nurse manager perceptions of the impact of process improvements by nurses. *Journal of Nursing Care Quality, 26*(3), 226–235. doi:10.1097/NCQ.0b013e318213a607Mel

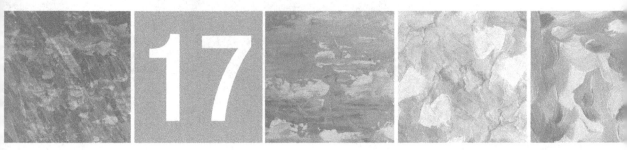

TRANSITION FROM STUDENT NURSE TO LEADERSHIP AND MANAGEMENT OF YOUR FUTURE AS A REGISTERED NURSE

Jodi L. Boling and Patricia Kelly

A caring environment is one that offers the development of potential while allowing the person to choose the best action for himself or herself at a given point in time. People feel more cared for when they are empowered to make their own choices about healthcare.

—Jean Watson

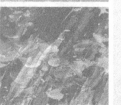

Upon completion of this chapter, the reader should be able to

1. Transition from student nurse to leadership and management of their future as an RN.

2. Implement a study plan for the National Council Licensure Examination (NCLEX) using NCLEX test question practice, nursing knowledge review, and test anxiety management.

3. Describe how to manage your job search with preparation of a resume and good interview techniques.

4. Begin working as a nursing leader and manager of your nursing career.

5. Develop a plan for additional nursing education and certification.

6. Discuss the importance of physical, emotional, and spiritual health.

7. Describe preparation for buying a home.

8. Discuss saving for a future retirement.

R achel will graduate from nursing school in 6 weeks. She completed her university's exit exam and developed her National Council Licensure Examination (NCLEX) study plan, using the exit exam's results to guide her. Rachel also will apply for a nursing position as she waits for her test day to approach.

1. *How many hours per day should she study for the NCLEX?*
2. *How should Rachel use her exit exam results to design her study plan?*
3. *When should Rachel apply for a job before or after she takes the NCLEX?*

Transitioning from student nurse to nurse leader and manager of your future as a RN starts with preparing for the NCLEX and getting a job as a happy and successful RN. This chapter discusses implementing a study plan for the NCLEX using NCLEX test question practice, nursing knowledge review, and test anxiety management. It describes how to manage your job search with preparation of a job resume and good interview techniques. The chapter discusses beginning your work as a nursing leader and manager of your nursing career and developing a plan for additional nursing education and certification. It discusses the importance of physical, emotional, and spiritual health and describes preparation for buying a home. Finally, the chapter discusses saving for future retirement.

The National Council for State Boards of Nursing (NCSBN) has identified the RN NCLEX Test Plan, available at www.ncsbn.org/testplans.htm (Table 17.1). Review this test plan during the early phases of your studying to help with your planning, identify what you will need to focus on, and what study areas you need to address more attention. There are four major categories in the NCLEX Test Plan, that is, Safe and Effective Care Environment, Health Promotion and Maintenance, Psychosocial Integrity, and Physiological Integrity.

NCSBN is responsible for developing the NCLEX licensure exam based on this plan. The NCLEX exam tests the knowledge that is essential to providing safe and effective nursing care to patients. In preparing for the NCLEX, the new graduate will find it useful to focus preparation in three areas: NCLEX test question practice, NCLEX knowledge review, and NCLEX test anxiety management. Students should develop a plan to deal with all three of these areas in preparation for the NCLEX.

NCLEX TEST QUESTION PRACTICE, KNOWLEDGE REVIEW, AND TEST ANXIETY MANAGEMENT

Many nursing schools across the United States have incorporated an end-of-curriculum exit exam that tests student knowledge and may help to predict a student's performance on the NCLEX. One of the aims of exit exams is to provide the future RN with an idea of NCLEX content areas requiring more review prior to scheduling the nursing licensure exam. It is in the best interest of students to review findings from an exit exam or other comprehensive nursing exams and use these exam findings as one of the bases for an NCLEX study plan.

In preparation for your NCLEX, complete Self-Analysis of NCLEX-RN Preparation Needs (Table 17.2) to identify areas that you need to review. Based on this Self-Analysis, plan to answer 60 to 100 NCLEX style questions daily for 25 days ($60 \times 25 = 1,500$ questions) in preparation for the exam. Set up a daily schedule for NCLEX knowledge review and test question practice (Table 17.3). Practice test questions and review NCLEX knowledge when you are most alert daily. The literature

TABLE 17.1 NCLEX-RN® DETAILED TEST PLAN

CLIENT NEEDS	PERCENTAGE OF TEST ITEMS FROM EACH CATEGORY/SUBCATEGORY
Safe and effective care environment	
• Management of care	17%–23%
• Safety and infection control	9%–15%
Health promotion and maintenance	6%–12%
Psychosocial integrity	6%–12%
Physiological integrity	
• Basic care and comfort	6%–12%
• Pharmacological and parenteral therapies	12%–18%
• Reduction of risk potential	9%–15%
• Physiological adaptation	11%–17%

Source: NCLEX-RN® detailed test plan. (2016). *The National Council of State Boards of Nursing*. RN Test Plans Effective April 1, 2016 through March 31, 2019. Retrieved from www.ncsbn.org/testplans.htm

TABLE 17.2 SELF-ANALYSIS OF NCLEX-RN® PREPARATION NEEDS

Anxiety level (circle)   1   2   3   4   5   6   7   8   9   10

Weak knowledge areas identified in NCLEX Test Plan in Table 17.1 or on an exit exam or comprehensive exam

Nursing courses below grade of B:

Weak knowledge areas identified in leading causes of health problems in the United States:

- Mental health, e.g., schizophrenia, bipolar disorders, anxiety, personality disorders, suicide, eating disorders, substance abuse, and so on
- Women's health, e.g., antepartum care, intrapartum care, postpartum care, newborn care, and so on
- Adult health, e.g., cancer, myocardial infarction, diabetes, pneumonia, HIV, hepatitis, cholecystectomy, cerebrovascular accident, nephrectomy, renal failure, thyroidectomy, shock, appendectomy, and so on
- Children's health, e.g., leukemia, cardiovascular surgery, fractures, cancer, diabetes, asthma, cleft palate, and so on

Weak knowledge areas identified in any of the following areas:

- Therapeutic communication
- Growth and development (developmental milestones and toys)
- Management and priority setting
- Medications (see Table 17.4)
- Defense mechanisms
- Immunization schedules
- Diagnostic tests and laboratory values

suggests practicing 60 to 100 questions daily (Ng, Lilyquist, Sanders, & Parsh, 2015). The more you practice test questions, the less test anxiety you may have come test day. Review the rationales for the all the questions answered and review any weak NCLEX knowledge areas. Also, study Table 17.4 as a guideline for identifying medications for NCLEX. Keep your nursing textbooks handy and when you run into NCLEX knowledge you do not know, look it up!

TABLE 17.3 NCLEX STUDY SCHEDULE (PRACTICE 60 TO 100 QUESTIONS DAILY)

Time	M	T	W	T	F	S	S
8–9	60	60	60	60	60		
9–10							
10–11							
11–12							
12–1							
1–2							
2–3							
3–4							
4–5							
5–6							
6–7							
7–8							
8–9							
9–10							

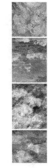

CASE STUDY 17.1

Paul is studying for his NCLEX examination, when he gets a call from friends to attend a local sports team home football game. It is the season opener, a game he has been waiting for. The NCLEX test date is 7 days away. Paul has been practicing 50 NCLEX questions every few days and reviewing some rationales.

1. *What would you recommend Paul do at this point?*
2. *Does Paul have enough time in his testing plan to make up for missing a study day?*

TABLE 17.4 STARTER MEDICATION LIST—GENERIC AND TRADE NAME STEMS OF A FEW COMMON MEDICATIONS (ADD TO THIS LIST AS YOU STUDY)

PREFIX, ROOT, SUFFIX	EXAMPLES	ACTION	NURSING IMPLICATIONS
-asone	Betamethasone (Celestone) Dexamethasone (Decadron)	Steroid Anti-inflammatory	Many side effects, e g., increased sodium, increased sugar, decreased potassium —Must wean patients off steroids to avoid adrenal crisis —Slow wound healing, mood swings, depression

(continued)

TABLE 17.4 STARTER MEDICATION LIST—GENERIC AND TRADE NAME STEMS OF A FEW COMMON MEDICATIONS (ADD TO THIS LIST AS YOU STUDY) (*continued*)

PREFIX, ROOT, SUFFIX	EXAMPLES	ACTION	NURSING IMPLICATIONS
-olol	atenolol (Tenormin) propranolol (Inderal)		
-asone	betamethasone (Celestone) dexamethasone (Decadron)		
-olol	atenolol (Tenormin) propranolol (Inderal)		
-parin	enoxaparin (Lovenox) heparin		
-dipine	nifedipine (Procardia) amlodipine (Norvasc)		
-pril	enalapril (Vasotec) captopril (Capoten)		
-ide	chlorothiazide (Diuril) furosemide (Lasix)		
-statin	lovastatin (Mevacor)		
-mycin	gentamicin (Garamycin) vancomycin (Vancocin)		
-cycline	doxycycline (Vibramycin)		
-pam	diazepam (Valium) lorazepam (Ativan)		
-sartan	candesartan (Atacand) irbesartan (Avapro)		
-zosin	doxazosin mesylate (Cardura) prazosin hydrochloride (Minipress)		

(continued)

TABLE 17.4 STARTER MEDICATION LIST—GENERIC AND TRADE NAME STEMS OF A FEW COMMON MEDICATIONS (ADD TO THIS LIST AS YOU STUDY) (*continued*)

PREFIX, ROOT, SUFFIX	EXAMPLES	ACTION	NURSING IMPLICATIONS
-floxacin	levofloxacin (Levaquin)		
-tidine	ranitidine omeprazole (Prilosec)		

Source: U.S. Food and Drug Administration (FDA). (2017). Retrieved from http://www.takerx.com/class.html

ORGANIZE YOUR NCLEX REVIEW

Your study schedule could look like the following, depending on the feedback from your self-analysis:

Day 1: Practice 60 to 100 questions in weak NCLEX knowledge area identified earlier. Score the test, analyze your performance, and review test question rationales and knowledge weaknesses. Practice deep breathing, relaxation exercises, and positive thinking.

Day 2: Practice 60 to 100 questions in weak NCLEX knowledge area identified earlier. Repeat earlier process.

Day 3: Practice 60 to 100 questions in weak NCLEX knowledge area identified earlier. Repeat earlier process.

Day 4: Practice 60 to 100 questions in NCLEX knowledge area identified earlier. Repeat earlier process.

Day 5: Continue with test question practice and NCLEX knowledge review in all weak knowledge areas identified earlier. Practice deep breathing, journaling, relaxation exercises, and positive thinking. Continue this process until you are doing well in all areas of the NCLEX.

Study when you are most alert!

CRITICAL THINKING EXERCISE 17.1

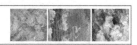

Visit www.vark-learn.com/the-vark-questionnaire/. Take the VARK questionnaire and explore the methodology that works best for your learning style. The VARK model of learning styles suggests that there are four main types of learners. These four types are visual learners, auditory learners, reading/writing learners, and kinesthetic learners. This site also provides information on the best way to take notes and improve your test performance. Utilizing learning methods that are effective for you can enhance the retention and comprehension of NCLEX material.

1. Was using the VARK questionnaire helpful?
2. What did you find out about your learning style?

(*continued*)

CRITICAL THINKING EXERCISE 17.1 (*continued*)

Consider when and where you study best. Are you a morning person? A night person? Study in a quiet environment, away from distractions with food, snacks, and water available at a time that works best for you. Remember, the NCLEX exam is one of the most important exams in your life. Do not cram for the exam. The results of your efforts will show and you want to give this your best. Consider your NCLEX preparation to be your FULL-time job. School is over. You are now managing your life in preparation for your new career.

Think positive, congratulate yourself on any exam areas in which you test well, and imagine your name with RN following it.

Many companies offer NCLEX review courses targeted toward newly graduating nurses. Often, NCLEX review companies will contact a school of nursing or the school's student nursing organization to advertise their products. Students can elect to participate in a NCLEX review course in a classroom live setting or in an online preparatory class. Students can also practice test questions online and study individually or in a group. NCSBN's Learning Extension website (www.learningext.com/) offers online access to 1,300 online exam questions and a Question of the Week, changed every Monday. There is also an NCLEX application, available at the website. You can also consider reviewing more NCLEX practice questions, available at www.nclexinfo.com/nclex-practice-questions-1-10/. There are many NCLEX review books and other test question banks, as well as NCLEX applications for mobile phones offering NCLEX-style exam questions. For example, Health Education Systems Incorporated (HESI) Q & A for the NCLEX-RN Exam, NCLEX Mastery, Saunders Mobile Review Questions for the NCLEX-RN Exam, and ATI-RN Mentor, www.chamberlain.edu/blog/4-apps-for-nclex-practice. Manage any anxiety you may have about the exam with good preparation, journaling, regular exercise, positive thinking, deep breathing exercises, and listening to relaxing music.

Preparation is key to NCLEX success. Practicing NCLEX-style questions, scoring them, and reviewing any practice questions you miss is important. Writing about your testing worries also boosts exam performance. Ramirez and Beilock (2011) found that students who were anxious about an exam and were given 10 minutes to write their feelings down on paper just before taking an important test performed much better than other students who either wrote about something unrelated to the test or did nothing at all. Consider this approach:

- Arrive at the testing center early, take out a piece of paper, and clear your mind by putting your thoughts and feelings into words.
- After you have cleared out every negative emotion, crumple the paper and symbolically toss those worries into the trash.

Take several deep breaths, feeling your heart rate slow; tell yourself, "I'm ready to conquer the NCLEX!" (www.learningext.com/suesblog/b/suesblog/posts/preparing-your-mind-for-nclex).

TEST ANXIETY

Note that some test anxiety may be normal and often helpful to stay mentally and physically alert. When one experiences too much anxiety, however, it can result in emotional and physical distress along with difficulty concentrating and worry. Some suggest that between 25% and 40% of students experience test anxiety (Cassady, 2010). Students who experience test anxiety tend to be easily distracted during a test, experience difficulty with comprehending relatively simple instructions, and have trouble organizing or recalling relevant information (Zeidner, 1998).

NCLEX APPLICATION

For information on the NCLEX application process, visit the following website: www.ncsbn.org/before-the-exam.htm. Before you can take the NCLEX, you will need an Authorization to Test. To get this, you will need to apply to your state board of nursing and then register with Pearson VUE. Start this process well in advance of your target date for taking the exam.

Make a trial run to the testing center the day before NCLEX so that you know how to get there. Anticipate traffic the day of the exam and leave an hour earlier than normal, especially if you live in an area with high traffic or construction. Eat healthy foods the day before the exam and drink plenty of water. Avoid alcohol or caffeinated beverages. Plan on getting 8 hours of sleep before the exam. Relax and spend time with family and friends. On the day of the exam, wake up at a decent time. Do not oversleep. If you normally exercise, do so and keep your day as normal as possible. Eat a well-balanced meal. Leave for the exam in plenty of time. Wear layered clothing to the exam and dress for success. If you feel successful, you will have a better mindset for the exam.

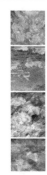

CASE STUDY 17.2

Visit the NCSBN website Before the Exam at www.ncsbn.org/before-the-exam.htm. This site discusses the steps required to register for the NCLEX. Review each of the areas, making sure to understand the necessary requirements for your state, province, or country. Review the areas on:

- *Authorization to test—This is received prior to being able to schedule your NCLEX; it is valid for 90 days.*
- *Application to your state nursing regulatory body*
- *Registration with Pearson Vue*

    1. *Did you understand the steps required?*
    2. *Do you know when to register with Pearson Vue?*

Computerized adaptive testing (CAT) is the method utilized for the NCLEX. There is a minimum of 75 questions and a maximum of 265 questions on the NCLEX. As a candidate takes the NCLEX, test items are selected based on the candidate's response to previous items. The exam ends when it can be determined with 95% confidence that a candidate's performance is either above or below the passing standard, regardless of the number of items answered or the amount of testing time elapsed. There is a 6-hour maximum period for the NCLEX-RN.

NCLEX

Question styles include:

- Multiple response items that require a candidate to select two or more responses
- Fill-in-the-blank items
- Hot spot items that ask a candidate to identify one or more area(s) on a picture or graphic
- Chart/exhibit format
- Ordered response items
- Audio item format
- Graphic options that present the candidate with graphics instead of text for the answer options

Test item formats, including standard multiple choice items, may include multimedia, charts, tables, or graphic images. Examples of each alternate item format can be found in the NCLEX Tutorial at www.ncsbn.org/9010.htm.

SAMPLES OF TWO TYPES OF NCLEX QUESTIONS

Test Question 1. Multiple response item.
 The nurse is assessing a patient with respiratory acidosis. Which of the following does the nurse expect to find? Select all that apply.

_____A. Hypoventilation
_____B. Hyperventilation
_____C. Decreased level of consciousness
_____D. Increased CO_2 levels
_____E. Increased pH levels

Answer: The correct answers are A, C, and D.
 The patient with respiratory acidosis will be found to have hypoventilation and a decreased level of consciousness caused by increased CO_2 levels. Hyperventilation and increased pH levels are associated with respiratory alkalosis.

Test Question 2. Fill-in-the-blank item.
 Heparin is ordered to be infused at 1,800 Units/hr. On hand is 25,000 Units Heparin/250 mL NaCL. How many mL/hr will the nurse set the infusion pump at?
 mL/hr = 25,000 Units/250 mL × 1,800 units/hr. = 18 mL/hr.
 The nurse will set the infusion pump at 18 mL/hr.

REAL-WORLD INTERVIEW

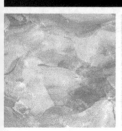

Focus your NCLEX studying on answering questions. I felt like practicing questions helped cement the information in my mind. I did 75 questions minimum every day. When I got a question wrong, I read the rationales and looked up additional content. The review course I took was also very helpful.

Rachael Kennedy-Bennet, MS, ASN, RN, Graduate May 20, 2017

MANAGING YOUR JOB SEARCH

Many institutions, clinics, agencies, and other facilities advertise open nursing positions in a variety of ways. There are job openings on their websites and on job search sites such as www.monster.com/jobs/search/?q=nursing or www.indeed.com/jobs?q=nursing%20rn&l. Job fairs are a great place to meet prospective employers. To find them locally, check for advertisements in the local paper or on institutional websites. When applying for a job, it is of great importance to look good online, on paper, and in person. Be sure all your social media accounts are professional. Employers may use social media to screen potential applicants when deciding who to schedule for an interview or who to hire.

Develop a resume that helps you stand out from other applicants. As you begin to work on your resume and cover letter to apply for jobs, note the Microsoft Word templates. To find the resume and cover letter templates on Microsoft Word, click on File, scroll down to New. Note the templates for designing your own resume and cover letters, as well as templates for other documents. Each resume should have a cover letter attached when submitted. A great resource to check for resume and cover letter review and often offers free assistance with building them is the student services center associated with your school or university.

CRITICAL THINKING EXERCISE 17.2

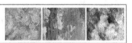

Go to www.monster.com/. Type in Nursing, and your location. Construct a resume using the Microsoft Word template. To find the templates on Microsoft Word, click on File, scroll down to New. Note the templates for designing your own resumes and cover letters, as well as templates for other documents.

1. What types of nursing positions did you find at the site?
2. Are you interested in applying for any of the nursing positions?

Prepare carefully for your first interview. Visit some websites, for example, www. thebalance.com/nurse-interview-questions-and-advice-2061215 for interviewing tips. Practice interview questions with a friend or family member. Review an organization's mission statement and goals, often found on its website, and be ready to comment on how your personal mission and goals align with the organization. Having open and honest communications with the interviewer creates an environment of sincerity (Martin, C., n.d).

Arriving on time or early is the first key to success for the interview. Dress in business attire; wearing scrubs to an interview is not appropriate. Smile, maintain good eye contact, and be friendly to the office staff and the interviewer. Be prepared to answer questions about what makes you the ideal candidate for the job and what are your best and weakest characteristics. Have some answers planned for these types of questions. One of the last things an interviewer often asks is, Do you have any questions for us? Some great questions for you to ask here are: Do you have a residency program or a traditional orientation program? How long is it? Note that orientation programs for graduate nurses are, at a minimum, 6 weeks to 1 year in length, not including the 1 to 2 weeks of general orientation to the facility itself (Green, 2016). Also ask, how are preceptors assigned? How does preceptor feedback occur? Does the orientation program offer formalized classes based on the specialty area of nursing that you are entering? How often are these classes offered? What do employees say are the most rewarding things about working here? What do employees find most challenging on the unit I would be working on? These types of questions may help you be successful in your interview.

Be sure to do your research before you accept a position. Check out, what do your peers and other nurses you know say about their experiences working at a facility? Would they recommend applying there as a graduate nurse if they had to do it again? First-hand testimony is often the best advice one can get. The 2016 Bureau of Labor and Statistics reported that the median salary for an RN was $68,450 per year (www. bls.gov/ooh/healthcare/registered-nurses.htm). This figure can vary with years of experience, location, shift differential, and so on. When inquiring about salary during the interview process, ask about shift pay differentials as well as weekend and holiday pay. Other considerations are what kind of retirement planning do they offer? Do they offer tuition reimbursement? How much sick and paid time off and vacation time is accrued during each pay period?

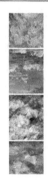

CASE STUDY 17.3

Jessica has an interview scheduled for a RN position at a local hospital. She has many friends who have recently been hired there. She feels comfortable in her interview skills. She states, "I feel that I am a good fit for this hospital and have two friends who work on the floor."

1. *What interview tips do you have for Jessica to prepare further for this interview? Is she adequately prepared?*
2. *What should she know about the organization?*

EVIDENCE FROM THE LITERATURE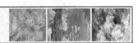

Twibell, R., & St. Pierre, J. (2012). Tripping over the welcome mat: Why new nurses don't stay and what the evidence says we can do about it. *American Nurse Today, 7*, 6.

DISCUSSION

Research evidence strongly supports nurse residency programs as a key strategy to retain new graduate nurses (NGNs). Residencies are longer than traditional orientation programs, ranging from 6 to 12 months. Key evidence-based elements of residency programs include the following:

- Clinical coaching by a preceptor matched for compatibility with the NGN
- Preceptors and NGNs on the same schedules as much as possible

(continued)

EVIDENCE FROM THE LITERATURE (*continued*)

- Evidence-based classroom curriculum with case studies and direct linkage to clinical experiences
- Hands-on learning of skills in a clinical setting or simulations
- Time spent in areas outside the NGN's home unit to understand overall system issues
- Participation in a support group of NGN peers
- High visibility of nurse leaders
- Professional socialization and opportunities for development

A frequently cited barrier to residency programs is the cost in nurses' time. Yet the cost of not retaining one NGN can fund a large portion of a residency program. One hospital reported saving over $2.7 million in 3 years following the initiation of a nurse residency program. If a residency program is not feasible, hospitals can capture many elements of the residencies in a well-designed, traditional orientation.

IMPLICATIONS

A nurse residency program can smooth the transition of a new nurse into practice. Note that orientation programs for graduate nurses are usually, at a minimum, 6 weeks to 1 year in length, not including the 1 to 2 weeks of general orientation to the facility itself.

FOLLOW-UP

It is customary and polite to send a thank you note to the persons with whom you interviewed. Send them EACH an individual separate email, thanking them for the time they spent interviewing you, as well as highlighting two of your personal characteristics that make you beneficial to the company. Remind them in the email how they can contact you to offer you the position. Be certain that your email address is professional and is not something that would reflect negatively on your image. Be positive and optimistic in your follow up. A thank you note sets you out positively from the crowd.

If the potential employer identified the deadline for deciding on the nursing position and that time has passed, contact the person from the Human Resources Department of the organization and ask if anything has been decided about the position. Usually upon completion of the interview, details are given as to when a job offer will be made. Many Human Resource Departments do not want daily or weekly phone calls as to whether the job has been filled. Wait for the deadline, then make a phone call or send an email.

Where Should I Apply?

Think about the type of nursing you want to practice. Is there a certain type of patient population you like to work with? Are you willing to commute? Do you want to work in a teaching hospital or a community hospital? Is the hospital a Magnet® hospital? Table 17.5 has a list of selected job opportunities for NGN employment. Once you apply to an agency, it is helpful to keep a running list of where and when you applied as well as for what position. Table 17.6 shows a Job Application Tracker for keeping this organized.

TABLE 17.5 SELECTED JOB OPPORTUNITIES FOR NURSES

Nurse on Medical Unit	Nurse on Maternity Unit
Emergency Department Nurse	Travel Nurse
Nursing Informatics	Nurse on Psychiatric Unit
Nurse Case Manager	Nurse Educator
Public Health Nurse	Nurse Practitioner
Nurse on Pediatric Unit	Clinical Nurse Specialist
Legal Nurse Consultant	Infection Control Specialist
Nurse on Surgical Unit	Mental Health Nurse
Home Health Nurse	School Nurse
Nurse Entrepreneur	Health and Wellness Coach
Telemedicine Nurse	Research Nurse

TABLE 17.6 JOB APPLICATION TRACKER

DATE APPLIED	ORGANIZATION	INTERVIEWED	THANK YOU SENT	RESPONSE?	FOLLOW-UP

Your First Job

You got the job! You will go through the organization's formal orientation program but you should also consider your own goals for leading and managing your career. Note there is a comprehensive five-course series for NGNs, the Transition to Practice Program, available at the NCSBN Learning Extension website (www.ncsbn.org/transition-to-practice.htm). Each of the five courses encourages reflection and enhances critical thinking skills. There's also a course for preceptors that integrates with the five core courses.

Your new employer's formal orientation program will include working with a preceptor and clinical coaching as well as opportunities for socialization and career development (Figure 17.1). As you start your new nursing role, review the following on your unit:

- Ten most common patient diagnoses
- Ten most common nursing diagnoses
- Ten most common medications and IV solutions
- Ten most common diagnostic tests
- Ten most common laboratory tests
- Ten most common nursing and medical interventions and treatments

You want to be up to date on caring for the patients on your unit. Assume leadership in developing your new nursing role. Begin to identify the names and contact information of all nursing, medical, and healthcare staff that you work with. Be sure to present yourself and dress as a professional nurse. Discuss delegation with your preceptor and observe how your preceptor delegates to others. Respect others and observe the impact of delegation on the person delegated to. Remember the golden rule: Do unto others as you would want them to do unto you.

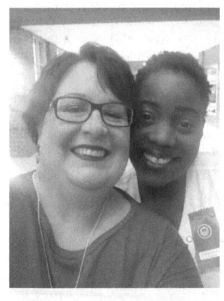

FIGURE 17.1 Meeting your new preceptor.

Consider how you will utilize the Quality and Safety Education for Nurses (QSEN) six competencies of patient-centered care: teamwork and collaboration, evidence-based practice, quality improvement, safety, and informatics to lead and manage your patient care. How can you make patient care better?

Recognize that, under the Nurse Practice Act, the RN holds the responsibility and accountability for nursing care. Develop a standardized unit routine for your patient care (Table 17.7). Practice assertiveness and work at being direct, open, honest, and kind in your nursing role. Hold others accountable and responsible for their duties as spelled out in their job description and be open to performance improvement feedback about your performance. Modify your communication approach to fit the needs of patients, staff, your boss, and yourself.

An important concept for all nurses to understand as they develop a new role is that when you meet the needs of patients, other staff, and your boss, you increase the likelihood that they will be happy. Hopefully this happiness will be contagious and spread to you and all (Table 17.8). This usually makes all lives happier, including yours.

CERTIFICATION

Initially, or after you have worked a while, you will want to consider becoming certified in your specialty area of practice. The American Nurses Credentialing Center has many certifications available at their website at www.nursecredentialing.org/Certification. aspx. Some of these are listed in Table 17.9. Other useful certifications, depending on your area of practice, include Advanced Cardiac Life Support (ACLS), Pediatric Advanced Life Support Course (PALS), Trauma Nursing Core Course (TNCC), Emergency Nursing Pediatric Course (ENPC), Neonatal Resuscitation Program (NRP), and so on.

BACK TO SCHOOL

There are many decisions to be made concerning when and if one decides to go back to school. The biggest questions are often: Will I have the time and the money? What

TABLE 17.7 STANDARDIZED DAY SHIFT ROUTINE FOR PATIENT CARE

Throughout the day shift, nursing and interprofessional staff and unit staff communicate and work together to deliver quality patient care.

7:00 a.m.	Patient handoff report from night shift to day shift; patient assignment sheet for all staff developed.
7:15 a.m.	Patient assessment, including vitals, lab work, IVs done; nursing standards, priorities, and goals identified; patient care assignments given by charge nurse to all nurses and unit staff. Monitor that all patient pain is managed and that patients are satisfied with their care.
7:30 a.m.	Breakfast served.
7:45 a.m.	Morning care with baths given following nursing care standard.
8:00 a.m.	Medications administered; patient care hourly rounds begun; patients sent for diagnostic tests; documentation begun; nursing care standards implemented to prevent patient complications, e.g., turn Q2H, ambulate TID, monitor IVs, give fresh water, complete routine dressing changes, monitor intake and output, review new provider orders, etc.
11:30 a.m.	Vital sign assessment.
12:00 p.m.	Lunch served; Medications administered.
2:00 p.m.	Intake and output reports completed; documentation completed.
3:00 p.m.	Patient handoff report from day shift to evening shift.

TABLE 17.8 HOW TO IMPROVE YOUR ABILITY TO WORK WITH THE BOSS

KNOW YOUR BOSS'S . . .
- Goals and objectives
- Pressures
- Strengths, weaknesses, and blind spots
- Working style

UNDERSTAND YOUR OWN . . .
- Objectives
- Pressures
- Strengths, weaknesses, and blind spots
- Working style
- Predisposition toward dependence on authority figures

DEVELOP A RELATIONSHIP WITH YOUR BOSS THAT . . .
- Meets both your objectives and styles
- Keeps your boss informed
- Is based on dependability and honesty
- Selectively uses your boss's time and resources

Source: Adapted from Gabarro, J. J., & Kotter, J. P. (1993, May-June). Managing your boss. *Harvard Business Review*, pp. 150–157.

TABLE 17.9 SAMPLE OF NURSING CERTIFICATIONS AVAILABLE FROM THE AMERICAN NURSES CREDENTIALING CENTER

INTERPROFESSIONAL CERTIFICATIONS, FOR EXAMPLE, NATIONAL HEALTHCARE DISASTER CERTIFICATION
Nurse Practitioner Certifications, e.g., Emergency NP Clincal Nurse Specialist Certifications, e.g., Pediatric CNS Specialty Certifications, e.g., Informatics Nursing

do I see myself doing in 3, 5, and 10 years? What are my career goals? Do I see myself at the bedside, in administration, education, research, working as an entrepreneur, or as the Surgeon General of the United States? Note that on April 21, 2017, Rear Admiral (RADM) Sylvia Trent-Adams, PhD, RN, FAAN, was named the current acting Surgeon General of the United States.

Nursing is a profession with many opportunities in a variety of areas and settings with unlimited potential. Nurses can join the ranks of clinical practice, administration, teaching, and so on. Taking the time to explore the area of practice in which you want to pursue an advanced degree is important prior to deciding which school to attend. Verify the accreditation of any programs you are considering and decide whether you prefer an online environment or prefer taking a seat at an actual university.

Financing your future education is something you should think of early. Do you plan to go to school full time or part time? How much does school cost per credit hour? Do they let you sit out for a session or semester without penalty in the event of a challenging life event? Does your employer offer tuition reimbursement? If so, what is the tuition reimbursement amount and is there a stipulation as to how long you must work for your employer upon completion of a degree? Can you finance school on your own? Will you have to take out additional loans? Are you able to get additional funding from low rate federal loans? Will you need a cosigner for a private loan? Are grants or scholarships available? What is the return on your education investment? Will there be a raise in salary significant enough to justify going back to school? Will you be able to manage work and school at the same time? Consider these things prior to deciding if you are going back to school. The next degree is often more time consuming than the last, including more reading and writing of papers. The rigor of education seems to increase with each degree level.

PHYSICAL, EMOTIONAL, AND SPIRITUAL FITNESS

Nurses care for others and can often forget to take care of themselves as well. Maintaining your physical, emotional, and spiritual fitness are safeguards to staying healthy.

Physical fitness is the first factor that one must consider. The Office of Disease Prevention and Health Promotion recommends that, for major health benefits, adults should do at least 150 minutes of moderate-intensity aerobic activity each week (Figure 17.2). In addition to this activity, muscle strengthening activities that are moderate or vigorous intensity should be included 2 or more days a week (Office of Disease Prevention and Health Promotion, 2018). Remember, prior to beginning any new health regimen, to obtain clearance from your healthcare provider.

Eating a healthy diet and developing good sleep habits are also part of physical fitness. The U.S. Department of Health and Human Services and the U.S. Department of Agriculture 2015–2020 Dietary Guidelines for Americans (2015) recommend eating a healthy diet throughout one's lifetime. The correct combination of food can help you become and remain healthier now and in the future. The guidelines have recommendations for healthy eating that incorporate how much to fill your plate with grains, fruits, vegetables, protein, and dairy. Limiting choices in sodium, saturated fats, and additional sugars will also place you on the correct path to a healthier lifestyle.

Adults normally spend 33% of life sleeping (National Sleep Foundation, 2017). The average young adult needs 7 to 9 hours of sleep per night. However, this sleep number varies from individual to individual. Stress can rob one of a good night's sleep, causing a pattern to be formed that may lead to higher risk of health problems. Having a set sleep routine is helpful and abiding by this nightly is important. To destress from your day or night shift of work prior to retiring to bed, write down any thoughts or uncompleted tasks in a journal by your bed to increase the likelihood that your last thoughts before sleep are happy. Spend some time doing progressive muscle relaxation or deep breathing before turning in for the night. It is also wise to develop a relaxing presleep ritual, for example, taking a warm bath or having a soothing cup of caffeine-free tea

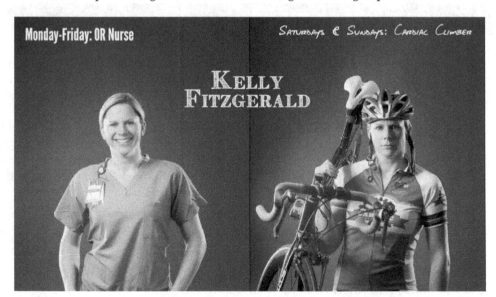

FIGURE 17.2 Kelly Fitzgerald: Monday through Friday, an OR nurse; Saturday and Sunday, mountain climber/biker on behalf of her cardiac patients.

Source: Children's Hospital Colorado Foundation. Retrieved from www.childrenscoloradofoundation.org/courage-classic/community/stories-from-the-road/courage-classic-stories/nurse-kelly-fitzgerald-rides-for-juniper.html.

that you use consistently to set yourself up for a good night's slumber, night after night (National Sleep Foundation, 2017).

Staying fit also incorporates emotional and spiritual health. Taking care of yourself emotionally, controlling stress, and finding a balance is important. Meditation, relaxation exercises, deep breathing, mindfulness, Yoga, Pilates, positive thinking, centering yourself, and finding a place where you can destress are all useful emotional health techniques. Spiritual health is often closely associated with religion; however, spiritual health also extends to include the feelings of love, meaning, hope, compassion, and connectedness (Baumsteiger & Chenneville, 2015). Evidence shows that incorporating spiritual assessment and interventions with patient care are also beneficial to patient outcomes (Pullen, McGuire, Famer, & Dodd, 2015).

If nurses take good of care of themselves emotionally and spiritually, the care environment for patients, as well as for the nurse personally, can improve. If at any time, a nurse is feeling overly stressed, the nurse can seek help from the healthcare provider or contact the Employee Assistance Program at work for counseling in stress reduction.

BUYING A HOME

Deciding to buy a home is a big decision. It is also often the basis of future financial security. Consider carefully where you want to live. Is the home in a safe area and surrounded by safe areas in all directions? No matter whether you have children, choose a home in a school district with a high ranking. This will help your home maintain and grow in value.

A mortgage preapproval by a realtor will give you an idea of how much you can pay for a new home and how much is needed for a down payment. You may often be offered the best mortgage interest rates if your credit score is excellent. One of the most well-known types of credit score are FICO Scores, which often range from 300 to 850. A FICO Score above 670 is considered a good credit score, and a score above 800 is usually perceived to be exceptional (www.experian.com/blogs/ask-experian/credit-education/score-basics/what-is-a-good-credit-score).

REAL-WORLD INTERVIEW

Buying a home is a huge decision and one not to be taken lightly. Look over your finances and make sure you have 6 months of income in savings to cover the unexpected. Obtain a preapproval for your mortgage to determine what range of home prices you can look at.

Make a list of your must haves and list three areas where you would like to live. Review the school districts within those areas and revamp your list as necessary. When you find a house you like, work within your budget, and work with your real estate agent to determine what is the best buy for you and your family. Take into consideration the commute and amenities that are within certain distances to the neighborhood. Good luck finding your dream home!

Laura Demaree
President/Employing Broker, Destination, Denver Realty, Denver, Colorado

RETIREMENT

It is important to maximize your retirement plan contributions from the first day of employment and never touch it. Doing this will allow you to develop your lifestyle with a set amount of money from the start of your employment and then continue to be able to have that same lifestyle when you retire. Consider your employer-matched retirement account at work. How much does your employer contribute to it? Does your employer contribute matching amounts to employee accounts, for example, 401(k) or 403(b)? As a new nurse, you want to maximize this financial opportunity. The money you contribute to this retirement account is usually a pretax contribution, therefore lowering your annual taxable income. Currently for 2017, an individual under age 50 cannot contribute more than $18,000 pretax to their employer-matched retirement account. The most common 401(k) match is $1 per $1 on the first 6% of employee contributions (Miller, 2013). Investing in your retirement early at work and diversifying your investments is key to having enough money to be happily retired without financial worry throughout retirement. To reiterate, invest the maximum amount of money that you can afford and do not touch it until retirement. Diversify the money you invest and stick with your plan for the long term, reviewing it annually.

REAL-WORLD INTERVIEW

If a 25-year-old nurse invests $100 every month in a retirement account at 6% compounded monthly, the account would be worth over $46,000 by the age of 45 and almost $200,000 by the age of 65.

Katie Fox, CFP®, CFA
TIAA, Chicago, Illinois

REAL-WORLD INTERVIEW

Start with creating a workable budget and then monitor your spending monthly to make sure you are staying on track. As part of this budget, you should be allocating between 10% and 15% of your income toward long-term retirement savings. Before you know it, you will be surprised and excited by how much you have accumulated in your retirement nest egg.

Identify and document your short-, medium-, and long-term savings goals and develop an action plan to make them a reality. Taking the time to document your goals and understanding the steps to reach them dramatically increases the probability that they will, in fact, be reached. Additionally, carve out some time in your schedule on an annual basis to revisit those savings goals and monitor your progress toward them. When you can see positive movement on even a short-term basis, you are likely to become even more committed to making your financial dreams a reality.

Take the time to educate yourself about the basics of financial planning including investment, tax, protection, retirement, and estate planning issues. If all this seems a bit daunting at first, seek the help of a financial professional, who is a CERTIFIED FINANCIAL PLANNER™, who has been trained to advise people in these areas and can help you develop a plan to reach your financial goals.

Douglas J. Hoover, CFP®, ChFC®, CDFA™
Vice President, Wealth Management
Strategic Financial Group

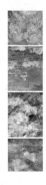

CASE STUDY 17.4

Calculate how much money you need to save to be able to retire at various ages. If you saved a little more each month, how would that affect your retirement savings? Visit Bankrate to calculate these numbers. The link is www.bankrate.com/calculators/retirement/retirement-plan-calculator.aspx. Think of the various scenarios of when you would like to retire. Plan ahead—being money savvy in your younger years will be beneficial in your older years.

1. *Will you change your retirement savings amount based on what you discovered on Bankrate?*
2. *What goals will you implement in order to achieve your retirement dreams?*

KEY CONCEPTS

- The National Council Licensure Examination (NCLEX) review courses are designed to assist the graduate nurse in preparation for the NCLEX.
- A graduate nurse can review the NCLEX Test Plan along with the summary results of their exit exam or other comprehensive exam to develop a NCLEX study plan.
- A consistent and dedicated study schedule is imperative in NCLEX preparation.
- Preparing a well-designed resume as well as preparing for a job interview are keys to success in your first job.
- Nursing certifications and going back to school for additional education may be part of a nurse's future.
- Setting up a retirement account early in one's career allows for financial rewards later in life, after a great career.
- Physical, emotional, and spiritual health are important personally and professionally to the career of the RN.
- A good credit score and identification of your personal home needs are key to buying your first home.

REVIEW QUESTIONS

1. Which statements concerning studying for the National Council Licensure Examination (NCLEX) are correct? Select all that apply.

   A. Study in your house with family present.
   B. Control your study environment.
   C. Review your exit exam study topics.
   D. Have a set study schedule.
   E. Schedule your NCLEX for 3 months after graduation.

2. Which of the following actions is important and courteous for the graduate nurse after an interview?

   A. Contact Human Resources to identify when the job will be filled.
   B. Send a thank you note or email to all persons involved in the interview.
   C. Call the interviewer and request a follow up interview.
   D. Do nothing as this is normal.

3. What are essential steps in maintaining a healthy diet? Select all that apply.

   A. Eat three small meals a day.
   B. Drink carbonated beverages.
   C. Avoid saturated fats.
   D. Avoid sugars.
   E. Fill your plate with fruits and vegetables.

4. Minimizing stress is a key component for the RN. Activities to control stress can include which of the following? Select all that apply.

   A. Meditation
   B. Exercise
   C. Binge eating
   D. Yoga
   E. Prayer

5. The National Sleep Foundation recommends that adults receive ____ hours of sleep per night?

   A. 4 to 6 hours
   B. 5 to 7 hours
   C. 6 to 8 hours
   D. 7 to 9 hours

6. Lack of sleep can lead to changes in healthcare conditions such as which of the following? Select all that apply.

   A. Anorexia
   B. Hyperactivity
   C. Depression
   D. Dental problems
   E. Heart disease

7. Key factors in deciding to purchase a home include which of the following? Select all that apply.

   A. Amount of down payment
   B. Number of bedrooms
   C. Proximity to friends
   D. Amount of mortgage
   E. Ranking of schools

8. Success on the National Council Licensure Examination (NCLEX) can be enhanced if the graduate nurse performs which of the following tasks daily?

   A. Answers NCLEX style test questions and reviews rationales
   B. Reviews course notes from nursing school

C. Takes time to regroup mentally

D. Reads the NCLEX candidate test plan

9. The amount of time recommended for the average adult to exercise per week is which of the following?

A. 60 minutes

B. 80 minutes

C. 120 minutes

D. 150 minutes

10. The type of questions on the National Council Licensure Examination (NCLEX) include which of the following? Select all that apply.

A. Multiple response

B. True/false

C. Essay

D. Ordered response

E. Drag and drop

REVIEW ACTIVITIES

1. Go to www.qsen.org/tic-tac-toe-abgs-interpretation-and-patient-safety/. Click on www.youtube.com/watch?v=URCS4t9aM5o, then watch the video, and take the test. Are you better able to solve arterial blood gas (ABG) problems now?
2. Design your study schedule to answer 60 to 100 National Council Licensure Examination (NCLEX) questions daily for 5 days a week, utilizing the schedule tool (Table 17.2) in this chapter. Identify where you are going to study. List any limitations you may have and how you plan to overcome them before the actual time to begin your NCLEX study.
3. Go to Microsoft Word, click on File, then click on New. Choose one of the resume styles and construct a resume. How does it look?
4. List three strengths and weaknesses of your work ethic. Describe them to a classmate, utilizing feedback from them on how you could improve as needed.

QSEN ACTIVITIES

1. Go to the QSEN website (www.qsen.org) and search for Health. Click on Safety, and then Leadership in Healthcare. Review the information there to improve your leadership skills.
2. Go to the QSEN website (www.qsen.org) and search for Safety. Click on Safety and note the Patient Safety America Newsletter, which is a monthly newsletter dedicated to educating patients and their care providers about new developments in patient safety. Review them to improve your patient's safety.

CRITICAL DISCUSSION POINTS

- What areas of the National Council Licensure Examination (NCLEX) content strength and weakness did you note on your exit exam or other comprehensive exam?
- Make a plan to exercise 150 minutes weekly. How can you fit this into your busy schedule?

- Note the certifications available at the website, www.nursecredentialing.org/Certification.aspx. Are any of them interesting to you? How can you plan to achieve this certification?
- How will increasing your knowledge base on the QSEN competencies help you develop your nursing leadership and management skills for your future?

EXPLORING THE WEB

1. Go to the National Council Licensure Examination (NCSBN) website, www.ncsbn.org/testplans.htm. Review the 2016 NCLEX RN Test Plan. Highlight the content areas that you need to focus on.
2. Visit these sites for creating a resume: www.monster.com and www.indeed.com (search for Nursing Jobs). What tips do they offer?
3. Go to www.choosemyplate.gov/. Click on Popular topics. Choose one and review it. What did you find?
4. Look up a financial stability calculator. Go to www.fistscore.com/do/home. Click on an area of interest to you. What did you find?

REFERENCES

Baumsteiger, R., & Chenneville, T. (2015). Challenges to the conceptualization and measurement of religiosity and spirituality in mental health research. *Journal of Religious Health, 54*(6), 2344–2354. doi:10.1007/s10943-015-0008-7

Cassady, J. C. (2010). Test anxiety: Contemporary theories and implications for learning. In J. C. Cassady (Ed.), *Anxiety in schools: The causes, consequences, and solutions for academic anxieties* (pp. 7–26). New York, NY: Peter Lang.

Gabarro, J., & Kotter, J. (1993). Managing your boss. *Harvard Business Review*, pp. 150–157.

Miller, S. (2013). *Employers boost 401(k) match contributions, relax eligibility.* Retrieved from www.shrm.org/ResourcesAndTools/hr-topics/benefits/Pages/401k-Match-Contributions.aspx

National Sleep Foundation. (2017). *3 Signs you are too stressed to sleep.* Retrieved from www.sleepfoundation.org/press-release/national-sleep-foundation-recommends-new-sleep-times/page/0/1

NCLEX-RN® detailed Test Plan. (2016, April). *The national council of state boards of nursing.* Retrieved from www.ncsbn.org/testplans.htm

Ng, P., Lilyquist, K., Sanders, S., & Parsh, B. (2015). Prepping for NCLEX? Eight tips to get you started. 2015. *Nursing, 45*(4), 19–20. doi:10.1097/01.NURSE.0000461840.63163.c2

Office of Disease Prevention and Health Promotion. (2018). Physical Activity Guidelines for Americans. Office of the Assistant Secretary for Health, Office of the Secretary, U.S. Department of Health and Human Services. Retrieved from https://health.gov/paguidelines/guidelines/default.aspx

Pullen, P., McGuire, S., Farmer, L., & Dodd, D. (2015). The relevance of spirituality to nursing practice and education. *Mental health practice, 18*(5), 14–16. doi:10.7748/mhp.18.5.14.e916

Twibell, R., & St. Pierre, J. (2012). Tripping over the welcome mat: Why new nurses don't stay and what the evidence says we can do about it. *American Nurse Today, 7*(6).

U.S. Department of Health and Human Services and U.S. Department of Agriculture. 2015–2020 Dietary Guidelines for Americans. Retrieved from https://health.gov/dietaryguidelines/2015/

U.S. Food and Drug Administration (FDA). (2017). Drug prefixes, roots, and suffixes. Retrieved from www.takerx.com/class.html

Zeidner, M. (1998). *Test anxiety: The state of the art.* New York, NY: Plenum.

SUGGESTED READINGS

Brewer, S. (2010). Landing a job in a tough economy. *American Journal of Nursing, 110* (Suppl. 1), 18–19.

Carter, E. (2017). *Why the traditional 401 (k) is underrated?* Forbes. Retrieved from https://www.forbes.com/sites/financialfinesse/2017/07/26/why-the-traditional-401k-is-actually-better-than-it-may-seem

Chen, H. C., & Bennett, S. (2016). Decision-tree analysis for predicting first-time pass/fail rates for the NCLEX-RN® in associate degree nursing students. *Journal of Nursing Education, 55*(8), 454–457. doi:10.3928/01484834-20160715-06

Fiske, E. (2017). Contemplative practices, self-efficacy, and NCLEX-RN success. *Nurse Educator, 42*(3), 159–161. doi:10.1097/NNE.0000000000000327

Foreman, S. (2017). The accuracy of state NCLEX-RN passing standards for nursing programs. *Nurse Educator Today, 52,* 81–86. doi:10.1016/j.nedt.2017.02.019

Green, VB. (2016). ENGAGE: A Different New Nurse Orientation Program. *J Contin Educ Nurs, 47*(1), 32–6. doi:10.3928/00220124-20151230-09

Hanna, K., Roberts, T., & Hurley, S. (2016). Collaborative testing as NCLEX enrichment. *Nurse Educator, 41*(4), 171–174.

Johnson, T., Sanderson, B., Wang, C. H., & Parker, F. (2017). Factors associated with first-time NCLEX-RN success: A descriptive research study. *Journal of Nursing Education, 56*(9), 542–545. doi:10.3928/01484834-20170817-05

Kaddoura, M. A., Flint, E. P., Van Dyke, O., Yang, Q., & Chiang, L. C. (2017). Academic and demographic predictors of NCLEX-RN pass rates in first- and second-degree accelerated BSN programs. *Journal of Professional Nursing, 33*(3), 229–240. doi:10.1016/j.profnurs.2016.09.005

Liu, X., & Mills, C. (2017). Assessing the construct congruence of the RN comprehensive predictor and NCLEX-RN test plan. *Journal of Nursing Education, 56*(7), 412–419. doi:10.3928/01484834-20170619-05

Lown, S. G., & Hawkins, L. A. (2017). Learning style as a predictor of first-time NCLEX-RN success: Implications for nurse educators. *Nurse Educator, 42*(4), 181–185. doi:10.1097/NNE.0000000000000344

Murray, T. A., Pole, D. C., Ciarlo, E. M., & Holmes, S. (2016). A nursing workforce diversity project: Strategies for recruitment, retention, graduation, and NCLEX-RN success. *Nursing Education Perspectives, 37*(3), 138–143.

National Heart Lung, Blood Institute. (2016). *Recommendations for physical activity.* Retrieved from www.nhlbi.nih.gov/health/health-topics/topics/phys/recommend

National Sleep Foundation. (2017). *How America sleeps.* Retrieved from www.sleepfoundation.org/sleep-health-index-2014-highlights

Pullen, R. (2017). A prescription for NCLEX-RN success. *Nursing, 47*(6), 19–24.

Ramirez, G., & Beilock, S. L. (2011). Writing about testing worries boosts exam performance in the classroom. *Science, 331*(6014), 211–213. doi:10.1126/science.1199427

Randolph, P. K. (2017). Standardized testing practices: Effect on graduation and NCLEX® pass rates. *Journal of Professional Nursing, 33*(3), 224–228. doi:10.1016/j.profnurs.2016.09.002

Shoemaker, J. R., Chavez, R. A., Keane, P., Butz, S., & Yowler, S. K. (2017). Effective utilization of computerized curricular assistive tools in improving NCLEX-RN pass rates for a baccalaureate nursing program. *Computer Informatics Nursing, 35*(4), 194–200. doi:10.1097/CIN.0000000000000311

Smith, J. (2013). How social media can help or hurt you in your job search. *Forbes.* Retrieved from https://www.forbes.com/sites/jacquelynsmith/2013/04/16/how-social-media-can-help-or-hurt-your-job-search

United Stated Department of Agriculture (USDA). (2017). *Dietary guidelines.* Retrieved from www.cnpp.usda.gov/dietary-guidelines

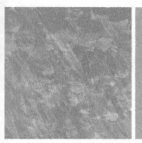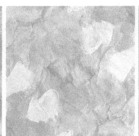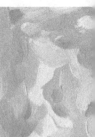

APPENDIX A
SELECTED REPORTS OF THE NATIONAL ACADEMIES OF SCIENCES, ENGINEERING, AND MEDICINE, FORMERLY THE INSTITUTE OF MEDICINE (IOM)

1st Annual Crossing the Quality Chasm Summit: A Focus on Communities. Released September 14, 2004

A Foundation for Evidence-Driven Practice: A Rapid Learning System for Cancer Care. Workshop summary released June 4, 2010

A Summary of the December 2009 Forum on the Future of Nursing: Care in the Community. Workshop summary released June 3, 2010

A Summary of the February 2010 Forum on the Future of Nursing: Education. Workshop summary released August 31, 2010

A Summary of the October 2009 Forum on the Future of Nursing: Acute Care. Workshop summary released April 14, 2010

Advancing the Science to Improve Population Health: Proceedings of a Workshop (2017).

Advancing the Science to Improve Population Health: Proceedings of a Workshop (2017).

Adverse Drug Event Reporting: The Roles of Consumers and Health Care Professionals. Workshop summary released April 12, 2007

Cancer Care for the Whole Patient: Meeting Psychosocial Health Needs. Released October 15, 2007

Certifying Personal Protective Technologies: Improving Worker Safety. Released November 11, 2010

Child and Adolescent Health and Health Care Quality: Measuring What Matters. Released April 25, 2011

Clinical Data as the Basic Staple of Health Learning. Workshop summary released February 3, 2011

Clinical Practice Guidelines We Can Trust. Released March 23, 2011

Creating a Business Case for Quality Improvement and Quality Improvement Research. Workshop summary released April 7, 2008

Crossing the Quality Chasm: A New Health System for the 21st Century. Released March 1, 2001.

Digital Infrastructure for the Learning Health System: The Foundation for Continuous Improvement in Health and Health Care. Workshop series summary released May 23, 2011

Emerging Safety Science. Workshop summary released April 9, 2008

Engineering a Learning Healthcare System: A Look at the Future. Workshop summary released July 8, 2011.

Evidence-Based Medicine and the Changing Nature of Healthcare. Released October 9, 2008

Exploring the Role of Accreditation in Enhancing Quality and Innovation in Health Professions Education (2017).

Finding What Works in Health Care: Standards for Systematic Reviews. Released March 23, 2011

Future Directions for the National Healthcare Quality and Disparities Reports. Released April 14, 2010

Global Health and the Future Role of the United States (2017).

Health IT and Patient Safety: Building Safer Systems for Better Care. Released November 8, 2011

Health Literacy Implications for Health Care Reform. Workshop summary released July 15, 2011

Health Professions Education: A Bridge to Quality. Released April 18, 2003

Initial National Priorities for Comparative Effectiveness Research. Released June 30, 2009

Innovations in Health Literacy Research. Workshop summary released March 10, 2011

Institute of Medicine of the National Academies, 2012. Accessed June 12, 2012.

Keeping Patients Safe: Transforming the Work Environment of Nurses. Released November 3, 2003

Key Capabilities of an Electronic Health Record System. Released July 31, 2003

Leadership by Example: Coordinating Government Roles in Improving Health Care Quality. Released October 30, 2002

Leadership Commitments to Improve Value in Healthcare: Toward Common Ground. Workshop summary released June 14, 2010

Learning What Works: Infrastructure Required for Comparative Effectiveness Research. Workshop summary released July 25, 2011

Medicare's Quality Improvement Organization Program: Maximizing Potential. Released March 9, 2006

Patient Safety: Achieving a New Standard for Care. Released November 20, 2003

Patient-Centered Cancer Treatment Planning: Improving the Quality of Oncology Care. Workshop summary released June 13, 2011

Patients Charting the Course: Citizen Engagement in the Learning Health System. Workshop summary released October 3, 2011

Performance Measurement: Accelerating Improvement. Released December 1, 2005

Preventing Medication Errors: Quality Chasm Series. Released July 20, 2006

Priority Areas for National Action: Transforming Health Care Quality. Released January 7, 2003

Public Health Effectiveness of the FDA 510(k) Clearance Process: Balancing Patient Safety and Innovation. Workshop report released October 14, 2010

Redesigning Continuing Education in the Health Professions. Released December 4, 2009

Redesigning the Clinical Effectiveness Research Paradigm: Innovation and Practice-Based Approaches. Workshop summary released December 6, 2010

Retooling for an Aging America: Building the Health Care Workforce. Released April 11, 2008

Rewarding Provider Performance: Aligning Incentives in Medicare. Released September 20, 2006

Standardizing Medication Labels: Confusing Patients Less. Workshop summary released April 22, 2008

The Future of Drug Safety: Promoting and Protecting the Health of the Public. Released September 22, 2006

The Future of Nursing: Leading Change, Advancing Health. Released October 5, 2010

The Healthcare Imperative: Lowering Costs and Improving Outcomes. Workshop series summary released February 24, 2011

The Learning Healthcare System. Released March 30, 2007

The Richard and Hinda Rosenthal Lecture 2002: Fostering Rapid Advances in Health Care. Released January 1, 2002

The Richard and Hinda Rosenthal Lecture 2003: Keeping Patients Safe. Released November 11, 2004

The Richard and Hinda Rosenthal Lecture 2005: Next Steps Toward Higher Quality Health Care. Released October 12, 2006

The Richard and Hinda Rosenthal Lecture 2011: New Frontiers in Patient Safety. Released October 5, 2011

The Richard and Hinda Rosenthal Lecture Spring 2001: Crossing the Quality Chasm. Released May 1, 2001

The Safe Use Initiative and Health Literacy. Workshop summary released December 1, 2010

The State of Quality Improvement and Implementation Research: Expert Views. Workshop summary released October 5, 2007

To Err Is Human: Building A Safer Health System. Released November 1, 1999

Value in Health Care: Accounting for Cost, Quality, Safety, Outcomes, and Innovation. Workshop summary released December 16, 2009

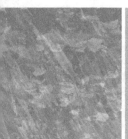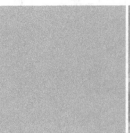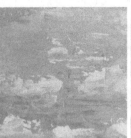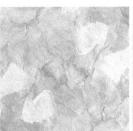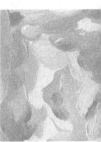

APPENDIX B
PRELICENSURE KNOWLEDGE, SKILLS, AND ATTITUDES

Listed in the following are the prelicensure Quality and Safety Education for Nurses (QSEN) competencies. The chapter of this textbook that has information related to the competency is also identified (see qsen.org/competencies/pre-licensure-ksas).

PATIENT-CENTERED CARE

Definition: Recognize the patient or designee as the source of control and full partner in providing compassionate and coordinated care based on respect for patient's preferences, values, and needs.

KNOWLEDGE	SKILLS	ATTITUDES
Integrate understanding of multiple dimensions of PCC: patient/family/community preferences, values coordination, and integration of care information, communication, and education physical comfort, and emotional support involvement of family and friends, transition, and continuity • Chapter 3 • Chapter 5 • Chapter 7	Elicit patient values, preferences, and expressed needs as part of clinical interview, implementation of care plan, and evaluation of care • Chapter 5 • Chapter 7 • Chapter 11 Communicate patient values, preferences, and expressed needs to other members of healthcare team • Chapter 6 • Chapter 7 • Chapter 11	Value seeing healthcare situations "through patients' eyes" • Chapter 3 • Chapter 6 • Chapter 7 • Chapter 12 Respect and encourage individual expression of patient values, preferences, and expressed needs • Chapter 5 • Chapter 7 • Chapter 11

(continued)

PATIENT-CENTERED CARE (*continued*)

KNOWLEDGE	SKILLS	ATTITUDES
Describe how diverse cultural, ethnic, and social backgrounds function as sources of patient, family, and community values • Chapter 7	Provide PCC with sensitivity and respect for the diversity of human experience • Chapter 7 • Chapter 11 • Chapter 12	Value the patient's expertise with own health and symptoms • Chapter 7 • Chapter 11 Seek learning opportunities with patients who represent all aspects of human diversity • Chapter 7 Recognize personally held attitudes about working with patients from different ethnic, cultural, and social backgrounds • Chapter 7 • Chapter 5 • Chapter 11 Willingly support patient-centered care for individuals and groups whose values differ from your own • Chapter 7 • Chapter 11
Demonstrate comprehensive understanding of the concepts of pain and suffering, including physiological models of pain and comfort • Chapter 7	Assess presence and extent of pain and suffering • Chapter 7 Assess levels of physical and emotional comfort • Chapter 7 Elicit expectations of patient and family for relief of pain, discomfort, or suffering • Chapter 7 Initiate effective treatments to relieve pain and suffering in light of patient values, preferences, and expressed needs • Chapter 7 • Chapter 12	Recognize personally held values and beliefs about the management of pain or suffering • Chapter 7 Appreciate the role of the nurse in relief of all types and sources of pain or suffering • Chapter 7 Recognize that patient expectations influence outcomes in management of pain or suffering • Chapter 7 • Chapter 11
Examine how the safety, quality, and cost effectiveness of healthcare can be improved through the active involvement of patients and families • Chapter 2 • Chapter 3 • Chapter 7 • Chapter 8 • Chapter 11	Remove barriers to presence of families and other designated surrogates based on patient preferences • Chapter 7 • Chapter 11 Assess level of patient's decisional conflict and provide access to resources • Chapter 7 • Chapter 11	Value active partnership with patients or designated surrogates in planning, implementation, and evaluation of care • Chapter 7 • Chapter 8 • Chapter 11

(continued)

PATIENT-CENTERED CARE (*continued*)

KNOWLEDGE	SKILLS	ATTITUDES
Examine common barriers to active involvement of patients in their own healthcare processes • Chapter 7 Describe strategies to empower patients or families in all aspects of the healthcare process • Chapter 7 • Chapter 8 • Chapter 12 Explore ethical and legal implications of PCC • Chapter 5 • Chapter 7 Describe the limits and boundaries of therapeutic PCC • Chapter 7	Engage patients or designated surrogates in active partnerships that promote health, safety and well-being, and self-care management • Chapter 7 • Chapter 8 • Chapter 11 • Chapter 12 Recognize the boundaries of therapeutic relationships • Chapter 7 Facilitate informed patient consent for care • Chapter 7	Respect patient preferences for degree of active engagement in care process • Chapter 7 • Chapter 11 Respect patient's right to access to personal health records • Chapter 7 • Chapter 9 Acknowledge the tension that may exist between patient rights and the organizational responsibility for professional, ethical care • Chapter 5 • Chapter 7 Appreciate shared decision making with empowered patients and families, even when conflicts occur • Chapter 7 • Chapter 11
Discuss principles of effective communication • Chapter 6 • Chapter 8 Describe basic principles of consensus building and conflict resolution • Chapter 6 • Chapter 8 Examine nursing roles in ensuring coordination, integration, and continuity of care • Chapter 3 • Chapter 4 • Chapter 6 • Chapter 8 • Chapter 12	Assess own level of communication skill in encounters with patients and families • Chapter 7 • Chapter 8 Participate in building consensus or resolving conflict in the context of patient care • Chapter 8 Communicate care provided and needed at each transition in care • Chapter 6 • Chapter 8	Value continuous improvement of own communication and conflict resolution skills • Chapter 5 • Chapter 6 • Chapter 7 • Chapter 8

PCC, patient-centered care.

TEAMWORK AND COLLABORATION

Definition: Function effectively within nursing and interprofessional teams, fostering open communication, mutual respect, and shared decision making to achieve quality patient care.

KNOWLEDGE	SKILLS	ATTITUDES
Describe own strengths, limitations, and values in functioning as a member of a team • Chapter 4 • Chapter 8 • Chapter 15 • Chapter 16 • Chapter 17	Demonstrate awareness of own strengths and limitations as a team member • Chapter 8 Initiate plan for self-development as a team member • Chapter 8 Act with integrity, consistency, and respect for differing views • Chapter 5 • Chapter 8	Acknowledge own potential to contribute to effective team functioning • Chapter 1 • Chapter 2 • Chapter 8 • Chapter 13 • Chapter 15 Appreciate importance of intra- and interprofessional collaboration • Chapter 8 • Chapter 15
Describe scopes of practice and roles of healthcare team members • Chapter 6 • Chapter 8 Describe strategies for identifying and managing overlaps in team member roles and accountabilities • Chapter 6 • Chapter 8 Recognize contributions of other individuals and groups in helping patient/family achieve health goals • Chapter 8	Function competently within own scope of practice as a member of the healthcare team • Chapter 3 • Chapter 6 • Chapter 8 Assume role of team member or leader based on the situation • Chapter 3 • Chapter 8 • Chapter 15 Initiate requests for help when appropriate to situation • Chapter 5 • Chapter 8 Clarify roles and accountabilities under conditions of potential overlap in team member functioning • Chapter 5 • Chapter 8 Integrate the contributions of others who play a role in helping patient/family achieve health goals • Chapter 8 • Chapter 15	Value the perspectives and expertise of all health team members • Chapter 1 • Chapter 2 • Chapter 3 • Chapter 6 • Chapter 8 • Chapter 13 • Chapter 15 Respect the centrality of the patient/family as core members of any healthcare team • Chapter 7 • Chapter 8 • Chapter 15 Respect the unique attributes that members bring to a team, including variations in professional orientations and accountabilities • Chapter 8 • Chapter 15

(continued)

TEAMWORK AND COLLABORATION (*continued*)

KNOWLEDGE	SKILLS	ATTITUDES
Analyze differences in communication style preferences among patients and families, nurses, and other members of the health team • Chapter 8 • Chapter 12	Communicate with team members, adapting own style of communicating to needs of the team and situation • Chapter 8 • Chapter 15 Demonstrate commitment to team goals • Chapter 8 • Chapter 15	Value teamwork and the relationships upon which it is based • Chapter 1 • Chapter 2 • Chapter 3 • Chapter 4 • Chapter 8 • Chapter 12 • Chapter 13
Describe impact of own communication style on others • Chapter 8 Discuss effective strategies for communicating and resolving conflict • Chapter 6 • Chapter 8	Solicit input from other team members to improve individual, as well as team, performance • Chapter 4 • Chapter 8 Initiate actions to resolve conflict • Chapter 5	Value different styles of communication used by patients, families, and healthcare providers • Chapter 7 • Chapter 8 Contribute to resolution of conflict and disagreement • Chapter 8
Describe examples of the impact of team functioning on safety and quality of care • Chapter 1 • Chapter 3 • Chapter 4 • Chapter 8 • Chapter 13 • Chapter 15 Explain how authority gradients influence teamwork and patient safety • Chapter 8	Follow communication practices that minimize risks associated with handoffs among providers and across transitions in care • Chapter 6 • Chapter 8 Assert own position/ perspective in discussions about patient care • Chapter 6 • Chapter 8 • Chapter 15 Choose communication styles that diminish the risks associated with authority gradients among team members • Chapter 8	Appreciate the risks associated with handoffs among providers and across transitions in care • Chapter 6 • Chapter 8
Identify system barriers and facilitators of effective team functioning • Chapter 3 • Chapter 8 • Chapter 13 • Chapter 15 Examine strategies for improving systems to support team functioning • Chapter 1 • Chapter 2 • Chapter 3 • Chapter 15	Participate in designing systems that support effective teamwork • Chapter 8 • Chapter 13 • Chapter 15	Value the influence of system solutions in achieving effective team functioning • Chapter 3 • Chapter 4 • Chapter 8 • Chapter 15

EVIDENCE-BASED PRACTICE (EBP)

Definition: Integrate best current evidence with clinical expertise and patient/family preferences and values for delivery of optimal healthcare.

KNOWLEDGE	SKILLS	ATTITUDES
Demonstrate knowledge of basic scientific methods and processes • Chapter 11 • Chapter 14	Participate effectively in appropriate data collection and other research activities • Chapter 14	Appreciate strengths and weaknesses of scientific bases for practice • Chapter 11 • Chapter 13 • Chapter 14
Describe EBP to include the components of research evidence, clinical expertise, and patient/family values • Chapter 11	Adhere to Institutional Review Board guidelines • Chapter 11 • Chapter 13 Base individualized care plan on patient values, clinical expertise, and evidence • Chapter 7 • Chapter 11 • Chapter 12	Value the need for ethical conduct of research and quality improvement • Chapter 5 • Chapter 11 • Chapter 13 Value the concept of EBP as integral to determining best clinical practice • Chapter 11
Differentiate clinical opinion from research and evidence summaries • Chapter 10 • Chapter 11 Describe reliable sources for locating evidence reports and clinical practice guidelines • Chapter 10 • Chapter 11	Read original research and evidence reports related to area of practice • Chapter 10 • Chapter 11 Locate evidence reports related to clinical practice topics and guidelines • Chapter 10 • Chapter 11	Appreciate the importance of regularly reading relevant professional journals • Chapter 10 • Chapter 11
Explain the role of evidence in determining best clinical practice • Chapter 10 • Chapter 11 Describe how the strength and relevance of available evidence influences the choice of interventions in provision of PCC • Chapter 7 • Chapter 10 • Chapter 11 • Chapter 13	Participate in structuring the work environment to facilitate integration of new evidence into standards of practice • Chapter 4 • Chapter 11 • Chapter 13 Question rationale for routine approaches to care that result in less-than-desired outcomes or adverse events • Chapter 11	Value the need for continuous improvement in clinical practice based on new knowledge • Chapter 4 • Chapter 11 • Chapter 12 • Chapter 13
Discriminate between valid and invalid reasons for modifying evidence-based clinical practice based on clinical expertise or patient/family preferences • Chapter 11 • Chapter 13	Consult with clinical experts before deciding to deviate from evidence-based protocols • Chapter 11	Acknowledge own limitations in knowledge and clinical expertise before determining when to deviate from evidence-based best practices • Chapter 11

QUALITY IMPROVEMENT (QI)

Definition: Use data to monitor the outcomes of care processes and use improvement methods to design and test changes to continuously improve the quality and safety of healthcare systems.

KNOWLEDGE	SKILLS	ATTITUDES
Describe strategies for learning about the outcomes of care in the setting in which one is engaged in clinical practice • Chapter 1 • Chapter 2 • Chapter 3 • Chapter 4 • Chapter 9 • Chapter 11 • Chapter 13 • Chapter 14 • Chapter 15	Seek information about outcomes of care for populations served in care setting • Chapter 13 • Chapter 14 • Chapter 15 Seek information about QI projects in the care setting • Chapter 4 • Chapter 13 • Chapter 15	Appreciate that continuous QI is an essential part of the daily work of all health professionals • Chapter 1 • Chapter 2 • Chapter 3 • Chapter 4 • Chapter 5 • Chapter 9 • Chapter 11 • Chapter 12 • Chapter 13 • Chapter 14 • Chapter 15 • Chapter 16
Recognize that nursing and other health professions students are parts of systems of care and care processes that affect outcomes for patients and families • Chapter 3 • Chapter 4 • Chapter 11 • Chapter 13 • Chapter 14 • Chapter 15 Give examples of the tension between professional autonomy and system functioning • Chapter 4 • Chapter 8 • Chapter 15	Use tools (such as flow charts, cause-effect diagrams) to make processes of care explicit • Chapter 13 • Chapter 14 • Chapter 15 Participate in a root cause analysis of a sentinel event • Chapter 4 • Chapter 13 • Chapter 14 • Chapter 15	Value own and others' contributions to outcomes of care in local care settings • Chapter 4 • Chapter 8 • Chapter 13 • Chapter 15
Explain the importance of variation and measurement in assessing quality of care • Chapter 14	Use quality measures to understand performance • Chapter 13 • Chapter 14 • Chapter 15 Use tools (such as control charts and run charts) that are helpful for understanding variation • Chapter 14 Identify gaps between local and best practice • Chapter 14	Appreciate how unwanted variation affects care • Chapter 14 Value measurement and its role in good patient care • Chapter 13 • Chapter 14 • Chapter 15

(continued)

QUALITY IMPROVEMENT (*continued*)

KNOWLEDGE	SKILLS	ATTITUDES
Describe approaches for changing processes of care • Chapter 4 • Chapter 11 • Chapter 13 • Chapter 14 • Chapter 15	Design a small test of change in daily work (using an experiential learning method such as Plan-Do-Study-Act) • Chapter 13 • Chapter 15 Practice aligning the aims, measures, and changes involved in improving care • Chapter 13 • Chapter 14 • Chapter 15 Use measures to evaluate the effect of change • Chapter 14	Value local change (in individual practice or team practice on a unit) and its role in creating joy in work • Chapter 13 • Chapter 14 • Chapter 15 Appreciate the value of what individuals and teams can do to improve care • Chapter 4 • Chapter 8 • Chapter 13 • Chapter 14 • Chapter 15

QI, quality improvement.

SAFETY

Definition: Minimizes risk of harm to patients and providers through both system effectiveness and individual performance.

KNOWLEDGE	SKILLS	ATTITUDES
Examine human factors and other basic safety design principles as well as commonly used unsafe practices (such as work-arounds and dangerous abbreviations) • Chapter 1 • Chapter 3 • Chapter 4 • Chapter 5 • Chapter 7 • Chapter 12 • Chapter 13 Describe the benefits and limitations of selected safety-enhancing technologies (such as barcodes, Computer Provider Order Entry, medication pumps, and automatic alerts/alarms) • Chapter 9 • Chapter 12 Discuss effective strategies to reduce reliance on memory • Chapter 9 • Chapter 12	Demonstrate effective use of technology and standardized practices that support safety and quality • Chapter 4 • Chapter 9 • Chapter 12 • Chapter 13 • Chapter 14 Demonstrate effective use of strategies to reduce risk of harm to self or others • Chapter 5 • Chapter 12 Use appropriate strategies to reduce reliance on memory (such as forcing functions, checklists) • Chapter 9 • Chapter 12	Value the contributions of standardization/reliability to safety • Chapter 4 • Chapter 12 • Chapter 13 • Chapter 14 Appreciate the cognitive and physical limits of human performance • Chapter 4

(*continued*)

SAFETY (*continued*)

KNOWLEDGE	SKILLS	ATTITUDES
Delineate general categories of errors and hazards in care • Chapter 12 Describe factors that create a culture of safety (such as open communication strategies and organizational error reporting systems) • Chapter 4 • Chapter 12	Communicate observations or concerns related to hazards and errors to patients, families, and the healthcare team • Chapter 4 • Chapter 12 Use organizational error reporting systems for near miss and error reporting • Chapter 4 • Chapter 9 • Chapter 12	Value own role in preventing errors • Chapter 4 • Chapter 12
Describe processes used in understanding causes of error and allocation of responsibility and accountability (such as root cause analysis and failure mode effects analysis) • Chapter 4 • Chapter 12 • Chapter 13	Participate appropriately in analyzing errors and designing system improvements • Chapter 4 • Chapter 12 • Chapter 13 • Chapter 15 Engage in root cause analysis rather than blaming when errors or near misses occur • Chapter 4 • Chapter 12 • Chapter 13	Value vigilance and monitoring (even of own performance of care activities) by patients, families, and other members of the healthcare team • Chapter 9 • Chapter 12 • Chapter 13
Discuss potential and actual impact of national patient safety resources, initiatives, and regulations • Chapter 1 • Chapter 2 • Chapter 3 • Chapter 4 • Chapter 12 • Chapter 13	Use national patient safety resources for own professional development and to focus attention on safety in care settings • Chapter 1 • Chapter 2 • Chapter 4 • Chapter 12 • Chapter 13	Value relationship between national safety campaigns and implementation in local practices and practice settings • Chapter 1 • Chapter 2 • Chapter 4 • Chapter 12 • Chapter 13

INFORMATICS

Definition: Use information and technology to communicate, manage knowledge, mitigate error, and support decision making.

KNOWLEDGE	SKILLS	ATTITUDES
Explain why information and technology skills are essential for safe patient care • Chapter 4 • Chapter 9 • Chapter 10	Seek education about how information is managed in care settings before providing care • Chapter 9 • Chapter 13 • Chapter 14 Apply technology and information management tools to support safe processes of care • Chapter 4 • Chapter 9 • Chapter 12	Appreciate the necessity for all health professionals to seek lifelong, continuous learning of information technology skills • Chapter 1 • Chapter 2 • Chapter 9
Identify essential information that must be available in a common database to support patient care • Chapter 9 Contrast benefits and limitations of different communication technologies and their impact on safety and quality • Chapter 9	Navigate the electronic health record • Chapter 9 Document and plan patient care in an electronic health record • Chapter 9 Employ communication technologies to coordinate care for patients • Chapter 7 • Chapter 9 • Chapter 12	Value technologies that support clinical decision making, error prevention, and care coordination • Chapter 9 Protect confidentiality of protected health information in electronic health records • Chapter 9
Describe examples of how technology and information management are related to the quality and safety of patient care • Chapter 1 • Chapter 2 • Chapter 4 • Chapter 7 • Chapter 9 • Chapter 13 Recognize the time, effort, and skill required for computers, databases, and other technologies to become reliable and effective tools for patient care • Chapter 9	Respond appropriately to clinical decision-making supports and alerts • Chapter 9 • Chapter 12 Use information management tools to monitor outcomes of care processes • Chapter 9 • Chapter 13 Use high-quality electronic sources of healthcare information • Chapter 9 • Chapter 13	Value nurses' involvement in design, selection, implementation, and evaluation of information technologies to support patient care • Chapter 9

Source: Reprinted from Cronenwett, L., Sherwood, G., Barnsteiner, J. Disch, J., Johnson, J., Mitchell, P., ... Warren, J. (2007, May–June). Quality and safety education for nurses. *Nursing Outlook, 55*(3), 122–131, with permission from Elsevier.

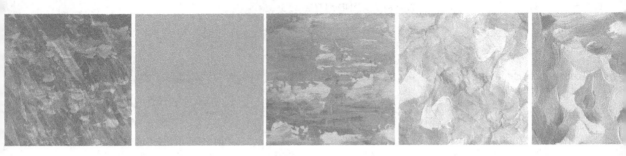

APPENDIX C
CRITICAL THINKING EXTRAS

CRITICAL THINKING C.1

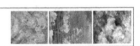

You are concerned with improvement of your nursing practice of the Quality and Safety Education for Nurses (QSEN) competencies. Review all the competencies and knowledge, skills, and attitudes (KSAs) in Appendix B. Identify a personal goal for your development of one of the competencies in each of the six areas. What do you think a patient's wish for quality care might be in each of the competencies? Do you think there are differences in a patient's wishes depending on the care setting? For example, would a patient have different wishes for patient-centered care (PCC) in a hospital clinic, an ambulatory surgery center, a primary care office, or an inpatient nursing unit?

QSEN COMPETENCY	PERSONAL FUTURE GOAL	PATIENT'S WISH
Patient-centered care		
Safety		
Quality improvement		
Evidence-based practice		
Informatics		
Teamwork and collaboration		

CRITICAL THINKING C.2

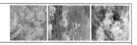

You are a new nurse just out of orientation on a 30-bed medical patient-care unit. Many of the patients on this unit are elderly and suffer from various cardiac and respiratory healthcare conditions. Staffing for the patients on this unit is usually one RN to five patients. There are two nurse aides on the unit also, in addition to a charge nurse. You arrive for your evening shift and begin to plan your patient care.

- Identify which healthcare structures and processes you will assess early in your shift to ensure patient safety and quality. Incorporate these into your patient care, as needed. Refer to Table 12.1 when necessary.
- What patient outcomes should be monitored on these patients?
- What criteria will you use to assess this patient staffing situation from a safety perspective?
- What actions will you take if you feel this is an unsafe staffing situation?

CRITICAL THINKING C.3

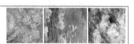

You have just been named to an interprofessional healthcare team to design a future patient care unit for your medicql nursing patients. Identify which structure and process quality elements you will incorporate into the new unit for patient-centered safe care. What health care quality outcomes will you monitor? Which interprofessional health care team members could help on this team? Be sure to identify and plan for which types of medical patients will be cared for on this nursing unit. What is their acuity level? Review the evidence-based literature and benchmark with other organizations on lengths of stay and care modalities for your identified medical patient population (e.g., pneumonia, chronic obstructive lung disease). Consider how to include necessary interprofessional service units, for example, medicine, physical therapy, respiratory, pharmacy, dietary, laboratory, housekeeping, in the planning. Plan to monitor medical infection rates for each patient population. Also, plan to monitor the elements in the Institute for Healthcare Improvement (IHI) Global Trigger Tool (app.ihi.org/webex/gtt/ihiglobaltriggertoolwhitepaper2009.pdf). Refer to Table 12.1 as needed. How will you ensure that the Quality and Safety Education for Nurses (QSEN) elements are built into this future unit? Give at least one example of each of the structure and process elements, one example of the outcomes, and one example of the QSEN elements you will monitor in the table that follows for this future unit. Identify one to two elements from the IHI Global Trigger Tool in Chapter 12 that you will also monitor. We did some parts below for you. Add to the chart, as needed.

(continued)

CRITICAL THINKING C.3 *(continued)*

QUALITY ELEMENTS	EXAMPLES OF ELEMENT
Structures	• Safe environment, e.g., side rails on beds • Staffing guidelines • Chain of command policy • High-reliability environment • Just culture • Assignment sheets • Informatics, e.g., computer availability
Processes	• Evidence-based patient-care medical standards, guidelines, bundles, etc. • Delegation policies and procedures • Routines for medication administration, IV monitoring, and bedfast patient care to prevent lung, leg, bowel, bladder, bleeding, and infection problems
Outcomes	Interprofessional team to review the following outcomes monthly • Patient-centered care • Patient satisfaction • Patient safety • Infection rates • Complication rates • Staff safety

QSEN ELEMENTS	
Team and collaboration	Include representatives from nursing, medicine, pharmacy, dietary, physical therapy, laboratory, etc., in planning of unit
Patient-centered care	Monitor patient satisfactions survey
Safety	

(continued)

CRITICAL THINKING C.3 (*continued*)

QUALITY ELEMENTS	EXAMPLES OF ELEMENT
Quality	
Informatics	
Evidence-based practice	

IHI GLOBAL TRIGGER	
Code	Cardiac or pulmonary arrest
Positive blood culture	Positive blood culture

Source: Patricia Kelly, unpublished manuscript.

CRITICAL THINKING C.4

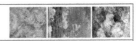

You are a new nurse just out of orientation on a 30-bed surgical patient-care unit. You have just arrived for your 7 a.m. to 7 p.m. shift. There are six RNs for the 30 patients. Based on the staffing classifications for patient acuity, you have been assigned five patients on this unit. There are three nurse aides on the unit. Identify how you will plan your day and the day of your fellow team members. Remember to consider, with all of this work, what requires the skills and knowledge of an RN and what could be safely delegated to another healthcare team member? Note the example of this patient-care routine on a surgical unit. How would you alter this routine on another unit?

06:45	ARRIVE ON UNIT; CHECK ASSIGNMENT SHEET
07:00–09:00	Receive shift handoff report. Delegate, as needed. Finalize assignments with staff. Make rounds on high-priority patients, e.g., patients with airway, breathing, bleeding, circulation, or safety needs.
	Check IV fluids, surgical dressings. Ensure that preoperative patients are ready for the operating room (consents, labs, NPO, etc.). Serve breakfast, feed patients as needed; complete vital signs, pass medications.
	Check vital signs. Turn, cough, and deep breathe surgical patients, check bleeding, bladder, dressings, lung and bowel sounds, ambulation, etc. Based on your patient assessments, determine the frequency needed for rounds on priority patients.
09:00–11:00	Work with nurse aides to complete a.m. care; review new orders regularly throughout shift, consult with interprofessional team as needed. Pass medications.
	Turn, cough, and deep breathe surgical patients, ambulate new surgical patients, give fresh drinking water to patients.
11:00–13:00	Check vital signs.
	Lunch, pass medications.
	Turn, cough, and deep breathe surgical patients, check bleeding, dressings, lung and bowel sounds, etc.
13:00–15:00	Turn, cough, and deep breathe surgical patients.
	Patient reassessment as indicated based on patient's condition.
15:00–17:00	Check vital signs, pass medications.
	Turn, cough, and deep breathe surgical patients, ambulate new surgical patients.
	Patient reassessment as indicated based on patient's condition.
18:00–19:00	Check vital signs.
	Turn, cough, and deep breathe surgical patients, check bleeding, dressing, lung and bowel sounds, etc.
	Prepare and give shift handoff report to oncoming staff.

CRITICAL THINKING C.5

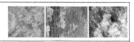

Take a look at your nursing unit's policy and procedure book. Pick a policy and examine the type of evidence used as a reference for the policy. Use the pyramid of evidence sources in the evidence-based practice chapter (Chapter 11) to evaluate the types of evidence used to support the policy. Is the evidence appropriate? If possible, can you tell how the evidence was evaluated? Why is it important to evaluate the evidence used to support the policy?

CRITICAL THINKING C.6

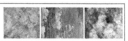

You are a professional RN on an interprofessional team at your hospital. Sometimes you notice that nursing's input into decisions does not seem to be respected. Some of the team members are dismissive and condescending to the nursing team members.

How can you work to change this and build respect for the profession of nursing as skilled practitioners with much to bring to patient care?
Does the way you dress, introduce yourself as an RN, and communicate with patients and other members of the interprofessional team convey that you expect to be respected?
How do other members of the interprofessional team dress, communicate, and introduce themselves to patients and to you?

CRITICAL THINKING C.7

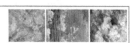

In an effort to make healthcare more affordable and accountable, data are being released by the Centers for Medicare and Medicaid Services (CMS) that show significant variation across the country in what healthcare providers charge for common services. See https://www.cms.gov/Research-Statistics-Data-and-Systems/Statistics-Trends-and-Reports/Medicare-Provider-Charge-Data/index.html. These data include information comparing the charges for the 100 most common inpatient services and 30 common outpatient services. Compare the average covered charges and the average total payment for a diagnostic related group (DRG) with a large number of total discharges at two of the hospitals in your state. What did you see there? Can you make some decisions about quality care using this information?

CRITICAL THINKING C.8

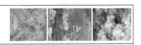

Have you asked a patient, "What is patient-centered care (PCC)?" Have you considered what outcomes you should monitor to evaluate PCC? Do you get any patient feedback that allows you to examine patient satisfaction with respect, caring, timeliness of service, and so on, offered to them? Should nurses be concerned with patient satisfaction or is it enough to focus just on ensuring high-quality physical outcomes?

CRITICAL THINKING C.9

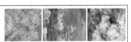

Look at how informatics is used at a hospital where you have clinical experience. Has an electronic patient care record documentation system been developed? Is informatics used to improve clinical decision making, medication safety, evidence-based care, and so on? How does informatics improve patient care?

CRITICAL THINKING C.10

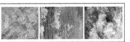

The Affordable Care Act (ACA) was proposed to increase the quality and affordability of health insurance, lower the uninsured rate by expanding public and private insurance coverage, and reduce the costs of healthcare for individuals and the government. In addition, an aim of the ACA is to increase transparency of healthcare and empowering of patients. There is some uncertainty of the future of the ACA, which can result in confusion for many Americans. Review the U.S. Department of Health and Human Services website on Empowering Patients (https://www.hhs.gov/healthcare/empowering-patients/index.html). How can you use this information to help your patients understand their rights and coverage under the ACA or other healthcare reform?

CRITICAL THINKING C.11

During your next clinical experience pay attention to how nurses use the electronic clinical documentation for more than charting. How does the documentation system support the nursing informatics framework of data, information, knowledge, and wisdom? Can the electronic documentation system improve the nurse's clinical decision-making skills? Does informatics improve patient care and communication among the various healthcare professionals working with patients?

CRITICAL THINKING C.12

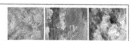

Read through the quality improvement (QI) methodology provided by the Department of Health and Human Services at https://www.hrsa.gov/sites/default/files/quality/ toolbox/pdfs/introductionandoverview.pdf. Identify a quality problem during a clinical experience. Work as a group or individually to use the steps provided in the QI methodology to address the quality problem. While working on the project, reflect on the need for nurses to be involved in the QI process.

CRITICAL THINKING C.13

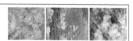

Read through the quality improvement (QI) measures at qualityindicators.ahrq.gov. Select one of the four groups of QI measures and read about the identification of indicators, the measurement of indicators, the development of clinical practice guidelines, and the creation of pathways to support compliance and support for sustaining improvement. Identify where nurses are affected by the measures. How do the QI measures affect interprofessional team members? How do interprofessional team members affect the measures? Why is it important to have representation from a variety of healthcare professions involved in the development of QI measures?

CRITICAL THINKING C.14

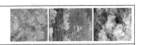

Complete the Institute for Healthcare Improvement (IHI) Open School courses at app. ihi.org/lms/onlinelearning.aspx. You will need to register for the free courses. Once all the modules are completed, you will receive a certificate of completion. After each course, reflect on what you have learned. Think about your most recent clinical experience. Do you see any of what you have learned being used in clinical practice? Do you see opportunities to use what you have learned in clinical practice? Use the following table to document your reflections for each IHI Open School course completed.

IHI OPEN SCHOOL COURSE	CLINICAL EXPERIENCE THAT REFLECTED THE COURSE TEACHINGS	CLINICAL PRACTICE THAT DID NOT REFLECT THE COURSE TEACHINGS	OPPORTUNITIES FOR USE IN THE CLINICAL SETTING (YOUR SUGGESTIONS FOR USING THE COURSE TEACHINGS)
Patient safety			
Leadership			
Improvement capability			
Patient- and family-centered care			
Quality cost and value			
Triple aim for populations			
Overall thoughts			

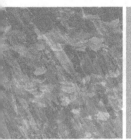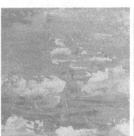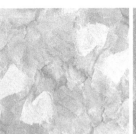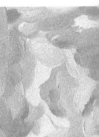

GLOSSARY

Accountability is defined as "to be answerable to oneself and others for one's own choices, decisions and actions as measured against a standard such as that established by the *Code of Ethics for Nurses with Interpretive Statements*" (ANA, 2015).

Accountable Care Organizations (ACOs) are a group of care providers who assume risk in order to manage the full continuum of care and are accountable for overall costs and quality of care for a defined group of patients.

Adverse event is an incident that results in harm to the patient. An adverse event that may be considered either preventable or not, is defined as any undesirable experience in which harm resulted to a person receiving healthcare that "requires additional monitoring, treatment, or hospitalization, or that results in death" (IOM, 1999).

Agency for Healthcare Research and Quality (AHRQ) is a government entity organized to produce evidence to make healthcare safer, higher in quality, more accessible, equitable, and affordable, and to work with the U.S. Department of Health and Human Services and with other partners to make sure that research findings are understood and used.

Aggregate data are the summary of data collected. Data are grouped together based on the process under measurement. It may be aggregated by minute, hour, day, week, month, year, or multiple years depending on the variable. Aggregate data are commonly presented in a table format.

Assignment is the routine care, activities, and procedures that are within the authorized scope of practice of the RN or licensed practical nurse (LPN)/licensed vocational nurse (LVN) or part of the routine functions of the unlicensed assistive personnel (UAP; NCSBN, 2016).

Attitude is a behavior or point of view.

Authority is the right to act or to command the action of others. Authority comes with the job and is required for a nurse to take action.

Authority gradient refers to positions within a group or profession, such as a direct care nurse and the nurse manager or a medical resident and the attending physician (Institute of Medicine, 1999).

Baldrige Award recognizes organizations that have improved and sustained quality results. The purpose of the Baldrige Award is to challenge organizations to improve their effectiveness of care and healthcare outcomes to pursue excellence, which moves organizations toward becoming a high reliability organization (HRO; NIST, 2017).

Bar-code medication administration (BCMA) links the electronic medication administration record (eMAR) with medication-specific identification in the form of bar codes to help with compliance of the five "rights" of medication administration: right patient, right dose, right route, right time, and right medication (AHRQ, 2017).

Baseline data are the before, or preintervention, measurements that indicated the need for improvement. Without baseline data, there is no ability to assess if an improvement intervention succeeded or failed.

Best available evidence implies that someone must conduct a thorough search of the literature and then judge the quality of the evidence to determine if it truly is the "best available."

Bibliographic databases provide a basic record, or citation, for an article and often provide an abstract or brief summary of the article; they do not necessarily contain the complete text of the article itself.

Big data is a term for data sets that are so large or complex that traditional data processing application software is inadequate to deal with them.

A **breach in duty** occurs when a nurse or other healthcare professional has a duty of care toward another person but fails to live up to the accepted standard of care.

Clinical decision support system (CDSS) is an integrated database of clinical and scientific information to aid healthcare professionals in providing care (AHRQ, 2016).

Clinical expertise develops as the nurse tests and refines both theoretical and practical knowledge in actual clinical situations (Benner, 1984).

Collaboration is an interpersonal personal process characterized by healthcare professionals from multiple disciplines with shared objectives, decision making, responsibility, and power working together to solve patient care problems (Petri, 2010).

Commitment to zero harm means that the healthcare system has leaders that believe and commit to eliminating all patient harm, referred to as zero harm.

Common cause variation is the variability seen in a process that is inherent or expected to that process. When common cause variability exists within a process, that process is considered to be stable or "in control."

Common law is the body of law that has been created through the application of prior court decisions, that is, precedents, to a unique set of facts; it has been developed by judges, courts, and other special courts or tribunals appointed to deal with a particular problem.

Comorbidities are two or more coexisting medical conditions or disease processes that are additional to an initial diagnosis.

Computerized physician (provider) order entry is any system that allows the physician to directly transmit an order electronically to a recipient (AHRQ PSNet, 2017).

Control chart is a graphical display of data in a time-series design using the mean as the centerline. In addition, the control chart includes an upper control limit line. (3 standard deviations [SDs] above the mean) and a lower control limit line. (3 SDs below the mean). Using interpretation rules, common cause variation and special cause variation in a data set can be identified.

Cross monitoring is the process of monitoring the actions of other team members for the purpose of sharing the workload and reducing or avoiding errors (AHRQ, n.d. Retrieved from http://www.ahrq.gov/teamsteppstools/instructor/fundamentals/module4/slsitmonitor.pdf)

Culture of safety refers to the extent to which individuals and groups will commit to personal responsibility for safety; act to preserve, enhance, and communicate safety concerns; strive to actively learn, adapt, and modify both individual and organizational behavior based on lessons learned from mistakes; and strive to be honored in association with these values.

The Cumulative Index to Nursing and Allied Health Literature (CINAHL) is bibliographic database that indexes thousands of journals in the fields of nursing, biomedicine, alternative/complementary medicine, consumer health, and numerous allied health fields.

Daily safety huddle is a brief meeting that includes senior and operational leaders who meet at the start of each day to discuss safety concerns and resolve problems.

Data is a collection of numbers, characters, or facts that are named, collected, and organized according to a perceived need for analysis; discrete entities that are described objectively without interpretation. Another definition is a list of raw numbers or results collected to monitor a variety of processes within the organization or those provided the organization from an outside source. It is used to determine if performance meets the expected goal.

Data display refers to the visual picture or graphing of data that best illustrate the story you want that data to exhibit. It is important to display data in ways staff, patients, and families can understand them. Both graphs and tables are acceptable methods of displaying data.

Debriefing is recounting key events and analyzing why they occurred; include what worked, what did not work, leading to a discussion of lessons learned and how they will alter the plan next time (AHRQ, n.d. Retrieved from http://search.ahrq.gov/search?q=debriefing&output=xml_no_dtd&proxystylesheet=AHRQ_GOV&client=AHRQ_GOV&sort=date%3AD%3AL%3Ad1&entsp=a&oe=UTF-8&ie=UTF-8&ud=1&exclude_apps=1&site=default_collection).

De-escalation strategies in healthcare are actions that decrease aggressive behaviors during challenging communications, which include refocusing attention on the patient (Altmiller, 2012).

Delegation is allowing a delegatee to perform a specific nursing activity, skill, or procedure that is beyond the delegatee's traditional role and not routinely performed (NCSBN, 2016).

Descriptive statistics are useful when evaluating aggregate data sets. Several basic descriptive statistics commonly calculated when doing quality improvement activities include mean, median, mode, range, and standard deviations of a set of data.

Duty of care is the legal obligation of professionals to deliver a certain standard of care when performing acts, which could directly or indirectly harm others.

DynaMed (www.dynamed.com/home/) is an evidence-based point-of-care reference database for nurses, nurse practitioners, physicians, residents, and other healthcare professionals.

eHealth (electronic health) are health services and information delivered through communication technologies to improve the quality of healthcare, thus empowering patients to take an active role in their care management.

Electronic clinical decision support (CDS) tools or systems provide nurses with knowledge and patient-specific information, intelligently filtered and presented at appropriate times.

Electronic health record (EHR) is a longitudinal electronic record of patient health information generated by one or more encounters in any care delivery setting (CMS, 2012).

Electronic medical record (EMR) is a legal record of what happened to a patient during one care encounter at a healthcare organization (HIMSS, 2006).

Empathetic communication is a process by which we seek to appreciate or understand the perspective of the person first and then convey meaning in an attempt to create a shared understanding.

E-patient is a healthcare consumer who is equipped, enabled, empowered, and engaged in his or her health and healthcare decisions.

Error are defined as "an act of commission (doing something wrong) or omission (failing to do the right thing) leading to an undesirable outcome or significant potential for such an outcome" (Wilson et al., 1999).

Evidence implementation involves the evolving and imperfect science of moving evidence into practice (Pearson, 2010).

Evidence-based practice (EBP) is the delivery of optimal healthcare through the integration of best current evidence, clinical expertise, and patient/family values (QSEN, 2012).

Executive branch of the federal government consists of the office of the president of the United States.

External data are those data provided to the organization from those outside the organization.

Failure mode and effect analysis (FMEA) is a proactive approach to mitigate harm that involves a comprehensive risk assessment of a select high-risk process that the organization has identified. The goal of the team is to improve the high-risk processes before an adverse event occurs.

Failure to rescue occurs when clinicians fail to notice patient symptoms or fail to respond adequately or quickly enough to clinical signs that may indicate that a patient is dying of preventable complications in a hospital.

The **Federal Anti-Kickback Statute** is a law that prohibits the payment or receipt of any gift or remuneration in exchange for federal healthcare referrals to Medicare patients.

Financial performance reflects the income and the expenses of a healthcare organization.

Flow map, sometimes referred to as a process map, allows the team to visualize or diagram the actual flow or sequence of a process from the beginning to the end of that process.

Follower is an individual who supports and is guided by another person who usually functions as a leader. However, a good follower is not blindly led but rather exhibits traits of discernment, commitment, and trustworthiness; that is, exhibits similar traits of a leader.

Full-text databases provide the complete text of an article as well as the article citation.

Gantt chart is a graph depicting the phases of a project as they are planned over the projects time frame and are periodically reviewed by the team in determining if the team is staying on schedule.

Handoff is the process of one healthcare professional updating another on the status of one or more patients for the purpose of taking over their care (AHRQ, n.d.. Retrieved from http://www.psnet.ahrq.gov/glossary.aspx?indexLetter=H).

The **Health Insurance Portability and Accountability Act (HIPAA)** was passed in 1996 to set national standards for the protection of patient information. It is a federal law requiring healthcare providers to use several privacy protections for patients and their records (Department of Health and Human Services, 2013).

Health literacy is the degree to which individuals have the capacity to obtain, process, and understand basic health information and services they need to make health decisions.

Healthcare Failure Mode and Effect Analysis (HFMEA™) is a proactive approach to mitigate harm that involves a comprehensive risk assessment of a select high-risk process that the organization has identified. The goal of the team is to improve the high-risk processes before an adverse event occurs. It is a proactive step-by-step process that examines activities having a high possibility of a negative outcome.

Healthcare quality is defined as "the degree to which healthcare services for individuals and populations increase the likelihood of desired health outcomes and are consistent with current professional knowledge" (IOM, 2001).

Healthcare value is achieving the best health outcomes (quality + experience) at the lowest cost (Scheurer, Crabtree, & Cawley, 2016).

Hierarchies of evidence (also known as levels of evidence) provide a visual representation of evidence from the least reliable (at the bottom) to the most reliable (at the top; Ingham-Broomfield, 2016).

Hierarchy refers to perceived level of power across groups, such as a housekeeper and a direct care nurse, or a direct care nurse and a physician.

High-quality care is defined as care that is safe, timely, effective, efficient, equitable, and patient centered (also referred to as STEEEP) with no disparities between racial or ethnic groups (IOM, 2001).

High-reliability organizations (HROs) are healthcare organizations that establish and maintain high quality and safety expectations for patient care and keep quality and safety error rates near zero (Weick & Sutcliffe, 2007).

Histogram is a bar graph that displays the frequency distribution of a process or event. Data displayed using a histogram allow for easier visualization of large, aggregate data sets.

HITECH Act is a federal law that provides money to healthcare providers, institutions, and organizations to encourage the use of electronic health records (Department of Health and Human Services, 2017).

Home healthcare is the provision of limited healthcare services by a nurse or other healthcare professional in the home of the patient.

Hospital Value-Based Purchasing is an incentive payment system that rewards healthcare providers for the quality of care outcomes their patients achieve; it adjusts the Centers for Medicaid and Medicare Services (CMS) reimbursement to hospitals who either demonstrate improvement in performance of quality measures from a baseline or achievement of benchmarks.

Huddle is a structured tool designed to gather a team together to plan for a future event or set of events (such as a preview of an operating room day); it ensures a common understanding of the work to be accomplished and potential risks to be aware of, such as a high-volume day or the high acuity of certain patients.

Implementation science is a science that investigates the adoption and integration of evidence-based findings, including identification of barriers and facilitators, to successfully integrate the evidence into routine healthcare (www.implementationscience.biomedcentral.com/about).

Incidence is the actual counts of every event that occurred. For example, falls incidence data include the actual number of falls that occurred over a specific timeframe.

Informatics calls for the use of information and technology to communicate, manage knowledge, mitigate (prevent) error, and support decision making.

Information is collected and analyzed data, such as trends in blood pressure that is used to take action. It is data that have been interpreted, organized, or structured

Institute for Healthcare Improvement (IHI) uses the science of improvement approach to work with health systems, countries, and other organizations on improving quality, safety, and value in healthcare.

Institute for Safe Medication Practices (ISMP) is an organization that pushes initiatives to improve safe medication practices, which are built upon a nonpunitive approach and system-based solutions these initiatives fall into five key areas: knowledge, analysis, education, cooperation, and communication.

Internal data are those data generated by staff within the organization.

Interprofessional education is when two or more professions learn with, from, and about each other to improve collaboration and the quality of care (Barr, 2002).

Interrater reliability is a process used that provides evidence that those collecting the data are doing so following the same procedures. When interrater reliability exists, the data are considered more reliable because data are collected in a consistent manner.

Judicial branch of the federal government has the responsibility of interpreting federal laws and ensuring that the laws are in compliance with the U.S. Constitution.

Just culture is where all healthcare team members are treated equally and fairly for their actions based on the situation they are placed in and the behavioral choices they make in that situation.

Keyword is a search term that uses your own personal natural language to search the literature.

Knowledge is information that is synthesized so that relationships are identified and formalized, based on a logical process of analysis; it provides order to thoughts and ideas.

Knowledge-based performance occurs when clinicians solve a problem by applying their knowledge in a new and unfamiliar situation.

Knowledge-focused triggers are triggers that stem from the research literature, a new philosophy of care, new national standards, or from professional guidelines (Titler et al., 2001).

Leadership is the ability to lead or command a person or group of people. Within this perspective, anyone who leads and facilitates change by speaking up, providing education, role modeling, and/or coaching resulting in changed behavior of an individual or group is a leader.

Lean thinking, originating from the Toyota Motor Corporation, strives to eliminate forms of waste within a process to increase efficiency while enhancing effectiveness. There are eight identified sources of waste in organizations that include unused human potential, waiting, transportation, defects, inventory, motion, overproduction, and processing.

Learning culture is a culture where all team members recognize that they have a duty to continuously learn and change, for the betterment of themselves, their patients, and the healthcare system in which they work.

Legislative branch of the federal government has the responsibility under the U.S. Constitution to make laws.

Lippincott's Nursing Advisor (lippincottsolutions.com/solutions/advisor) is a point-of-care tool developed specifically for nursing; it includes drug information, patient education handouts, evidence-based care guidelines, and care plans.

Lower control limit is the line three standard deviationss below the mean on a control chart. If a data point falls below this line, special cause variability is occurring in the process under study.

Magnet® designation recognizes that an excellent infrastructure must result in positive outcomes in order to create a culture of excellence and innovation with the result of high nurse retention and better patient outcomes.

Malpractice is one form of negligence and is improper, illegal, or negligent professional activity or treatment by a healthcare practitioner, lawyer, or public official.

Manager is someone who is responsible for controlling all or parts of an organization. Their focus is getting the work of their designated group or unit done effectively.

Mean is a descriptive statistic that is the average of a set of data points. To calculate the mean, add the data points together and divide by the number of data points in the data set.

Median is a descriptive statistic that represents the data point exactly in the middle of a set of data. To calculate the median, the data are sorted from lowest to highest values, thus dividing the data into two groups.

MEDLINE is the U.S. National Library of Medicine's (NLM) bibliographic database, indexing thousands of journals in the fields of medicine, nursing, dentistry, veterinary medicine, healthcare systems, and the preclinical sciences.

mHealth (mobile health) is the use of mobile devices to collect data, provide health services, and educate patients about preventive healthcare. mHealth is part of eHealth.

Mindfulness is staying focused with the ability to see the significance of early and weak signals and to take strong and decisive action to prevent harm (Weick & Sutcliff, 2001).

Misuse of healthcare services is when incorrect diagnoses, medical errors, and avoidable healthcare complications occur.

Mode is a descriptive statistic that is the value repeated most frequently in a set of data, the "typical" value observed.

Mosby's Nursing Consult (www.clinicalkey.com/nursing/) is a point-of-care tool developed specifically for nursing; it includes drug information, patient education handouts, evidence-based care guidelines, and care plans.

Mutual support is the ability to anticipate team members' needs and provide assistance as needed through accurate knowledge about their workloads and responsibilities to enhance teamwork.

National Quality Forum (NQF) convenes panels and other educational forums to work with quality measure developers and others in healthcare to help understand measurement gaps and encourage strategies to fill them.

Near miss is an event or situation that did not produce a patient injury but only because of chance; considered a *close call* (AHRQ, n.d. Retrieved from http://www.psnet.ahrq.gov/glossary.aspx?indexLetter=N).

Near miss safety event occurs when an error or safety event is caught before it reaches the patient because it is caught either by chance or because the process was engineered with a detection barrier.

Negligence is a failure to exercise the care that a reasonably prudent person would exercise in like circumstances.

Nurse practice acts (NPAs) are laws that have been enacted by state governments to protect the public's health, safety, and welfare by overseeing and ensuring the safe practice of nursing.

Objective (patient) data are what the healthcare worker can see or measure, such as the patient's blood pressure or glucose results, and is collected and analyzed to make conclusions about whether the patient is getting better, worse, or if the data require physician notification.

Operational definition is a clear, unambiguous definition that specifies measurement methods and the conditions in which that variable is measured or not.

Organizational culture is the shared values and beliefs of individuals in a group or organization (Schein, 2004).

Outcomes refer to the "changes (desirable or undesirable) in individuals and populations that can be attributed to healthcare" such as patient satisfaction results or outcomes of care (Donabedian, 2003, p. 46).

Outliers are findings that are not expected and are outside of normal findings.

Overuse of healthcare services is when a healthcare service is provided even though it is not justified by the patient's healthcare needs.

P4 Medicine (i.e., medicine that is predictive, preventive, personalized, and participatory) is emerging out of the convergence of systems biology, the increasing activation of networked consumers, and the digital revolution in communications and information technology (P4 Medicine Institute, 2012).

Pareto chart is a type of bar graph, similar to the histogram because it depicts a frequency distribution. The Pareto chart orders findings in a descending order with the most frequent issue contributing to the results farthest to the left of the *x*-axis. Visualizing results from high to low allows for prioritizing as to what data are most impacting the variable in question.

Participatory medicine is a model of care that supports a cooperative approach by all members of the healthcare team across the full continuum of care.

Patient acuity refers to the degree of healthcare service complexity needed by a patient related to their physical or mental status.

Patient advocacy are actions directed at decision makers to support and promote patients' healthcare rights, enhance community health and policy initiatives, and focus on the availability, safety, and quality of care.

Patient- and family-centered care is an approach to the planning, delivery, and evaluation of healthcare that is grounded in mutually beneficial partnerships among healthcare providers, patients, and families (IPFCC, 2017).

Patient-centered care (PCC) emphasizes recognition of the patient or designee as the source of control and full partner in providing compassionate and coordinated care based on respect for the patient's preferences, values and needs.

Patient-centered medical homes are a team-based care delivery model whereby patient treatment is led by a healthcare provider and provides comprehensive patient care with the goal of achieving maximal health outcomes in the patient's home, a hospice, or other ambulatory setting, or by telehealth.

Patient experience is "the sum of all interaction, shaped by an organization's culture, that influence patient perceptions, across the continuum of care" (The Beryl Institute, 2017).

Patient handoff is the transfer of responsibility for a patient from one clinician to another and involves sharing current information that is pertinent to the patient's care with time allowed for discussion, questions, and clarification.

Patient preferences refer to the involvement of the patient and family with a consideration of their values and beliefs in clinical shared decisions (Hopp & Rittenmeyer, 2012).

Patient Safety Organization (PSO) is a group, institution, or association that improves patient care by reducing errors, allowing organizations to learn from their own safety events and the safety events of others (Patient Safety and Quality Improvement Act of 2005).

Person approach to safety in when we only blame the person at the end of the long chain of errors for making an error that caused an adverse event from overuse, underuse, or misuse of healthcare services.

Personal representative is a person that is legally authorized to make healthcare decisions on an individual's behalf or to act for a deceased individual or an estate (such as under a power of attorney or guardian).

PICOT model is an effective way to systematically identify and retrieve nursing and healthcare published studies (see Table 10.1); the "P" represents the patient or population of interest, "I" represents the intervention of interest, "C" represents the comparison of interest, "O" represents the desired outcome of interest, and "T" represents the amount of time the outcome will be observed.

Plan-Do-Study-Act (PDSA) incorporates knowledge of engineering, operations, and management with the goal of improving accuracy, reducing costs, increasing efficiency and safety. It is composed of four parts: (a) appreciation for a system, (b) understanding process variation, (c) applying theory of knowledge, and (d) using psychology.

Pluralistic approach considers all the literature when searching for evidence (Pearson, Wiechula, Court, & Lockwood, 2007).

Point-of-care databases contain evidence summaries, literature reviews, and enhanced content such as pictures, videos, and patient education materials.

Population-focused healthcare is care based on the health status and needs assessment of a target group of individuals who have one or more personal or environmental characteristics in common.

Population health is an approach to healthcare that aims to improve the health of an entire human population, not just individual patients.

Postintervention data are collected after an intervention is applied to confirm the success or failure of the intervention.

Practice guidelines are summaries of information developed by practitioners, professional organizations, expert groups, and others who synthesize information about a clinical topic, procedure, or scenario and make recommendations for clinical practice.

Precision medicine is a medical model that proposes the customization of healthcare, with medical decisions, practices, or products being tailored to the individual patient (Lu, Goldstein, Angrist, & Cavalleri, 2014); in this model, molecular diagnostics, imaging, and analytics are often employed for selecting appropriate and optimal therapies based on the context of a patient's genetic content.

Precursor safety events occur when a healthcare error reaches the patient and results in no harm or minimal detectable harm.

Predictive analytics (PA) uses technology and statistical methods to search through massive amounts of information, analyzing it to predict outcomes for individual patients (Elsevier, 2017).

Prevalence measures are the collection of data taken on one single day.

Problem-focused triggers are triggers that stem from internal identification of a clinical problem or local data (Titler et al., 2001).

Process refers to "the activities that constitute healthcare" such as healthcare policies and standards of care (Donabedian, 2003, p. 46).

Project management (PM), as defined by the Project Management Institute (PMI), is "the application of knowledge, skills, tools, and techniques to project activities to meet the project requirements" (PMI, 2017).

PubMed provides free Internet access to MEDLINE citations and abstracts, access to citations from journal articles not indexed within the MEDLINE database, citations from journals before the MEDLINE database began indexing the journal, articles from journals that submit their full text directly to PubMed Central, and citations for National Center for Biotechnology Information (NCBI) books.

Quality is the degree to which health services for individuals and populations increases the likelihood of desired health outcomes and is consistent with current professional knowledge (Institute of Medicine, 2011).

Quality improvement is the use of data to monitor the outcomes of care processes and the use of improvement methods to design and test changes to continuously improve the quality and safety of healthcare systems (QSEN, 2005).

Radio frequency identification (RFID) is technology that uses radio waves to transfer data from an electronic tag to an object for the purpose of identifying and tracking the object (Ajami & Rajabzadeh, 2013).

Range is a descriptive statistic that represents the lowest and highest values within the data points.

Rapid response team is an interprofessional team of healthcare providers summoned to a bedside when a patient demonstrates signs of imminent deterioration to assess and treat the patient with the goal of preventing adverse clinical outcomes (AHRQ, n.d. Retrieved from http://www.psnet.ahrq.gov/glossary.aspx?indexLetter=R).

Read back is a tool designed to teach healthcare professionals to state, out loud, what they just heard from another team member; it is used primarily in situations where critical information is being verbally transferred between healthcare providers, such as when reporting a critical lab value or a medication request during a code.

Reliability is the probability of failure-free performance over a specified timeframe (Morrow, 2016).

Reporting culture is where all care team members know how to report and feel comfortable reporting all harm, near misses, and unsafe conditions.

Responsibility is the obligation involved when a person accepts an assignment.

Role is a position or part the position fulfills within an organization, such as a CEO or Vice President of Nursing. Depending on the formal position, appropriate responsibilities will be delegated or assigned.

Root cause analysis (RCA) is an investigative approach of what caused a problem and why the problem occurred. A root cause is a system or process finding that has redesign capability to reduce the risk of a repeat error. The Joint Commission requires that a RCA take place whenever a sentinel event occurs (TJC, 2017). It is an error analysis tool in healthcare whose central tenet is to identify the underlying problems that increase the likelihood of errors while avoiding the trap of focusing on mistakes of individuals (AHRQ, n.d.. Retrieved from http://www.psnet.ahrq.gov/glossary.aspx?indexLetter=R).

Rule-based performance is when the clinician has learned a rule and applies it in appropriate situations. The delivery of healthcare is largely based on rules, often called protocols.

Run chart is a graphical display of data in a time-series design using a median as the centerline. Using interpretation rules, common cause variation in a data set can be identified from special cause variation.

Safety minimizes risk of harm to patients and providers through both system effectiveness and individual performance. It has to do with lack of harm and focuses on avoiding bad events. Safety makes it less likely that mistakes and errors will happen (Institute of Medicine, 2001).

Safety initiatives are programs that use standardized clinical practice tools and strategies and focus on reducing healthcare errors and improving patient safety in selected areas of healthcare.

Safety science uses scientific methods and theoretical frameworks to achieve a trustworthy system of healthcare delivery. Safety science helps to describe how safety errors and near misses are recognized and reported, ways to manage human factors that impact safe healthcare delivery and the competencies required for health professionals to provide safe care.

SBAR is an acronym designed to standardize the transfer of patient information between team members; SBAR stands for "Situation, Background, Assessment, Recommendation."

Scatter plot diagrams display relationships between two variables. Scatter plots provide a visual means to test the strength of the relationship between the two variables.

Scope of a project is the work to be completed in order to achieve the goal (PMI, 2017).

Self-concept is the conception an individual holds about his or her own particular traits, aptitudes, and unique characteristics; it typically includes physical, social, and personal components.

Sentinel events (or "never events") are defined as any unanticipated event in a healthcare setting resulting in "death, permanent harm, or severe temporary harm and requiring intervention to sustain life" (Joint Commission, 2017d).

Separation of powers is a government system with checks and balances that allows one branch of government to limit another and that ensures that no one single branch of government can ever have total control or power.

Shared decision making is an approach that involves both clinicians and patients in considering the best available evidence to make healthcare decisions where patients are empowered, engaged, and supported to make autonomous decisions about healthcare (Truglio-Londrigan et al., 2014).

The term **sharp end** has been used to identify the important and significant direct contact role that nurses at the bedside, closest to clinical activities, play in recognizing the need for and potential impact of practice changes.

Simplification of work processes is the act of reducing a work process to its basic components and, in so doing, making it easier to complete the work and to understand it.

Situational awareness is the degree to which one's perception of a situation matches reality; that is, fatigue and stress of team members, environmental factors that threaten safety, deteriorating status of the patient (AHRQ, n.d. Retrieved from http://www.psnet.ahrq.gov/glossary.aspx?indexLetter=S).

Six Sigma methodologies, adopted by healthcare organizations from the business sector, encompass interventions with the goal to reduce variation in existing processes. Six Sigma incorporates several problem-solving steps to reduce variation in the process referred to as DMAIC (define, measure, analyze, improve, and control).

Skills is the "hands on" or physical skills that one applies to his or her work.

Skill-based performance is used for routine, familiar tasks that can be done without thinking about them.

Special cause variation may occur when a change in a process occurs. It is unexpected variation within a process. Special cause variability signals that something happened, that the process changed for the better or worse, or that the process is "out of control."

Stakeholders can include persons, groups or organizations who have an interest in, are affected by, or can affect a practice change (RNAO, 2012).

Standard deviation (SD) is a common statistical method used to describe variation of a data set. It is sometimes referred to as sigma and may be represented by the Greek letter for sigma: σ. SD represents the square root of the variance. Variance is defined as the average of the squared difference from the mean.

Standardization of simplified work processes uses a single set of terms, definitions, and/or practices to reduce variation in patient-care delivery.

The **Stark Law** prohibits a physician from making a Medicare or Medicaid referral to a healthcare provider or organization with whom the physician or his or her family member has a financial relationship.

Statistical process control is a type of statistic that when applied demonstrates a statistical approach to quality improvement decision making. Statistical process control is used to monitor a process over time (time-series design) but adds the ability to scientifically identify variation within that process by plotting data points within a run or control chart.

Statutory laws are written laws that derive from a legislative body, for example, written laws from the U.S. Congress, a state legislative body, or a municipal board of trustees of a city or town.

Stratification is the process of breaking the data down into subsets to better interpret what is happening. It can help focus improvement efforts on specific areas where problems are found.

Structure refers to "the conditions under which care is provided," such as nursing staff ratios, supplies available to provide patient care, and so on (Donabedian, 2003, p. 46).

Subject heading is a search term or phrase, which represents a concept used consistently for data organization and retrieval.

Subjective (patient) data may include the patients' descriptions of how they feel. For example, patients may state they feel dizzy, hot, or lightheaded.

Supervision is the provision of guidance or direction, evaluation, and follow-up by the licensed nurse for accomplishment of a nursing task delegated to the UAP (NCSBN, 1995).

System approach to safety looks at the total context in which the adverse event took place, and considers how to prevent future occurrences through improvement in the total healthcare system.

Systems thinking is the ability to recognize, understand, and synthesize the interactions and interdependencies in a set of components designed for a specific purpose and understand how the components of a complex healthcare system influence the care of an individual patient.

TeamSTEPPS is a teamwork system designed to improve communication skills among healthcare professionals (AHRQ, 2017).

Teamwork and collaboration emphasize healthcare providers functioning effectively within nursing and interprofessional teams, fostering open communication, mutual respect, and shared decision making to achieve quality patient care.

Telehealth is the use of electronic information and communications technologies to support and facilitate clinical- and population-based healthcare, patient health education, and health administration from long distances (HRSA, 2015).

TIGER is a national plan to enable practicing nurses and nursing students to fully engage in the unfolding digital electronic era in healthcare (TIGER, 2012).

Tracer methodology is a process used by The Joint Commission when conducting an onsite survey. The surveyor will use information from the organization to trace an individual patient or a system to determine if staff is following defined policies and procedures while providing care and services. The surveyor will speak with the intraprofessional teams the patient encountered across all settings starting with the current team. The patient's care and services are traced back until the surveyor concludes the tracer after speaking with the team where the patient accessed the organization (TJC, 2017).

Translation science examines variables affecting adoption of evidence-based changes by individuals or organizations designed to improve healthcare decision making (Titler, 2008).

Transparency is the open sharing of errors and other aspects of performance, making them visible to everyone so that others can learn from the errors and improve quality (Makary & Daniel, 2016).

Underuse of healthcare services is when a healthcare service is not provided even though it would have benefited the patient.

Upper control limit is defined as the line three standard deviations above the mean on a control chart. If a data point falls above this line, special cause variability is occurring in the process under study.

Utilization management is a process of patient case management using evidence-based and standardized criteria to evaluate a patient's level of care from hospital admission to discharge.

Variability of data refers to the spread of the data. Determining the high and low values within a data set (range) is one way to assess for variability. There are more sophisticated statistical process control methods in assessing for variation in data points.

Wearables are mobile electronic devices that can be worn by patients as part of clothing or as an accessory; collects biometric variables that communicate with a patient's electronic health record (EHR).

Wisdom is the use of data, information, and knowledge in making decisions and implementing appropriate interprofessional team actions.

Work-arounds occur when nurses and other clinicians use short cuts in an effort to streamline care and they occur when one does not follow the rules and/or works around the rules or correct actions of a patient care process or a work process in order to save time.

Workforce bullying refers to ongoing negative behaviors and negative verbal and nonverbal communications.

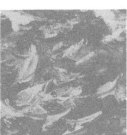

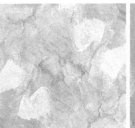
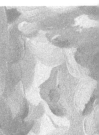

INDEX

INTRODUCTION TO QUALITY AND SAFETY EDUCATION FOR NURSES

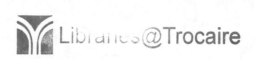